ENT
SECRETS

ENT SECRETS

BRUCE W. JAFEK, MD
Professor and Chairman
Department of Otolaryngology–Head and Neck Surgery
University of Colorado Health Sciences Center
Denver, Colorado

ANNE K. STARK, MD
Clinical Fellow
Department of Otolaryngology–Head and Neck Surgery
University of Colorado Health Sciences Center
Denver, Colorado

HANLEY & BELFUS, INC./ Philadelphia

Publisher: HANLEY & BELFUS
              210 S. 13th Street
              Philadelphia, PA 19107
              (215) 546-7293
              FAX (215) 790-9330

Library of Congress Cataloging-in-Publication Data

Jafek, Bruce W.
    ENT Secrets / Bruce W. Jafek, Anne K. Stark.
        p.   cm. — (The Secrets Series®).
    Includes bibliographical references and index.
    ISBN 1-56053-159-2 (alk. paper)
        1. Otolaryngology—Examinations, questions, etc.   I. Stark, Anne
K., 1968–   .   II. Title.   III. Series.
        [DNLM: 1. Otorhinolaryngologic Diseases—examination questions.
WV 18.2 J23e 1996]
RF57.J34   1996
617.5'1'0076—dc20
DNLM/DLC
for Library of Congress   96-19319
                                                             CIP

ENT SECRETS   ISBN 1-56053-159-2

Last digit is the print number: 9   8   7   6   5   4   3   2

CONTENTS

I. INTRODUCTION

    1. Introduction to Otolaryngology 1
       Bruce W. Jafek, M.D.

    2. The Head and Neck Examination 3
       Anne K. Stark, M.D.

II. OTOLOGY

    3. Anatomy and Physiology of the Ear 9
       Bruce W. Murrow, M.D., Ph.D.

    4. The Hearing Evaluation 12
       Catherine Winslow, M.D., and Jerry L. Northern, Ph.D.

    5. Conductive Hearing Loss 21
       Bruce W. Murrow, M.D., Ph.D.

    6. Sensorineural Hearing Loss 24
       Nicolas G. Slenkovich, M.D.

    7. Hearing Aids and Cochlear Implants 29
       Kent E. Gardner, M.D., and Jerry L. Northern, Ph.D.

    8. Diseases of the External Ear and Tympanic Membrane 34
       Douglas M. Sorensen, M.D., and Catherine Winslow, M.D.

    9. Otitis Media and Associated Complications 39
       Douglas H. Todd, M.D., and Sylvan E. Stool, M.D.

   10. Diseases of the Middle Ear 43
       Douglas M. Sorensen, M.D.

   11. Evaluation of the Dizzy Patient 47
       Anne K. Stark, M.D., and Carol Foster, M.D.

   12. Vestibular Disorders 53
       Anne K. Stark, M.D., and Carol Foster, M.D.

   13. Tinnitus 58
       Mark A. Voss, M.D.

   14. Ear Injuries After Flying and Diving 62
       Mark R. Mount, M.D., and Philip E. Asmar, M.D., M.M.Sc.

   15. Neuro-otology 68
       Cameron Shaw, M.D., and Anne K. Stark, M.D.

III. THE NOSE AND SINUSES

   16. Anatomy and Physiology of the Nose 77
       Bruce W. Jafek, M.D.

   17. Nasal Septal Abnormalities 83
       Abilio Muñoz, M.D., and Michael Leo Lepore, M.D.

   18. Rhinitis 86
       Bruce Murrow, M.D., Ph.D.

Contents

19. Sinus Anatomy and Function 90
    Kent E. Gardner, M.D.

20. Sinusitis 96
    Tyler M. Lewark, M.D.

21. Medical Management of Sinusitis 102
    Tyler M. Lewark, M.D.

22. Surgical Management of Sinusitis 107
    Nicolas G. Slenkovich, M.D.

IV. GENERAL OTOLARYNGOLOGY

23. Temporomandibular Joint Disease 113
    Steven B. Aragon, M.D., D.D.S.

24. Oral Lesions 118
    Thomas D. MacKenzie, M.D., and Michael L. Lepore, M.D.

25. Facial Nerve Disorders 123
    Shawna Harris Abbey

26. Esophageal Disorders 131
    Michael F. Spafford, M.D.

27. The Thyroid and Parathyroid Glands 136
    Catherine Winslow, M.D.

28. Salivary Gland Disorders 137
    Bruce W. Jafek, M.D.

29. Deep Space Neck Infections 141
    Ethan Lazarus, M.D.

30. Sleep Apnea and Snoring 144
    Abilio Muñoz, M.D.

31. The Hoarse Patient 149
    Abilio Muñoz, M.D.

32. Otolaryngologic Manifestations of AIDS 153
    Daniel W. Watson, M.D.

33. Antimicrobial Therapy in Otolaryngology 158
    Tyler M. Lewark, M.D.

34. Pharmacology of Otolaryngology 164
    Erik Vinge and Stephen Batuello, M.D.

V. ENDOSCOPY

35. Laryngoscopy 169
    Bruce W. Jafek, M.D.

36. Esophagoscopy 172
    Stephen G. Batuello, M.D.

37. Broncoscopy 176
    Bruce W. Jafek, M.D.

38. Mediastinoscopy 181
    Bruce W. Jafek, M.D., and Marv Pomerantz, M.D.

VI. TUMORS

    39. Salivary Gland Tumors 189
        Bruce W. Jafek, M.D.

    40. Tumors of the Oral Cavity and Pharynx 193
        Vincent D. Eusterman, M.D., D.D.S.

    41. Odontogenic Cysts, Tumors, and Related Jaw Lesions 200
        Ethan Lazarus, M.D., and R. Casey Strahan, M.D.

    42. Tumors of the Nose and Paranasal Sinuses 204
        Mark R. Mount, M.D.

    43. Laryngeal Cancer 208
        Vincent D. Eusterman, M.D., D.D.S., and Mark R. Mount, M.D.

    44. Tumors of the Trachea and Tracheobronchial Tree 214
        Douglas M. Sorensen, M.D.

    45. Tumors of the Esophagus 217
        John P. Campana, M.D.

    46. Thyroid and Parathyroid Tumors 222
        Catherine Winslow, M.D., and Margaret K.T. Squier, M.D.

    47. Vascular Tumors of the Head and Neck 227
        Catherine Winslow, M.D.

    48. Cutaneous Neoplasms of the Head and Neck 229
        Tyler M. Lewark, M.D.

    49. Radiation Therapy for Head and Neck Cancer 237
        Rachel Rabinovitch, M.D.

    50. Chemotherapy for Head and Neck Cancer 240
        Allen L. Cohn, M.D.

VII. FACIAL PLASTIC SURGERY

    51. Principles of Grafts and Flaps 245
        Gregory E. Krause, M.D., and Michael L. Lepore, M.D.

    52. Principles of Skin Resurfacing 251
        Arlen D. Meyers, M.D., M.B.A.

    53. Rhinoplasty 254
        David A. Hendrick, M.D.

    54. Blepharoplasty 262
        R. Casey Strahan, M.D.

    55. Otoplasty 268
        David A. Hendrick, M.D.

    56. Rhytidectomy 274
        Richard A. Mouchantat, M.D.

VIII. TRAUMA AND EMERGENCIES

    57. Principles of Trauma 283
        James F. Benson, Jr., M.D.

58. Epistaxis 286
    Anne K. Stark, M.D.

59. Nasal Trauma 290
    James F. Benson, Jr., M.D.

60. Penetrating Neck and Facial Trauma 293
    James F. Benson, Jr., M.D.

61. Upper Airway Obstruction 296
    Tyler M. Lewark, M.D.

62. The Mandibular Fracture 302
    Kent E. Gardner, M.D., and Steven B. Aragon, M.D., D.D.S.

63. Zygomatic, Maxillary, and Orbital Fractures 309
    Philip C. Fitzpatrick, M.D., and R. Casey Strahan, M.D.

64. Temporal Bone Trauma 314
    Kent E. Gardner, M.D., Mark Mount, M.D., and Ethan Lazarus, M.D.

IX. PEDIATRIC OTOLARYNGOLOGY

65. The Pediatric Airway 321
    Tyler M. Lewark, M.D., and Marshall E. Smith, M.D.

66. Tonsils and Adenoids 325
    Robert Pearson, M.D.

67. Congenital Malformations 329
    Michelle R. Kuntz, M.S., and Kenny H. Chan, M.D.

68. Genetic Issues in Otolaryngology. 333
    Katie J. Hanson, M.S., and Anne L. Matthews, R.N., Ph.D.

69. Cleft Lip and Palate 338
    David A. Hendrick, M.D.

X. RELATED SPECIALTIES

70. Taste and Smell. 345
    Miriam R.I. Linschoten, Ph.D., Pamela M. Eller, M.S.,
    and Anne K. Stark, M.D.

71. Allergy and Immunology 349
    Monique L. McCray, Betty Luce, B.S.N., M.A., and William H. Wilson, M.D.

72. Radiology of the Head and Neck 353
    Caroline L. Hollingsworth, M.D., David Rubinstein, M.D.
    and B. Burton Putegnat, M.D.

73. Anesthesia in Otolaryngology 365
    Kathryn Beauchamp, M.D., and Matthew Flaherty, M.D.

74. The Eye and Orbit. 370
    David M. Kleinman, M.D., David W. Johnson, M.D.,
    and Jon M. Braverman, MD

75. Cost-Effective Otolaryngology. 378
    Arlen D. Meyers, M.D., M.B.A.

XI. CRITICAL CARE ISSUES

76. Fluid and Electrolyte Management.. 381
    Anne K. Stark, M.D.

77. Acid-Base Disturbances 384
    Anne K. Stark, M.D.

78. Nutritional Assessment and Therapy 389
    Anne K. Stark, M.D.

79. Blood Products and Coagulation 393
    Chitra Rajagopalan, M.D.

80. Wound Healing and Dehiscence... 396
    Cara Hyman Dawson

81. Tracheotomy... 398
    Anne K. Stark, M.D.

82. Mechanical Ventilation 402
    Michael F. Spafford, M.D., Catherine P. Winslow, M.D.,
    and Joel H. Witter, M.D.

83. Cardiopulmonary Resuscitation and Advanced Cardiac Life Support........... 408
    Terry G. Murphy, R.N., C.C.R.N., M.S.

84. Shock 413
    Gregory J. Martin

85. Fever in the Critical Care Patient 418
    John W. Hollingsworth, M.D.

XII. CONCLUSION

86. Minutiae in Otolaryngology (Things You Shouldn't Really Be Expected
    to Know, But Will Really Impress the Attending on Rounds or
    in Conferences).. 425
    Bruce W. Jafek, M.D., and Anne K. Stark, M.D.

INDEX 431

CONTRIBUTORS

Shawna Harris Abbey
Third-year medical student, University of Colorado Health Sciences Center, Denver, Colorado

Steven B. Aragon, M.D., D.D.S.
Department of Otolaryngology–Head and Neck Surgery, University of Colorado Health Sciences Center, Denver, Colorado

Philip Elias Asmar, M.D., M.M.Sc.
Medical College of Georgia, Augusta, Georgia

Stephen G. Batuello, M.D.
Resident in Otolaryngology–Head and Neck Surgery, University of Colorado Health Sciences Center, Denver, Colorado

Kathryn Beauchamp, M.D.
Resident, Department of Anesthesiology, University of Colorado Health Sciences Center, Denver, Colorado

James F. Benson, Jr., M.D.
Department of Otolaryngology–Head and Neck Surgery, University of Colorado Health Sciences Center, Denver, Colorado

Jon M. Braverman, M.D.
Assistant Professor, Department of Ophthalmology, University of Colorado Health Sciences Center, Denver, Colorado

John P. Campana, M.D.
Clinical Instructor, Department of Otolaryngology–Head and Neck Surgery, University of Colorado Health Sciences Center, Denver, Colorado

Kenny H. Chan, M.D.
Associate Professor, Pediatric Otolaryngology, The Children's Hospital, Denver, Colorado

Allen L. Cohn, M.D.
Assistant Professor, Division of Medical Oncology, Department of Medicine, University of Colorado Health Sciences Center, Denver, Colorado

Cara Hyman Dawson
Fourth-year medical student, University of Colorado Health Sciences Center, Denver, Colorado

Pamela M. Eller, M.S.
Research Associate, Rocky Mountain Taste and Smell Center, University of Colorado Health Sciences Center, Denver, Colorado

Vincent D. Eusterman, M.D., D.D.S.
Assistant Professor, Department of Otolaryngology–Head and Neck Surgery, University of Colorado–Fitzsimons Army Medical Center, Denver, Colorado

Philip C. Fitzpatrick, M.D.
Department of Otolaryngology–Head and Neck Surgery, Tulane University School of Medicine, New Orleans, Louisiana

Matthew Flaherty, M.D.
Assistant Professor, Department of Anesthesiology, University of Colorado Health Sciences Center, Denver, Colorado

Carol Ann Foster, M.D.
Assistant Professor, Department of Otolaryngology–Head and Neck Surgery, University of Colorado Health Sciences Center, Denver, Colorado

Kent Eric Gardner, M.D.
Resident, Department of Otolaryngology–Head and Neck Surgery, University of Colorado Health Sciences Center, Denver, Colorado

Katie J. Hanson, M.S.
Genetic Counselor, Department of Pediatrics, University of Colorado Health Sciences Center, Denver, Colorado

David A. Hendrick, M.D.
Chief Resident, Department of Otolaryngology–Head and Neck Surgery, University of Colorado Health Sciences Center, Denver, Colorado

Caroline L. Hollingsworth, M.D.
Resident, Department of Radiology, University of Texas Medical Branch, Galveston, Texas

John Hollingsworth, M.D.
Department of Internal Medicine, University of Texas Medical Branch, Galveston, Texas

Bruce W. Jafek, M.D., F.A.C.S., F.R.S.M.
Professor and Chairman, Department of Otolaryngology–Head and Neck Surgery, University of Colorado Health Sciences Center, Denver, Colorado

David W. Johnson, M.D.
Assistant Professor, Department of Ophthalmology, University of Colorado Health Sciences Center, Denver, Colorado

David M. Kleinman, M.D.
Resident in Ophthalmology, University of Colorado Health Sciences Center, Denver, Colorado

Gregory E. Krause, M.D.
Resident, Department of Otolaryngology–Head and Neck Surgery, University of Colorado Health Sciences Center, Denver, Colorado

Michelle R. Kuntz, M.S.
Third-year medical student, University of Colorado Health Sciences Center, Denver, Colorado

Ethan Lazarus, M.D.
Resident, Department of Family Practice, John Peter Smith Hospital, Fort Worth, Texas

Michael Leo Lepore, M.D.
Professor, Vice Chairman of Academic Affairs, and Program Director, Department of Otolaryngology–Head and Neck Surgery, University of Colorado Health Sciences Center, Denver, Colorado

Tyler M. Lewark, M.D.
Clinical Fellow, Department of Otolaryngology–Head and Neck Surgery, University of Colorado Health Sciences Center, Denver, Colorado

Miriam R.I. Linschoten, Ph.D.
Instructor, Rocky Mountain Taste and Smell Center, University of Colorado Health Sciences Center, Denver, Colorado

Betty Luce, B.S.N., M.A.
Clinical Nurse, Department of Otolaryngeal Allergy, University of Colorado Health Sciences Center, Denver, Colorado

Thomas D. MacKenzie, M.D.
Private Practice, Internal Medicine, Denver, Colorado

Gregory J. Martin
Medical student, University of Colorado Health Sciences Center, Denver, Colorado

Anne L. Matthews, R.N., Ph.D.
Assistant Professor of Pediatrics, and Associate Director, Graduate Program in Genetic Counseling, University of Colorado Health Sciences Center, Denver, Colorado

Monique L. McCray
Medical student, University of Colorado Health Sciences Center, Denver, Colorado

Arlen D. Meyers, M.D., M.B.A.
Professor and Vice-Chairman, Department of Otolaryngology–Head and Neck Surgery, University of Colorado Health Sciences Center, Denver; Chief of Otolaryngology, Veterans Affairs Medical Center, Denver, Colorado

Richard A. Mouchantat, M.D.
Division of Plastic and Hand Surgery, University of Colorado Health Sciences Center, Denver, Colorado

Mark R. Mount, M.D., CPT–MC
Department of Otolaryngology–Head and Neck Surgery, University of Colorado Health Sciences Center, Denver, Colorado

Abilio Muñoz, M.D.
Resident, Department of Family Medicine, University of Texas Health Sciences Center, San Antonio, Texas

Terry G. Murphy, R.N., C.C.R.N., M.S.
Fourth-year medical student, University of Colorado Health Sciences Center, Denver, Colorado

Bruce W. Murrow, M.D., Ph.D.
Resident, Department of Otolaryngology–Head and Neck Surgery, University of Colorado Health Sciences Center, Denver, Colorado

Jerry L. Northern, Ph.D.
Professor and Head, Audiology Services, Department of Otolaryngology–Head and Neck Surgery, University of Colorado Health Sciences Center, Denver, Colorado

Robert D. Pearson, M.D.
Resident, Department of Otolaryngology–Head and Neck Surgery, University of Colorado Health Sciences Center, Denver, Colorado

Marv Pomerantz, M.D.
Professor of Surgery, University of Colorado Health Sciences Center, Denver, Colorado

B. Burton Putegnat, M.D.
Resident, Department of Radiology, University of Texas Medical Branch, Galveston, Texas

Rachel Rabinovitch, M.D.
Assistant Professor, Department of Radiation Oncology, University of Colorado Health Sciences Center, Denver, Colorado

Chitra Rajagopalan, M.D.
Professor of Clinical Pathology, University of Colorado Health Sciences Center, Veterans Affairs Medical Center, Denver, Colorado

David Rubinstein, M.D.
Associate Professor, Department of Radiology, University of Colorado Health Sciences Center, Denver, Colorado

Cameron Shaw, M.D.
Assitant Professor of Neuro-otology, University of Colorado Health Sciences Center, Denver; Swedish Medical Center, Littleton, Colorado

Nicolas George Slenkovich, M.D.
Resident, Department of Otolaryngology–Head and Neck Surgery, University of Colorado Health Sciences Center, Denver, Colorado

Marshall E. Smith, M.D.
Assistant Professor, Pediatric Otolaryngology, The Children's Hospital, Denver, Colorado

Douglas M. Sorensen, M.D.
Resident, Department of Otolaryngology–Head and Neck Surgery, University of Colorado Health Sciences Center, Denver, Colorado

Michael Frederick Spafford, M.D.
Chief Resident, Department of Otolaryngology–Head and Neck Surgery, University of Colorado Health Sciences Center, Denver, Colorado

Margaret K.T. Squier, M.D.
Department of Otolaryngology–Head and Neck Surgery, University of Colorado Health Sciences Center, Denver, Colorado

Anne K. Stark, M.D.
Clinical Fellow, Department of Otolaryngology–Head and Neck Surgery, University of Colorado Health Sciences Center, Denver, Colorado

Sylvan E. Stool, M.D.
Senior Educator, Pediatric Otolaryngology, The Children's Hospital, Denver, Colorado

R. Casey Strahan, M.D.
Associate Clinical Professor, Department of Otolaryngology–Head and Neck Surgery, University of Colorado Health Sciences Center, Denver, Colorado

Douglas H. Todd, M.D.
Chief Resident, Department of Otolaryngology–Head and Neck Surgery, University of Colorado Health Sciences Center, The Children's Hospital, Denver, Colorado

Erik Vinge
Medical student, University of Colorado Health Sciences Center, Denver, Colorado

Mark A. Voss, M.D.
Resident, Department of Otolaryngology–Head and Neck Surgery, University of Colorado Health Sciences Center, Denver, Colorado

Daniel W. Watson, M.D.
Resident, Department of Otolaryngology–Head and Neck Surgery, University of Colorado Health Sciences Center, Denver, Colorado

William H. Wilson, M.D.
Clinical Professor Emeritus, Department of Otolaryngology–Head and Neck Surgery, University of Colorado Health Sciences Center, Denver, Colorado

Catherine P. Winslow, M.D.
Resident, Department of Otolaryngology–Head and Neck Surgery, University of Colorado Health Sciences Center, Denver, Colorado

Joel Hoefer Witter, M.D.
Chief Medical Resident, Department of Medicine, University of Colorado Health Sciences Center, Denver, Colorado

PREFACE

Daily, the physician is asked to make decisions in the face of inadequate data. Asking questions and investigating possibilities are intuitive processes for the accomplished physician. In addition to explicating details and specifics, training should refine the student's ability to formulate the appropriate questions. *ENT Secrets*, in the Socratic spirit, should guide the reader toward questions that stimulate discussion and sharpen the focus of inquiry.

Because otolaryngology involves perhaps the most challenging surgical anatomy, *ENT Secrets* addresses this complexity, as well as its broad scope of practice, in an approachable manner suitable for the medical student. *ENT Secrets* is also appropriate for otolaryngology residents, presenting broad practical concepts and "bullets" of information that may be used in the operating room, in the clinics, and on the wards. *ENT Secrets* should also be useful for primary care practitioners, as the evolution of medicine dictates that these providers become increasingly proficient in all specialties.

We hope this book will stimulate the reader to investigate more comprehensive textbooks and current literature pertaining to the immense field of otolaryngology.

Bruce W. Jafek, M.D.
Anne K. Stark, M.D.

I. Introduction

I. INTRODUCTION TO OTOLARYNGOLOGY

Bruce W. Jafek, M.D.

1. What is otolaryngology?

Otolaryngology, pronounced with an initial long $\bar{o}$ (ōtolaryngology, **not** autolaryngology) is the specialty that deals with diseases of the head and neck region, or in simplified terms, the region from the eyebrows to the collarbones. As one of the earliest specialties, otolaryngology saw the establishment of the American Academy of Ophthalmology and Otolaryngology in 1896, and American board certification examination and recognition followed approximately 25 years later. Originally, the specialty was commonly identified as EENT (eyes, ears, nose, throat), also including ophthalmology. However, in recognition of the explosion of medical knowledge, the two disciplines split many years ago, and few physicians presently practice in both areas. Calling an otolaryngologist an "ENT" is no more appropriate than calling a cardiologist a "heart" or an oncologist a "cancer." The American Academy of Otolaryngology recognized this expanded breadth and adopted a more anglicized qualification when it changed the name to "otolaryngology–head and neck surgery." Of course, not even this qualification solves the problem, but it improves the definition of the specialty.

2. What subdivisions exist within the specialty?

Initially, otology, laryngology, rhinology, and bronchoesophagology were recognized. With increased medical knowledge, however, pediatric otolaryngology, otolaryngologic allergy, facial plastic and reconstructive surgery, and "head and neck" (primarily cancer) surgery have been identified. "Otology" has been expanded to include otology, neurotology, and skull-base surgery. Even this is not all-encompassing, as otolaryngologists are interested in neurolaryngology, microvascular surgery, chemosensation (taste and smell disorders), audiology, and speech disorders. Truly, the specialty deals with the comprehensive management of all diseases of the head and neck region, including the manifestations of systemic processes affecting this area.

3. Is otolaryngology a medical or surgical specialty?

Actually, it is both. Many conditions are managed medically and require no surgery, while others require surgery. In common practice, for every 13 patients needing medical care, 1 will require surgery. Therefore, otolaryngology is both a medical and a surgical specialty. The otolaryngology specialist cares for adults and children, males and females, young and old. The breadth of the field and the complexity of the patients make it both challenging and stimulating, as well as extremely satisfying for the practitioner.

4. Why is the otolaryngology match an "early match"?

Resident positions are coordinated through the Otolaryngology Matching Program, a separate program from the "general match." Medical students who are interested in otolaryngology should complete their applications no later than September of their senior year. Interviews are usually conducted in November and December. Rank lists are due the first week in January, and the match is in mid-January. However, internships are determined through the general match. Because the otolaryngology match is so competitive, it is an "early match." Those who do not find a position have time to find another position in the "general match."

5. How many students and graduates are interested in otolaryngology?

In 1996, 727 medical students and graduates applied to the otolaryngology match. Each applicant subsequently applied to an average of 36 otolaryngology programs and received an average of 7.5 interviews.

6. How many resident positions exist in the United States?

There are about 1000 otolaryngology residents in the United States. In 1996, 241 resident positions were available at a postgraduate year 2 (PGY-2) level. All positions consistently and competitively fill with the match.

7. Overall, what is the likelihood of a match?

In 1996, of those who submitted a rank list, 62% of U.S. seniors matched. Fifty percent of U.S. graduates matched (i.e., those students who graduated and started a preliminary surgical internship, etc.) and 10% of foreign medical graduates matched.

8. How do I request an application for the otolaryngology match?
Write to:
Central Application Service of the Otolaryngology Matching Program
P.O. Box 7999
San Francisco, CA 94120-7999

9. Have these statistics remained stable with the present changes in the health care system?

Although many students are considering primary care today, otolaryngology remains a highly desirable and competitive field. In general, these statistics have not fluctuated significantly in the last 10 years.

10. What kind of training does an otolaryngologist–head and neck surgeon receive?

To qualify for board examination, the otolaryngologist first completes 1 year of preliminary training, or internship (postgraduate year 1), in general surgery, followed by 4 years of training in otolaryngology–head and neck surgery, for a total of 5 years of training. Some programs are longer, but this defines the minimum training necessary to sit for the certification examination.

11. How about subspecialization?

Fellowships are offered in pediatric otolaryngology; head and neck surgery; rhinology and sinus surgery; otolaryngologic allergy; and otology, neurotology and skull-base surgery.

12. How long are subspecialization training programs?

One or 2 years of additional training are offered. Many programs are currently moving toward 2-year training periods.

13. Do these programs lead to subcertification?

Subspecialty certification is not currently offered by either the American Board of Medical Specialties or the American Board of Otolaryngology–Head and Neck Surgery. Award of a "Certificate of Added Qualification" is, however, currently being considered by the latter organization.

2. THE HEAD AND NECK EXAMINATION

Anne K. Stark, M.D.

1. Should the head and neck examination be performed in a specific order?

It is not necessary to follow a strict exam order. However, unlike many exams, a complete head and neck examination requires several instruments, including an otoscope, head mirror, light source, and various speculums. Much of the examination requires practice and patience. Become familiar with the otolaryngologic instruments, organizing them before you begin the exam. Establishing a comfortable routine for yourself will ensure that you do not miss any portion of the exam on any patient.

2. What size speculum is used in the otologic examination?

Select the largest speculum that will fit comfortably into the patient's ear. This ensures optimal visualization and a tight seal for pneumatic otoscopy.

3. Describe the proper technique of otoscopic examination.

The patient's head should be tilted toward the opposite shoulder. With a firm but gentle grasp on the auricle, retract the auricle upward and backward while inserting the speculum. This maneuver straightens the auditory canal and provides the best visualization of the tympanic membrane (TM). The auditory canal is inspected from the meatus to the TM, checking for discharge, scaling, erythema, lesions, foreign bodies, and cerumen. The speculum should be inserted carefully 1.0–1.5 cm. If the inner two-thirds of the auditory canal (i.e., the bony portion) is touched with the speculum during the exam, it will be exquisitely painful to the patient. Once the speculum is comfortably in place, the direction of the light should be varied so that the entire TM can be inspected.

4. Describe the appearance of a normal tympanic membrane.

The normal TM (eardrum) is oval, pearly gray, and translucent. The **manubrium** of the malleus is the TM's most prominent landmark. It appears as a white streak running down the center of the eardrum. The **short process** of the malleus is a small superior projection. From this process, the TM has two folds, the **malleolar folds**, which stretch anteriorly and posteriorly. Above these two folds, the TM is known as the **pars flaccida**. The contour of the TM membrane is conical, with the center attached to the **umbo** of the malleus.

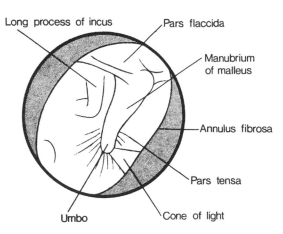

Structural landmarks of the normal tympanic membrane. (From Marshall KG, Attia EL: Disorders of the Ear: Diagnosis and Management. Boston, John Wright, PSG Inc., 1983, p 4, with permission.)

Long process of incus — Pars flaccida

Manubrium of malleus

Annulus fibrosa

Pars tensa

Umbo — Cone of light

3

5. What is pneumatic otoscopy?

The pneumatic attachment to the otoscope may be used to evaluate the mobility of the TM. The speculum must form a tight seal between the canal and instrument. Gentle puffs of alternating positive and negative pressure applied to the normal TM cause the structure to shift slightly. Positive pressure causes the TM to retract inward, toward the patient, and negative pressure causes the TM to bulge outward, toward the examiner. If a middle ear is under negative pressure, applied positive pressure will not shift the TM, but applied negative pressure will cause it to bulge outward. If a middle ear is under positive pressure from a Valsalva maneuver or acute otitis media, the TM will move with applied positive pressure but not with applied negative pressure.

6. How do you properly use a head mirror?

The otolaryngologic head mirror is a valuable tool in the examination of the nasal cavity, oral cavity, larynx, and nasopharynx. If you are a right-handed examiner, sit in front of the patient or to the patient's right side. Secure the head mirror around your head so that the back of the mirror is as close to your left eye as possible. You should be able to see clearly through the hole in the mirror with your left eye, even if your right eye is closed. A concentrated light source placed over the patient's shoulder is directed into your mirror. The examining chair should be raised so that the light source, head mirror, and patient are all at the same horizontal level. Position the patient so that he or she is leaning forward with the chin extended. Most mirrors have a focal length of approximately 20 cm. The light is reflected from your mirror onto the patient's face. Often, moving the patient toward you will help to focus the beam. Adjust the patient, light source, and your mirror so that the point of maximally focused light is on the area to be examined. Always examine with both eyes open.

7. What should the clinician look for when examining the external nose?

The nose should be inspected for evidence of previous trauma, such as scars or deformities. Often, a bend in the external nose is associated with a septal deformity. The skin should be examined for lesions. The nares and columella are examined for symmetry. A septal bend near the columella may be associated with a septal bend deep in the nose.

8. How do you properly use a nasal speculum?

Position the patient and focus the light of the mirror. With the nasal speculum in your left hand, put your right hand on top of the patient's head. With the speculum closed, insert it into the nasal cavity. Lift the ala, and gently open the speculum vertically. Avoid touching the septum with the speculum, as this will cause discomfort. Rotate the patient's head to view inside the nasal cavity. Remove the speculum while it is open (otherwise you will pull out nasal hairs). Without changing hands, inspect the other side.

9. Describe the examination of the internal nose.

With the speculum in place, the examiner should first focus on the nasal septum and nasal cavities. The cavities should be fairly symmetrical, and the inferior septum should be without spurs. A deviated septum may produce asymmetry of the posterior nasal cavities. Evaluate the septum for any perforations. When examining a patient with a history of epistaxis, special attention should be given to enlarged anterior blood vessels or crusting.

The examiner then focuses on the turbinates, inspecting the mucosa for color, discharge, masses, lesions, and swelling. The turbinates are rarely the same size due to the normal nasal cycle; however, excessive deformities should be noted. Only the inferior and middle turbinates are easily visualized. With the patient's head in the erect position, examine the vestibule and inferior nasal turbinate. Then tilt the patient's head back to more clearly visualize the middle meatus and middle turbinate. Turbinates should be firm and the same color as the surrounding mucosa. Swollen boggy turbinates which are bluish gray or pale pink are often associated with allergies. Polyps may appear as round or elongated masses protruding from the middle meatus.

10. What should the examination include concerning the lips?
Normally, the lips should be smooth and without lesions. The lips should be evaluated for all lesions, including plaques, vesicles, nodules, and ulcerations, which may be associated with infection or skin cancer.

11. How is a tongue blade used to examine the oral cavity?
Position the patient so that the headlight is focused on the oral cavity. Stand on the patient's right side, and put your right hand on the top of the patient's head. Do not ask the patient to stick out the tongue, as this maneuver only exposes more of the gag area. With the tongue blade in your left hand, place the tip of the blade in the center of the tongue, depressing it and gently pulling forward. Focus the light on the oropharynx. To view the entire oral cavity, move the patient's head into the path of the light. Do not move your head since this will defocus the light.

12. Describe the oropharyngeal exam.
With the tongue blade in place, observe the tonsillar pillars and note the size of the tonsils. The tonsillar mucosa should be the same pink color as the surrounding pharyngeal mucosa. The tonsils normally do not project beyond the tonsillar pillars. Crypts may be present on the tonsils where debris may collect. Infected tonsils may appear erythematous, hypertrophied, or covered with exudate. The posterior wall should be smooth and without lesions. Postnasal drip may be associated with a yellowish mucoid film running down the back of the pharynx. By touching the posterior wall of the pharynx, you can elicit the gag reflex (cranial nerve IX and X).

13. Describe the physical examination of the tongue.
First inspect the dorsum of the tongue for smoothness, color, and health of the papillae. Ask the patient to stick out the tongue, and inspect it for symmetry as 12th nerve lesions and cancer may cause an asymmetric protrusion. Cancer most commonly occurs on the sides of the tongue and at the base, where lesions may not be easily identified. With a gloved hand and a gauze, gently pull the tongue to either side to inspect for lesions. Firmly palpate the entire tongue, including its base, evaluating for any suspicious induration.

14. How should the buccal mucosa, teeth, and gums be examined?
Initially ask the patient to clench the teeth and smile. This maneuver simultaneously evaluates for facial nerve (VII) function and occlusion of the teeth. Ask the patient to remove all dental appliances in order to inspect the buccal mucosa, gums, and teeth fully. The mucosal surface should be pink, smooth, moist, and free of masses or lesions. Patchy, dark pigmentation may be a normal variation in dark-skinned people. With a gloved hand, palpate the gums for lesions, induration, tenderness, or masses. Note loose, missing, or carious teeth. Finally, do not forget to inspect and palpate the soft palate.

15. How do you use a laryngeal mirror?
Warm a #4 laryngeal mirror (this prevents fogging). Position the patient so that he or she is leaning slightly forward with the head slightly extended. Ask the patient to stick out the tongue. With gauze in your left hand, grasp the tongue. With the laryngeal mirror in your right hand and your hand stabilized against the patient's chin, place the mirror against the soft palate. Focus the light of your head mirror onto the laryngeal mirror. Firmly slide the mirror back along the soft palate, rotating the mirror until the larynx is visualized. If the patient gags, spray the pharynx with 10% lidocaine and try again after a few minutes.

16. How do you use a nasopharyngeal mirror?
The nasopharyngeal exam is one of the most technically difficult examinations and is done to assess the nasopharynx for adenoid hypertrophy, nasopharyngeal tumors, or posterior nasal polyps. Again, optimally position the patient. Depress the tongue with a tongue blade held in

your left hand and expose the oropharynx. Grasp a warmed #0 nasopharyngeal mirror with the thumb and index finger of your right hand. Stabilize your hand against the patient's chin. With the patient breathing through the nose, slip the mirror behind the soft palate, focus your head mirror, and view the nasopharynx and posterior choanae. This examination has largely been replaced by the use of rigid and flexible fiberoptic scopes.

17. Your attending tells you to prepare the patient for fiberoptic laryngoscopy. What do you do?

Tell the patient that you will be spraying two solutions into the nose, a topical decongestant and a topical anesthetic. These solutions may taste bitter and may produce a numb tongue. The patient may feel as if he or she cannot swallow or talk, but both functions are unaffected. Repeating the technique used for the nasal exam, decide which nasal cavity is the most patent. Hold the nasal speculum in place and tilt the patient's head back. Your solutions are in atomizers. Attach these bottles to the air compressor. Apply 0.5% phenylephrine followed by 4% lidocaine. These solutions take several minutes to kick in. Go get the scope (and don't forget to attach the teaching head).

18. Identify the structures visualized as the scope is advanced on fiberoptic laryngoscopy.

Upon insertion of the scope, you visualize the entire nasal cavity. This includes the inferior and middle turbinates, superior nasal cavity, eustachian tube orifice, and adenoids. As the scope is advanced, the oropharynx is visible, including the soft palate, uvula, posterior pharyngeal wall, and base of the tongue. As the scope reaches the hypopharynx, the valleculae and epiglottis appear. The epiglottic folds, arytenoids, and piriform fossa are visualized. Finally, as the scope is advanced deep into the larynx, the false vocal cords, ventricles, and true vocal cords are seen. At this point, the patient is asked to phonate, and vocal cord motion is evaluated.

19. How are the sinuses evaluated on physical examination?

When the nasal examination reveals polyps or drainage suggestive of sinus disease, the sinuses should be thoroughly evaluated. The evaluation includes direct examination, palpation, percussion, and transillumination of sinus walls. Walls that are directly available for examination include the maxillary floor (from the palate), anterior maxillary wall (from the cheek), lateral ethmoid wall (from the medial canthus), frontal floor (from the roof of the orbit), and anterior frontal wall (from the supraorbital skull). Palpation and percussion of these areas may demonstrate tenderness in the presence of acute inflammation. However, discomfort is rarely elicited in the presence of chronic sinusitis.

20. How is transillumination of the nasal sinuses performed?

Transillumination is used to assess the health of the maxillary and frontal sinuses. In a darkened examination room, the maxillary sinus is evaluated by illuminating it with a light placed medial to the nose and then inspecting the palate. The frontal sinus is illuminated by placing the light at the upper and inner angle of the orbit. Comparing the sinuses bilaterally, decreased brightness on one side suggests sinus disease. Mucosal disease may be present where the least light transmission is appreciated.

21. What are the 10 classic lymph node groups?

Your examination should note the size, consistency, shape, and tenderness of palpable lymph nodes. It is important to determine if the nodes are discrete, fixed, or matted. The 10 groups of lymph nodes include:

1. Preauricular
2. Posterior auricular (postauricular)
3. Occipital
4. Tonsillar
5. Submaxillary
6. Submental
7. Superficial cervical
8. Posterior cervical chain
9. Deep cervical chain
10. Supraclavicular

22. Explain the physical examination of the trachea and thyroid.

The Adam's apple, or thyroid notch, is the most prominent landmark. Inferior to this landmark lies the cricoid, which may be felt as a firm ring. Inferior to the cricoid, the tracheal rings are palpable. Deviation of these rings is suggestive of a mass. The thyroid isthmus lies between the cricoid cartilage and the sternal notch. Asking the patient to swallow may allow the identification of the isthmus as it moves up and down with the trachea. The thyroid may be palpated on either side of the trachea just superior to the sternal notch. It may be difficult to feel the thyroid distinctly, although asymmetric masses or nodules suggest pathology.

23. How does the head and neck examination differ in children from that in adults?

In newborns, the ears, nose, mouth, and throat are common areas of congenital malformations and therefore require thorough evaluation for deformities, skin tags, and clefts. In older children, the key to a successful pediatric examination is trust. The examination may be more effective if the clinician dispenses with the use of many of the otolaryngologic instruments. Often a child's ears and nose may be successfully examined without speculums. The ear may be examined by gently retracting the pinna backward while drawing the tragus forward, and the nose may be examined by slightly lifting the nasal tip.

CONTROVERSIES

24. What is the diagnostic significance of an otologic "light reflex"?

A light reflex is often described in the normal ear as a cone of light that reflects from the umbo of the malleus upon otoscopic examination. While some feel that an aberrance of this finding signifies disease, the light reflex generally has no diagnostic importance. This finding may be present in a severely diseased ear, while it may be absent or abnormal in a normal ear.

25. Who should perform fiberoptic laryngoscopy?

Traditionally, otolaryngologists remain experts at the evaluation of the larynx and may be the most experienced with fiberoptic laryngoscopy. However, primary care physicians and emergency medicine physicians may be trained to perform this examination safely and effectively. Most emergency departments possess a fiberoptic laryngoscope, and the physicians find them useful in their practice. Complex problems, however, may necessitate an otolaryngologist.

BIBLIOGRAPHY

1. Bates B : The head and neck. In Bates B (ed): A Guide to Physical Examination, 3rd ed. Philadelphia, J.B. Lippincott, 1983, pp 95–124.
2. Coleman BH: Diseases of the external ear. In Diseases of the Nose, Throat and Ear, and Head and Neck, 14th ed. Edinburgh, Churchill-Livingstone, 1992, pp 209–220.
3. Upchurn DT: Otolaryngology. Oradell, NJ, Medical Economics Books, 1989, pp 1–65.

II. Otology

3. ANATOMY AND PHYSIOLOGY OF THE EAR

Bruce W. Murrow, M.D., Ph.D.

1. What structures compose the external ear?

The external ear consists of the pinna and external auditory canal and is bounded medially by the tympanic membrane. The lateral, cartilaginous part of the canal has hair follicles and ceruminous glands, while the inner, bony part is free of accessory structures. The external ear serves to collect and direct the sound toward the tympanic membrane. The length of the external canal, about 2.5 cm in adults, gives it a resonant frequency of 3.0–4.0 kHz.

2. What is the middle ear?

The middle ear is a 1–2-cm³ air-filled cavity that houses the ossicles, chorda tympani nerve (parasympathetic to submandibular and sublingual glands, and taste to posterior tongue), and stapedius and tensor tympani muscles. It is bounded laterally by the tympanic membrane and medially by the lateral wall of the inner ear (labyrinth capsule). It is continuous with the mastoid air cells and eustachian tube. The facial nerve runs in a bony canal very close to the middle ear and consequently can be affected by middle ear pathology. The tympanic membrane and ossicular chain most efficiently transmit frequencies between 500–3000 Hz with a resonance around 1 kHz.

3. Name the three ossicles in the middle ear.

The malleus, incus, and stapes form the ossicular chain. The malleus is positioned between the tympanic membrane and the incus. The incus is connected to the stapes. The stapes subsequently connects to the oval window of the inner ear.

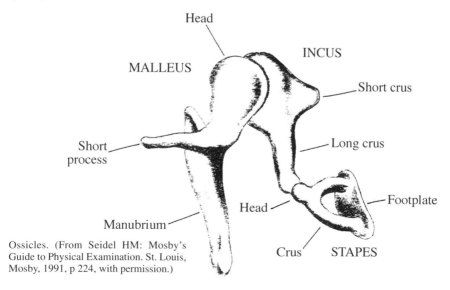

Ossicles. (From Seidel HM: Mosby's Guide to Physical Examination. St. Louis, Mosby, 1991, p 224, with permission.)

4. What role does the tensor tympani and stapedius muscles play?

The tensor tympani and stapedius muscles dampen middle ear mechanics. Loud sounds (about 80 dB) cause the stapedius muscle to contract, which limits the movement of the stapes. While the acoustic reflex may provide a protective role, it also may serve as a gain-control mechanism to keep cochlear input more constant and expand the dynamic range of the system. Alternatively, contraction of the stapedius muscle has been noted with chewing and vocalization, and thus, it may reduce self-generated noise.

5. Which structure provides aeration of the middle ear?

The eustachian tube, by its connection to the nasopharynx, aerates and drains the middle ear. Its dysfunction can cause otitis media. The immature function of the eustachian tube predisposes children to ear infections.

6. How does the middle ear maximize the transfer of sound stimuli to the cochlea?

As sound travels from air to a fluid medium, the final stimuli is greatly diminished because of impedance mismatching. The middle ear minimizes this problem by the **area effect** of the tympanic membrane and the **lever action** of the ossicular chain. The effective vibrating area of the tympanic membrane is about 17 times the area of the stapes footplate, resulting in a 17-fold increase in sound energy. The handle of the malleus is about 1.3 times the length of the short process of the incus, so the force at the stapes is increased by 1.3-fold. The combination of these two effects creates a 22:1 mechanical advantage, which provides a 25-dB increase in sound energy arriving to the cochlea.

7. What is the inner ear?

The inner ear is a membranous labyrinth system embedded in bone. This system consists of the auditory end organ (cochlea) and the vestibular end organs (utricle, saccule, and semicircular canals).

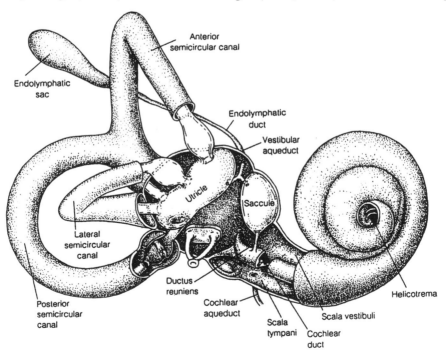

The membranous labyrinth. (From Pender DJ: Practical Otology. Philadelphia, J.B. Lippincott, 1992, p 7, with permission.)

8. Describe the tonotopic organization of the cochlea.

A tonotopic gradient exists in the cochlea. Higher-frequency sounds are detected at the base of the cochlea, while lower-frequency sounds are detected at the apex. The mechanical properties of the basilar membrane shape this tonotopic gradient.

9. What is the "traveling wave"?

G. von Bekesy is credited with describing the pattern of movement of the basilar membrane (traveling wave) in response to sinusoidal sound. Each point on the basilar membrane moves at the same frequency as the stimulus. However, the amplitude and phase differ considerably along the length of the cochlea. As a result, the movement of the basilar membrane appears as a traveling wave moving from the base to the apex. The tonotopic map of the basilar membrane determines where the largest peak of the wave occurs.

10. What structures are key to the receptor cells of the inner ear?

Receptor cells have evaginations of the membrane on their apical surfaces called **stereocilia**. Stereocilia appear as hairs at lower magnification.

11. Describe the anatomy of the cochlea.

The cochlea is a snail-like tube that is divided along its length into three compartments: the **scala vestibuli** (top), **scala media** (middle) and **scala tympani** (bottom). **Reissner's membrane** separates the scala vestibuli from the scala media. The **basilar membrane** separates the scala media from the scala tympani. **Perilymph**, a fluid similar to extracellular fluid, fills the scala vestibuli and tympani, while **endolymph**, a fluid similar to intracellular fluid, fills the scala media. The scala media houses the **organ of Corti**.

12. What is the organ of Corti?

The organ of Corti contains hair cells that sit on the basilar membrane and are overlaid by the tectorial membrane. There are two types of hair cells in the cochlea, inner hair cells and outer hair cells. One row of inner hair cells spirals up the cochlea near the central axis, while 3–4 rows of adjacent outer hair cells spiral up the cochlea further from the central axis.

13. How are the cochlear hair cells stimulated?

The tectorial and basilar membranes are connected centrally. Sound moves these two structures differentially, producing a shear force that bends the stereocilia. Movement of the stereocilia opens and closes ion channels, producing a receptor potential in the inner hair cell. The receptor potential in turn releases neurotransmitters onto afferent nerve fibers, essentially signaling the brain to the presence of a specific sound frequency. The specific hair cells which are stimulated by a given sound depend on the tonotopic map of the basilar membrane.

14. How do inner and outer hair cells differ?

Inner hair cells are thought to be the classic auditory receptor cells that are responsible for signaling the brain as to the presence of specific sound frequencies. The **outer hair cells** are located further from the central axis. More recently, the outer hair cells have been shown to shorten and lengthen when stimulated by sound. This movement is thought to affect the inner hair cells by altering the basilar membrane motion and increasing the sensitivity and frequency selectivity of the cochlear output.

15. How does the innervation of inner and outer hair cells differ?

Inner hair cells are predominantly **afferently** innervated. Afferent nerve fibers carry information from the hair cells to the brain. In contrast, outer hair cells are predominantly **efferently** innervated. Efferent fibers carry information from the brain to the hair cells. Efferent stimulation of the outer hair cells may be responsible for decreasing the responsiveness of the cochlea.

16. Trace the neural sound pathway from the cochlea to the brain.
Stimulation begins at the hair cells and travels through the afferent nerves, cochlear nuclei, superior olive, lateral lemniscus, inferior colliculus, and medial geniculate body to arrive in the auditory cortex.

17. Name the five vestibular end organs and their stimuli.
One utricle, one saccule, and three semicircular canals. The semicircular canals each detect angular acceleration such as head rotation. The utricle has receptor cells in a horizontal plane, and the saccule has receptor cells in the vertical plane. The utricle and saccule detect linear acceleration, such as gravity and straight line motion.

18. How are the receptor cells in the semicircular canals, utricle, and saccule stimulated?
In each semicircular canal are hair cells with stereocilia embedded in the jelly-like substance of the cupola. This substance has the same density of endolymph. Angular motion moves the endolymph, as well as the cupola, bending the stereocilia and stimulating the hair cell. The saccule and the macule of the utricle contain hair cells that are overlaid by an otolithic membrane made of calcium carbonate crystals. This otolithic membrane is denser than the endolymph. Therefore, gravity and linear acceleration move the membrane relative to the hair cells, bending the cells' stereocilia and causing stimulation.

19. Why are vestibular reflexes important?
These reflexes link the vestibular system with a number of other systems (i.e., vestibulo-ocular reflex, vestibulospinal reflex, cerebellovestibular reflex). Vestibular reflexes contribute to maintaining posture and muscle tone. In addition, they generate transient muscle contractions which contribute to equilibrium and eye stability while moving.

BIBLIOGRAPHY
1. Ashmore JF: The G.L. Brown Prize Lecture: The cellular machinery of the cochlea. Exp Physiol 79: 113–134, 1994.
2. Ashmore JF, Kolston PJ: Hair cell based amplification in the cochlea. Curr Opin Neurobiol 4:503–508, 1994.
3. Becker W, Naumann HH, Pfaltz CR: Ear, Nose, and Throat Diseases, 2nd ed. Stuttgart, Georg Thieme, 1994.
4. Bekesy GV: Experiments in Hearing. New York, McGraw-Hill, 1960.
5. Cummings CW (ed): Otolaryngology–Head and Neck Surgery, 2nd ed. (vol. 4). St. Louis, Mosby Year Book, 1993.
6. Lee KJ: Essential Otolaryngology: Head & Neck Surgery, 6th ed. Norwalk, CT, Appleton & Lange, 1995.
7. Pender DJ: Practical Otology. Philadelphia, J. B. Lippincott, 1992.
8. Pickles JO: Recent advances in cochlear physiology. Prog Neurobiol 24:1-42, 1985.
9. Yates GK, Johnstone BM, Patuzzi RB, Robertson D: Mechanical processing in the mammalian cochlea. Trends Neurosci 15:57–61, 1992.

4. THE HEARING EVALUATION

Catherine Winslow, M.D., and Jerry L. Northern, Ph.D.

1. Describe the two general types of hearing loss. How are they different?
1. **Conductive hearing loss** (CHL) results from any disruption in the passage of sound from the external ear to the oval window. Anatomically, this pathway includes the ear canal, tympanic membrane, and ossicles. Such a loss may be due to cerumen impaction, tympanic membrane perforation, otitis media, or otosclerosis. Conductive losses are often correctable with medical or surgical treatment.

2. **Sensorineural hearing loss** (SNHL) results from otologic abnormalities beyond the oval window. Such abnormalities may affect the sensory cells of the cochlea or the neural fibers of the eighth nerve. Presbycusis is an example of a sensorineural hearing loss. Eighth nerve tumors may also lead to such a loss. Sensorineural losses are generally permanent and more difficult to manage medically. Patients may also have a mixed hearing loss (e.g., resulting from chronic otitis media coexistent with cochlear damage).

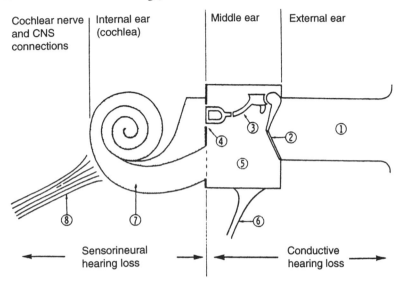

Conductive and sensorineural hearing loss. Examples of (1) wax, inflammatory swelling; (2) perforated eardrum; (3) necrosed or immobile ossicles; (4) stapes fixation by otosclerosis; (5) otitis media; (6) eustachian tube block; (7) sensory presbycusis, mumps, noise injury; (8) neural presbycusis, acoustic tumors. (From Coleman BH: Diseases of the Nose, Throat and Ear, and Head and Neck. Edinburgh, Churchill Livingstone, 1992, p 196, with permission.)

2. What type of tuning fork is used in the basic clinical examination?
A **512-Hz fork** should be used when performing tuning fork tests. It is essential that the fork be sounded gently. Overtones with excessive vibration lead to inaccurate results.

3. What is the Weber tuning fork test? How is it performed and interpreted?
The Weber test is a basic test of hearing. In the Weber test, the tuning fork is struck, and its base is placed midline on the patient's skull. The patient is asked where the tone is perceived and if the tone is louder in one ear or the other. In a conductive loss, the tone is louder and localizes to the poorer hearing, affected ear. In a sensorineural hearing loss, the patient perceives the tone to be louder in the better hearing or unaffected ear. Patients with equal hearing or bilaterally symmetrical hearing problems will localize the sound to the skull midline.

4. What is the Rinne tuning fork test? How is it done?
The Rinne test is also used to differentiate between conductive and sensorineural hearing losses. The test is performed by alternately placing the prongs of a vibrating tuning fork at the patient's ear canal and the base of the tuning fork on the patient's mastoid bone. The patient is asked whether the tone is heard louder at the ear canal or on the mastoid. In the patient with normal hearing and normal middle ear status, the tuning fork is heard louder at the ear canal or equally loud in both positions. Similar findings are expected from a patient with a sensorineural hearing loss. Patients with conductive loss, however, hear the tuning fork sound louder at the mastoid position (a **negative** Rinne test result). A negative test is obtained when the hearing loss is at least 25 dB HL.

5. Describe the Schwabach tuning fork test.

The Schwabach test is a crude estimation of sensorineural hearing deficit. The base of a vibrating tuning fork is placed on the patient's mastoid bone. When the tone decays to the point that the patient is unable to perceive it, the examiner quickly transfers the tuning fork to his or her own mastoid. If the examiner is able to hear the tone, the test indicates that the patient has a sensorineural hearing loss. The test result is then reported as "diminished," reflecting the patient's hearing status. This test, of course, requires that the examiner have hearing within normal limits.

6. What is an audiogram?

An audiogram is a graphic representation of auditory threshold responses which are obtained from testing a patient's hearing with pure-tone stimuli. The parameters of the audiogram are **frequency**, as measured in cycles per second (Hz), and **intensity**, as measured in decibels (dB). The typical audiogram is determined by establishing hearing thresholds for single-frequency sounds at 250, 500, 1000, 2000, 4000, and 8000 Hz.

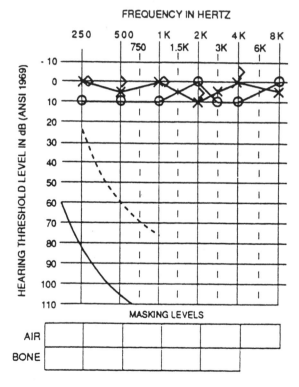

Commonly Used Audiogram Symbols

LEFT EAR (BLUE)	INTERPRETATION	RIGHT EAR (RED)
x	Unmasked air conduction	O
n	Masked air conduction	Δ
>	Unmasked bone conduction	<
]	Masked bone conduction	[
↘	No response	↙

A normal audiogram. (From Lee KJ: Essential Otolaryngology–Head and Neck Surgery. Norwalk, CT, Appleton & Lange, 1995, p 37, with permission.)

7. How wide is the frequency range for normal hearing?
   The human ear reportedly can detect sound in the frequency range of 20–20,000 Hz. However, the typical adult can only detect frequencies between 200–10,000 Hz. The speech frequency spectrum ranges from 400–3000 Hz.

8. What is a decibel?
   A decibel is an arbitrary unit of measurement that is logarithmic in nature. Several decibel scales are used to measure sounds and hearing, and it is necessary to identify each reference scale when presenting a value in decibels. For example, hearing is measured on a biologic scale in Decibels Hearing Level (dB HL), while environmental sounds are measured on a physical scale in Decibels Sound Pressure Level (dB SPL).

9. Does "0 dB HL" mean silence or deafness?
   Neither. The normal human ear is not equally sensitive to all frequencies, and it is able to hear high frequencies better than low frequencies. For example, normal hearing at 125 Hz is about 45 dB SPL, but normal hearing at 1000 Hz is about 7 dB SPL. Therefore, a reference level is needed. "0 dB HL" is a reference level on the audiogram that represents normal hearing across the entire frequency spectrum. Therefore, normal hearing at 124 Hz may be 0 dB HL, and normal hearing at 1000 Hz may also be 0 dB HL.

10. What is normal hearing?
   Practically speaking, normal adult hearing is represented as a biologic range between –10 and 20 dB HL. The measurement of hearing is based on threshold responses, with a threshold defined as that point at which a patient perceives a sound stimulus 50% of the time. Patients with hearing loss have audiograms with poorer thresholds (larger numbers in decibels) at the involved frequencies.

11. How much of a hearing loss can a patient have and still have "normal" hearing?
   A hearing threshold level (HTL) of < 20 dB is considered to be within the normal hearing range.

Hearing Threshold Levels

< 20 dB HTL	Normal hearing
20–40 dB HTL	Mild hearing loss
40–60 dB HTL	Moderate hearing loss
60–80 dB HTL	Severe hearing loss
> 80 dB HTL	Profound hearing loss

12. What is the pure-tone average?
   The pure-tone average is an estimate of the patient's ability to hear within the speech frequencies. The value is calculated by averaging the air conduction hearing thresholds at 500, 1000, and 2000 Hz.

13. What is masking?
   Sound that is presented to the test ear can travel via bone conduction through the head and be perceived in the opposite, nontest ear. This phenomenon, called **crossover**, can obscure measurement results in the test ear. Therefore, the nontested ear must be eliminated from the test. Air conduction sounds crossover when a 50-dB difference exists between the air conduction threshold of the test ear and the bone conduction threshold of the nontest ear. However, bone conduction sounds may crossover when as little as 0-dB difference

exists between the bone conduction thresholds of the two ears. **Masking** is the presentation of sound to the nontest ear and serves to prevent the nontest ear from interfering with true sound perception in the test ear.

14. How does the audiologist distinguish between air and bone conduction deficits?

In measurements of air conduction hearing thresholds, headphones deliver sound to the patient. If a hearing loss is noted on testing air conduction, bone conduction hearing thresholds are subsequently performed. Bone conduction is tested by placing a vibrating device behind the ear on the mastoid. This vibrating device presents the sound to the inner ear, thus bypassing the middle ear system. Patients with sensorineural hearing loss have equal hearing thresholds by air and bone conduction measurements. Patients with conductive hearing loss have normal cochlear function; therefore, they show normal hearing thresholds by bone conduction but poor hearing thresholds by air conduction.

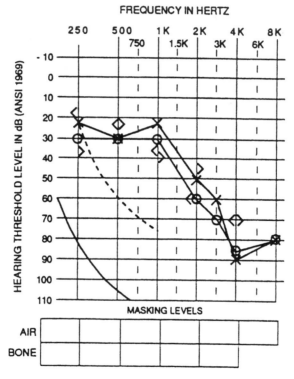

Audiogram showing sensorineural hearing loss. (From Lee KJ: Essential Otolaryngology–Head and Neck Surgery. Norwalk, CT, Appleton & Lange, 1995, p 38, with permission.)

15. What is an air-bone gap?

An air-bone gap is the difference in decibels between the hearing threshold levels for air and bone conduction. Significant air-bone gaps represent conductive hearing loss. Because the patient hears better through bone conduction than with headphones, a gap exists between the two measurements. With normal hearing, the air and bone conduction thresholds are approximately equal (< 15 dB HTL). With sensorineural hearing loss, the air and bone conduction thresholds are approximately equal but, overall, show a deficit.

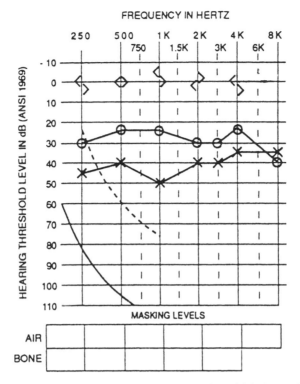

Air-bone gap typical of a conductive hearing loss. (From Lee KJ: Essential Otolaryngology–Head and Neck Surgery. Norwalk, CT, Appleton & Lange, 1995, p 37, with permission.)

16. What is the speech reception threshold (SRT) test?

This test is performed to confirm the pure-tone threshold findings. A specific set of bisyllabic words, known as **spondees**, are presented to the patient at decreasing intensities. Spondees are two-syllable compound words that are pronounced with equal emphasis on each syllable—e.g., oatmeal, popcorn, shipwreck. The SRT is the lowest intensity at which the patient correctly identifies the word in 50% of the presentations. The SRT should be within ± 6 dB of the three-frequency pure-tone average.

17. Describe the speech discrimination test.

The speech discrimination test utilizes word recognition to assess the patient's understanding of speech. A standardized list of single-syllable words are presented 30–40 dB above the SRT. The patient repeats each word, and the score is determined according to the percentage of words that are correctly identified. For example, a patient may understand the test word *knee* as *me*. A score > 90% is considered to represent normal word recognition and speech understanding.

18. Which is the "gold standard" test, the audiogram or tuning fork test?

The answer lies primarily in the skill of the tester. A carefully performed Weber tuning fork test can detect a 3-dB difference between the two ears. However, the tuning fork is easily misused. A "null point" exists 45° from the head where the fork cannot be optimally heard. Therefore, perpendicular placement must be used. The usefulness and consistency of the audiogram are determined by the patience and skill of the tester. On an emergency basis, the audiogram is disadvantageous because it is often difficult to obtain both the proper equipment and a skilled tester. Ideally, the patient should be tested by correlating the results of *both* the tuning fork tests and the audiogram.

19. If the audiogram disagrees with the findings on the physical exam and tuning fork tests, what should you do next?

A number of factors should be considered. Has the audiometry equipment recently been producing questionable results? Do both headphones work? Is the examiner properly using the tuning forks? Is the examiner comfortable with the anatomy? Does the patient understand the instructions? Does the patient have a secondary gain? If available, old audiograms should be obtained for comparison. Re-testing the patient in the presence of both the otolaryngologist and audiologist may help to identify the cause of the discrepancy. Most importantly, the inconsistency needs to be resolved.

20. What is the immittance test battery?

The immittance test battery is not a hearing test, per se, but rather an electroacoustic testing procedure that is used to evaluate the status of the auditory system. The test battery typically includes tympanometry, the physical volume measurement of the ear canal, and ipsilateral and contralateral acoustic reflex measurements.

21. What is tympanometry?

Tympanometry can be thought of as electronic pneumatic otoscopy. Tympanometry is an objective test that measures the mobility, or compliance, of the tympanic membrane and the middle ear system. A seal is formed between the instrument probe and the external canal. Air pressure is manipulated into the space bound by the probe, the external ear canal, and the tympanic membrane. Tympanometry results are represented by air pressure/compliance graphs known as tympanograms. The compliance of the tympanic membrane is at its maximum when air pressure on both sides of the eardrum is equal. The **peak** air pressure of the tympanogram is equal to the patient's middle ear pressure. The range of normal middle ear pressures is between 0 and -150 mm H_2O and represents normal eustachian tube function. Middle ear pressures that are more negative than -150 mm H_2O are indicative of poor eustachian tube function.

22. How are tympanograms classified?

Tympanograms are classified into five general configurations:

Type A	Normal middle ear function
Type A_s	Tympanic membrane is stiffer than normal (lower compliance) in the presence of normal middle ear pressures (e.g., otosclerosis)
Type A_d	Tympanic membrane is more flaccid than normal (higher compliance) in the presence of normal middle ear pressure (e.g., ossicular discontinuity)
Type B ("flat" tympanogram)	Shows no pressure peak and indicates nonmobility of the tympanic membrane (e.g., middle ear effusion or perforated tympanic membrane)
Type C	Shows a peak in the negative pressure range (< -150 mm H_2O); indicates poor eustachian tube function

23. What is the ear canal physical volume test?

This test is conducted with an immittance meter and measures the volume that is medial to a hermetically sealed probe. The result, typically reported in cm^3, is the absolute volume of the ear canal when the tympanic membrane is normal. However, in situations where the tympanic membrane is perforated or nonintact, the measurement is quite large as the volume of the middle ear space is also included. Pressure equalization tubes will therefore result in a large volume measurement.

24. What is the function of the stapedius muscle?

The stapedius muscle, attached to the posterior crus of the stapes, contracts reflexively at the onset of a loud sound. The muscle contracts bilaterally, even when only one ear is stimulated. The stapedius muscle can provide some protection to the inner ear in the presence of potentially damaging intense sound. The acoustic reflex causes immediate stiffening of the ossicles and increased compliance of the middle ear system and tympanic membrane. Testing the contraction of the stapedius muscle and the acoustic reflex is an important part of the immittance test battery.

25. Describe the acoustic reflex neural pathways.

The acoustic reflex has both an ipsilateral and contralateral pathway. The majority of neurons run through the ipsilateral pathway. The **ipsilateral** pathway begins at the cochlea and proceeds through the eighth nerve, cochlear nucleus, trapezoid body, superior olivary complex, and facial motor nucleus to the ipsilateral stapedial muscle. The **contralateral** pathway crosses the brainstem to continue to the opposite cochlear nucleus, trapezoid body, contralateral olivary complex, motor nucleus of the facial nerve, and opposite stapedius muscle.

26. How is the acoustic reflex measured?

The acoustic reflex is measured with the **immittance meter**. The change in compliance of the middle ear is caused by contraction of the stapedial reflex and is time-locked to the presence of a loud acoustic stimulus. When the ipsilateral reflex is measured, the stimulus is presented through a sealed probe. When the contralateral reflex is measured, the stimulus is presented through an earphone on the opposite ear. Measurement of the acoustic reflex is a valuable screening technique that is used to determine the integrity of the neural pathways. It is also used to detect eighth nerve tumors, sensory cell impairment of the cochlea, and loudness tolerance for patients with sensorineural hearing loss.

27. What is auditory brainstem response audiometry?

Auditory brainstem response (ABR) is an objective, physiologic measurement of hearing. This computerized audiometric test is also useful in the identification of retrocochlear pathology and can detect lesions that interfere with the main neural hearing pathways (e.g., tumors of the eighth nerve, internal auditory meatus, and cerebellopontine angle). An ABR is conducted by using scalp electrodes to pick up the minute electroencephalographic activity created when sound is perceived. A series of clicks are delivered to the patient through earphones. When an acoustic signal stimulates the ear, it elicits ("evokes") a series of small electrical events ("potentials") along the entire peripheral and central auditory pathway. This minute electrical activity is picked up by the electrodes, amplified, and averaged with a computer. The electrical activity is displayed as a waveform with five latency-specific wave peaks. The latency of each wave peak corresponds to sites in the neural auditory pathway. In basic terms, each peak represents one anatomic structure in the auditory pathway. A tumor will slow the neural circuit and delay the waveform at the site of the lesion. The ABR may also be used to determine hearing thresholds. By decreasing the amplitude of the stimulus click, the peaks of the waveform will eventually disappear. The ABR test is especially useful in testing hearing in infants and young children who are unable to be tested by conventional methods.

28. How do you interpret an ABR?

The mnemonic, **E COLI**, will help you to remember which structure corresponds to each wave form.

Wave I	—**E**ighth nerve action potential
Wave II	—**C**ochlear nucleus
Wave III	—**O**livary complex (superior)
Wave IV	—**L**ateral lemniscus
Wave V	—**I**nferior colliculus

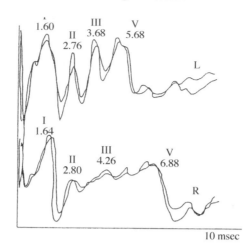

Normal and abnormal ABRs. ABR tracing from left ear *(top)* is normal. Right ear *(bottom)* is abnormal. (From Glasscock ME, Cueva RA, Thedinger BA: Handbook of Vertigo. New York, Raven Press, 1990, p 24, with permission.)

29. Why use so many different types of auditory tests?

The auditory system is the most complex sensory pathway, with numerous bilateral ascending and descending routes for neural transmission. Accordingly, the various types of hearing tests are used to form a differential diagnosis and to help localize the specific site of an auditory lesion. It is not uncommon for patients with central lesions to have a pure-tone hearing test which is within normal limits.

30. How do you evaluate hearing in a pediatric patient?

The hearing evaluation of infants and children poses a challenge. Audiologists use special techniques, adapted to the age level of the child, to obtain valid and reliable test results.

1. In **behavioral observation audiometry**, sounds are presented to the child at various intensity levels, and an audiologist watches for a movement or reaction. Positive reinforcement is typically incorporated into the test procedure. For example, when the child reacts appropriately to the presence of the auditory stimulus, a visual reinforcement is utilized, such as a lighted toy. An older infant or young child may be conditioned to look toward the source of sound where they expect to see the illuminated toy.

2. During **play audiometry**, used for children over 3 years of age, a game is incorporated into the test. Each time the child hears the stimulus tone, the child responds by picking a marble out of a bucket, putting a peg into a board, or performing another simple but fun task.

3. In **speech audiometry**, the audiologist presents spondee words along with pictures, and the child points to the appropriate picture. The intensity level of the spondee word is adjusted to determine the speech reception threshold.

4. Objective tests, such as immittance measurements and ABRs, are of particular value in determining the hearing status of young children who are difficult to test with conventional methods.

31. What are the pediatric high-risk factors commonly associated with hearing loss?

1. Family history of childhood hearing impairment
2. Congenital perinatal infection (e.g., cytomegalovirus, rubella, herpes, toxoplasmosis, syphilis)
3. Anatomic malformation of head or neck
4. Birth < 1500 gm

5. Hyperbilirubinemia at level exceeding indications for exchange transfusion
6. Bacterial meningitis, especially *Haemophilus influenzae*
7. Severe asphyxia, including infants with Apgar scores of 0–3 who fail to institute spontaneous respiration by 10 min and those with hypotonia persisting to 2 hr of age

High-risk newborns should be screened for hearing with ABR prior to hospital discharge.

(Above criteria are from Lee KJ: Essential Otolaryngology–Head and Neck Surgery, 6th ed. Norwalk, CT, Appleton and Lange, 1995, p 57, with permission.)

32. When should a primary care physician be concerned about a patient's hearing complaint?

Always. All patients with hearing loss need further evaluation. Often patients with conductive hearing problems may be successfully treated by medical or surgical means. Patients with sensorineural hearing loss need to be medically evaluated prior to audiologic fitting with hearing aids. Patients with a history of sudden-onset hearing loss, trauma, infection associated with the loss, or asymmetrical hearing loss should be given thorough hearing tests and concurrent otolaryngologic evaluation. Symptoms of tinnitus, aural fullness, vertigo, or ear drainage also necessitate complete otolaryngologic evaluation.

BIBLIOGRAPHY

1. Bluestone CD: Physiology of the middle ear and eustachian tube. In Paparella MM (ed): Otolaryngology. Philadelphia, W.B. Saunders, 1991, pp 163–197.
2. Carhart R, Jerger J: Preferred method for clinical determination of pure tone thresholds. J Speech Hear Dis 24:330–345, 1959.
3. Katz J: Handbook of Clinical Audiology, 4th ed. Baltimore, Williams & Wilkins, 1994.
4. Litton WB: Epithelial migration over tympanic membrane and external canal. Arch Otolaryngol 77:254–257, 1963.
5. Martin FN: Clinical audiometry and masking. New York, Bobbs-Merrill, 1972.
6. Northern J (ed): Hearing Disorders, 3rd ed. Needham Heights, MA, Allyn & Bacon, 1995.
7. Northern JL, Downs MP: Hearing in Children, 4th ed. Baltimore, Williams & Wilkins, 1991.
8. Yanagisawa K, Lee KJ: Audiology. In Lee KJ (ed): Essential Otolaryngology. East Norwalk, CT, Appleton & Lange, 1991, pp 25–60.
9. Yellin MW: Hearing measurement in adults. In Paparella MM (ed): Otolaryngology. Philadelphia, W.B. Saunders, 1991, pp 961–975.
10. Zwislocki J: Normal function of the middle ear and its measurement. Audiology 21:4–14, 1988.

5. CONDUCTIVE HEARING LOSS

Bruce W. Murrow, M.D., Ph.D.

1. What is conductive hearing loss?

A conductive hearing loss involves pathology located between the opening of the external auditory canal and the hair cells of the cochlea—i.e., the ear canal, tympanic membrane, or ossicles. Essentially, the conduction of the auditory stimulus is hindered from reaching the cochlear receptor cells.

2. In the evaluation of a conductive hearing loss, what should the history and physical exam address?

History: age of onset; progression of hearing loss; unilateral versus bilateral; family history; ear fullness; tinnitus; vertigo/dizziness; medications; trauma; visual, speech, or other neurologic problems; ear pain; and ear discharge.

Physical exam: complete head and neck exam with focus on the external ear, tympanic membrane, and middle ear; pneumatic otoscopy; tuning fork tests.

3. Describe the results of tuning fork tests in a purely conductive hearing loss.

In the Weber test, the sound "lateralizes" toward the ear with the conductive hearing loss. If the conductive hearing loss is > 20 dB, the Rinne test will demonstrate bone conduction louder than air conduction.

4. What are the typical audiometric findings of a conductive hearing loss?

On an audiogram, an air-bone gap is often present. This gap represents a response discrepancy between air- and bone-conducted stimuli. The bone-conducted stimuli, placed directly on the mastoid, bypasses the conductive mechanisms of the external and middle ear. Air-conducted stimuli must pass through these structures. For example, a patient has a conductive hearing loss if he or she exhibits a deficit with air conduction but a normal response with bone conduction.

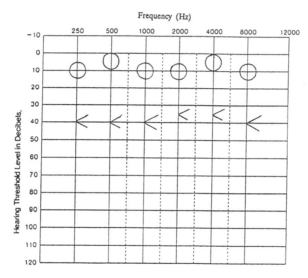

Audiogram of a right ear with pure conductive hearing loss. The difference between the air conductive response *(circles)* and the bone conductive response *(arrows)* is referred to as the air-bone gap. (From Lee KJ: Essential Otolaryngology–Head and Neck Surgery, 6th ed. Norwalk, CT, Appleton & Lange, 1995, with permission.)

5. What is the greatest loss that a conductive hearing loss can produce?

A pure and complete conductive hearing loss can result in a 60–70-dB deficit. Ossicular discontinuity should be considered with losses > 50 dB.

6. How do other audiometric tests aid in the diagnosis of conductive hearing loss?

In the absence of tympanic membrane pathology, low compliance (type A_s) occurs with fixation of the ossicles, as in otosclerosis, while high compliance (type A_d) is found with ossicular discontinuity. The tympanogram in cases of otitis media also has decreased compliance (type B or C) due to the fluid in the middle ear. The stapedial reflex is often absent in conductive hearing loss.

7. List the pathologies of the external ear that produce conductive hearing loss.

Impacted cerumen	Exostosis (bony projections into the canal)
Foreign bodies	Osteomas
External otitis	Tumors
Congenital aplasia or stenosis	Cysts

8. **List the pathologies of the middle ear that produce conductive hearing loss.**

Tympanic membrane perforations	Hemotympanum
Tympanosclerosis	Otitis media
Retracted tympanic membranes	Tumors
Ossicular malformations	Cholesteatoma
Ossicular discontinuity	Previous ear surgery
Otosclerosis	Eustachian tube dysfunction

9. **Which is the most common cause of conductive hearing loss?**
   Cerumen impaction is probably the most prevalent cause of conductive hearing loss. Excluding cerumen, the most common cause between the ages 15 and 50 is otosclerosis. Approximately 1% of the population is affected by otosclerosis.

10. **Which is the most common cause of conductive hearing loss in children?**
    Otitis media with effusion.

11. **What amount of hearing loss can be attributed to cerumen impaction?**
    Impacted cerumen that completely occludes the canal may lead to a 30–40 dB hearing loss.

12. **What is otosclerosis? How does it cause conductive hearing loss?**
    Otosclerosis is an abnormality of bone metabolism and turnover affecting the otic capsule of the ossicles. Stiffening and fixation of the stapes footplate occur secondary to the dense sclerosis and cause a conductive hearing loss. Stapedectomy has a 90–95% success rate for improving hearing.

13. **How do tympanic membrane perforations cause conductive hearing loss?**
    The efficiency of transferring sound from the external auditory canal to the cochlea relies heavily on the larger surface area of the tympanic membrane in relation to the area of the stapes footplate. This physical advantage is reduced by a perforation, which decreases the sound-receiving area of the tympanic membrane. Sound distortion from the edge of the perforation and a phase difference from sound arriving at the oval and round windows at similar times add to the hearing loss.

14. **How do temporal bone fractures result in conductive hearing loss?**
    Longitudinal fractures through the temporal bone tend to produce bloody otorrhea and conductive hearing loss by perforating the tympanic membrane and disrupting the ossicular chain and external auditory canal. Transverse fractures are likely to produce a hemotympanum and cochlear damage. The hemotympanum initially produces a component of conductive loss but, more significantly, eventually results in a sensorineural hearing deficit.

15. **How does a cholesteatoma produce conductive hearing loss?**
    A cholesteatoma is a nest of epithelial cell growth that can occur in the middle ear. It causes conductive hearing loss by a mass effect which impairs movement of the ossicles. If untreated, cholesteatoma can erode the ossicles, leading to ossicular dysfunction or discontinuity.

16. **What procedure is commonly undertaken to offset conductive hearing loss due to otitis media?**
    Myringotomy and placement of **tympanostomy tubes** are often employed in patients with a conductive hearing loss due to otitis media. A tympanostomy tube is also known as a pressure equalization tube (PET). A small incision (myringotomy) is made in the anterior-inferior or anterior-superior quadrant of the tympanic membrane, and a tube is placed into the incision. This tube allows for drainage and aeration of the middle ear space.

17. What other surgical treatments are used for conductive hearing loss?

1. **Myringoplasty** involves the closure of the tympanic membrane perforation with a tissue graft, most often temporalis fascia. Small perforations can be closed with a paper patch, allowing reepithelialization over the perforation.

2. If repair of the ossicles is needed, as in ossicular discontinuity, an **ossiculoplasty** is performed.

3. Stiffening and fixation of the stapes footplate in otosclerosis are surgically treated with a **stapedectomy**, which involves replacement of the stapes with a prosthesis. Alternatively, a **stapeotomy** involves drilling a hole through the stapes footplate and placing a movable prosthesis through the hole.

4. Treatment of cholesteatoma requires removal of the offending material and reconstruction of the damaged middle ear structures via a **mastoidectomy** and **tympanoplasty**.

BIBLIOGRAPHY

1. Austin DF: Acoustic mechanisms in middle ear sound transfer. Otolaryngol Clin North Am 27:641–654, 1994.
2. Bailey BJ (eds): Head and Neck Surgery–Otolaryngology, vol 2. Philadelphia, J. B. Lippincott, 1993.
3. Bluestone CD, Stool SE, Scheetz MD: Pediatric Otolaryngology, 2nd ed (vol 1). Philadelphia, W. B. Saunders, 1990.
4. Briggs RJS, Luxford WM: Correction of conductive hearing loss in children. Otolaryngol Clin North Am 27:607–620, 1994.
5. Goodwin WJ Jr: Temporal bone fractures. Otolaryngol Clin North Am 16:651–659, 1983.
6. Hannley MT: Audiologic characteristics of the patient with otosclerosis. Otolaryngol Clin North Am 26:373–386, 1993.
7. Harris JP, Cueva RA: Conductive hearing loss: Inflammatory and noninflammatory causes. In Meyerhoff WL, Rice DH (eds): Otolaryngology–Head and Neck Surgery. Philadelphia, W. B. Saunders, 1992.
8. Katz J: Handbook of Clinical Audiology, 4th ed. Baltimore, Williams & Wilkins, 1994.
9. Lee KJ: Essential Otolaryngology–Head and Neck Surgery, 6th ed. Norwalk, CT, Appleton & Lange, 1995.
10. Nadol JB Jr: Hearing loss. N Engl J Med 329:1092–1102, 1993.
11. Pensak ML, Adelman RA: Conductive hearing loss. In Cummings CW (ed): Otolaryngology–Head and Neck Surgery, 2nd ed (vol 4). St. Louis, Mosby, 1993.
12. Sataloff RT, Sataloff J: Hearing Loss, 3rd ed. New York, Marcel Dekker, 1993.
13. Schuller DE, Schleuning AJ: DeWeese and Saunders' Otolaryngology–Head and Neck Surgery, 8th ed. St. Louis, Mosby, 1994.

6. SENSORINEURAL HEARING LOSS

Nicolas G. Slenkovich, M.D.

1. What is sensorineural hearing loss?

Sensorineural hearing loss (SNHL) is due to defects either in the **sensory** end-organ of the cochlea or in **neural** transmission to the CNS. A defect exists either in the conversion of acoustic energy by the sense organ of the inner ear or in the transmission of neural impulses centrally.

2. Describe the audiogram in sensorineural hearing loss.

An audiogram in SNHL shows similar air and bone conduction lines, which are both below normal hearing thresholds. Pure SNHL shows no air-bone gap.

3. What are the major etiologies of sensorineural hearing loss?

Ototoxicity	Hereditary
Meniere's disease	Noise-induced
Presbycusis	Syphilis
Sudden idiopathic hearing loss	Multiple sclerosis
Trauma	Diabetes mellitus

4. What pathophysiologic mechanisms are responsible for sensorineural hearing loss?

Sensory loss can be due to degenerative, toxic, immune-mediated, infectious, or traumatic damage to the cochlea, as well as genetic or vasculopathic etiologies. **Neural transmission impairment** is most commonly due to either traumatic nerve damage or nerve impingement from a neoplastic lesion. Central neural transmission includes bilateral pathways from each ear. Central defects, therefore, are difficult to detect and generally cause subtle findings, such as impaired sound localization.

5. List the essential elements of the history and physical exam for patients presenting with hearing loss.

1. Elicit a history that includes events surrounding the hearing loss, such as infection, trauma, strain, and medication usage.

2. Assess the nature of the onset of symptoms, including the timing, side involved, and fluctuation, as well as associated otologic symptoms of pain, discharge, tinnitus, vertigo, and cranial nerve or other neurologic disturbance.

3. Obtain a history regarding prior hearing loss, otologic surgery, noise exposure, and family history of hearing loss.

4. Physical examination includes a complete head and neck evaluation, including cranial nerves, pneumatic otoscopy, and tuning fork tests.

5. A neurologic exam is performed when indicated.

6. What treatments are available for sensorineural hearing loss?

SNHL is most commonly treated with hearing aids. Directed treatment is undertaken when possible, such as patching of a perilymphatic fistula, surgical excision of an acoustic neuroma, or antibiotic and corticosteroid therapy for a syphilitic infection. Steroid therapy is advocated for cases of suspected immune-mediated hearing loss and for idiopathic sudden SNHL. Cochlear implantation is an option in cases of profound sensorineural deafness.

7. Name the major cause of preventable hearing loss in the United States.

Noise-induced hearing loss. Noise, either occupational or recreational, can cause permanent hearing loss due to hair cell damage within the cochlea. There are no medical or surgical treatments that can reverse noise-induced hearing loss.

8. What symptoms suggest that a person is receiving potentially hazardous noise levels?

People with noise-induced hearing loss may complain that they need to shout to converse in their workplace. They may have symptoms of aural fullness, tinnitus, or muffled hearing after work.

9. How does acoustic trauma cause sensorineural hearing loss?

Damage to the stereocilia of hair cells within the organ of Corti in the cochlea is implicated. Outer hair cells are damaged first, followed by inner hair cells and neural degeneration.

10. What is the most common nonoccupational cause of noise-induced hearing loss?

Gunfire. An audiogram typically documents a hearing loss in the 4000-Hz range. A right-handed rifle or shotgun shooter tends to sustain a left-sided hearing loss, since the right ear is semiprotected by being tucked to the shoulder while the rifle is aimed and fired.

11. What is the dB A scale?

The dB A scale is a noise-level scale weighted toward high-frequency noises (1000–5000 Hz), as high-frequency noises tend to cause more hearing damage than equivalent levels of low-frequency noise. Workplace exposures > 85 dB A are concerning if these levels are sustained for long periods. Federal occupational regulations require hearing protection for workers who are exposed to 90 dB A for 8-hour periods each day.

12. Define presbycusis.

Presbycusis is a slowly progressive, symmetric SNHL presenting in people over age 60. More than one-third of persons over age 75 are affected by presbycusis. Although studies have attempted to link noise, ototoxicity, diet, metabolism, arteriosclerosis, and hereditary factors to this disorder, the cause remains unclear. Hearing loss is usually greatest in frequencies > 2000 Hz and tends to be accompanied by a significant decrease in speech discrimination. Often patients can hear conversation but are unable to interpret the words, regardless of how loud the speech is presented. Hearing aids may be helpful.

13. Which drugs lead to ototoxic hearing loss?

Salicylates, aminoglycosides (gentamicin, tobramycin, amikacin), erythromycin, and loop diuretics (furosemide, ethacrynic acid, bumetanide) are commonly used drugs associated with hearing loss. Hearing loss is typically bilateral and can be permanent.

14. Who is at special risk for ototoxicity?

Patients receiving more than one ototoxic drug or patients with compromised renal function are at increased risk of hearing loss. Prevention of hearing loss in these patients requires special care in administering known ototoxic drugs. Such a patient should undergo serum drug level monitoring in addition to serial audiometric evaluations. Any patient with elevated peak and trough ototoxic drug levels, for either nonintentional or therapeutic reasons, must be strictly monitored for hearing loss.

15. Describe the mechanism of ototoxic drugs.

Aminoglycosides damage cochlear hair cells, whereas loop diuretics damage the stria vascularis. The stria vascularis is a region of specialized epithelium in the organ of Corti which is responsible for maintaining ionic balance.

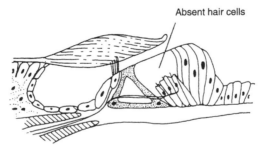

Aminoglycoside toxicity causing outer hair cell loss within the organ of Corti. (From Pender DJ: Practical Otology. Philadelphia, J.B. Lippincott Co., 1992, p 145, with permission.)

16. What are the symptoms of aminoglycoside ototoxicity?

Patients with acute damage initially suffer from tinnitus. Hearing is first affected in the high frequencies, reflecting damage to hair cells in the basal turn of the cochlea. Hearing loss in the lower frequencies follows as damage progresses toward the cochlear apex.

17. What are common genetic causes of hearing loss?

Genetically influenced hearing loss is believed to be responsible for a major portion of SNHL, including deafness. Mid- or high-frequency loss is most commonly described, and hearing loss can be congenital or late-onset, progressive or stable. SNHL has been described in Waardenburg's syndrome, Alport's syndrome, and Usher's syndrome. In addition, it is described in association with abnormalities of the external ear, skin, eye, CNS, musculoskeletal system, kidneys, and other organs.

18. Which immune-mediated disorders can cause sensorineural hearing loss?

Immune-mediated hearing loss is poorly understood. Systemic and locally mediated immune disorders have been implicated in SNHL, including Cogan's syndrome, Wegener's granulomatosis, Behçet's disease, and systemic lupus erythematosus. Additionally, multiple sclerosis causes SNHL resulting from demyelination in central auditory pathways.

19. What signs and symptoms suggest immune-mediated SNHL?

Immune-mediated SNHL most often presents as an unexplained, bilateral, rapidly progressive hearing loss in the 20–50-year-old age group. Patients may exhibit coexistent systemic immune disease. Otoscopic exam is typically normal. The audiogram is variable, often with poor speech discrimination relative to the hearing loss.

20. How is immune-mediated SNHL diagnosed?

Although histopathologic temporal bone study has demonstrated inflammatory vasculitis and infiltration in patients with these disorders, it is difficult to make a definitive diagnosis in clinical cases. Serologic tests to rule out syphilis are obtained. Cellular and humoral antigen-specific immune lab tests, such as lymphocyte transformation testing and Western blot, may be more helpful than nonspecific immune testing.

21. How is immune-mediated hearing loss treated?

Steroid therapy is indicated in most cases. Cytotoxic drugs and plasmapheresis may be indicated when hearing loss progresses despite steroids.

22. What are the causes of sudden sensorineural hearing (SSNHL) loss?

Only 10–15% of sudden hearing loss cases are found to have a specific etiology. Most cases are attributed to **infectious** causes, **vascular** causes, or **otologic membrane rupture**. Patients have a high rate of seroconversion to viruses such as mumps, rubeola, varicella zoster, cytomegalovirus, and influenza B. One-third of patients report symptoms of upper respiratory infection within 1 month of the hearing loss. Rare infectious causes of SSNHL include otosyphilis and Lyme disease.

Because the cochlea receives its entire blood supply from the cerebellar artery, vascular compromise may lead to SSNHL. Vascular associations include embolic events during cardiopulmonary surgery and hypercoagulable states. However, it is notable that the population of SSNHL patients is not skewed toward persons with vascular risk factors.

Cochlear membrane rupture can be caused by external barotrauma from diving or ascending to altitude rapidly or from a rapid increase in cerebrospinal fluid (CSF) pressure from straining. Fistulas of the oval or round window cause a leak of perilymphatic fluid. Rupture of Reissner's membrane or the basilar membrane causes ionic fluid imbalance from mixing of perilymphatic and endolymphatic fluids. Acoustic neuromas, causing impingement of cranial nerve VIII within the internal auditory canal, are rare causes of SSNHL but should be kept in the differential diagnosis.

23. Do any factors influence the prognosis in SSNHL?

It is reported that 40–70% of patients with SSNHL experience recovery of hearing without treatment.

Good Prognostic Factors	*Poor Prognostic Factors*
Minimal hearing loss	Old age
Low-frequency loss	Presentation with total deafness
Lack of vestibular symptoms	Objective vestibular symptoms
Early treatment referral	Vascular risk factors
	Delayed treatment

24. Should SSNHL be evaluated differently from hearing loss of gradual onset?

Yes. In addition to standard audiometric evaluation, the work-up for SSNHL should include studies to rule out the possibility of an acoustic neuroma in the internal auditory canal. Either an auditory evoked brainstem response test (ABR) or, in cases of high suspicion, a gadolinium-enhanced magnetic resonance imaging (MRI) of the internal auditory canal is performed. About 1–3% of sudden hearing loss is due to acoustic neuroma. Roughly 10% of acoustic neuromas present with sudden hearing loss. Additionally, electronystagmometry (ENG) with a fistula test to document vestibular findings and a screen for a perilymphatic fistula is performed.

25. Describe traumatic causes of sensorineural hearing loss.

Barotrauma, blunt trauma, and penetrating trauma can all cause hearing loss. Barotrauma can cause sufficient pressure transmission to cause rupture of the oval or round windows and a leak of perilymphatic fluid from the inner ear. Additionally, an acute increase in CSF pressure from physical strain is thought to be capable of causing inner-cochlear membrane rupture via pressure transmission through the cochlear aqueduct. Trauma to the temporal bone can cause a conductive hearing loss by disrupting the external canal, tympanic membrane, or ossicular chain or by creating a hemotympanum. Sensorineural loss occurs from damage to the cochlea or auditory nerve.

26. Describe the infectious causes of SNHL.

Infections may impair the cochlear labyrinth or eighth nerve. Bacterial meningitis, spread of otitis media, congenital and acquired syphilis, and viral infections have all been implicated in infectious labyrinthitis or neuritis leading to hearing loss. Additionally, opportunistic infections of the temporal bone or cerebellopontine angle in immunocompromised patients may cause SNHL.

CONTROVERSIES

27. Are any additional diagnostic tests merited in patients with SSNHL?

Hematologic studies, viral studies, syphilis serologies, and metabolic and autoimmune work-up are controversial in terms of cost-effectiveness and usefulness in changing outcomes.

28. How should sudden hearing loss be treated?

To date, only corticosteroid therapy has been proved efficacious for idiopathic SSNHL. A number of other treatments have been advocated, including antivirals, carbogen (5% carbon dioxide in oxygen), vasodilators, diuretics, anticoagulants, thrombolytics, plasma expanders, and intravenous contrast therapy. When specific lesions are suspected or diagnosed, such as when history suggests oval or round window rupture, then directed surgical or other treatments may be indicated.

BIBLIOGRAPHY

1. Ciesla CJ, Lee KJ: Audiology. In Lee KJ (ed): Essential Otolaryngology, 6th ed. Norwalk, CT, Appleton & Lange, 1995, pp 25–70.
2. Dobie RA: Noise-induced hearing loss. In Bailey BJ (ed): Head and Neck Surgery–Otolaryngology. Philadelphia, J.B. Lippincott Co., 1993, pp 1782–1792.
3. Hugher GB, Barna BP, Calabrese LH, Koo A: Immunologic disorders of the inner ear. In Bailey BJ (ed): Head and Neck Surgery–Otolaryngology. Philadelphia, J.B. Lippincott Co., 1993, pp 1833–1842.
4. Konigsmark BW: Hereditary deafness in man. N Engl J Med 281:713–20, 1969.
5. Mills JH, Adkins WY: Anatomy and physiology of hearing. In Bailey BJ (ed.): Head and Neck Surgery–Otolaryngology. Philadelphia, J.B. Lippincott Co., 1993, pp 1441–1461.
6. Nadol JB: Hearing loss. N Engl J Med 329:1092–1102, 1993.
7. Paparrella MM: Review of sensorineural hearing loss. Am J Otol 5:311–314, 1984.
8. Shikowitz MJ. Sudden sensorineural hearing loss. Med Clin North Am 75(6):1239–1250, 1991.

7. HEARING AIDS AND COCHLEAR IMPLANTS

Kent E. Gardner, M.D., and Jerry L. Northern, Ph.D.

1. Name the major components of a hearing aid. How do these components work?

A traditional hearing aid consists of five main components: a microphone, amplifier, receiver, volume control, and battery power source. The function of a hearing aid is to amplify acoustic signals, which it accomplishes in three basic stages that correspond to the major hearing aid components. In the first stage, the diaphragm of the microphone converts acoustic energy, or sound, into mechanical energy. The microphone then converts this energy into electrical energy. The second stage involves the amplifier, which boosts the electrical signal. In the final stage, the receiver transforms the boosted electrical signal back into an acoustic signal which is then broadcast into the ear.

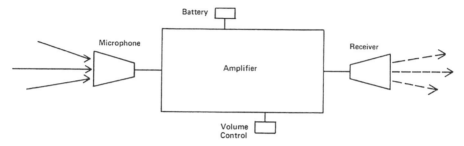

Block diagram of a simple hearing aid. (From Pollack MC (ed): Amplification for the Hearing impaired, 3rd ed. Orlando, Grune and Stratton, Inc., 1988, p 25, with permission.

2. When does a patient with a hearing loss need a hearing aid?

Patients with hearing loss who manifest communication difficulties, either objectively or subjectively, may benefit from hearing amplification. Because of current technology, audiologists are able to fit almost all patients with variable types and degrees of hearing loss.

3. Define saturation sound pressure level, acoustic gain, frequency response, and distortion.

These terms describe the different electroacoustic properties of a hearing aid. **Saturation sound pressure level** (SSPL) is the maximum amount of sound pressure output, or power, that a hearing aid can produce. **Acoustic gain** refers to the difference in the output of a hearing aid relative to its input. For example, if a tone at 1000 Hz is presented to the microphone at 60 dB, and if the measured output is 100 dB, then the gain of the hearing aid at this frequency is 40 dB. **Frequency response** refers to the gain of a hearing aid across a range of frequencies. **Distortion** refers to the clarity of signal produced by a hearing aid.

4. What is meant by an analog hearing aid?

Traditional hearing aids are *analog* devices. These aids convert acoustic and mechanical energy into electric waveforms which are similar in shape, or *analogous*, to actual sound waves. In the future, *digital* hearing aids may be available. Using technology much like that used in compact discs, digital aids may convert electrical signals to a series of signals that are coded by binary numbers. These aids will theoretically be programmed specifically to a patient's individual needs.

5. Name the seven common types of hearing aids.

(1) Behind-the-ear (BTE) aids, (2) in-the-ear (ITE) aids, (3) in-the-canal (ITC) aids, (4) completely-in-the-canal (CIC) aids, (5) body aids, (6) eyeglass aids, and (7) CROS aids.

6. **What are the advantages and disadvantages of behind-the-ear (BTE) hearing aids?**
Advantages
   1. They generate enough power to adequately accommodate a patient with severe to profound hearing loss.
   2. These aids are more cosmetically appealing than body aids.
   3. These devices are large enough to accommodate multiple controls for electroacoustic properties, allowing for adjustment flexibility.
   4. The microphone and receiver are more easily separated in BTE aids than in ITE and ITC models, which allows for less feedback.
Disadvantages
   1. In patients with severe to profound hearing loss, the earpiece must fit tightly in the canal to eliminate feedback problems.
   2. More manual dexterity is required than with body aids.
   3. BTE aids require a relatively normal pinna, are easily affected by perspiration, and may be less cosmetically appealing than ITE and ITC aids.

7. **What are the advantages and disadvantages of in-the-ear (ITE) hearing aids?**
Advantages
   1. More cosmetically appealing than BTE aids
   2. Increased amplification provided by the pinna boosts gain in high frequencies
   3. Improve localization of sound sources
   4. Comprised of only one component
Disadvantages
   1. Amount of gain is limited due to problems with acoustic feedback
   2. Appropriate only for patients with mild, moderate, and moderately severe hearing loss
   3. Small size limits the number of adjustment controls
   4. More fragile than BTE aids.

8. **List the advantages and disadvantages of in-the-canal (ITC) hearing aids.**
Advantages
   1. More cosmetically appealing than most hearing aids
   2. Increased amplification provided by the pinna to boosts gain in high frequencies
   3. Placement of microphone improves sound localization
Disadvantages
   1. Only appropriate for patients with mild to moderate hearing loss
   2. Models are fragile and difficult to use for patients with manual dexterity problems
   3. Small size limits the number of controls for adjustments
   4. Limited venting options.

9. **And for completely-in-the-canal (CIC) hearing aids?**
Advantages
   1. CIC aids are barely noticeable because they are placed deep in the canal
   2. Provide full or partial resolution of the occlusion effect
   3. Improved use with telephones because they do not need a vent
   4. Resolves wind-noise problem
   5. Improve gain in high frequencies due to pinna effect
   6. Secure fit, reduced acoustic feedback due to minimal venting, and good sound localization
Disadvantages
   1. Provide adequate amplification only for patients with mild to moderate hearing loss
   2. Fragile aids that need frequent repairs, and shell modifications are expensive
   3. More extensive counseling is required to teach use
   4. Some dispensers are reluctant to perform deep canal impressions
   5. Small batteries are difficult for patients with inadequate dexterity

6. Can develop feedback with jaw movement

7. Cannot be used in patients with unfavorable external auditory canals

10. What is a CROS-type hearing aid?

CROS stands for **contralateral routing of signals**. These hearing aids are used in individuals with usable hearing in one ear but no hearing, very poor hearing, or unaidable hearing in the other ear. A microphone is placed on the side of the patient's poorer ear. The signal received through this microphone is routed to the opposite ear and amplified. The signal is routed by either an electrical cord worn behind the head and neck or by wireless FM radio signals. These aids improve the patient's ability to hear sounds that originate on the side of the poorer-hearing ear.

11. What are the advantages and disadvantages of body-type hearing aids?

Body hearing aids yield high output for patients with profound hearing loss. They also are very easy to use for patients with manual dexterity problems. However, these aids are rarely used because they are cosmetically unappealing and bulky. Clothes rub against the microphone and cause excessive aberrant noise.

12. Explain the occlusion effect.

The occlusion effect occurs when the body of the hearing aid blocks the external auditory canal. To the patient, this occlusion causes a muffled sensation due to a shift in the peak of the natural resonance of the ear canal. The result of this shift is an increase in low-frequency amplification. In individuals with normal low-frequency hearing, this amplification is not desired. The occlusion is lessened by using aids that do not occlude the canal, which contain a vent, or which have electronic filtering of low frequencies.

13. How does acoustic feedback occur?

Acoustic feedback results when amplified sound leaks from the receiver back into the microphone. The result is an unpleasant high-pitched squeal. Short microphone-to-receiver distance, wax in the canal, vents, and poor hearing aid fit are all associated with increased feedback problems. ITE or ITC hearing aids are more likely to have these problems than BTE aids.

14. What is loudness compression?

Hearing aids are not tolerated if they amplify sound beyond a level that is comfortable to the patient. Compression means that as the hearing input increases, the amount of gain is automatically reduced to avoid reaching an uncomfortable output level. This concept can be applied across the entire frequency range (single-band compression) or can be applied to specific frequencies at which the patient experiences recruitment or loudness discomfort (multiple-channel compression).

15. Are patients with sensorineural hearing loss candidates for hearing aids?

Yes. Until the last few decades, it was felt that only patients with conductive hearing losses were candidates for hearing amplification. It was thought that boosting the volume would not improve clarity or speech discrimination. It is now well accepted that patients with sensorineural hearing loss benefit from hearing aids. Although the processing component of a sensorineural hearing loss cannot be overcome, the heightened volume increases audibility and reduces the strain of understanding sound in daily listening situations.

16. Do patients with bilateral hearing loss need monaural or binaural amplification?

In most cases, patients with bilateral hearing losses do better with binaural amplification. Binaural amplification is advantageous because it eliminates the "head shadow" effect—i.e., the 6-dB loss in sound intensity that occurs when sound has to cross the head to the contralateral ear. This effect is amplified in a noisy environment. Additional benefits include better speech discrimination, improved ease of listening, heightened speech localization, and avoidance of sensory deprivation. Retrospective studies have shown that when only one ear is aided, the unaided ear suffers a reduction in word-recognition score.

17. What are assistive listening devices (ALDs)? Why are they needed?

ALDs assist the hearing impaired in specific "difficult listening situations" (i.e., lecture halls, theaters, television, etc.). Most of these difficult listening situations involve a sound source that is located far from the listener. The intensity of a sound signal decreases by 6 dB each time the distance between the listener and the sound source doubles. This leads to a decreased **signal-to-noise ratio**. Some ALDs maintain a normal signal-to-noise ratio by transferring the sound signal, at the original intensity level, directly to the listener or hearing aid microphone via FM, infrared, or inductance loop transmission devices. Other available ALDs include telephone amplifiers, vibrating alarm clocks, TV closed-caption decoders, and visual alarm systems.

18. What is the earliest age at which a child can benefit from hearing amplification?

When needed, children should be fitted for hearing aids at the earliest possible age, even during infancy. Although determining the exact nature of an infant's hearing loss is challenging, an infant can be fitted initially with a nonspecific hearing aid based on available audiometric data. Hearing amplification can be adjusted as the child grows and more reliable testing can be performed. Caution should be exercised in infants to prevent further hearing damage with over-amplification. Infants with congenital atresia or microtia of the pinna may be fit as young as 2 months of age.

19. How do prelingual and postlingual hearing loss differ?

Prelingual deafness refers to hearing loss prior to the development of basic spoken language skills. **Postlingual deafness** refers to the loss of hearing after the development of basic language skills. The development of basic spoken language skills usually occurs at 2–3 years of age. The classification of patients into prelingual and postlingual categories has prognostic significance when predicting how a patient will respond to cochlear implantation.

20. What is a cochlear implant?

A cochlear implant is a highly sophisticated listening device that can restore auditory abilities to deafened individuals who do not benefit from hearing aids. The first device was developed for clinical use in Australia in the 1970s. Early cochlear implants were single electrode devices. Current implants tend to have multiple electrodes which transmit more sound information. These devices require surgical implantation and extensive postoperative therapy.

21. Name the components of a cochlear implant.

Cochlear implants have internal and external components. The internal components consist of a receiver/stimulator, magnet, an antenna placed under the skin, and electrode probe placed into the scala tympani of the cochlea. The external components consist of a cigarette-pack-sized speech processor (which is usually worn on the belt), a behind-the-ear microphone, and transmitter placed over the mastoid. These components are connected by wires. The transmitter is magnetically secured over the mastoid to the magnet in the implanted portion of the device.

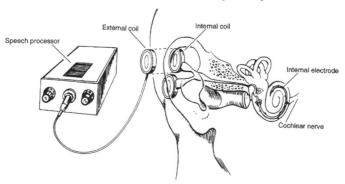

The cochlear implant system. (From Cummings CW, et al (eds): Otolaryngology–Head and Neck Surgery. St. Louis, Mosby, 1986, p 3270, with permission.)

22. Who can benefit from cochlear implantation?
Cochlear implants are currently indicated for patients over 2 years of age who have profound binaural sensorineural hearing loss, have intact eighth cranial nerve function, and show little or no benefit from hearing aids. However, several other patient populations will likely be approved for cochlear implantation in the near future. Postlingual patients tend to do better than prelingual ones. Other important prognostic variables include general health, level of motivation, expectations, and quality of the patient's support group.

23. How do cochlear implants work?
The behind-the-ear microphone receives sound and converts it into electrical signals. These signals are delivered to the external signal processor worn on the belt. The signal processor modifies the signal and delivers it to the transmitter over the mastoid. The transmitter then delivers the signal to the implanted receiver/stimulator either directly or indirectly. Directly, the signal may be carried via a hard-wired percutaneous connector. Indirectly, the signal may be carried by an FM radio frequency or magnetic induction. The receiver/stimulator, implanted under the skin in the mastoid, further modifies the signal and delivers it to electrodes implanted in the scala tympani. These electrodes stimulate the remaining neural tissue, usually spiral ganglion cells, in the cochlea.

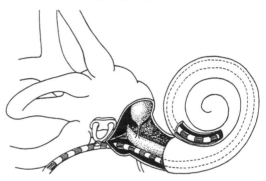

Internal view of cochlear implant. (From Pender DJ: Practical Otology. Philadelphia, J.B. Lippincott, 1992, p 65, with permission.)

24. How is sound perceived by a patient with a cochlear implant?
Sounds produced by cochlear implants are not like normal hearing. The electrical stimulation provided by the implant is perceived as auditory sensations that vary in pitch and loudness. The speech processor of the implant selects out specific characteristics of sound that are important for speech understanding. The quality of these sounds is such that most patients are able to develop improved communication skills. A few patients are even able to understand speech without visual cues.

25. How much does cochlear implantation cost?
In 1995, cochlear implantation costs $30,000–50,000. This cost includes surgery, the device, hospitalization, fitting, and aural rehabilitation.

BIBLIOGRAPHY

1. Balkany T, Telischi FF, Hodges AV: Cochlear implant basics. In Jackler RK, Brackman DE (eds): Neurotology. St. Louis, Mosby, 1994.
2. Boothroyd A: Profound deafness. In Tyler RS (ed): Cochlear Implants. San Diego, Singular Publishing Group, 1993.
3. De Chicchis AR, Bess FH: Hearing aids and assistive listening devices. In Bailey BJ (ed): Head and Neck Surgery–Otolaryngology. Philadelphia, J.B. Lippincott, 1993.
4. Harford ER: Hearing aid selection for adults. In Pollack MC (ed): Amplification for the Hearing Impaired, 3rd ed. Orlando, FL, Grune & Stratton, 1988.
5. Northern JL, Downs MP: Hearing in Children, 4th ed. Baltimore, Williams & Wilkins, 1991.
6. Sweetlow RW: Hearing aids and assistive listening devices. In Jackler RK, Brackman DE (ed): Neurotology. St. Louis, Mosby, 1994.
7. Zazove P, Kileny PR: Devices for the hearing impaired. Am Fam Physician 46:851–858, 1992.

8. DISEASES OF THE EXTERNAL EAR AND TYMPANIC MEMBRANE

Douglas M. Sorensen, M.D., and Catherine Winslow, M.D.

1. Identify the parts of the auricle.

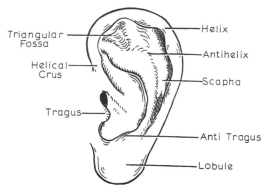

Triangular Fossa — Helix — Antihelix

Helical Crus — Scapha

Tragus — Anti Tragus — Lobule

Anatomy of the auricle. (From Lee KJ: Essential Otolaryngology–Head and Neck Surgery. Norwalk, CT, Appleton & Lange, 1995, p 2, with permission.)

2. Name the six hillocks of His. What is their clinical significance?

In the embryo, the first and second branchial arches each give rise to three hillocks. The first arch gives rise to the first three hillocks which form the tragus, helical crus, and helix. The second arch gives rise to the second three hillocks which form the antihelix, scapha, and lobule. If these primitive ear hillocks fail to fuse, preauricular pits result. Preauricular pits may become recurrently infected, requiring excision.

3. What are the complications of an auricular hematoma if left untreated?

This blunt injury commonly occurs in wrestlers and boxers. Characteristically, as the ear swells to become large and blue, it loses the outline of its conchal folds. Because an auricular hematoma accumulates between the cartilage and perichondrium, the proper name for this injury is **subperichondrial hematoma**. This hematoma deprives the cartilage of nutrients and predisposes the ear to necrosis and infection. The principal complication is the "**cauliflower ear**" deformity, which results from cartilage loss. More subtle ear deformities may result from an infection or fibrosis.

4. How should an auricular hematoma be managed?

The goal of management is to prevent deformity. First, the skin overlying the hematoma should be anesthetized with 1% lidocaine. The clinician should then evacuate the hematoma by making an incision with a no. 15 scalpel. Next, the cavity should be irrigated with saline. Finally, this evacuated space should be bolstered with 4–0 nylon suture and dental rolls. The dental rolls compress the wound and prevent reaccumulation of blood. An antistaphylococcal antibiotic should be prescribed, and the rolls should be left in place for 1 week.

5. What is perichondritis of the auricle? How is it treated?

Perichondritis and **chondritis** are infections that involve the perichondrium and cartilage of the auricle, respectively. Invariably, these infections result from an auricle laceration, although

34

noninfectious causes, such as relapsing polychondritis, may also lead to this disorder. These infections may present with diffuse swelling of the auricle. Deflection of the pinna may produce exquisite tenderness. Treatment begins with surgical debridement of the devitalized cartilage, and intravenous antibiotics that cover aerobic and anaerobic bacteria should be administered.

6. What is keratitis obturans?

Keratitis obturans, also known as cholesteatoma of the external auditory canal, is a rare condition. Pain is due to bony erosion of the external auditory canal from a cholesteatoma. This condition is frequently associated with disorders such as chronic obstructive pulmonary disease (COPD), bronchiectasis, and sinusitis. Treatment is aimed at the removal of debris.

7. Describe the clinical signs and symptoms of frostbite to the external auricle.

Frostbite may progress clinically from cyanosis to ischemia with pallor, edema with vesicle formation, and finally, tissue necrosis. Temperatures which are $< 10°C$ block sensory nerve conduction and therefore pain. Treatment involves rapid rewarming.

8. What is otitis externa?

Otitis externa is a common inflammatory condition involving the skin of the external auditory canal. A history of antecedent ear canal trauma or water exposure is common, hence the term "swimmer's ear." Symptoms include otalgia, pruritus, and foul-smelling otorrhea. The ear canal may appear mildly erythematous. If the infection is severe, edema may completely obstruct the canal. The ear and its canal may be exquisitely tender. *Pseudomonas aeruginosa* and *Staphylococcus aureus* are the primary pathogenic organisms. Treatment begins with local debridement and the administration of antibiotic steroid drops. In cases of severe canal swelling, an anti-inflammatory impregnated wick should be placed carefully in the canal and left there for 2–7 days.

9. How are exostoses differentiated from an auditory canal osteoma?

Exostoses are benign periosteal outgrowths that occur in the bony canal. They are associated with multiple exposures to swimming in cold water. Clinically, they appear as nodules next to the annulus and frequently are multiple and bilateral. Exostoses are usually small enough that they do not obstruct the canal, although a patient may suffer from secondary otitis externa. An **osteoma** is usually single and unilateral, often occurring at the bony cartilaginous junction of the tympanomastoid suture line.

10. An elderly insulin-dependent diabetic woman with a history of chronic otitis externa presents to your clinic with severe otalgia and auricle edema. Examination shows granulation tissue at the external auditory meatus. What is your diagnosis and what treatment do you prescribe?

Malignant otitis externa refers to a progressive and necrosing *Pseudomonas* infection of the ear. This infection does not remain localized to the skin of the ear canal, but instead it extends to the deeper tissues and invades medially along the floor of the ear canal. This medial and posterior extension leads to invasion of the mastoid, facial nerve, and base of the skull. The typical patient is elderly, diabetic, and has severe otalgia. Management begins with gaining control of the patient's diabetes. Local ear canal debridement or mastoidectomy may be necessary. Intravenous antipseudomonal antibiotics should be given early.

11. How is otomycosis recognized and managed?

Otomycosis, or externa mycotica, refers to a fungal or candidal infection of the external auditory canal. Symptoms are similar to those of otitis externa; however, pruritus is a more common symptom than otalgia. Upon examination of the ear canal, the disease may be recognized easily by visualization of the fungal mycelia. Moisture, high temperature, poor hygiene, and immunosuppression appear to contribute to the development of this condition. The offending organisms usually are *Aspergillus albicans, A. niger,* and *Candida albicans.* Treatment begins with debridement of the ear canal. A topical fungicide, such as nystatin powder, cresylate, 4% boric acid powder, or 1% gentian violet, should be applied. Applying Cortisporin drops or other antimicrobials may exacerbate otomycosis.

12. What is Ramsay Hunt syndrome?

Ramsay Hunt syndrome, also known as **herpes zoster otiticus**, is due to infection of the geniculate ganglion and other cranial nerve ganglia, probably by the chickenpox virus. The chief symptom stems from painful herpetic lesions in the external auditory meatus and auricle. If the virus affects the seventh nerve, cutaneous herpes and ipsilateral facial paralysis (Bell's palsy) may result. If the virus affects the eighth nerve, vomiting, vertigo, nystagmus, and hearing loss may result.

13. What is microtia?

Microtia is a term used to describe hypoplasia of the external ear, often associated with atresia of the external auditory canal. Microtia typically presents as a rudimentary auricle with maldeveloped cartilage. In the place of a normal ear, an S-shaped skin fold is often positioned vertically. This external ear anomaly presents a challenge to the reconstructive surgeon.

14. What is aural atresia?

Aural atresia is a congenital deformity of the auricle and middle ear and is accompanied by inner ear deformity in 10% of cases. Atresia is more commonly unilateral, occurs more often in males, and is more common on the right. The degree of abnormality may be minor, moderate, or severe. Treatment involves fitting the patient with bone-conduction hearing aids until the patient is old enough for surgery.

15. Where do keloids develop?

A keloid is a common benign tumor often affecting the auricle that commonly forms after ear-piercing, trauma, or surgical ear procedures. Often, these tumors do not develop until long after the initial insult to the ear. Keloids present a difficult problem because their surgical excision usually results in a larger, more-deforming tumor recurrence. Keloids are often treated with intralesional steroids.

16. How do you clean a cerumen impaction?

Because cerumen has an acidic pH, it is bacteriostatic and fungistatic. If the tympanic membrane is obscured by cerumen, the canal must be cleaned for proper evaluation. Cleaning with **warm water irrigation** is often the preferable approach, especially in children. However, if you suspect a tympanic membrane perforation, the ear should never be irrigated. You should consider a perforation based on a suspicious history, odor, blood, or discharge within the auditory canal. A cerumen spoon may also be used; however, the skin of the auditory canal is fragile and bleeds easily. Small abrasions may cause the patient significant pain. If you are unable to remove tightly impacted cerumen, you may advise the patient to use mineral oil or Cortisporin drops daily for 1 week to soften the impaction. Such impactions may need removal with the aid of an otolaryngologist's working microscope.

17. A 3-year-old child presents with a small calculator battery in his right ear. The child is crying and upset. What is the proper management?

Foreign bodies of the ear are usually confined to children. Management can be divided into two categories—those cases that should be irrigated, and those that should not. Most foreign bodies can be removed easily with gentle syringe irrigation. However, in certain cases, irrigation is contraindicated. Small batteries, such as calculator and watch batteries, are dangerous because they may leak acid into the ear. Irrigation of this acid only aggravates the problem. Batteries should be removed with the aid of a microscope and a small hook. Often children insert peas or other vegetable material into their ears. Irrigation in these cases is also inappropriate, as water will cause the vegetables to swell, leading to excruciating pain. Again, this material should be removed with a small hook. Occasionally, removal is inhibited when the child is extremely upset. General anesthetic is reserved for very small or uncooperative children with deeply embedded foreign bodies.

18. Describe abnormal signs that may be found on examination of the tympanic membrane and their associated conditions.

Tympanic Membrane Signs and Associated Conditions

SIGNS	ASSOCIATED CONDITIONS
Mobility	
Bulging, no mobility	Fluid or pus in middle ear
Retracted, no mobility	Obstruction of eustachian tube
Mobility on negative pressure only	Obstruction of eustachian tube
Excessive mobility in one small area	Healed perforation
Color	
Amber	Serous fluid in middle ear
Blue or deep red	Blood in middle ear
White	Infection in middle ear
Red (with crying)	Infection in middle ear
Dullness	Fibrosis
White plaques	Healed inflammation
Contents	
Air bubbles	Serous fluid in middle ear

Adapted from Seidel HM: Ears, nose, and throat. In Seidel HM (ed): Mosby's Guide to Physical Examination. St. Louis, Mosby, 1991, p 236.

19. What are the causes of traumatic tympanic membrane perforations?

Perforations may be caused by foreign bodies, such as hairpins or Q-tips. Trauma to the ear may cause sufficient air compression in the external meatus to rupture the drum. Gunfire may also cause sufficient air displacement, leading to tympanic membrane rupture. The drum generally heals spontaneously, but residual perforations may be repaired with surgery.

20. Where is Prussak's space?

Prussak's space, or the superior recess of the tympanic membrane, is an area behind the tympanic membrane. It is bound laterally by the flaccid portion of the tympanic membrane, or the pars flaccida, and medially by the neck of the malleus. Prussak's space is enclosed by the lateral malleolar fold in the middle ear.

21. Why is Prussak's space significant?

A retraction or perforation in the pars flaccida may allow keratinous debris to enter the middle ear space, resulting in infection, osteitis, and erosion. This leads to the progression of a cholesteatoma.

22. In patients with chronic otitis media, how are tympanic membrane perforations classified?

Perforations resulting from chronic otitis media are classified as central or marginal. In **central** perforations, the fibrous annulus remains unaffected, and the tympanic membrane circumscribes the entire intact ring. In **marginal** perforations, the fibrous annulus is involved. In these cases, the defect is usually seen posteriorly on the drum. Occasionally, destruction of the drum's margin leads to abnormal epithelial growth. If squamous epithelium grows into the middle ear cavity, a subsequent cholesteatoma may form. Marginal perforations are generally more difficult to repair than central perforations.

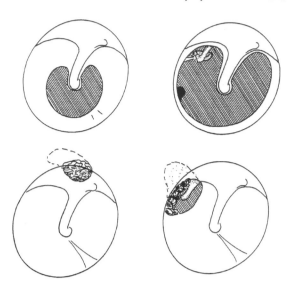

Tympanic membrane perforations. *Top,* Central perforations. There is a margin of eardrum around the periphery. The perforation may be small or subtotal. It may be posterior, inferior, or anterior. *Bottom,* Marginal perforations. An attic perforation *(left)* may harbor a small or large cholesteatoma. In the posteromarginal defect *(right)* granulations are present, and the incus will soon necrose. Again, there may be a small or large cholesteatoma. (From Coleman BH: Diseases of the Nose, Throat, and Ear, and Head and Neck. Edinburgh, Churchill Livingstone, 1922, p 220, with permission.)

23. Can the tympanic membrane heal after perforations?

Tympanic membrane perforations usually heal well, although not all perforations heal. Epithelial migration proceeds from the umbo outward at a rate of 0.05 mm/day.

24. Name the three layers of the tympanic membrane.

The outermost layer, or the **lateral squamous layer**, is continuous with the skin of the external auditory meatus. Directly under it lies the **middle fibrous layer**, also known as the lamina propria. Finally, the **medial mucosal layer** is continuous with the mucosa of the tympanic cavity.

25. Which tympanic membrane layers will regenerate after a perforation?

The epithelial and endothelial layers will regenerate to seal the perforation. However, the fibrous mesothelial layer does not regenerate. Although the new membrane has two layers, the newly formed membrane is called a **monomeric membrane**. Occasionally, the new membrane will be very translucent and resemble a perforation to the untrained eye. On pneumoscopy, the monomeric membrane appears hypermobile with positive and negative pressure.

26. How do you "paper patch" a tympanic membrane?

For small to moderate-sized perforations which will not heal spontaneously, a paper patch may be applied to the tympanic membrane. This patch acts as a scaffold for the re-epithelization process. Prior to the procedure, the ear must be dry with no infection or exudate. The edges of the perforation can be abraded with an instrument or with chemical cautery to stimulate migration. A circular patch of cigarette or ricepaper is made with a paper punch and is placed over the opening. Because the patch is frequently displaced with the resultant epithelial migration, the patient should be followed monthly, and the procedure should be repeated as necessary.

27. A whitish plaque is seen on the tympanic membrane of an otherwise normal ear. Is further evaluation needed?

In **myringosclerosis**, also known as tympanosclerosis, whitish plaques form in the fibrous layer of the tympanic membrane in response to infection or inflammation. Alone, this process generally does not lead to a hearing loss. However, a concurrent otitis may certainly lead to a conductive deficit.

28. What is bullous myringitis?

Bullous myringitis is a viral infection that involves the tympanic membrane and its adjacent deep canal. This condition is associated with viral upper respiratory tract infections. Severe otalgia is usually present. Examination of the tympanic membrane reveals reddish vesicles on the surface that enlarge to form bullae. The causative organism is unknown. Treatment includes antibiotic steroid drops, oral antibiotics, and analgesics.

BIBLIOGRAPHY

1. Chandler JR: Malignant external otitis and osteomyelitis of the base of the skull. Am J Otol 10:108–110, 1989.
2. Coleman BH: Diseases of the external ear. In Coleman BH (ed): Diseases of the Nose, Throat and Ear, and Head and Neck. Edinburgh, Churchill Livingstone, 1992, pp 209–220.
3. Grandis RG, Kamerer DB: External otitis. In Gates GA (ed): Current Therapy in Otolaryngology–Head and Neck Surgery. St. Louis, Mosby, 1994, pp 1–3.
4. Hirsch BE: Infections of the external ear. Am J Otol 13:145–155, 1992.
5. Jahn AF, Hawke M: Infections of the external ear. In Cummings CW (ed): Otolaryngology–Head and Neck Surgery. St. Louis, Mosby, 1993, pp 2787–2794.
6. Seidel HM: Mosby's Guide to Physical Examination. St. Louis, Mosby Year Book, 1991, pp 233–234.

9. OTITIS MEDIA AND ASSOCIATED COMPLICATIONS

Douglas H. Todd, M.D., and Sylvan E. Stool, M.D.

1. Explain the terminology used to describe ear infections.

Historically, the terminology used to describe ear infections has been confusing and has resulted in miscommunication among patients and physicians. When describing infections of the ear, the terminology should define the anatomic location of the process and its chronicity.

Otitis externa—inflammatory process of the external auditory canal or auricle

Myringitis—inflammatory process of the tympanic membrane

Otitis media—inflammatory process of the middle ear space. The presence or absence of a middle ear effusion should be noted.

Mastoiditis—inflammatory process of the mastoid cavity

Labyrinthitis—inflammatory process of the inner ear

Acute processes last < 3 weeks. **Subacute** processes last between 3 weeks and 3 months. **Chronic** processes persist > 3 months.

2. What are the functions of the eustachian tube?

The eustachian tube may be considered as a valve that connects the middle ear cleft to the nasopharynx. This structure ventilates the middle ear and protects the middle ear from nasopharyngeal secretions. Fluid that collects in the middle ear is usually drained by the eustachian tube. Conditions that alter eustachian tube function may lead to the accumulation of fluid in the middle ear and mastoid. This accumulation may subsequently lead to infection, resulting in otitis media and mastoiditis.

3. Which organisms are most commonly found in otitis media?

The most common organisms found in **acute otitis media** are *Streptococcus pneumoniae*, *Haemophilus influenzae*, and *Moraxella (Branhamella) catarrhalis*. Although rare in older patients, gram-negative enteric bacilli are isolated in 20% of infants with middle ear effusions. Viruses can be isolated in approximately 4% of middle ear effusions, with respiratory syncytial virus and influenza virus being the most common. The most commonly isolated bacterial organisms in **chronic otitis media** vary considerably. The predominant organisms are gram-negative bacilli, such as *Pseudomonas aeruginosa*, *Proteus* spp., and *Escherichia coli*, and anaerobes such as *Bacteroides fragilis*.

4. What organisms are found in mastoiditis?

Mastoiditis is the inflammation of the mastoid cavity. **Acute mastoiditis** is most likely caused by the same organisms that cause acute otitis media, including *S. pneumoniae*, *S. pyrogenes*, and *S. aureus*. *H. influenzae* is less common. **Chronic mastoiditis** is most likely to be caused by the organisms that cause chronic otitis media.

5. How is otitis media diagnosed?

Common signs and symptoms of acute otitis media may include **otalgia**, often associated with ear tugging or irritability, **otorrhea**, indicating perforation or patent tympanostomy tubes, and **fever**, indicating an acute infection. Less commonly seen are postauricular swelling, facial paralysis, vertigo, and tinnitus. Pneumatic otoscopy is the "gold standard" for the diagnosis of otitis media. The tympanic membrane should be evaluated for position, mobility, and color. Decreased mobility indicates an effusion or perforation, and erythema indicates infection. Perforation, retraction pockets, or other pathology should be noted and documented.

6. How is tympanometry used in the diagnosis of otitis media?

Tympanometry measures the mobility or compliance of the tympanic membrane. It is an objective measure that requires little patient cooperation. Five patterns are seen on tympanograms:

Type A indicates normal middle ear pressure.

Type B demonstrates flattening of the normal curve, indicating decreased tympanic membrane mobility. A type B tympanogram may be seen with a middle ear effusion or perforation. If a large volume of air is utilized in the test, a perforation is confirmed.

Type C demonstrates a curve with a peak < 100 mm H_2O, indicating a retracted eardrum.

Type A_S is a shallow type A tympanogram, suggesting restricted mobility as seen in ossicular chain fixation or severe myringosclerosis.

Type A_d is a deep type A tympanogram with a higher amplitude, indicating a hypermobile tympanic membrane such as seen in ossicular chain discontinuity.

7. What type of hearing loss is expected with otitis media with effusion?

In otitis media with effusion, the middle ear cleft contains fluid which decreases tympanic membrane mobility. This results in a conductive hearing loss with a type B tympanogram and normal external auditory canal volume.

8. Why are younger children predisposed to otitis media?

At birth, the eustachian tube is in a horizontal plane and has a relatively small lumen. In adults, this structure is at a 45-degree angle with the ear. The adult eustachian tube is higher than the nose and has a relatively large lumen. Children are predisposed to otitis media because secretions from the nasopharynx can readily pass through a horizontal patent eustachian tube, introducing pathogens into the middle ear. Additionally, a small amount of inflammation can obstruct a child's already small lumen, aggravating the infectious process.

9. What is the appropriate medical management for acute otitis media?

Treatment options for otitis media are controversial and include antimicrobials, decongestants, antihistamines, corticosteroids, immunizations, and allergy hyposensitization. Standard medical therapy for acute otitis media includes antimicrobial agents given for 10–14 days. Amoxicillin has been considered the drug of choice, although multiple effective agents are readily available. The selected agent should be active against *Streptococcus pneumoniae*, *Haemophilus influenzae*, and *Moraxella catarrhalis*. It should also have a convenient dosing schedule, produce minimal side effects, be cost-effective, and taste good.

10. Describe the medical management for chronic otitis media with effusion.

Medical management of otitis media with effusion initially includes watchful waiting, control of environmental risk factors, and antimicrobial therapy. Research indicates that middle ear effusions following acute otitis media usually resolve within 3–6 months. Therefore, watchful waiting may be appropriate therapy. Other studies indicate that antibiotics help about 15% of children to hasten clearance of effusion within a 1-month period. Corticosteroid therapy remains controversial. Antihistamines and decongestants are not recommended for isolated otitis media with effusion.

11. What environmental risk factors are associated with otitis media with effusion?

1. Bottle-feeding of infants instead of breast-feeding
2. Propping a bottle in a supine infant's mouth (resulting in milk reflux into the middle ear through the eustachian tube)
3. Passive smoking
4. Attendance in a child care facility

12. How long can middle ear effusions persist after an episode of otitis media?

Research has shown that in 80% of children aged 2–6 years old, otitis media with effusion clears within 2 months. Without medical intervention, approximately 60% of children recover within 3 months.

13. What are tympanocentesis and myringotomy?

Tympanocentesis is needle aspiration of fluid from the middle ear space. It is utilized to identify organisms in middle ear effusions of children who are toxic-appearing or unresponsive to antimicrobial therapy. **Myringotomy** is an incision into the tympanic membrane which allows drainage of middle ear secretions. It is usually preceded by tympanocentesis. Indications for myringotomy include complications of purulent otitis media, such as severe otalgia, meningitis, or facial paralysis.

14. What are the surgical options for treatment of otitis media?

Surgical options include tympanocentesis, myringotomy, and tympanostomy tube insertion (pressure equalization tube, PET). Complications from otitis media may necessitate tympanoplasty, ossiculoplasty, and mastoidectomy.

15. List the indications for myringotomy and tympanostomy tube insertion.

- History of severe otitis media
- Chronic otitis media with effusion (present for > 3 months with associated hearing loss of > 30 dB in the better ear)
- Poor response to antibiotic therapy
- Impending complication of otitis media
- Recurrent acute otitis media (3 episodes in 6 months or 4 episodes in 12 months)
- Chronic retraction pockets of the tympanic membrane or tympanic membrane atelectasis
- Barotitis media
- Autophony secondary to eustachian tube dysfunction

16. Are there any potential complications of tympanostomy tube insertion?

Complications from tympanostomy tube insertion are uncommon with experienced surgeons. Potential morbidity can include external auditory canal laceration, persistent otorrhea, granuloma formation, cholesteatoma, and chronic tympanic membrane perforation. Structural changes, such as tympanic membrane retraction, flaccidity, and myringosclerosis, may also occur. Myringosclerosis is felt to be of little clinical or functional importance. Tympanostomy tube insertion into the posterior superior quadrant should be avoided, as this is the most compliant part of the pars tensa and may result in chronic perforation, atrophic scarring, or retraction. Likewise, injury to the ossicles may occur. Insertion of a tube under the tympanic annulus may result in cholesteatoma.

17. At what age is adenoidectomy useful in the treatment of otitis media with effusion?

Adenoidectomy decreases the morbidity of otitis media in children 4 years of age or older. Adenoidectomies in younger children have not been demonstrated to control otitis media and are generally not recommended.

18. What are the intratemporal complications of untreated otitis media?

Conductive hearing loss	Mastoiditis
Sensorineural hearing loss	Petrositis
Tympanic membrane perforation	Labyrinthitis
Retraction pocket	Perilymphatic fistula
Cholesteatoma	Facial paralysis
Tympanosclerosis	Cholesterol granuloma
Ossicular chain fixation or discontinuity	

19. List intracranial complications of untreated otitis media.

Meningitis	Brain abscess
Extradural abscess	Lateral sinus thrombosis
Subdural empyema	Otitic hydrocephalus
Focal otitic encephalitis	

20. What is the significance of unilateral otitis media in an adult?

Unilateral otitis media in the adult may indicate the presence of a nasopharyngeal mass obstructing the eustachian tube orifice. Unilateral otitis media in the adult should be considered neoplastic until proved otherwise by examination of the nasopharynx.

CONTROVERSY

21. Is steroid therapy useful in the treatment of otitis media with effusion?

Although this is a controversial treatment, the literature regarding the use of corticosteroid agents is growing rapidly. Currently, steroids are not recommended for the treatment of otitis media in children of any age.

BIBLIOGRAPHY

1. Bluestone CD, Klein JO: Otitis Media in Infants and Children. Philadelphia, W.B. Saunders, 1995.
2. Casselbrant ML, Brostoff LM, Cantekin EI, et al: Otitis media with effusion in preschool children. Laryngoscope 95:428–436, 1985.
3. Gates GA, Avery CA, Cooper JC, Prihoda TJ: Chronic secretory otitis media: Effects of surgical management. Ann Otol Rhinol Laryngol Suppl 138:2–32, 1989.
4. Lee KJ. Essential Otolaryngology. New Haven, CT, Medical Examination Publishing Co., 1995.
5. Maw AR, Bawden R: Spontaneous resolution of severe chronic glue ear in children and the effect of adenoidectomy, tonsillectomy and insertion of ventilation tubes. BMJ 306:756–760, 1993.
6. Stool SE, Berg AO, Berman S, et al. Otitis Media with Effusion in Young Children. [Clinical Practice Guideline, no. 12.] Rockville, MD, Agency for Health Care Policy and Research, Public Health Service, U.S. Department of Health and Human Services, July 1994, p 41. [AHCPR Publication no. 94-0622.]

7. Todd DH, Stool SE: Otitis media with effusion: A condensed review. Ambul Child Health 1:44–54, 1995.
8. Zielhuis GA, Straatman H, Rach GH, van den Broek P:. Analysis and presentation of data on the natural course of otitis media with effusion in children. Int J Epidemiol 19:1037–1044, 1990.

10. DISEASES OF THE MIDDLE EAR

Douglas M. Sorensen, M.D.

1. What are the signs and symptoms of eustachian tube dysfunction?
The three classic functions of the eustachian tube are aeration, clearance, and protection of the middle ear. The hallmark of eustachian tube dysfunction is a **middle ear effusion**. However, the signs and symptoms vary from patient to patient. Patients may experience intermittent ear popping in the absence of middle ear effusion. Those with middle ear effusions may report otalgia, fullness in the ear, hearing loss, or vertigo. Patients may even be asymptomatic. Signs of middle ear effusion include limited mobility on pneumatic otoscopy and loss of normal landmarks.

2. What is a retraction pocket?
A retraction pocket is an invagination of the tympanic membrane that usually occurs in the pars flaccida, or posterosuperior quadrant. It may appear to be a perforation to the untrained eye. This disorder is due to negative middle-ear pressure which is often secondary to otitis media and its associated inflammation. As a retraction pocket deepens, desquamated keratin cannot be cleared from the recess and a cholesteatoma results. Specifically, this type of cholesteatoma is termed a **primary acquired cholesteatoma**.

3. What is a cholesteatoma? Where do they occur?
A cholesteatoma is an epithelial cyst that contains desquamated keratin. It is located medial to the normal position of the tympanic membrane. The suffix *oma* may suggest that it is a tumor, but this is not the case. However, as more debris accumulates in the cyst, the cholesteatoma expands.

4. Name the two basic types of cholesteatoma.
Congenital and acquired.

5. Describe a congenital cholesteatoma.
A congenital cholesteatoma is generally discovered in children. Potential sites include the middle ear, petrous apex, and cerebellopontine angle. Most congenital cholesteatomas are visible behind the tympanic membrane.

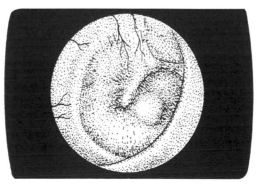

Congenital cholesteatoma pearl. (From Pender DJ: Practical Otology. Philadelphia, J.B. Lippincott, 1992, p 168, with permission.)

6. What are the two types of acquired cholesteatoma?

An acquired cholesteatoma generally occurs as a consequence of otitis media and eustachian tube dysfunction. The accumulation of keratin debris within the middle ear may be associated with a conductive hearing loss or chronic otorrhea.

1. A **primary acquired cholesteatoma** occurs as the consequence of a retraction pocket of the tympanic membrane and negative pressure within the middle ear. Once the retraction pocket invaginates so deeply that keratin fails to clear from the pocket, the debris accumulates.

2. A **secondary acquired cholesteatoma** occurs with the ingrowth of squamous epithelium from the margin of a perforation. Such a perforation is most commonly caused by an infectious process.

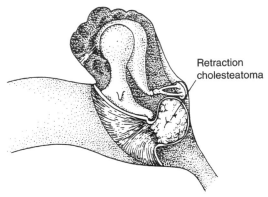

Retraction cholesteatoma

Retraction cholesteatoma. (From Pender DJ: Practical Otology. Philadelphia, J.B. Lippincott, 1992, p 156, with permission.)

7. How do patients with cholesteatomas present clinically?

Patients with a cholesteatoma generally present with repeated infections or progressive conductive hearing loss. Infection of the keratin debris is usually due to *Pseudomonas aeruginosa*. When infection is present, a mucopurulent, malodorous discharge can be detected. A primary acquired cholesteatoma usually presents as an invagination in the superior region of the tympanic membrane.

8. What are the complications of cholesteatomas?

Cholesteatomas destroy bone. Therefore, any bony structure in or near the middle ear and mastoid cavity may be eroded and subsequently infected. Complications include:
Semicircular canal erosion/fistula and dizziness
Extradural or perisinus abscess
Serous or suppurative labyrinthitis
Facial nerve paralysis
Meningitis
Epidural, subdural, or parenchymal brain abscess
Sigmoid sinus thrombosis/phlebitis

9. How are cholesteatomas managed?

Treatment is primarily surgical. Surgery is directed at eradication of the entrapped keratinizing epithelium and keratin from the middle ear and mastoid spaces. Medical management is indicated in preparation for a definitive surgical procedure. Infections should be controlled preoperatively with microscopic debridement of the ear canal and topical antibiotic solutions, such as tobramycin and gentamicin. The primary goal of surgery is to create a disease-free, or "safe," ear. Reconstruction of the hearing mechanism is secondary.

10. What is a cholesterol granuloma of the middle ear?

The hallmark of a cholesterol granuloma is **idiopathic hemotympanum**, or a dark bluish discoloration of the tympanic membrane that is not associated with antecedent trauma. Cholesterol crystals cause a foreign-body reaction of the temporal bone. An initial hemorrhage in the middle ear is followed by drainage interference and leads to this foreign-body reaction. Bony erosion is rare in the setting of a cholesterol granuloma.

11. What is glomus tympanicum?

A **glomus tympanicum** is a tiny tumor that usually presents as pulsatile tinnitus. It is otoscopically visualized as a reddish-blue mass behind the tympanic membrane. It may be difficult to differentiate a glomus tympanicum from a larger **glomus jugulare** which has extended into the middle ear cavity. CT scans may be obtained to distinguish these two tumors. A glomus tympanicum is exclusively contained within the middle ear cavity. This tumor is usually small enough to be excised surgically without embolization.

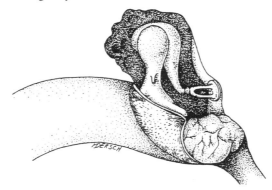

Glomus tympanicum. (From Pender DJ: Practical Otology. Philadelphia, J.B. Lippincott, 1992, p 160, with permission.)

12. What are the clinical features of otosclerosis?

Otosclerosis is due to the fixation of the stapes where it articulates with the oval window. Hearing loss is the major symptom, with the initial conductive hearing loss progressing over months to years. Fixation of the stapes may result in a maximum 50–60 dB air-bone gap. Vertigo may occur in up to 50% of patients with otosclerosis. Audiologic features include a conductive hearing loss which is frequently unilateral, normal speech discrimination, and absence of recruitment. Physical examination is usually normal. **Schwartze's sign**, visualized through the tympanic membrane, is hyperemia of the promontory mucosa which is due to increased vascularity. However, this physical sign is present in only a minority of patients.

13. How frequently does otosclerosis occur?

In autopsy studies, otosclerotic disease is found in temporal bones of 7.3% of white males and 10.3% of white females. Therefore, for every person with a hearing loss caused by otosclerosis, approximately 9 people have asymptomatic histologic disease. In blacks, otosclerosis is found in only 1% of temporal bones. Overall, the female-to-male ratio of patients with symptomatic otosclerosis is about 2:1. The disease usually presents in patients aged 30–49 years. Patients usually delay seeking medical advice for an average of 2–3 years after symptomatic hearing loss begins.

14. Describe the classic audiogram associated with otosclerosis.

The predominant audiometric finding in a patient with otosclerosis is a conductive hearing loss. Early in the disease process, these conductive losses typically involve the low frequencies. As the disease progresses, conductive losses in the higher frequencies become evident. Sensorineural losses may also develop with advanced disease. The bone conduction curve often demonstrates a distinctive notch with a maximum hearing loss at 2000 Hz. This notch is referred to as the **Carhart notch** and is felt to be associated with mechanical impedance changes in the middle ear transformer due to stiffness, friction, and the mass effect of an otosclerotic lesion.

15. What is cochlear reserve?

Otosclerosis falsely decreases sensorineural levels on audiometry. These deceptive levels often show that a patient has greater sensorineural losses than are truly present. We know that this is true because of the surprising audiogram results after otosclerosis surgery. Surgery on the stapes is intended to improve only the conductive defects, but sensorineural levels may also improve or return to normal. Cochlear reserve refers to the true sensorineural thresholds in a patient with otosclerosis prior to surgery. The true sensorineural levels prior to surgery may be estimated by adding 0 dB at 250 Hz, 5 dB at 500 Hz, 10 dB at 1000 Hz, 15 dB at 2000 Hz, and 10 dB at 4000 Hz to the obscured sensorineural levels.

16. If a parent has otosclerosis, what is the chance that his or her child will develop the disease?

The child of a parent with otosclerosis has a 20% chance of developing the disease. Some feel that otosclerosis is transmitted in an autosomal recessive pattern, while others feel that it is transmitted in an autosomal dominant pattern with variable penetrance. A positive family history can be obtained in over 50% of patients with otosclerosis. In women, pregnancy tends to exacerbate the development and progression of otosclerosis and hearing loss.

17. What are the signs and symptoms of ossicular dysfunction?

The hallmark of ossicular dysfunction is **hearing loss**. Physical findings may be normal, except in those cases in which tympanic membrane perforation has occurred with ossicular damage. The Weber tuning fork test lateralizes to the side of the conductive hearing loss. In the case of ossicular discontinuity, a maximum conductive hearing loss of 55–65 dB may be present.

18. What are the possible etiologies of ossicular dysfunction?

There are many **congenital malformations** involving the ossicles: malleus ankylosis; congenital stapes fixation; malformation of the malleus, incus, and stapes; and incudostapedial joint disruption. **Ossicular fixation** physically restricts normal ossicular motion and is associated with otosclerosis, hyalinized connective tissue in tympanosclerosis, and scar tissue after surgery or infection. **Ossicular discontinuity** occurs when the incudostapedial joint is separated completely. In this condition, maximal conductive hearing loss occurs when the tympanic membrane is intact. In general, ossicular dissociation presents as a flat conductive loss. The incudostapedial joint is at risk of devascularization when trauma or infection occurs.

19. In a patient with ossicular discontinuity, does the patient have better hearing with or without a perforated tympanic membrane? Why?

A patient with ossicular diarticulation will have a maximal conductive hearing loss when the tympanic membrane is intact. However, the patient will have better hearing if a perforation is present. This is due to the preservation of a phase difference between the oval and round windows.

20. How can you reconstruct the ossicular chain?

The goal of functional ossicular reconstruction is to obtain permanent restoration of hearing. When the stapes is normal, a carefully fitted ossicular prosthesis may be implemented. The **incus** is the most readily available ossicle. The incus (shaped or sculptured) may be placed between the handle of the malleus and the head of the stapes. **Cartilage** may also be used. A TORP or PORP may be used if an autograft is neither available nor appropriate.

21. What is a PORP?

Partial ossicular reconstruction prosthesis. Prostheses are composed of porous plastipore which is bioinert. If a stapes arch exists, the PORP is interposed between the capitulum of the stapes and the posterior tympanic membrane. To decrease the likelihood of extrusion, cartilage is used to cover the platform of the prosthesis.

22. What is a TORP?

Total ossicular reconstruction prosthesis. A TORP is used when the stapes suprastructure is missing. The TORP can be placed directly from the mobile footplate to the tympanic membrane. A cartilage interface may also prevent extrusion through the tympanic membrane.

23. How do you place a pressure equalization tube (PET) in an adult?

In contrast to children, adults rarely require general anesthesia for PET insertion. The adult patient is placed in the supine position under the clinic microscope. Prior to the myringotomy, local anesthesia can be achieved with either 1% lidocaine injections or topical phenol on the tympanic membrane. A four-quadrant injection with 1% lidocaine is performed at the external auditory meatus. After successful local anesthesia has been obtained, a myringotomy is placed in either the anteroinferior or posteroinferior quadrant. If middle ear fluid is present, gentle suctioning is performed. The ventilation tube is inserted, and the procedure is complete.

CONTROVERSY

24. Can sodium fluoride therapy help to treat otosclerosis?

Sodium fluoride (with calcium and vitamin D) is used as a controversial treatment for otosclerosis. Although otosclerosis tends to cause a conductive hearing loss, it may also cause a sensorineural hearing loss. Sodium fluoride appears to retard the development of this sensorineural component. Because most patients with otosclerosis do not have a significant sensorineural component, sodium fluoride is usually not indicated. Sensorineural hearing loss or vestibular symptoms are the primary indications for the use of sodium fluoride in otosclerosis.

BIBLIOGRAPHY

1. Chole RA: Cellular and subcellular events of bone resorption in human and experimental cholesteatoma: The role of osteoclasts. Laryngoscope. 94:76–95, 1984.
2. Chole RA: Chronic otitis media, mastoiditis and petrositis. In Cummings CW (ed): Otolaryngology–Head and Neck Surgery. St. Louis, Mosby, 1993, pp 2883–2837.
3. Chole RA: Cholesteatoma. In Gates GA (ed): Current Therapy in Otolaryngology–Head and Neck Surgery. St. Louis, Mosby, 1994, pp 21–25.
4. Coleman BH: Chronic infections of the tympano-mastoid. In Coleman BH (ed): Diseases of the Nose, Throat and Ear, and Head and Neck. Edinburgh, Churchill Livingstone, 1992, pp 231–240.

11. EVALUATION OF THE DIZZY PATIENT

Anne K. Stark, M.D., and Carol Foster, M.D.

1. What are the major categories of dizziness?

When you are evaluating a dizzy patient, it is important to try to define the site of the lesion. Dizziness may be categorized as vestibular or nonvestibular. A vestibular lesion may be located in the peripheral vestibular system or central vestibular system. Nonvestibular processes may be the result of systemic disease or anxiety.

2. Which lesions should be recognized as emergent cases necessitating urgent treatment?

CNS hemorrhages and infarcts are the most serious emergent causes of dizziness and necessitate early recognition. Trauma to the inner ear or temporal bone, bacterial labyrinthitis, otosyphilis, autoimmune hearing loss, and acute perilymphatic fistulas should also be considered emergent cases which need urgent treatment. Your evaluation should be structured around ruling out these processes immediately.

3. List the main peripheral vestibular disorders that commonly cause dizziness.
Most common: benign positional vertigo, viral neurolabyrinthitis
Common: trauma to labyrinth, Meniere's disease
Uncommon: bacterial infections, otoxic drug exposure, autoimmune disease

4. What are the main central vestibular disorders causing dizziness?
Migraines are the most common central disturbances associated with dizziness. Other central processes include vertebrobasilar transient ischemic attacks (TIAs), cerebrovascular accidents, CNS vaculitides, and CNS lesions as seen in multiple sclerosis and neoplastic disease. Acoustic neuromas are an important cause of dizziness associated with hearing loss.

5. As you proceed with your diagnostic workup, how should you control the vertigo?
An antihistamine-type drug, such as meclizine (25 mg or more, three or four times daily), may control mild vertigo. Promethazine (25 mg four times daily) may control severe vertigo or vertigo that is associated with vomiting. Small doses of diazepam (2 mg two or three times daily) can be used to control vertigo with a central origin.

6. Your patient claims he is "dizzy." How should you explore this word during your history?
Vertigo is the illusion that the patient's body or environment is spinning or tumbling. Often, patients use the word *dizzy* to describe a general sensation of altered spacial orientation, such as unsteadiness, disequilibrium, or lightheadedness. In your history, it is important to distinguish this general unsteadiness from a rotational sensation. For example, upon standing quickly, an elderly patient is probably experiencing dizziness due to an orthostatic problem, not vestibular disease. Vertigo usually indicates vestibular disease. However, the sensation of tilting or falling can also be vestibular in origin.

7. Which elements of your history are useful in diagnosing lesions of the peripheral vestibular system?
A history of a chronic draining ear, previous ear surgeries, hearing loss, or barotrauma may suggest a peripheral lesion. Acute viral infections can cause peripheral vertigo. Usually, positional vertigo is also due to peripheral disease. Patients with a history of collagen disease should be evaluated for autoimmune disease affecting the inner ear.

8. Which elements of your history evaluate for central vestibular disorders?
When a CNS lesion is suspected, you should inquire about headaches and prior visual, sensory, or motor losses. Drop attacks, or syncope, followed by changes in normal thought processes suggest a central problem. The patient with a central lesion may also relay a history of dizziness during exposure to flashing lights or quickly changing peripheral scenes. In older patients with hypertensive cardiovascular disease, a TIA may be a cause of vertigo.

9. What elements of your history evaluate for systemic disease?
You should obtain a detailed drug history. Neuroleptics, antihypertensives, and street drugs commonly cause dizziness. An irregular heartbeat, faintness, fatigue, or irregular thought processes in combination with the dizzy episodes suggest a systemic problem. Extreme hypertension may cause dizziness in association with a severe headache, while hypotension can cause presyncopal dizziness. Nonspecific dizziness is often the chief complaint when a patient is experiencing hypoglycemia.

10. What elements of the history evaluate for anxiety?
These patients often have a history of panic attacks or phobias. They rarely describe true vertigo, but may describe a floating, detached feeling. If you suspect that the patient's dizziness is

associated with anxiety, you should not immediately rule out vestibular disease. A patient may suffer from both vestibular disease and anxiety.

11. You know very little about the dizzy patient in your examination room, but your attending wants the diagnosis now. You have time for only one more question in your history. What should you ask?

Of course, there is no excuse for an incomplete evaluation, and a diagnosis is never based on the reply from one question. However, knowing the duration of symptoms often helps the clinician broadly categorize the cause of vertigo. Therefore, it is important to ask, "How long do your dizzy spells last?"

Duration of Common Causes of Vertigo

Seconds	Benign positional vertigo
Minutes	Vertebrobasilar insufficiency, migraine
Hours	Meniere's disease
Days	Vestibular neuritis, infarct of the labyrinth

From Baloh RW, Honrubia V: Clinical Neurophysiology of the Vestibular System. Philadelphia, F.A. Davis Co., 1990, p. 92, with permission.

12. When evaluating a dizzy patient, what should your neurologic examination include?

A complete neurologic exam should always be performed and includes an evaluation of cranial nerves, cerebellar function, nystagmus, and hearing. The neck should be evaluated for carotid artery bruits. Also, the clinician should always perform a Dix-Hallpike maneuver.

13. How do you properly evaluate a patient for spontaneous and gaze-evoked nystagmus?

Nystagmus has slow and quick components. The slow component is generated by the vestibular system and causes the eye to deviate slowly. The fast phase represents a corrective response which quickly returns the eyes to the last field of gaze. By convention, the direction of the nystagmus is named by its fast component.

When testing a patient for **gaze-evoked nystagmus**, the examiner should not bring the patient's eyes to the extremes of lateral gaze, as this frequently induces normal "end-point nystagmus." Instead, the patient should be evaluated with the eyes in straight-ahead gaze, then 20–30° to the left, and 20–30° to the right. **First-degree nystagmus** is present if the nystagmus beats only in one direction of lateral gaze. **Second-degree nystagmus** is present if the nystagmus is present on straight-ahead gaze and on gaze in the direction of the fast component. **Third-degree nystagmus** is present if there is nystagmus in all three directions of gaze.

14. Name the four general categories of nystagmus.

1. **Gaze-evoked nystagmus** is present if the nystagmus begins when the patient looks to the left and right or up and down.
2. **Positional nystagmus** occurs with certain head or body positions.
3. **Spontaneous nystagmus** occurs without stimulation.
4. **Induced nystagmus** is elicited by stimulation with caloric or rotational tests.

15. What are Frenzl lenses?

Because labyrinthine nystagmus is suppressed with visual fixation, Frenzl lenses are placed on the patient. When worn, these 20-diopter lenses prevent the patient from visually fixating, and their magnification assists the examiner in detecting nystagmus.

16. How is the Dix-Hallpike maneuver performed?

The Dix-Hallpike maneuver is a test for benign paroxysmal positional vertigo (BPPV). The patient is seated lengthwise on the examination table and reassured that he or she will not fall during

50 Evaluation of the Dizzy Patient

the dizzy spell. Emphasize that the patient is to keep his or her eyes open throughout the maneuver, so that you can observe the eyes for nystagmus. The examiner holds the patient's head turned 45° to the right and then swiftly moves the person into the supine position until the head overhangs the table edge. The examiner should support the patient's head throughout the test. After several seconds, assist the patient in resuming the sitting position. The test is then repeated on the left.

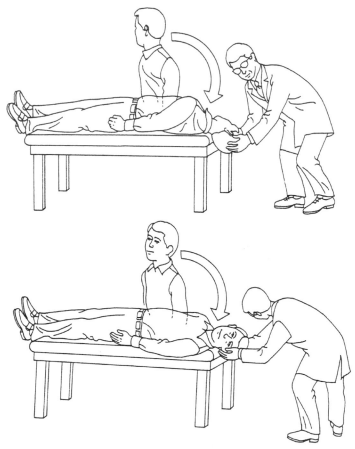

Dix-Hallpike Maneuver. (From Cummings CW, et al (eds): Otolaryngology–Head and Neck Surgery. St. Louis, Mosby, 1986, p 2751, with permission.)

17. What constitutes an abnormal Dix-Hallpike maneuver?

Although this test has many implications, it is most valuable when used to diagnose BPPV. A rotatory nystagmus and sensation of vertigo that begins several seconds after assuming the head-hanging position is characteristic of benign positional vertigo. The nystagmus fades after < 1 minute, reverses direction upon sitting, and "fatigues" with repeated testing. For example, if the patient has a left pathologic ear, he or she will manifest a clockwise rotatory nystagmus when positioned with the left ear down, and the upper pole of the eyes will appear to beat toward the floor.

18. Do other disorders cause nystagmus with the Dix-Hallpike maneuver?

Other disorders of central or peripheral vestibular pathways may cause positional nystagmus. This kind of nystagmus usually does not fade away while the head remains in the hanging position, nor does it fatigue on repeated testing. The nystagmus may be vertical, lacking the torsional component that is found in BPPV.

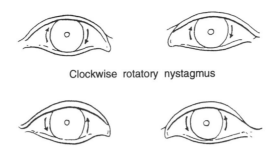

Clockwise rotatory nystagmus

Counterclockwise rotatory nystagmus

Rotatory nystagmus. (From Lee KJ: The vestibular system and its disorders. In Lee KJ (ed): Essential Otolaryngology–Head and Neck Surgery. Norwalk, CT, Appleton & Lange, 1995, p 97, with permission.)

19. Describe the doll's eye test.

This test of the vestibular system uses quick head rotation to demonstrate vestibular lesions in awake or comatose patients. Awake patients should be asked to stare into the examiner's eyes. The examiner faces the patient while holding the patient's head and then briskly turns the head to the right and to the left. Normally, the patient's gaze remains "locked" straight ahead on the examiner's eyes. The test is abnormal if the patient's gaze can be jerked off the examiner's eyes by the quick head turn. In patients with lesions, a series of "catch-up" saccades may occur as the eyes attempt to regain focus on the examiner. If the patient has an abnormal response with a right head turn, the patient has right vestibular loss. If the patient has an abnormal response with a left head turn, the patient has left vestibular loss.

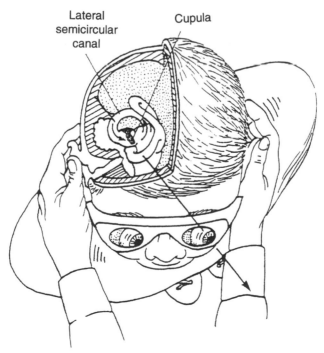

Doll's eye test. (From Pender DJ: Practical Otology. Philadelphia, J.B. Lippincott Co., 1992, p 108, with permission.)

20. On physical exam, what findings suggest a peripheral lesion?

An acute otitis media with a discharge, an attic perforation with a cholesteatoma, or hearing loss should lead the clinician to suspect a peripheral lesion. Viral inner ear infections are frequently associated with a concurrent upper respiratory infection, but nystagmus, although present initially, often disappears before the patient is evaluated.

21. What physical findings suggest a central lesion?

A central vestibular lesion causing dizziness without other neurologic findings is rare. Such lesions usually exhibit some type of neurologic deficit, such as cranial nerve abnormalities, smooth pursuit difficulties, motor deficits, or sensory deficits. In contrast to peripheral lesions, central lesions frequently exhibit persistent and odd nystagmus. Nystagmus may be vertical, caloric response may be extreme, and eye movements may be dissociated.

22. Should other systems be checked in patients with dysequilibrium?

Vision and proprioception assist the vestibular system in maintaining balance. Macular degeneration, cataracts, and abnormalities of ocular tracking can worsen dizziness and imbalance. Peripheral neuropathy with diminished sensation of proprioception in the legs and feet also worsens balance.

23. What studies should be performed on the dizzy patient?

Initially, an audiogram and an electronystagmogram should be obtained. If either of these studies or the neurologic examination shows an asymmetric or localizing finding, further studies are indicated. At this point, the clinician should consider obtaining an auditory-evoked brainstem response test or magnetic resonance image (MRI). In cases of suspected central vestibular lesions, an MRI with gadolinium contrast is the radiographic technique of choice. If a congenital disorder of the temporal bone is suspected, an enhanced fine-cut computed tomographic (CT) scan without contrast would be the most useful study. In cases of recurrent vertigo, laboratory studies may be beneficial, including a complete blood count, sedimentation rate, and test for tertiary syphilis. A lipid panel may be helpful in patients with suspected atherosclerotic disease.

24. What is an electronystagmogram (ENG)?

This is an electronic method of evaluating the visual tracking and vestibular systems. Electrodes on the patient's face record eye movements by measuring the changing electrical potential between the cornea and retina. Abnormal eye movements may be demonstrated when the patient is subjected to a series of visual tracking tests, caloric irrigation, and positional maneuvers.

25. Describe normal caloric responses.

Normally, when the left ear is stimulated with water that is cooler than body temperature, a right beating nystagmus results. When the left ear is stimulated with water that is warmer than body temperature, a left beating nystagmus results. The opposite is true for the right ear. You can remember the expected direction of nystagmus with the helpful mnemonic **COWS**:

$$\text{Cold} = \text{Opposite}$$
$$\text{Warm} = \text{Same}$$

CONTROVERSIES

26. What is the significance of positional nystagmus on an ENG?

Positional nystagmus is often found when the patient is reclining with the head or body turned to one side. This **static** positional nystagmus, which remains as long as the position is maintained, is sometimes mistaken for BPPV. However, this static positional nystagmus is nonlocalizing. It can result from either central or peripheral vestibular abnormalities and does not indicate BPPV.

27. When is posturography indicated in the workup of dizziness?

Posturography is a test of the vestibulospinal system in which standing sway is measured with a force plate. Although it has been advocated as a means of diagnosing vestibular disorders, it is not able to localize disease precisely to the central or peripheral vestibular system. It has proved most useful in following the recovery of balance in vestibular rehabilitation programs.

BIBLIOGRAPHY

1. Baloh RW, Honrubia V: Clinical Neurophysiology of the Vestibular System. Philadelphia, F.A. Davis Co., 1990.
2. Foster CA, Baloh RW: Episodic vertigo. In Rachel RE (ed): Conn's Current Therapy. Philadelphia, W.B. Saunders, 1995, pp 837–841.
3. Glasscock ME, Cueva RA, Thedinger BA: Handbook of Vertigo. New York, Raven Press, 1990.
4. Hart CW: Diagnosis and management of vertigo. Compr Ther 14(10):47–50, 1988.
5. Kumar A, Petchenik L: The diagnosis and management of vertigo. Compr Ther 16(12):56–66, 1990.
6. Lee KJ: The vestibular system and its disorders. In Lee KJ (ed): Essential Otolaryngology–Head and Neck Surgery. Norwalk, CT, Appleton & Lange, 1995, pp 93–124.
7. Singleton GT: Evaluation of the dizzy patient. In Bailey BJ (ed): Head and Neck Surgery–Otolaryngology. Philadelphia, J. B. Lippincott Co., 1993, pp 1870–1876.
8. Stringer SP, Meyerhoff WL: Diagnosis, causes, and management of vertigo. Compr Ther 16(3):34–41, 1990.

12. VESTIBULAR DISORDERS

Anne K. Stark, M.D., and Carol Foster, M.D.

1. What is the most common treatable cause of vertigo?

Benign paroxysmal positional vertigo (BPPV). Characteristically, sudden episodes of vertigo are precipitated by specific head movements, often those involving neck extension and rotation. For example, the patient may complain of vertigo precipitated by rolling over in bed or by looking upward. These brief episodes last < 1 minute. Hearing loss, aural fullness, and tinnitus are not typical. Although BPPV occurs most commonly in the elderly, it can occur in any age group. This condition is usually self-limited and resolves spontaneously over weeks to months. Treatment maneuvers can result in immediate resolution of symptoms.

2. How is BPPV treated?

BPPV is caused by the presence of heavy particles in one of the semicircular canals, possibly otoliths that have been displaced from the utricle. Movement of these particles with gravity causes stimulation of the canal. Since the canal only senses spinning motion, gravity is misinterpreted as spinning. Although this disorder usually disappears without treatment over a few weeks, the course can often be shortened dramatically by using therapeutic head maneuvers designed to rotate the particles out of the affected canal. The **Epley maneuver**, also called the canalith repositioning procedure, has proved very useful, with a success rate near 90%. Vestibular rehabilitation programs in which patients repeatedly trigger attacks of vertigo have also proved effective. If none of these procedures help, surgical ablation of the ear or blockage of the affected canal will stop the spells.

3. What is Meniere's triad?

In its classic form, the triad of Meniere's disease includes (1) a fluctuating, low-tone, **sensorineural hearing loss**, (2) fluctuating **tinnitus**, and (3) **episodic vertigo**. A feeling of aural fullness is also common.

The frequency of the attacks is variable, and long remissions from the symptoms occur. The episodes are most commonly preceded by a sense of fullness in the affected ear, followed by increasing tinnitus and hearing loss. Vertigo is usually the most distressing feature to patients; it can range in severity from episodic impaired balance to the intense illusion of spinning surroundings. The onset of vertigo is usually sudden, reaching a maximum intensity within minutes. Also distressing is the character of the tinnitus, which is often described as roaring or buzzing. The symptoms may last from 30 minutes to several hours, typically subsiding completely after the episode. The patient may, however, experience a sense of unsteadiness for hours or days. The attacks may occur anywhere at any time and may even waken the patient from sleep. As the disease progresses, the tinnitus may become constant and often is so irritating that this symptom becomes the chief complaint. Severe, permanent hearing loss may eventually develop in the affected ear, and the vertigo often ceases when this occurs. About one-third of patients go on to develop bilateral disease. If bilateral disease does develop, it usually occurs within the first few years.

4. Describe the pathophysiology of Meniere's disease.

The episodic symptoms of Meniere's disease are related to the fluctuating volume/pressure changes within a closed fluid system. Normally, endolymph moves from the cochlea, where it is produced, to the endolymphatic sac, where it is absorbed. Any disruption in this process can result in the accumulation of fluid within the membranous labyrinth and cochlea. The resulting endolymphatic hydrops distorts the cochlear duct and produces the various hearing symptoms. Vertigo results from pressure changes in the labyrinth and/or from changes in the chemical composition of the endolymph fluid that affect neural transmission.

5. Can Meniere's disease be treated medically?

Because it is impossible to predict when Meniere's disease will go into remission, several medical therapies are employed. Medical therapy is directed at slowing the progression of hearing loss and alleviating the uncomfortable symptoms. Traditional treatment has included dietary sodium restriction and the use of a diuretic. Vertigo spells may be treated with vestibular suppressors such as promethazine, diazepam, or meclizine.

6. When is Meniere's disease treated surgically?

About 10% of patients with Meniere's disease become severely disabled because of recurrent vertigo, despite medical management. Although controlling vertigo is the primary goal of treatment, hearing preservation is the secondary goal. Most surgeries destroy vestibular function in the affected ear. When the patient has no residual hearing, a labyrinthectomy is extremely effective in abolishing the debilitating episodes. When the patient has useful hearing, common effective surgeries include vestibular nerve section and transtympanic aminoglycoside treatment to the inner ear. Conservative procedures to decompress the hydropic endolymphatic sac have been used with variable results.

7. What is viral neurolabyrinthitis?

This vestibular disorder is usually preceded by a nonspecific viral illness. Within hours to days, the patient experiences the sudden onset of vertigo. This vertigo reaches a peak rapidly and then gradually declines over a few days to weeks. Cochlear symptoms are variable, ranging from normal hearing to a mild high-frequency hearing loss to sudden profound deafness. If there is no hearing loss, the disease is called **vestibular neuritis**. Total destruction of all auditory and vestibular function can occur after certain viral infections, such as measles, mumps, or herpes zoster. After the severe symptoms have subsided, the patient may experience mild lightheadedness with sudden movement. These mild symptoms may persist for months. However, with time, the patient's vestibular system compensates and the dizziness usually clears.

8. How are viral inner ear infections treated?

If hearing loss does not occur, most patients are managed symptomatically. Vestibular suppressant medication, such as meclizine, diazepam, or promethazine, are used to control vomiting. These medications should be discontinued after a week because they interfere with the normal process of compensation to vestibular injuries. Patients who are still symptomatic at that time are good candidates for vestibular rehabilitation. If hearing loss occurs, steroids are often given in an attempt to prevent deafness in the affected ear.

9. What is a perilymphatic fistula?

A perilymphatic fistula is any disruption in the limiting membranes of the labyrinth that allows communication of perilymph into the middle ear space. Most commonly, these fistulas occur in the round or oval windows of the middle ear. Classically, the patient gives a history of head trauma, a penetrating injury to the tympanic membrane, or barotrauma to the ears. During the precipitating event, the patient often experiences a "pop" in the ear. The subsequent symptoms may include vertigo, hearing loss, and tinnitus. Often subsiding at rest, these symptoms may be precipitated with straining, such as sneezing or nose blowing.

On physical examination, hematotympanum may be observed after trauma. The audiogram may demonstrate a mixed or sensorineural hearing loss, usually affecting the high frequencies more than low frequencies. An electronystagmogram may be normal, show nonspecific changes, or reflect a unilateral weakness in the affected ear. A fistula test, in which pressure is raised in the external auditory canal, may cause dizziness. Initial diagnosis, however, is strongly based on the patient's history. A definitive diagnosis cannot be made until the time of surgical exploration.

10. How should a perilymphatic fistula be treated?

Most fistulae spontaneously close. Conservative management involves bedrest, sedation, and activity modification. The patient should keep the affected ear above the level of the heart and elevate the head of the bed 4 inches. Patients should avoid straining with coughing or bowel movements and should avoid lifting anything > 10 lbs. Patients with severe unresolving symptoms may require surgical exploration and treatment. The middle ear is explored by lifting a tympanomeatal flap. With gentle aspiration, the middle ear is dried and then observed for the reaccumulation of perilymphatic fluid. Surgical management includes packing the oval and round window areas. Fat, Gelfoam, fascia, or fibrous tissues are used as packing material. If clinical suspicion is high and a fistula is not demonstrated on exploration, the surgeon will still pack the ear.

11. Which commonly used aminoglycosides preferentially affect the vestibular system rather than the auditory system?

The use of aminoglycosides may lead to ototoxicity in 5–10% of cases. Such ototoxicity leads to sensorineural hearing loss, tinnitus, or vertigo. Amikacin and neomycin tend to cause cochlear toxicity, while gentamicin, tobramycin, and streptomycin tend to cause vestibular toxicity. Patients with aminoglycoside-induced vestibular damage may suffer specifically from disequilibrium and oscillopsia.

12. What is oscillopsia?

Oscillopsia is the illusion that the environment is moving. Objects may appear to "jump" or "bob" spontaneously or with head movement. Two mechanisms can lead to this symptom. After **vestibular injuries**, there may be impairment of the vestibulo-ocular reflex, leading to the inability of patients to successfully stabilize an image on the retina during head motion. Vision blurs with rapid head movement, like that of a video camera. This head-movement-dependent oscillopsia is a classic symptom of aminoglycoside toxicity. When a patient sees the room spinning because of nystagmus, he or she is also describing oscillopsia. In this case, oscillopsia is due to **abnormal spontaneous eye movement**.

13. You suspect that a patient's vestibular symptoms are due to migraine. On what grounds are you basing your diagnosis?

"...the head be whirled round with dizziness and the ears ring as from the sound of rivers rolling along with a great noise, or like the wind when it roars among sails, or like the clang of pipers or reeds or a rattling of a carriage, we call the affection *scotoma*..."

Aretaeus of Cappadocia (131 A.D.)

Migraine is a frequently encountered disorder. Although this disorder often has a benign course between attacks, it also causes serious debility. The age of onset is between 5–30 years in 85% of cases, and > 50% of patients have a positive family history. These patients may exhibit attacks of vertigo, dysarthria, ataxia, diplopia, paresthesia, scintillating scotomas, or other neurologic symptoms such as an "aura." A unilateral headache usually follows. Vertigo may occur as part of an aura, as part of the headache phase, or between the headaches.

14. How should the clinician treat vestibular symptoms due to migraine?

Migraine with vertigo can be treated with suppressants such as meclizine or promethazine if attacks are infrequent. However, prophylactic treatment with beta-blockers, antidepressants, calcium channel blockers, or acetazolamide is necessary if attacks are frequent.

15. How are permanent vestibular injuries treated?

A simple list of vestibular exercises, developed by Cawthorne in the 1940s, has been used successfully for years to assist patients recovering from vestibular injuries. However, physical therapy programs for vestibular rehabilitation are generally more effective in shortening the duration and severity of symptoms. These programs provide exercises aimed at improving balance and eye-head coordination. Exercises to habituate the patient to feelings of dizziness are also included. Balance and coordination are gradually retrained, beginning with very simple exercises that can be performed while sitting or supported, and progressing to more complex exercises as the patient improves. For uncomplicated vestibular injury in young adults, a course of 4–8 weeks is usually sufficient.

16. What are the symptoms of vertebrobasilar insufficiency?

Vertebrobasiliar insufficiency can cause transient vertigo which usually lasts for several minutes. The vertigo may be accompanied by other brainstem symptoms, such as headache, diplopia, loss of vision, hallucinations, perioral numbness, or dysarthria. The patient may experience a drop attack without loss of consciousness due to sudden weakness of the lower limbs. Such attacks often occur spontaneously. Occasionally, symptoms can be provoked by positional changes such as hyperextension of the neck. These attacks are referred to as transient ischemic attacks (TIAs).

17. Describe the pathophysiology of transient ischemic attacks.

TIAs are due to a transient decrease in cerebral blood flow, frequently attributed to atherosclerosis. Vestibular symptoms are due to ischemia of the lateral part of the medulla where the vestibular nuclei are situated, or they are due to ischemia involving the labyrinthine artery. Cerebellar ischemia can also result in vertigo. The terminal branches of the vertebral arteries supply the pyramidal decussation. Drop attacks may be attributed to ischemia in this area.

18. Which neoplastic diseases of the CNS may lead to vertigo?

Tumors of the cerebellopontine angle, such as acoustic neuromas, meningiomas, and epidermoid cysts, are associated with vestibular symptoms. Gliomas and secondary tumors of the brainstem or cerebellum may also lead to vestibular symptoms.

19. What causes motion sickness?

Motion sickness, or kinetosis, is a condition characterized by nausea, vomiting, pallor, and sweating. Motion sickness is not a disease but rather a physiologic response to a mismatch between vestibular and visual information about the moving environment. Motion sickness can be devastating to some patients, however. For short exposures to motion, preventive medication includes diphenhydrinate or diphenhydramine. For exposures longer than 1 day, meclizine or transdermal scopolamine may be needed.

20. What is Cogan's syndrome?

Cogan's syndrome is a systemic autoimmune disorder that preferentially affects the inner ear and eye. Vestibuloauditory symptoms are severe and bilateral and include fluctuating hearing loss, episodic vertigo, tinnitus, and aural fullness. Such symptoms closely precede or follow ocular inflammation. On vestibular evaluation, caloric responses are decreased or absent.

21. What is Behçet's disease?

Behçet's disease, also an autoimmune disorder, exhibits a clinical triad of oral and genital ulcers, iritis or uveitis, and progressive sensorineural hearing loss. Vertigo is often associated with this disease. An underlying vasculitis is thought to be responsible for these symptoms.

CONTROVERSIES

22. Discuss the pathophysiology of benign paroxysmal positional vertigo.

In 1969, Schucknecht described the underlying pathophysiology of BPPV to be **cupulolithiasis**. In his classic study of two diseased temporal bones, he found that otoconial material was lodged on the cupula of the posterior semicircular canal. To further support this theory, patients suffering from BPPV exhibited immediate relief upon sectioning of the posterior ampullary nerve.

This theory has been disputed, however. Some argue that such deposits resulted from postmortem changes. Others have pointed out that cupular deposits should cause long-lasting nystagmus, rather than paroxysmal positional nystagmus. A newer theory, **canalithiasis**, posits that debris is lodged in the lumen of the posterior semicircular canal and acts as a piston to cause paroxysmal nystagmus. Recent intraoperative findings of chalky material in the posterior canal lumen of affected patients support this theory.

23. Do vascular loops cause vertigo?

Controversy surrounds the relationship of vascular loops in the cerebellopontine angle and vestibular symptoms. A vascular loop may be formed by the anterior inferior cerebellar artery or a branch that intrudes into the internal auditory canal. This causes compression of the eighth nerve. However, vascular loops in this area are commonly found in normal individuals. There is also considerable overlap between the reported symptoms of vascular loop and other inner ear diseases, such as Meniere's. If patients who suffer from brief attacks of positional vertigo and tinnitus are responsive to carbamazepine, they are likely candidates for the diagnosis of vascular compression.

24. What is "whiplash vertigo"?

Also known as cervical vertigo, this condition was previously a common diagnosis given to people with concomitant neck pain and vertigo. This diagnosis has largely gone out of fashion. Injury to the cervical joints and muscle receptors of the neck may indeed lead to disruptions of the ascending sensory pathways to the vestibular and cerebellar systems; however, the vertiginous accident victim is often symptomatic from post-traumatic BPPV, concussion, deceleration injury, or direct trauma to the inner ear. Therefore, a clinician should not immediately attribute vertigo to joint or muscle receptor disruption. Once a cervical fracture is ruled out, a Dix-Hallpike examination, audiogram, electronystagmogram, and magnetic resonance image should be considered in the setting of trauma.

BIBLIOGRAPHY

1. Baloh RW, Honrubia V: Clinical Neurophysiology of the Vestibular System. Philadelphia, F. A. Davis, 1990.
2. Dix MR, Hood JD: Vertigo. Chichester, John Wiley and Sons, 1984.
3. Foster CA, Baloh RW: Episodic vertigo. In Rachel RE (ed): Conn's Current Therapy. Philadelphia, W.B. Saunders, 1995, pp 837–841.
4. Glasscock ME, Cueva RA, Thedinger BA: Handbook of Vertigo. New York, Raven Press, 1990.
5. Hart CW: Diagnosis and management of vertigo. Compr Ther 14(10):47–50, 1988.
6. Kumar A, Petchenik L: The diagnosis and management of vertigo. Compr Ther 16(12):56–66, 1990.
7. Lee KJ: The vestibular system and its disorders. In Lee KJ (eds): Essential Otolaryngology–Head and Neck Surgery. Norwalk, CT, Appleton & Lange, 1995, pp 93–124.
8. Stringer SP, Meyerhoff WL: Diagnosis, causes, and management of vertigo. Compr Ther 16(3):34–41, 1990.

13. TINNITUS

Mark A. Voss, M.D.

1. What is tinnitus?
Tinnitus comes from the latin word *tinnire*, which means "to ring." It is described as a sound sensation that originates in the head and is not attributable to any perceivable external sound.

2. Who was George Catlin?
Born in 1796 and educated as a lawyer, George Catlin is mostly remembered for his paintings of Southwestern Native Americans. His contribution to otolaryngology was his revealing descriptions of living with tinnitus and a progressive hearing loss:

> If it were only deafness that I have to submit to, I feel as if I could sit down in silence for the rest of my life and be content in my daily employment, but the disease is attended with the sound in the ear not unlike the drawing of a viola bow across one of the strings and not a pulse night or day has been there without the sound. What I wish to hear I cannot hear, and what I do not wish to hear I am compelled to hear.

3. How common is tinnitus?
As many as one-third (32%) of Americans experience tinnitus sometime in their lives. These data are supported by similar studies performed in Europe. Even 13% of audiometrically normal school-aged children experience at least transient tinnitus. It is estimated that approximately 18 million Americans seek medical attention for their tinnitus. Nine million report being seriously affected by their condition, and 2 million are disabled because of the elusive sounds.

4. How do you classify a patient's tinnitus?
A historical classification schema for tinnitus that persists in contemporary literature revolves around objective versus subjective tinnitus. **Objective tinnitus** refers to those uncommon conditions that produce tinnitus that can be heard by an observer. **Subjective tinnitus** encompasses all other patients who experience a sound that defies detection. A more useful classification schema which is finding favor among otolaryngologists focuses on categorizing tinnitus by its etiology. These categories are vascular, external and middle ear, myogenic, peripheral sensorineural, and central sensorineural.

5. What historical or physical findings would make you suspect a vascular etiology for tinnitus?
A pulsatile or throbbing quality that parallels the heartbeat should raise your index of suspicion. A reddish or blue mass behind the tympanic membrane may indicate a glomus tumor arising within the middle ear cleft or a dehiscence of the jugular bulb or carotid artery. A hemotympanum may follow a history of head trauma. Arteriovenous malformations are uncommon but may occur between the occipital artery (arising from the external carotid artery and passing medial to the mastoid process) and the transverse sinus. A venous hum may represent one of the more common causes of vascular tinnitus. It may signify impingement of the jugular vein by the second cervical vertebra or suggest an underlying high output cardiac condition (anemia, exercise, pregnancy, thyrotoxicosis). Compression of the ipsilateral jugular vein may help with the diagnosis.

6. Can foreign bodies in the external auditory canal cause tinnitus?
Yes. Cerumen, hair, or foreign bodies in contact with the tympanic membrane have been associated with tinnitus. The close proximity of the mandibular condyle with the external auditory canal should also be ruled out with a careful history and focused exam.

7. Palatal myoclonus is known to produce a tinnitus. What is the best way to detect this condition?

Using flexible nasopharyngoscopy in the awake clinic patient allows examination of the palate from a superior perch in the nasopharynx. Examining the palate from an oral cavity approach may lead to temporary extermination of the myoclonus while the mouth is stretched open. From a practical approach, both methods of exam should be employed.

8. What systemic diseases may be associated with myoclonus?

Multiple sclerosis, cerebrovascular accidents, intracranial neoplasms, and various psychogenic causes.

9. What is the association of tinnitus with hearing loss?

85% of tinnitus patients have audiometrically documented hearing loss in the 250–8000 Hz range. However, the presence of tinnitus does not absolutely imply hearing loss.

10. How is the ototoxicity caused by salicylates different from that due to aminoglycosides?

High serum concentrations of salicylates and some nonsteroidal anti-inflammatory drugs (NSAIDs) cause a flat, bilateral hearing loss and tinnitus. The hearing loss is a mild to moderate sensorineural hearing loss of about 20–40 dB. No otologic histopathology has been consistently demonstrated. Both the hearing loss and tinnitus are reversible within 24–72 hours of discontinuation of the offending medication. Aminoglycoside ototoxicity occurs in up to 15% of patients and can occur at therapeutic serum concentrations. Effects can include cochlear toxicity, yielding hearing loss and tinnitus, or vestibulotoxicity, yielding vertigo. Hearing loss is also heralded by tinnitus. Ototoxic effects that are still present 2–3 weeks after therapy termination are likely to be permanent.

11. Name some common medications that can cause tinnitus.

ACE inhibitors: enalapril, fosinopril (Monopril)

Anesthetics: dyclonine, bupivacaine (Marcaine, Sensorcaine), lidocaine

Antibiotics: aztreonam, ciprofloxacin, erythromycin estolate, erythromycin-ethylsuccinate/sulfisoxazole (Pediazole), gentamicin (Garamycin), imipenem-cilastatin (Primaxin), sulfisoxazole (Gantrisin), trimethoprim-sulfamethoxazole, vancomycin

Antidepressants: alprazolam (Xanax), amitriptyline (Elavil), desipramine, doxepin, fluoxetine (Prozac), imipramine (Tofranil), maprotiline (Ludiomil), nortriptyline (Pamelor)

Anithistamines: aspirin-promethazine-pseudoephedrine (Phenergan), chlorpheniramine-phenylpropanolamine (Triaminic), clemastine (Tavist), pseudoephedrine-chlorpheniramine (Deconamine), pseudoephedrine-triprolidine (Actifed)

Antimalarials: chloroquine, pyrimethamine-sulfadoxine (Fansidar)

Beta-blockers: betaxolol (Kerlone), carteolol (Cartrol), metoprolol (Lopressor), nadolol (Corgard), timolol (Timoptic)

Calcium channel blockers: diltiazem (Cardizem), nicardipine (Cardene), nifedipine (Procardia)

Diuretics: acetazolamide (Diamox), amiloride, ethacrynic acid

Narcotics: dezocine (Dalgan), pentazocine (Talwin)

NSAIDs: diclofenac (Voltaren), diflunisal (Dolobid), flurbiprofen (Ansaid), ibuprofen, indomethacin, meclofenamate (Meclomen), naproxen (Naprosyn), sulindac (Clinoril), tolmetin (Tolectin)

Sedatives/hypnotics/anxiolytics: azatadine (Optimine), buspirone (Buspar), chlorpheniramine-phenylpropanolomine (Ornade)

Miscellaneous: albuterol (Proventil), allopurinol, bismuth subsalicylate (Pepto-Bismol), carbamazepine (Tegretol), cyclobenzaprine (Flexeril), cyclosporine, diphenhydramine (Benadryl), flecainide, hydroxychloroquine (Plaquenil), iohexol (Omnipaque), isotretinoin (Accutane), lithium, methylergonovine (Methergine), nicotine polacrilex (Nicorette), prazosin, omeprazole (Prilosec), quinidine, recombinant hepatitis B vaccine (Recombivax), salicylates, sodium nitroprusside (Nipride), sulfasalazine (Azulfidine), tocainide

12. What percentage of patients with acoustic neuromas have tinnitus as the presenting symptom? How many will develop it?

Ten percent of these patients present with tinnitus. Over their lifetimes, this rate increases to 83%.

13. When evaluating a patient with tinnitus, what questions should you ask to facilitate the patient's description of the ringing?

Most patients are able to localize the tinnitus to one ear. **Quality** (popping, clicking, pulsing, pure or multiple tones) gives insight into possible vascular or myogenic origins. It is important to document **progression** and **frequency of symptoms** as a gauge of disease, as these patients are typically followed for months or years. Daily or monthly **cycling** as well as **associated events** or symptoms can give important clues for determining etiologies.

14. List the key topics in obtaining an otologic history.

Accompanying audiovestibular disease	Trauma
Noise exposure	Family history
Ototoxic chemical/medications	Systemic diseases
Infection (local, systemic)	Otologic surgery

15. What instruments would you place in your black bag before going to evaluate a patient with tinnitus?

A sharp eye and skillful hands are invaluable when performing a thorough head and neck exam, though you can't put these in your bag. A sphygmomanometer and stethoscope will help to detect a potential vascular etiology. Pneumotoscopy is mandatory when observing the external and middle ear. Tuning forks (512 and 1024 Hz) are used in performing the Weber and Rinne tests. An ophthalmoscope will help to rule out a carotid-cavernous fistula. Tongue blades are a must for examining the palate and dental occlusion in suspected myogenic or temporomandibular joint-related causes. A flexible nasopharyngoscope would be helpful (but expensive) when looking for myogenic etiologies. Depending on the size of your black bag, an audiometer, tympanometer, CT scanner, and/or a MRI unit would be useful adjunctive equipment to evaluate suspected peripheral or central sensorineural tinnitus. A peek at the contents of your patient's medicine cabinet is often quite revealing.

16. In attempts to define the extent of a patient's tinnitus, how much sound pressure should mask the symptoms?

Approximately 80% of patients will have their tinnitus masked with 6 dB or less of sound pressure.

17. What is white noise?

Patients often complain that they are most affected by tinnitus at night, when the sound of daily activity has ceased. Tinnitus may be relieved with white noise, or a nonidentifiable background sound that drowns out their symptoms. A radio set at a nonoperational frequency or the hum of a fan may help these patients at night.

18. How do anesthetics such as lidocaine act to decrease tinnitus?

Lidocaine and several related anesthetics act as CNS depressants by inhibiting the influx of sodium and therefore reduce the number of action potentials. One theory to explain tinnitus pertains to the high baseline spontaneous firing rate of the normal auditory system and the loss of its natural inhibitors. Anesthetics are thought to augment or replace this natural inhibition process, holding tinnitus in check. At present, intravenous lidocaine is the only medication that can reliably stop tinnitus in many patients. However, it is impractical because of the short duration of action and its method of administration.

19. What role does surgery play in tinnitus?

Only a few of the many causes of tinnitus lend themselves to surgical intervention: persistent middle ear effusion, foreign body of the external auditory canal, otosclerosis, Meniere's disease, and tumors of the cerebellopontine angle.

CONTROVERSIES

20. List some alternative nonsurgical treatments for tinnitus.

Several controversial treatments exist for the control of tinnitus. Hypnotherapy has been shown to improve coping skills in approximately one-third of patients. Control of inhalants and food allergies has alleviated tinnitus in approximately 30% of patients with these conditions. Biofeedback has a high success rate (70–90%) for improving patients' ability to cope with their disease. Acupuncture has not been shown to be beneficial. Tinnitus correlates with levels of stress, and therefore support groups and stress-reduction tactics play important therapeutic roles. The American Tinnitus Association produces a quarterly newsletter. Their address is P.O. Box 5, Portland, OR 97207.

21. What laboratory tests should you consider in the evaluation of the patient with tinnitus?

One or more of the following tests may be indicated if the history of tinnitus or a review of systems suggests a possible etiology. Except in highly suspicious cases, their limited cost-effectiveness makes their use controversial.

Complete blood count

Fluorescent treponemal antibody absorption test

Screening for ototoxic drugs and environmental pollutants (including heavy metals and carbon monoxide)

Thyroid stimulating hormone

Blood glucose

Cholesterol, lipid profile

Autoimmune screening (rheumatoid factor, antinuclear antibody, ANA, total complement)

BIBLIOGRAPHY

1. Hazell JW: Tinnitus II: Surgical management of conditions associated with tinnitus and somatosounds. J Otolaryngol 19:6–10, 1990.
2. Hazell JW: Tinnitus III: The practical management of sensorineural tinnitus. J Otolaryngol 19:11–18, 1990.
3. Jastreboff PJ, Sasaki CT: An animal model of tinnitus: A decade of development. Am J Otol 15:19-27, 1994.
4. Levine SB, Snow JB. Pulsatile tinnitus. Laryngoscope 97:401–406, 1987.
5. Mattox DE, Wilkins SA: Tinnitus. In The American Academy of Otolaryngology–Head and Neck Surgery Self-Instructional Package. Rochester, NY, Mosby, 1989.
6. Murai K, Tyler RS, Harker LA, Stouffer JL: Review of pharmacologic treatment of tinnitus. Am J Otol 13:454-464, 1992.
7. Remley KB, Harnsberger HR, Jacobs JM, Smoker WR: The radiologic evaluation of pulsatile tinnitus and the vascular tympanic membrane. Semin Ultrasound, CT, MR 10:236–250, 1989.
8. Schleuning AJ: Management of the patient with tinnitus. Med Clin North Am 75:1225–1237, 1991.
9. Vernon J, Griest S, Press L: Attributes of tinnitus and the acceptance of masking. Am J Otolaryngol 11:44–50, 1990.

14. EAR INJURIES AFTER FLYING AND DIVING

Mark R. Mount, M.D., and Philip E. Asmar, M.D., M.M.Sc.

1. What is Boyle's law?

Most otolaryngologic problems that are caused by scuba diving fall within the realm of Boyle's law and involve the air-occupied spaces in the middle ear and sinuses. Unlike air, water is incompressible. Boyle's law states that at a constant temperature, the volume of a gas is inversely proportional to pressure. In other words, volume decreases as pressure increases.

2. What other law of physics is important in diving?

Henry's law states that "at a given temperature, the mass of a gas dissolved in a given volume of solvent is proportional to the pressure of the gas with which it is in equilibrium." This application becomes important when considering the increased amount of nitrogen that dissolves in the body fluids and tissues during descent and is released during ascent.

3. What depth of water registers two atmospheres?

Sea-level pressure is doubled at 33 ft (10 m) below the surface. The pressure increases linearly, and so every 10 m of descent causes a pressure increase of 14.7 psi, or 100 kpa, or 1 atm.

4. What altitude above sea level registers one-half atmosphere or one-half of sea-level ambient pressure?

Air pressure at 18,000 ft is one-half of that at sea level. Pressure changes much more slowly in the air compared with underwater. However, a pressurized aircraft that suddenly loses pressurization may have an extremely rapid pressure change and cause problems similar to those associated with ascending too quickly from a dive.

5. Is the eustachian tube normally open or closed? Why is this important in diving?

Normally, the eustachian tube is closed, only opening when there is positive pressure in the nasopharynx or by muscular action of the tensor veli palatini, levator palatini, or salpingopharyngeus. However, it has been shown that as a diver descends, the eustachian tube acts as a flutter valve, which remains closed under pressure unless it is reflexively or voluntarily opened by the diver. If the tube fails to open, this may result in middle ear barotrauma or a "squeeze effect."

6. Which nerves supply sensation to the ear?

Innervation of the external canal is through three cranial nerves: the auriculotemporal (V3), the facial nerve (VII) through the tympanic plexus, and Arnold's nerve (auricular branch of X). The auriculotemporal nerve (V3) innervates the tympanic membrane. The middle ear is supplied by Jacobson's nerve (IX), the auriculotemporal nerve (V3), and Arnold's nerve (X).

7. Why does ear pain occur during changes in ambient pressure, such as during diving or flying?

Air spaces in the head, such as the middle ear and paranasal sinuses, must maintain pressure equilibrium with ambient air. According to Boyle's law, as pressure increases, gas volume decreases. Therefore, as the middle ear descends in air or water, the existing air shrinks. This shrinkage creates a negative pressure inside the cavity, causing pain. During ascent, the gas in the cavity expands and must ventilate, or it will cause pressure on the middle ear mucosa.

8. Other than middle ear barotrauma, what can cause ear pain during flying or diving?
External ear barotrauma or "canal squeeze" often occurs in divers with impacted cerumen. The air deep to the occlusion remains the same as the surface pressure, while the surrounding pressure and middle ear pressure increase as the diver descends. A relative vacuum develops, resulting in the development of ear pain and congestion of the canal skin and tympanic membrane.

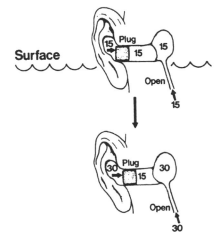

Canal squeeze, resulting from an ear plug in the external auditory canal. During descent, the pressure in the canal remains at seal-level pressure, whereas the middle ear and external to the ear are at ambient pressure. The resultant negative pressure in the canal pulls the plug inward and bulges the eardrum outward. A tympanic membrane perforation can occur if there is a great enough pressure differential. (From Reuter SH: Underwater medicine: Otolaryngologic considerations of the skin and scuba diver. In Paparella MM, Shumrick DA, Gluckman JL, Meyerhoff WL (eds): Otolaryngology. Philadelphia, W.B. Saunders, 1991, pp 3231–3257, with permission.)

9. What is meant by "reversed squeeze"?
On ascent, if the eustachian tube remains blocked, the pressure within the middle ear will increase as its volume of air expands. This results in severe ear pain, sometimes associated with dizziness. This "reversed squeeze" can be severe enough to result in rupture of the tympanic membrane, middle ear hemorrhage, and even permanent hearing loss.

10. At what depth do most divers terminate a dive because of pain?
Greater than 75% of divers terminate their dive within 33 ft of the surface. During the first 33 ft, the pressure doubles, demonstrating the greatest change in both density and pressure that the diver experiences.

11. Is it more common to have ear pain during ascent or during descent while flying?
During ascent, the relative pressure in the middle ear increases, causing the tympanic membrane to bulge out. Air escapes passively through the eustachian tube if the pressure differential is 15 mmHg or more. During descent, the relative pressure in the middle ear decreases, causing the tympanic membrane to bulge inward. Passive venting through the eustachian tube is more difficult, and passengers usually must take active measures to equalize pressure, such as the Valsalva maneuver. More people have trouble going down than up.

12. Is it ok to fly with myringotomy tubes in place?
Yes. The presence of myringotomy tubes or a tympanic membrane perforation creates an artificial pressure-equalization system that bypasses the eustachian tube. Therefore, no pressure buildup should occur. Anxious parents often need reassurance that tubes are ideal for flying. It is important, however, to ensure that the tubes are patent.

13. Should children fly when they have a cold?
Flying requires adequate eustachian tube function for equilibration of middle ear pressure. Because infants and young children have a poorly functioning tensor veli palatini as well as an already compromised eustachian tube during an upper respiratory infection, it is

recommended that they should *not* fly if they have a cold. However, if flying cannot be avoided, children should be encouraged to swallow repeatedly or chew gum (infants may be given a bottle) to maintain adequate operation of the eustachian tube in order to prevent severe pain and hearing loss.

14. At what pressure differential across the tympanic membrane does the membrane rupture during flying?

At an approximately 60-mmHg pressure differential, passengers begin to feel fullness within the middle ear. As the pressure differential increases to 90 mmHg, the eustachian tube becomes locked. Any attempts to equalize become futile. Finally, as the pressure differential increases between 100–500 mmHg, the tympanic membrane ruptures.

15. In a diver who develops ear pain, what is the significance of vertigo?

Divers are highly subject to disorientation due to several factors. Spatial orientation in humans depends on three sensory signals: visual signs, limb proprioception, and the vestibular apparatus. Underwater, darkness may inhibit visual signals, and near-loss of gravity prevents proprioception. Orientation thus relies on the vestibular system, but this is at risk to fail as well. Simple caloric stimulation as water enters the external canals at different times (because of cerumen or tight hoods) can cause temporary physiologic vertigo. This is worse if a unilateral eardrum perforation is present. Rapid pressure changes or failing to use the Valsalva maneuver during descent may cause a perilymphatic fistula, causing progressive vertigo. Some divers experience **alternobaric vertigo**, which is unequal pressures in the middle ears during ascent. This causes asymmetric stimulation of the vestibular apparatus.

In short, the differential diagnosis of vertigo in a diver includes simple disorientation, perilymphatic fistula, unequal plugging of the ears, perforated tympanic membrane, and alternobaric vertigo. Divers should know how to prevent vertigo and recognize its significance. Spatial disorientation underwater can be fatal. Divers know to observe their air bubbles whenever they become disoriented—air always goes up.

16. Besides unequal pressures in the middle ear, can other factors cause alternobaric vertigo?

Alternobaric vertigo can result from unequal signals to the vestibular nuclei as gas expands equally in the middle ears. The most common cause is end-organ damage on one side, which is usually seen in older divers. Divers who experience this type of vertigo should not participate in this sport.

17. What is a perilymphatic fistula?

Rapid changes in relative pressure of the middle ear space produce implosive or explosive forces on the various membranes, i.e., the tympanic membrane, oval window, and round window. Any of these structures may rupture, causing vertigo and/or hearing loss. Rupture of the round or oval windows produces a fistula, allowing perilymph to leak into the space. This rupture damages the cochlea or vestibular apparatus, causing hearing loss or vertigo.

18. Describe the pathophysiology involved in explosive and implosive mechanisms causing oval and round window ruptures.

Explosive mechanism: On descent, inadequate ear-clearing occurs, which causes a negative pressure (relative to the intralabyrinthine fluid pressure) to develop. As a result, the diver performs a Valsalva maneuver in an attempt to equalize the pressure. An increase in CSF pressure is then transmitted to the inner ear through the cochlear duct, further increasing the pressure differential across the inner ear membranes. This results in outward bulging of the round window and rupture.

Implosive mechanism: During descent, a relative negative pressure develops in the middle ear space, which causes the tympanic membrane to bulge inward. If a sudden forceful Valsalva maneuver is attempted, the eardrum suddenly approaches a neutral position, and the outward force is transmitted to the stapes. As a result, a relative negative pressure develops in the inner ear fluid, causing the round window to bulge inward and rupture.

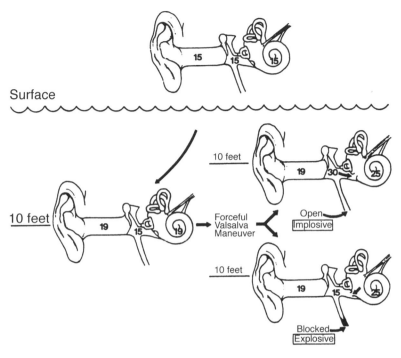

Implosive and explosive mechanisms. A forceful Valsalva maneuver can lead to a round window rupture (perilymphatic fistula). In *implosion*, sudden opening of the eustachian tube overinflates the middle ear, which may produce an inward rupture of the round window membranes. In *explosion*, the eustachian tube remains blocked with an increase in the CSF pressure, which is transmitted to the inner ear and may produce an outward rupture of the round window membrane. (From Reuter SH: Underwater medicine: Otolaryngologic considerations of the skin and scuba diver. In Paparella MM, Shumrick DA, Gluckman JL, Meyerhoff WL (eds): Otolaryngology. Philadelphia, W.B. Saunders, 1991, pp 3231-3257, with permission.)

19. Can a perilymphatic fistula cause conductive or sensorineural hearing loss?

Oval window fistula often accompanies ossicular disruption, or "uncorking" of the stapedial footplate resting on the oval window. Therefore, both conductive and sensorineural hearing loss may be present. Symptoms may be rapid or insidious in onset, depending on the size of the hole. Emergent surgery through a tympanotomy approach may be indicated to patch the fistula and possibly prevent permanent hearing loss.

20. What is a fistula test?

A fistula test involves applying positive pressure (via an otoscope) to the middle ear. In the presence of a perilymphatic fistula, positive pressure will cause nystagmus. Unfortunately, the fistula test is neither very sensitive nor specific.

21. What is the significance of hemotympanum after flying or diving?

Hemotympanum presents as a purplish hue to the tympanic membrane and results from ruptured blood vessels in the middle ear space by barotrauma. Also known as **barotitis media**, this condition is usually self-limiting and clears itself. Treatment includes use of an oral and topical decongestant for a few days, and divers should abstain until the condition clears. Middle ear barotrauma is the most common disorder in divers.

22. How does one diagnose a perforated tympanic membrane?

A practitioner can usually diagnose tympanic membrane perforation in the diver or flyer by pneumotoscopy. Often, the perforation is large enough to be obvious, but it should be confirmed with an insufflation bulb. A perforated drum does not move on insufflation.

23. How should one manage an acute perforated eardrum secondary to barotrauma?

A simple perforation needs no treatment. Most holes spontaneously heal within 8 weeks. The patient should be careful to keep soapy and dirty water out of the ear. The patient should not dive. If pus or drainage develops, antibiotic eardrops are indicated. If the perforation does not heal within 3 months, a paper patch may be applied in the office. The patch serves as a bridge under which epithelial cells migrate to repair the defect. If a paper patch fails, the patient should undergo formal tympanoplasty in the operating room.

24. Can a diver continue to dive after repair of a diving-related labyrinthine window fistula?

A recreational scuba diver suffering from inner ear injury should strongly consider giving up this activity. However, a diver determined to return to the sport should allow at least 3 months of recovery. If the individual has completely recovered from the hearing loss (with the exception of high-frequency loss), has a normal electronystagmogram, and can equilibrate middle ear pressures without difficulty, diving may be resumed. In addition, future diving practices should be altered to allow for proper equalization, avoid rapid descents, and avoid diving with upper respiratory symptoms. By actively practicing the above precautions, the diver may prevent further inner ear injury. Such injury could be fatal if disorientation or drowning occurs as a result of vertigo, nausea, and/or vomiting while diving.

25. Describe inner ear decompression sickness, and name the treatment of choice.

Decompression sickness involves the development of nitrogen bubbles in the microvasculature, causing blockage of venous circulation in the stria vascularis, spiral ligament, and semicircular canals. This accumulation results in the development of hemorrhages and the formation of protein exudates, as well as irritation of the endosteum of the bony semicircular canals. The treatment of choice is hyperbaric oxygen.

26. Why is it important, when treating a diver with inner ear symptoms, to be accurate and rapid in the diagnosis of inner ear barotrauma versus inner ear decompression sickness?

Hyperbaric treatment is essential for inner ear decompression symptoms, but it would be extremely harmful to the inner ear after barotrauma. Because hyperbaric treatment simulates the events that can result in barotrauma, subjecting the diver to this type of treatment could potentiate the damaging event.

27. What follow-up is recommended for divers after inner ear decompression sickness?

Histopathologic changes initiated by primary decompression insult may develop slowly over several months. In addition, vestibular function deficits are often masked in activities of daily living by the central vestibular compensatory mechanism. Therefore, long-term vestibular function follow-up is recommended and includes specific vestibular tests, such as electronystagmography and/or rotary chair examination.

28. Describe the signs and symptoms of inner ear barotrauma.

The signs and symptoms of inner ear barotrauma include persistent vertigo, sensorineural hearing loss, and/or loud tinnitus following dives in which decompression sickness is unlikely. However, inner ear decompression sickness may present with similar symptoms and should be considered due to the potential severity of the injury.

29. Which types of hearing-frequency losses have been associated with inner ear barotrauma?

The most common hearing losses are either high-frequency or total frequency types. The high-frequency losses are usually in the 4000–8000-Hz range.

30. Why is it important to do a thorough nasal exam on divers?

It is essential to have patent nasal airways as well as absence of nasal and sinus symptoms in order to prevent inner and middle ear barotrauma. Any condition blocking the nasal airway, such as nasal polyps, anatomic defect, or swollen turbinates, can hinder middle ear equalization.

31. Is short-term use of decongestants contraindicated in diving?

No. Short-term use of decongestants is not contraindicated. Experienced divers report that they are better able to equalize if the medications are used immediately before diving. However, rebound from topical decongestants can occur, or topical decongestants may cause tachycardia or hypertension. If these drugs are to be used, they should be tested first on nondiving days. In addition, these drugs should not be used so that an individual with an upper respiratory infection may dive (due to the risk of severe ear squeeze).

CONTROVERSIES

32. Which muscles are involved in the mechanism of eustachian tube dilatation?

The tensor veli palatini, levator veli palatini, salpingopharyngeus, and tensor tympani all have been associated directly or indirectly with tubal function. Although controversial, most anatomic physiologic evidence supports the tensor veli palatini muscle as being solely responsible for active tubal dilatation.

33. How is a perilymphatic fistula diagnosed and treated?

Early surgical exploration: No noninvasive tests have proven effective in accurately diagnosing a perilymphatic fistula. By exploring acutely dizzy patients early, one can both make the diagnosis and treat adequately in a timely fashion. Delay may result in permanent labyrinthine dysfunction and deafness. Especially in the patient with sudden hearing loss, surgery should not be delayed.

Noninvasive testing and observation: The diagnosis of perilymphatic fistula is difficult, even during surgery in some cases. The incidence of fistula due to indirect trauma is extremely low. Conservative therapy usually involves bedrest for 1–2 weeks with the head elevated. Many existing fistulas will heal spontaneously. Patients whose symptoms worsen should have surgery. A conservative approach will save many patients from surgery and the risk of complications.

BIBLIOGRAPHY

1. Adkisson GH, Meredith AP: Inner ear decompression sickness combined with a fistula of the round window. Ann Otol Rhinol Laryngol 99:733–737, 1990.
2. Bluestone CD, Klein JO: Otitis media, atelectasis, and eustachian tube dysfunction. In Bluestone CD, Stool SE, Scheetz MD (eds): Pediatric Otolaryngology, 2nd ed. Philadelphia, W.B. Saunders, 1990, pp 320–486.
3. Brown TP: Middle ear symptoms while flying. Postgrad Med 96(2):135–142, 1994.
4. Butler FK Jr, Thalmann ED: Report of an isolated mid-frequency hearing loss following inner ear barotrauma. Undersea Biomed Res 10(2):131–134, 1983.
5. Desforges J: Medical problems associated with underwater diving. N Engl JMed 326:30–35, 1992.
6. Farmer JC, Gillespie CA: Otologic medicine and surgery of exposures to aerospace, diving, and compressed gases. In Alberti PW, Ruben RJ (eds): Otologic Medicine and Surgery. New York, Churchill Livingstone, 1988, pp 1753–1802.
7. Freeman P, Edmonds C: Inner ear barotrauma. Arch Otolaryngol 95:556–563, 1972.
8. Head PW: Vertigo and barotrauma. In Dix MR, Hood JD (eds): Vertigo. Chichester, John Wiley & Sons, 1984.
9. Jerrard DA: Diving medicine. Emerg Med Clin North Am 10:329–339, 1992.

10. Lee KJ (ed): Essential Otolaryngology–Head and Neck Surgery, 6th ed. Norwalk, CT, Appleton & Lange, 1995.
11. Molvaer OI, Natrud E: Ear damage due to diving. Acta Otolarygol Suppl 360:187–189, 1979.
12. Money KE, Buckingham IP, Calder IM, et al: Damage to the middle ear and inner ear in underwater divers. Undersea Biomed Res 12:77–84, 1985.
13. Neblett LM: Otolaryngology and sport scuba diving update and guidelines. Ann Otol Rhinol Laryngol Suppl 115:1–12, 1985.
14. Parisier SC: Injuries of the ear and temporal bone. In Bluestone CD, Stool SE, Scheetz MD (eds): Pediatric Otolaryngology, 2nd ed. Philadelphia, W.B. Saunders, 1990, pp 578–595.
15. Reissman P, Shupak A, Nachum Z, Melamed Y: Inner ear decompression sickness following a shallow scuba dive. Aviat Space Environ Med 61:563–566, 1990.
16. Reuter SH: Underwater medicine: Otolaryngologic considerations of the skin and scuba diver. In Paparella MM, Shumrick DA, Gluckman JL, Meyerhoff WL (eds): Otolaryngology. Philadelphia, W.B. Saunders, 1991, pp 3231–3257.
17. Shupak A, Doweck I, Greenberg E, et al: Diving-related inner ear injuries. Laryngoscope 101:173–179, 1991.
18. Vartiainen E, Nuutinen J, Karjalainen S, Nykanen K: Perilymph fistula—A diagnostic dilemma. J Laryngol Otol 105:270–273, 1991.
19. Wall C III, Rauch SD: Perilymph fistula: Pathophysiology. Otolaryngol Head Neck Surg 112:145–153, 1995.

15. NEURO-OTOLOGY

Cameron Shaw, M.D., and Anne K. Stark, M.D.

1. Tumors of the ear may masquerade as what common otologic problem?
A neoplasm of the ear often presents with classic signs and symptoms of a **chronic ear infection**. The clinician should always consider neoplastic disease when evaluating these patients.

2. Name the three most common neoplasms of the auricle.
Basal cell carcinomas
Squamous cell carcinomas
Melanomas
Six percent of all skin cancers are auricular. Sebaceous cysts are a common benign neoplasm of the auricle.

3. Name the four most common *true* neoplasms of the temporal bone and external ear canal.
Fibrous dysplasia
Langerhans' cell histiocytosis
Leukemia
Sarcomas
These neoplasms are uncommon and account for < 0.05% of head and neck malignancies. Etiologic factors include a history of head and neck radiation or chronic ear inflammation. Osteomas/exostoses are very common benign lesions which generally need no treatment. Aural polyps are not uncommonly associated with perforations or cholesteatomas.

4. What percentage of leukemic patients eventually have leukemic involvement in the ear or temporal bone?
20%. Such involvement may present as mucosal ulceration or bleeding from the external auditory canal. The tympanic membrane and middle ear mucosa may become irregular and thickened. Leukemic patients may eventually exhibit deficits of cranial nerves VII and VIII.

5. What is the most common true neoplasm of the middle ear?

Glomus tumors, or paragangliomas. They are most often found in middle-aged Caucasians. Pulsatile tinnitus is the most common presenting symptom. On pneumatic otoscopy, positive pressure may cause blanching of the pulsating mass under the tympanic membrane (Brown's sign). Because of their appearance, these neoplasms may be mistaken for a high-riding jugular bulb or an aberrant carotid artery. Glomus tumors may grow to a significant size before becoming symptomatic with cranial nerve palsies. While a conductive hearing loss may be an early sign of a glomus tumor, sensorineural hearing is often normal. These tumors are usually benign neoplasms and carry a < 3% malignancy rate. Also, < 1% of these tumors are associated with catecholamine secretion.

6. Which vascular anomalies may present as tumors of the middle ear?

A dehiscent jugular bulb or an aberrant internal carotid artery may appear as a tumor of the middle ear.

7. What other tumors affect the middle ear?

Cholesteatomas are the most common tumor growth in the middle ear and mastoid. Hemangiomas, squamous cell carcinomas, and rhabdomyosarcomas may also affect the middle ear.

8. Name three tumors that affect the jugular foramen.
1. Paragangliomas
2. Nerve sheath tumors
3. Sarcomas

9. What is jugular foramen syndrome?

Jugular foramen syndrome may be due to lymphadenopathy, tumors, or skull fractures that involve the jugular foramen. This syndrome is associated with paralysis of cranial nerves (CN) IX, X, and XI. CN XII is spared because it runs through the hypoglossal canal.

10. What lesions affect the petrous apex?

Inflammatory: cholesterol granuloma, cholesteatoma, mucocele

Infectious: petrous apicitis or osteomyelitis

Neoplastic: schwannoma, meningioma, glomus tumor, chordoma, chondrosarcoma, nasopharyngeal carcinoma, or metastases from distant malignancies

Variants of normal: asymmetric bone marrow or air cell pattern

Aneurysm: aneurysm of the intrapetrous carotid artery

11. What is a cholesterol granuloma?

A cholesterol granuloma is an infrequently encountered temporal bone inflammatory lesion associated with a giant cell reaction. It may also be associated with otitis media, trauma, possibly barotrauma, or prior cholesteatoma. A cholesterol granuloma may present with pain and dysfunction of CN VII or VIII.

12. Are epidermoid cysts ever malignant?

In the temporal bone, an epidermoid is an aggressive but benign lesion. It consists of stratified squamous epithelium and collagen and contains keratin debris and cholesterol crystals. This lesion may appear at the cerebellopontine angle or elsewhere intracranially. An epidermoid is slow-growing and avascular and has little inflammatory effect. Rather, the lesion's progressive compression on neural structures leads to associated signs and symptoms.

13. Describe the common contemporary operations used to control balance disorders.

Vestibular nerve section: very high efficacy, spares hearing, and can be done best through middle fossa or retrolabyrinthine approaches; considered highly selectively destructive.

Labyrinthectomy: high efficacy, always destroys hearing, less frequently performed currently; may be considered when intractable tinnitus is also an issue; considered a permanently destructive technique.

Endolymphatic shunt: controversial; less efficacy, can also relieve inner ear symptoms of aural pressure and tinnitus associated with Meniere's disease; considered nondestructive.

Chemical vestibular ablation: a recently popular, less demanding technique; in a variety of methods, various aminoglycoside antibiotics can be introduced to the round window; permanently destroys vestibular hair cells with some degree of selectivity while hopefully preserving cochlear hair cell function; considered destructive.

Repair of oval or round window fistulas: controversial, but should be considered especially when there is an antecedent history of ossicular surgery (especially stapes surgery), serious head trauma, or physical exertion; the predictive value of all preoperative and intraoperative testing for the existence of fistulas remains an enigma for neuro-otologists.

14. Describe the six anatomic segments of the facial nerve.

Intracranial: from brainstem to internal auditory canal

Meatal: from fundus of internal auditory canal to meatal foramen (narrowest aperture of facial nerve's bony canaliculus)

Labyrinthine (narrowest segment of the facial nerve): from meatal foramen to geniculate ganglion (which may be dehiscent). The nerve is surrounded by an extension of the subarachnoid space and cerebrospinal fluid. The geniculate ganglion is the "first genu" of the facial nerve, and here it gives off its first branch (superficial petrosal nerve).

Tympanic: after the geniculate ganglion, coursing adjacent to the oval window of the stapes, to the pyramidal eminence of the stapedius tendon ("second genu"); 15–30% of normal nerves may be dehiscent in this segment.

Mastoid ("vertical segment"): from second genu to stylomastoid foramen

Extratemporal: from stylomastoid foramen to innervated facial mimetic muscles

15. Before operating on a patient with a facial nerve paralysis, how do you determine the site of the lesion ?

Depending on the etiology of the paralysis, surgery is directed to the site of the lesion. For temporal bone or skull-base trauma, a high-resolution CT scan is obtained, and the site of the lesion is anatomically correlated. In transverse or longitudinal temporal bone fractures, a direct disruption may be identified with a CT scan. In longitudinal fractures of the temporal bone without direct facial nerve disruption, the most likely site of injury is the perigeniculate ganglion. For iatrogenic injury, the most common site is the tympanic segment; however, during mastoid surgery, the site may be the vertical segment. For Ramsay Hunt (herpes zoster oticus), or less frequently Bell's palsy, the site of the lesion is always the labyrinthine segment and meatal foramen.

16. How do you decide whether a paralyzed facial nerve should be explored for decompression or repair?

The **Hilger** facial nerve stimulator should be used for any paresis that is obvious. The threshold and maximum stimulation tests are performed and may easily be repeated on subsequent office visits. When there is no significant visible motion of the face or when the exact onset of the paralysis is unclear, a more precise method to quantify the residual activity of the paretic face should be employed, i.e., electroneuronography (ENOG). ENOG is an evoked electromyographic response of the facial muscles. This test can also be repeated periodically.

If and when the testing indicates progressive nerve weakness that is > 90%, the nerve is at high risk of incomplete recovery. Surgical intervention for facial nerve decompression (for severe Ramsay Hunt, Bell's palsy, or perigeniculate neural injury due to trauma) should be performed at the earliest convenience. For other discrete trauma to the nerve, the site of lesion should be clarified by imaging (unless iatrogenic, in which case the site should be suspect from the history). In situations with unclear etiology (including Bell's), the course of the nerve should be imaged with CT and/or MRI to clarify the diagnosis. Tumors or other temporal bone processes should be identified.

17. By which approaches are facial nerve injuries surgically treated?

Facial nerve decompression of the labyrinthine and meatal segments is best approached via the middle fossa technique. The transmastoid facial recess approach can be used to decompresss the tympanic segment, but this procedure also can be done via the middle fossa. In both cases, the incus must be removed and an ossiculoplasty performed to gain access of the tympanic segment. The mastoid segment is, of course, best visualized with a mastoidectomy. The parotid gland needs to be dissected for access to the extratemporal distal nerve pes and branches. Most proximally, the middle fossa approach, in which the dura is opened, can be used to gain access to the facial nerve as it exits the brainstem. Likewise, a retrolabyrinthine approach can show the brainstem exit of the facial nerve, but the exposure to the IAC is lacking. For traumatic facial nerve paralysis with total deafness, a translabyrinthine approach may be indicated.

18. How are traumatized facial nerve injuries repaired?

No matter where the site of the lesion, end-to-end anastomosis for lacerations is appropriate if there is no residual tension on the nerve stumps across the anastomosis. Nerves that are physically damaged or have missing portions may be repaired with an interposition graft. Such a graft is taken from the greater auricular or sural nerves. Hypoglossal-facial nerve anastomosis can give acceptable results when the proximal facial nerve stump cannot be identified.

19. What is congenital aural atresia?

Congenital aural atresia ("congenital ear deformity") is embryonic failure or anomalous development of the middle ear, tympanic membrane, and external auditory canal. It usually manifests with some degree of external cosmetic auricular malformations, ranging from microtia to anotia.

20. What middle ear otologic anomalies are associated with congenital aural atresia?

The facial nerve tympanic segment and the vertical segments are often aberrant in location. The motor facial nerve rarely may be congenitally absent (Moebius syndrome) in association with congenital ear deformity. The chorda tympani nerve may contain motor fibers of the facial nerve. The stapedial artery may be persistent. The ossicular deformities range from malformation or absence of the stapes superstructure or crura, to fibrous unions of the ossicular linkages, to fusion of the malleus and incus into a single ossicle. The lateral ossicular component is usually fused to a plate of bone or soft tissue ("the atretic plate") that is located where the tympanic membrane would normally develop.

21. What are the significant findings and considerations for successful otologic surgery for congenital aural atresia?

On audiometry there is usually a significant or maximal conductive component to the hearing loss, but there also may be a sensorineural component. CT scanning is used to decide whether the patient's anatomy is favorable or unfavorable for surgery. Favorable features include well-pneumatized mastoid with normal inner ear structures. Unilateral cases in children are usually operated only when the child is old enough to participate in the decision to undergo surgery. A facial plastic and reconstructive surgeon (or general plastic surgeon) who has successful experience with reconstruction of the pinna should be consulted to coordinate any staged procedures. Finally the family and patient must be committed to frequent (sometimes every 1 to 4 weeks) clinical followup for a period of months to a few years.

22. What are the features and landmarks for otologic surgery for congenital aural atresia?

With absence of the external auditory canal, the space for reconstruction is limited by: retroposition of the mandible condyle, inferiorly positioned tegmen, anteriorly positioned sigmoid sinus, and, most importantly, the facial nerve. The facial nerve may be located anywhere. With absent or poor development of the mastoid tip, the facial nerve is often superficial, making it the limiting landmark both inferiorly and posteriorly, but it can limit the dissection in any direction.

23. What are the potential risks and complications of congenital aural atresia otologic surgery?

Such operations are some of the most demanding for the otologic surgeon. Operative complications may include facial nerve paralysis; intraoperative monitoring is mandatory. Injury to the inner ear is possible as result of manipulation of the ossicles, and throughout the procedure an especially delicate touch is essential. When there is microtia or anotia, the design of the otologic approach incisions may be important to the successful auricular reconstruction of the pinna. Postoperative complications include infections and particularly stenosis of the newly-made external auditory canal. This latter point is the reason why careful followup is so important for success.

24. What is the technique for cochlear implant surgery?

The selection for candidates for cochlear implant surgery is addressed in another chapter. Briefly, a generous postauricular incision is made and a standard mastoidectomy is performed. The external cortex of the retromastoid cranial bone is carved to accommodate the implant components without violating the inner cortex of bone. A generous facial recess approach is used to visualize the middle ear through the mastoid cavity. The round window niche is drilled to reveal the membrane. A cochleostomy is drilled adjacent to the lateral aspect of the wound window membrane, so the electrode may be inserted into the scala tympani as fully as possible, and it is advantageous for intraoperative testing of the device. When preoperative CT scanning indicates membranous cochlear obliteration, the implant may be successful with even a partial insertion, but a complete "drill-out" of the cochlea at the promontory may be necessary in order to lay the device into the cochlea. The wound is closed.

25. What are risks of cochlear implant surgery?

Infection, tissue breakdown at the incision or flap, implant stimulation of the facial nerve, vertigo, and device failure are potential postoperative complications. Aural rehabilitation often requires more than 50 hours and is crucial for successful implant use.

26. Name the structures contained in the internal auditory canal.

If the IAC is divided into four cross-sectional quadrants, each quadrant contains one major structure:
    Anterior-superior quadrant: the facial nerve
    Anterior-inferior quadrant: the cochlear nerve
    Posterior-superior quadrant: the superior vestibular nerve
    Posterior-inferior quadrant: the inferior vestibular nerve

27. What is an acoustic neuroma?

Acoustic neuromas, or schwannomas, account for approximately 6% of all intracranial neoplasms. These lesions, arising in the IAC, are benign encapsulated tumors of the VIIIth nerve sheath of Schwann. They tend to arise on the vestibular nerve twice as often as on the auditory nerve. Seventy percent of acoustic neuromas grow slowly (i.e., over years), while 30% remain stable. Although most of these tumors grow slowly, over time they may erode bone of the internal auditory meatus. Acoustic neuromas occur in a female to male ratio of 3:2. Asymptomatic, clinically silent acoustic neuromas occur in approximately 2% of the population.

28. How do acoustic neuromas present?

The most common presenting symptoms include **tinnitus** and a progressive, unilateral, high-frequency **hearing loss**. Patients are often unable to localize the tinnitus to a specific ear. About

50% of patients complain of **disequilibrium**. Late manifestations develop as the tumor erodes into the internal canal and extends into the posterior cranial fossa. Facial nerve compression may lead to unilateral numbness and weakness. Cerebellar symptoms, such as dysarthria and ataxia, may arise eventually. Very late disease may cause trigeminal symptoms.

29. What is Hitselberger's sign?
Numbness of the posterior aspect of the concha. This area is innervated by sensory fibers of the facial nerve. Numbness suggests facial nerve compression due to a neoplasm such as an acoustic neuroma.

30. Most acoustic neuromas arise on the vestibular nerve. Why don't patients present with vertigo more often?
Rarely do patients with an acoustic neuroma present with sudden-onset rotatory vertigo. Because these tumors grow slowly, the vestibular system adapts to their presence. More commonly, patients complain of mild disequilibrium.

31. What do audiometric tests show in a patient with an acoustic neuroma?
Although 5% of patients with an acoustic neuroma will have a normal audiogram, most patients have characteristic audiometric abnormalities. These patients often exhibit a loss of discrimination that is disproportionate to the pure-tone results. Sixty-five percent of patients exhibit a high-frequency sensorineural hearing loss. Unilateral hearing loss is a suspicious finding. Any patient with a 20-dB asymmetry at one frequency or a 10-dB asymmetry at two or more frequencies should undergo further evaluation. In addition, almost 90% of patients have no stapedial reflex. Therefore, impedance audiometry should be done if a patient has a suspicious audiogram. Auditory brainstem response (ABR) is a valuable tool when evaluating patients for acoustic neuromas. ABR's sensitivity in this setting approaches 95%, and yields a false-positive rate of 10%. In the presence of an acoustic neuroma, wave V may be absent or prolonged.

32. What is the "gold standard" study for an acoustic neuroma?
Thin-section MRI with gadolinium enhancement can detect very small acoustic neuromas of only a few millimeters in size in the temporal bones. It is currently the best study but generally too expensive to use as a routine screening test.

33. Are acoustic neuromas associated with a genetic disease?
Although 95% of acoustic neuromas occur spontaneously without any genetic associations, 5% of patients have **neurofibromatosis** (NF), also known as **von Recklinghausen disease**. In contrast to the spontaneously occurring acoustic neuroma, NF-associated tumors are unencapsulated and may be multiple or bilateral. In addition, they are more aggressive and tend to invade surrounding axons. Rarely, such schwannomas in NF patients undergo malignant transformation.

34. What are the standard treatment options for a patient with an acoustic neuroma?
In general, acoustic neuromas are surgically excised. However, because these tumors are slow-growing, elderly patients or patients with serious medical problems may choose a more conservative approach, foregoing surgery and electing observation.

35. Describe the anatomy of the cerebellopontine angle (CPA).
The CPA is a potential space in the posterior fossa. *Anteriorly*, the CPA is bound by the temporal bone. *Posteriorly*, it is bound by the cerebellum. The cerebellar tonsil is located *inferior* to the CPA, and the pons and cerebellar peduncles are located *superior* to the CPA.
Cranial nerves also are anatomically associated with the CPA. *CN VII* and *VIII* travel superiorly and laterally through the CPA and into the IAC. *CN V* is located superior to the CPA. *CN IX, X,* and *XI* are located inferior to the CPA.

36. What is the differential diagnosis of tumors of the CPA?

Acoustic neuromas, or schwannomas, account for 80% of all angle lesions. Other lesions in this area (in decreasing order) include meningiomas, lipomas, epidermoids, cholesterol granulomas, cholesteatomas, arachnoid cysts, aneurysms, and metastatic malignant tumors.

37. Name four surgical approaches to the cerebellopontine angle.

The CPA and skull base can be approached with several surgical techniques:
1. Translabyrinthine
2. Retrolabyrinthine
3. Middle fossa
4. Suboccipital

38. What does a translabyrinthine approach involve?

The translabyrinthine approach is a common approach to the CPA used for angle lesions that are < 3 cm. The approach is initiated in the postauricular area. The surgeon performs a mastoidectomy and labyrinthectomy, sparing the facial nerve. This provides direct access to the IAC. Bone overlying the posterior fossa, middle fossa, and sigmoid sinus is removed, exposing the dura. The IAC is opened, and the dura over the posterior fossa is incised and tumor is removed. The dura is closed, and a fat graft taken from the abdomen is used to obliterate the space.

39. Outline the advantages and disadvantages of the translabyrinthine approach.

This approach is advantageous because it allows a direct approach to the IAC and preserves the VIIth nerve. The approach also requires minimal cerebellar retraction.

Advantages: familiar approach for neurotologists, allowing access to contents of entire IAC. Variations include the transotic and transcochlear approaches which extend exposure anteriorly.

Disadvantages: complete hearing loss. However, "hearing-sparing" translabyrinthine techniques may be attempted which, in some cases, may preserve hearing.

Exposure limits: sigmoid sinus, facial nerve, dura of middle fossa.

40. What is the retrolabyrinthine approach?

The retrolabyrinthine approach to the IAC is an extension of a mastoidectomy. With this approach, the labyrinth remains intact. The CPA medial to the porus of the IAC may be visualized, and here, the vestibular nerve may be sectioned. If a tumor is small and does not extend into the IAC, it may be removed. The dura between the sigmoid sinus and labyrinth is opened, and the necessary surgery is performed.

Advantages: familiar approach for most neurotologists.

Disadvantages: no access to lateral intracanalicular IAC. As such, the indications for this approach are somewhat narrower.

Exposure limits: otic capsule, sigmoid sinus (a variant which transsects the sigmoid sinus can expand the operative field significantly), dura and brain in middle fossa.

41. What does the middle fossa approach involve?

The middle fossa or transtemporal supralabyrinthine approach is used for small intracanalicular tumors which are < 1 cm in size. An incision is made in the scalp above the auricle. A temporal craniotomy is performed, and the temporal lobe is minimally retracted extradurally. The superior aspect of the temporal bone is drilled, preserving the labyrinth. The facial nerve is identified in its meatal and labyrinthine segments. The bony canal is opened and the tumor is removed. Lastly, the wound is closed.

Advantages: may preserve hearing; can identify the entire course of the facial nerve in the IAC, meatal, labyrinthine, geniculate, and tympanic segments. As such, this approach is ideal for facial nerve decompression or repair, or vestibular nerve section. Any dural incision is limited.

Disadvantages: less familiar approach for many neurotologists, and more technically exacting; tumors must be smaller.

Exposure limits: the cochlea and superior semicircular canal are major landmarks that may be blue-lined but which must be preserved; retraction of the middle fossa is less forgiving and must be done minimally.

42. Describe the suboccipital/retrosigmoid approach.

The suboccipital approach allows access to the CPA from a posterior approach and may be used for quite large tumors in the region (> 3 cm). A craniotomy behind the ear is made below the sigmoid sinus. The dura is opened, and the cerebellum is retracted. A large tumor is evident. The majority of the tumor is debulked to expose the posterior aspect of the temporal bone at the porus of the IAC. The posterior aspect of the temporal bone is drilled, preserving the contents of the IAC, and the posterior semicircular canal is the lateral limit of dissection to preserve the labyrinth. The tumor in the IAC is removed, preserving the facial nerve. Any remaining tumor medial and anterior to the IAC is removed as well. The wound is closed.

Advantages: may remove very large tumors with brainstem compression; may be used to attempt hearing preservation when appropriate.

Disadvantages: less familiar approach for many neurotologists, great exposure of brain.

Exposure limits: cerebellum and brainstem, blue-line of posterior semicircular canal (unless hearing cannot be preserved).

43. What are the potential postoperative sequelae of neuro-otologic skull-base surgery?

In general, the patient should know that surgery may result in sensorineural hearing loss, temporary (infrequently permanent) balance problems, temporary (infrequently permanent) facial nerve paralysis, CSF leak, and meningitis. Intracranial hemorrhage, air embolus, cerebellar ataxia, stroke, and death are very rare complications.

44. Of these complications, which are emergencies? How should they be handled?

Altered mental status (obtundation), asymmetric pupils, hemiplegia, seizures, or severe hypertension may be associated with postoperative emergencies. Intracranial hemorrhage, strokes, CSF leaks, meningitis, and pneumocephalus are emergencies. In the case of intracranial hemorrhage or stroke, the patient may require emergency return to the operating room to control hemorrhage. A CSF shunt may be necessary. Dressings should be removed and the wound opened to allow for decompression of the brainstem. The patient should be taken to the operating room to further control hemorrhage. If meningitis is suspected, a lumbar puncture should be obtained and sent for culture and sensitivities. Frank wound infections should be treated aggressively. Leaks that persist should be closed surgically. If an unstable patient has pneumocephalus, an emergency burr-hole may be necessary to remove air.

45. How is the integrity of salvageable cranial nerves maintained in neuro-otologic skull-base surgery?

Intraoperative cranial nerve monitoring and somatosensory monitoring have become essential tools and require specialized equipment. In any case with potential facial nerve exposure, the nerve may be monitored using EMG techniques. ABR or electrocochleography can monitor the cochlear nerve. Practically all of the remaining cranial nerves can be monitored with sophisticated techniques when appropriate.

CONTROVERSIES

46. Can an acoustic neuroma be cured with "radiosurgery"?

Stereotactic gamma-irradiation therapy ("gamma knife") or linear accelerator (LINAC) are recent treatment modalities used in selected patients. Considerable controversy exists around the efficacy of such radiosurgery. It is currently applied to tumors that are < 3 cm. In principle, a high dose of ionizing radiation is delivered to the target tissue, while the surrounding structures are spared. This technique claims a low rate of facial nerve damage and hearing loss. In the United States, long-term results are presently unknown.

47. Can glomus tumors be cured with radiosurgery or radiation therapy?

No. The only indication for radiation therapy for glomus tumors is in those patients with contraindications to surgery. Such contraindications may be associated a patient's poor medical health. If the extent of disease makes a surgical attempt at complete or near-total removal impossible, radiation therapy may also be recommended. Radiation may slow or halt the growth of the tumor, but this is controversial. In addition, radiation therapy is not without risks.

48. Is there a role for chemotherapy in the treatment of the benign tumors of the skull base or CPA?

No.

49. What are the controversies surrounding otologic reconstructive surgery for congenital aural atresia?

The candidates for surgery are often children who may have mentally adjusted to a congenital imperfection such as unilateral atresia. It is sometimes debated whether such children should have elective surgery that entails the potential for serious risks. Furthermore, it is uncommon to achieve perfect closure of the hearing air-bone gap. More often the hearing results, while improved, are not spectacular. Delayed postoperative stenosis of the ear canal may occur and necessitate reoperation of the canal to maintian patency.

50. What is the biggest controversy surrounding cochlear implant surgery?

Surprisingly, members of the deaf community are often against the use of cochlear implant surgery, particularly in children. Many members of this community feel that these devices are experimental and unproven, and threaten to diminish the population of the deaf community by giving an otherwise deaf person the ability to hear. History and experience have proved to most unbiased observers that cochlear implant surgery generally has significant potential benefits and may enrich the quality of life and increase the standard of living in selected patients.

BIBLIOGRAPHY

1. Bailey BJ (ed): Head and Neck Surgery–Otolaryngology. Philadelphia, J.B. Lippincott, 1993.
2. Lee KJ (ed): Essential Otolaryngology–Head and Neck Surgery. Norwalk, CT, Appleton & Lange, 1995.
3. Jackler RK, Brackmann DE (eds): Neurotology. St. Louis, Mosby, 1994.
4. Fisch U, Mattox D: Microsurgery of the Skull Base. Stuttgart, Thieme, 1988.

III. The Nose and Sinuses

16. ANATOMY AND PHYSIOLOGY OF THE NOSE

Bruce W. Jafek, M.D.

1. Developmentally, which structures form the external nose?

The mesenchymal frontonasal process grows downward in the midline, above the roof of the stomodeum, to merge with the maxillary processes. The maxillary processes originate from the dorsal ends of the first visceral (mandibular) arch and the lateral nasal processes. The olfactory placode, an ectodermal thickening, invaginates as a pit between the medial portion of the frontonasal process and the lateral nasal process. The frontonasal process then continues to elongate, forming the median nasal process and fetal philtrum. The lateral nasal processes form the lateral portion of the adult nose (e.g., lower lateral cartilage and lobule). The olfactory placode finally comes to rest high in the nose as the anlage of the olfactory epithelium.

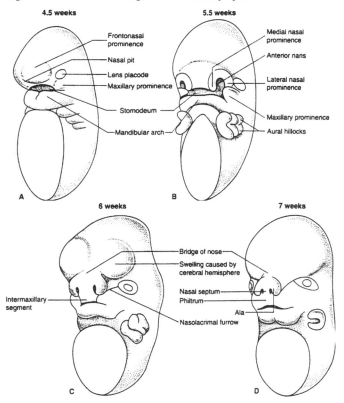

Nasal embryology. Development of the face. (From Fitzgerald MJT, Fitzgerald M: Human Embryology. London, Bailliere Tindall, 1994, pp 169–170, with permission.)

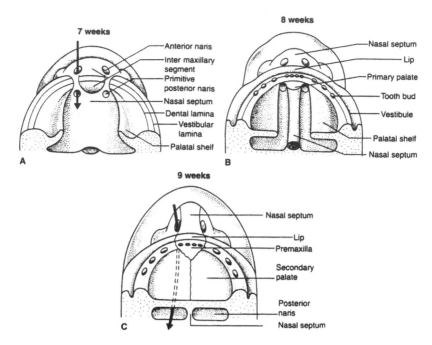

Nasal embryology. Head region, viewed from below, showing development of the palate. In (A) and (C), an arrow is passing along the nasal passage on one side. (From Fitzgerald MJT, Fitzgerald M: Human Embryology. London, Bailliere Tindall, 1994, pp 169–170, with permission.)

2. How does the internal nose form?

As the apices of the maxillary processes fuse with the median nasal process around the invaginating olfactory placode, primitive anterior nares form. This invagination leads posteriorly into an anterior (superior) nasal cavity. Posteriorly and inferiorly, a posterior nasal cavity (communicating with the anterior cavity superiorly) forms as the inner aspects of the maxillary processes. This gives rise to the palatine processes, which fuse in the midline to form the palate. Anteriorly, this fusion is completed, as these processes fuse with the premaxilla from the median nasal process and then "zip" posteriorly. Arrest of this process may cause a cleft soft palate, submucous cleft palate, or bifid uvula. The septum, a divider between the two nasal cavities, is thought to arise because of the dual origin of the olfactory placodes. This division produces side-by-side nasal pits. In the midline, the mesenchyme grows downward from the roof of the nose, dividing the nasal cavity in half. The primitive openings of the nasal cavity, the posterior choanae, are initially closed by the bucconasal membrane. This plug of epithelial cells usually ruptures at the end of the fourth embryonic week. Failure to rupture, unilaterally or bilaterally, leads to choanal atresia.

3. Describe the nasal bones and cartilages.

Several bones and cartilages give the external nose its characteristic pyramidal shape. The **nasal bones** articulate with the nasal processes of the frontal bone superiorly and the nasal processes of the maxilla laterally. The nasal bones are attached inferiorly to the upper lateral cartilages, which then attach inferiorly to the lower lateral cartilages. Medially, the lateral cartilages attach to the **cartilaginous septum**. Small rudimentary cartilages known as **sesamoid cartilages** or **alar cartilages**, give additional support to the lateral **nasal ala**, where the lower lateral cartilage extends to meet the cheek. The fibrofatty tissue of the lower lateral cartilage which contains the sesamoid cartilages is known as the **lobule**.

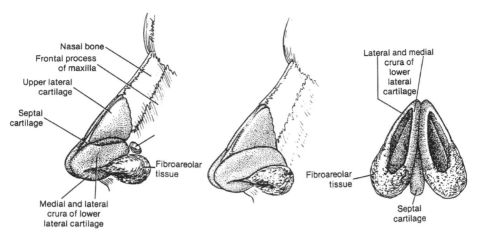

Nasal cartilages. (From Cummings CW, et al (eds): Otolaryngology–Head and Neck Surgery. St. Louis, Mosby, 1986, p 514, with permission.)

4. The internal nose has five areas that are susceptible to nasal airflow obstruction. What are these five areas?

The internal nose, as described by Maurice Cottle, has five areas in which narrowing may lead to airflow obstruction. Each area of obstruction is corrected differently.

1. **Anterior nare**, or nostril. This structure may be constricted congenitally or traumatically. For example, burns may constrict the anterior nare.

2. **Nasal valve**. This is the area of greatest constriction throughout the entire respiratory tract. This structure is limited medially by the septum, inferiorly by the floor of the nose, and by the junction between the cephalic lower lateral cartilage and caudal upper lateral cartilage. Further weakness, as might occur with injudicious resection of the lateral nasal cartilages in this area (e.g., unsuccessful rhinoplasty), produces collapse of the nose on inspiration and maximal "obstruction."

3 and 4. Upper and lower halves of the internal **nasal vestibule**. Either may be obstructed by nasal septal deviation.

5. Posterior passage of the nose, or **posterior choanae**

5. Which arteries provide the vascular supply to the nose?

The nose and sinuses are supplied by branches of the external and internal carotid arteries. The posterior inferior part of the internal nose is supplied by the external carotid artery and terminal branches of the internal maxillary artery (e.g., the sphenopalatine and greater palatine arteries). The anterior inferior nasal cavity is supplied by branches of the facial artery. The superior part of the nasal cavity is supplied by branches of the ophthalmic artery from the internal carotid artery. These branches include the anterior and posterior ethmoid arteries. Vascular distributions are important in the evaluation and treatment of nosebleeds.

6. Where do these vessels drain?

Nasal venous drainage nomenclature corresponds to arterial nomenclature. For example, drainage occurs through the sphenopalatine, ophthalmic, and anterior facial veins.

7. What is the "danger triangle?"

The danger triangle, also known as the danger area, is a triangle from the "nasion" (where the nose joins the forehead superiorly) to the lateral corners of the mouth, where the venous supply of the nose drains intracranially. From the angular vein, blood drains into the inferior ophthalmic vein and then into the cavernous sinus. This vascular supply provides cutaneous nasal infections (e.g., streptococci) with a potential route to spread intracranially.

8. Discuss the various nasal functions.

In addition to smelling and breathing, the nose warms, humidifies, and cleanses the inspired air. The temperature of the inspired air increases to nearly body temperature by the time it reaches the pharynx. Similarly, the humidity increases to 100%, regardless of the ambient humidity. Upon expiration, the nose removes water from the expired air, thus maintaining hydration, and removes heat, thus preventing hypothermia. Larger particulate matter in inspired air is removed anteriorly by the vibrissae. Progressively smaller particles are removed inside the nasal vestibule by direct impaction or electrostatic attraction with the nasal mucous blanket. The cilia move the mucus posteriorly, like a conveyor belt, causing the mucous blanket with inlaid particulate matter to empty into the stomach.

9. How is the nose innervated?

The muscles of the nose are innervated by the facial (seventh cranial) nerve. The external skin is innervated by the first and second branches of the trigeminal (fifth cranial) nerve. The trigeminal also supplies general sensory innervation (touch) to the internal nose and general chemosensation (e.g., irritation from acrid odors). Olfactory (first cranial) fibers are located in the superior portion of the internal nose and serve to smell. The sympathetic innervation originates from the hypothalamus, passes through the thoracolumbar region of the spinal cord, and synapses in the superior cervical ganglion in the neck. Postganglionic fibers then extend through the sphenopalatine ganglion to reach the nose. Additional fibers that run along blood vessels also extend from the carotid plexus to the nose. The parasympathetic supply originates in the facial nucleus of the brain, is relayed to the sphenopalatine ganglion, and finally reaches the nose via the posterior nasal nerve. The posterior nasal nerve also carries most of the postganglionic sympathetics.

10. What is the nasal reflex?

Clinical observations suggest the existence of poorly characterized reflex pathways between the upper and lower respiratory passages. Strong stimuli produce profound and widespread cardiopulmonary responses, including breathing cessation and bradycardia. Such responses may be the basis for some characteristics of sleep apnea syndrome. Milder stimuli may produce expulsion of the noxious stimulus with sneezing. A finger under the nose may actually abort a sneeze by blocking the nasal reflex!

11. What is the electro-olfactogram?

Recorded by an electrode placed on the olfactory epithelium, an electro-olfactogram (EOG) is a slow, negative, purely monophasic potential in response to odorants. Analogous to an electroretinogram of the eye, an EOG is thought to represent a "generator potential" from the olfactory epithelium.

12. Where do the lymphatics of the nose and paranasal sinuses form and drain?

The lymphatics of the nose and paranasal sinuses arise from the superficial portion of the mucous membrane and travel posteriorly to the retropharyngeal lymph nodes. Anteriorly, the lymphatics drain into the submandibular lymph nodes or the upper deep cervical nodes.

13. Describe the epithelial lining of the nose.

The respiratory tract, with the exception of the pharynx, is generally lined by specialized respiratory epithelium (pseudostratified, columnar, ciliated epithelium with interspersed goblet cells). The same epithelium lines the paranasal sinuses and eustachian tubes, but here the epithelium is somewhat flattened. In contrast, the nares are lined with stratified squamous epithelium, and the superior aspect of the internal nose is lined with olfactory epithelium. Beneath this surface epithelium on the lateral aspect of the nose are both racemose and tubular glands that provide serous and mucous secretions for the surface mucous blanket. Deeper yet, there is a specialized vascular plexus, consisting of arterioles, capillaries, vascular sinusoids, venous plexuses, and venules. This plexus forms erectile tissue, most prominently over the inferior turbinates, adjacent septum, and posterior middle turbinates, that assists the nose in its physiologic function.

14. How do the cilia function?

In mammals, cilia beat 10–20 times per second at room temperature. This beat has a characteristic biphasic motion, with a rapid "effective stroke" and a slower "recovery stroke." During the effective stroke, the extended cilium reaches a superficial, viscous mucous layer. During the recovery stroke, the cilium bends to travel in the other direction through the thinner periciliary layer. Thus, the mucous layer is conveyed in the direction of the effective stroke.

15. What is Kartagener's syndrome?

Kartagener's syndrome, or immotile cilia syndrome, is due to absence of the dynein arm on the peripheral ciliary microtubules. The cilia are unable to beat effectively. This syndrome produces a characteristic triad of chronic rhinosinusitis, bronchiectasis, and situs inversus. Clinically, nasal examination shows mucous or mucous accumulation.

16. What factors inhibit normal ciliary activity?

Normally, cilia beat 10–20 times/second. Drying (possibly produced by localized deflections or turbulence within the nasal cavity), drugs (e.g., cocaine, adrenaline), excessive heat or cold, hypertonic or hypotonic solutions, smoking (nicotine), infections (viral or bacterial), and noxious fumes (e.g., sulfur dioxide, carbon monoxide) all inhibit the normal ciliary beat.

17. What is the mucous blanket?

The goblet cells and submucosal glands of the nose produce mucus that forms a continuous blanket throughout the nose and sinuses. This blanket is composed of a superficial, thick, "mucous" layer and a deep, thin, "periciliary" layer. It collects dust, bacteria, viruses, and pollens. Ciliary action then carries the blanket to the pharynx, where it is swallowed into the stomach and digested. About 1–1.5 pints of mucus are produced each day. Lysozyme, an important enzyme of the mucus, initiates bacterial destruction. Both ciliary and lysozyme activity are optimal at pH 7.0. Anything that interferes with pH (e.g., medication, infection) interferes with nasal function.

18. Describe the function of the nasal submucosal vascular plexus.

Many of the mechanisms controlling the nasal vasculature remain incompletely understood. It is clear, however, that the blood vessel system resembles that of the erectile tissue of the genitalia. It is therefore possible to vary the flow of blood through the nasal mucosal surfaces independent of the variations in submucosal vascular engorgement. This deeper vasculature is under the control of the autonomic nervous system, but the precise receptor-reflex arcs have not yet been fully identified. Stimulation of sympathetic nerves causes noradrenaline release and vasoconstriction, while parasympathetic stimulation releases acetylcholine, resulting in vasodilatation and a watery nasal discharge. Mild mechanical or chemical stimulation of the internal nose produces sneezing, while stronger stimulation may result in apnea or bradycardia. Variations in nasal airflow are measured by rhinomanometry.

19. What is rhinomanometry?

Rhinomanometry is a measure of transnasal pressure and resultant airflow. Initially measured with water columns and mechanical devices, this pressure is now measured with electronic techniques and computers. Widely used in research, it has not yet achieved the clinical status of audiometric or vestibular function assessment.

20. Clinically, how is mucociliary flow measured?

Mucous transport can be measured clinically with the **indigo carmine/saccharin sodium test**. The test can be performed easily, without need for sophisticated equipment. A drop of indigo carmine (8 mg/ml) and a drop of saccharin sodium (3 mg/ml) are placed in the anterior nasal cavity, at the bottom of the inferior nasal meatus on the mucosa just behind the internal ostium. After 3 minutes, the patient is instructed to swallow every 30 seconds and to report any perception of sweet taste. The posterior pharynx is also inspected at these intervals for the presence of the blue dye. In general, the lag between the perception of a sweet taste and the appearance of the blue dye in the pharynx may be minimal or it may be several minutes. The lag, or mucous transport time (MTT), is normally 12–15 minutes. This normal MTT tends to correlate with a ciliary beat frequency of 10/second and a transit time of 6 mm/minute. A MTT of > 30 minutes is considered significantly abnormal.

Ciliary beat frequency can also be measured with a photoelectric-registration device, as well as by other methods. The MTT may also be measured by radioactive particle transit observed by gamma camera or multicollimator detectors. These latter methods, however, require sophisticated equipment and are not generally available.

21. What is the nasal cycle?

The nasal cycle was first described by Kayser in 1895 and has been studied with a variety of techniques, most notably by rhinomanometry. The total resistance to nasal airflow remains relatively constant because of the reciprocal relationship between the resistance of each nasal passage. It is observed in up to 80% of normal subjects, most of whom are unaware of the alteration in airflow since the total resistance remains constant. The alternating cycles of congestion and decongestion on each side of the nose are thought to be under the control of the autonomic innervation of the nose, possibly primarily the adrenergic innervation, through action on the specialized vascular plexus described previously. It is also observed in children and animals.

22. Name the standard x-ray views of the nose and sinuses.

Previously four standard views were used.

1. The **Waters view** tips the occiput down so that the maxillary and frontal sinuses are well seen.

2. The **Caldwell view**, or posteroanterior view, offers a superior view of the frontal and ethmoid sinuses.

3. The **lateral view** provides superior visualization of the sphenoid sinus and posterior frontal sinus wall.

4. The **submentovertex view** provides a superior view of the sphenoid sinuses.

Because of the difficulty in visualizing the sinuses through the overlying bone, the most frequently used study is the **limited CT of the ethmoid sinuses**. In this study, 3–5-mm cuts, without contrast, are obtained of the ethmoid sinuses in the coronal view. This technique allows visualization of all sinuses, especially the osteomeatal complex.

CONTROVERSIES

23. What is the function of the organ of Jacobson?

The vomeronasal organ (VNO), or organ of Jacobson, is an accessory concentration of olfactory tissue. In animals, the VMO primarily functions in mating behavior. Thought to be vestigial in humans, its existence in the adult has been described recently. Located in a 1–3-mm tubule with an oval orifice, this structure is approximately 1 cm posterior from the caudal septum and 2–4 mm off the floor of the nose. Its pale yellowish mucosa distinguishes it from the surrounding pinkish respiratory mucosa. An electrovomerogram has recently been recorded from the vomeronasal region in response to specific odorants. Whether the VMO has a similar function in human mating is a subject of ongoing research, but as yet the function of this organ in humans remains unknown.

24. How do you measure nasal obstruction?

Rhinometry, a measurement of nasal airflow, would seemingly be an inverse measurement of obstruction. However, airflow measurements correlate poorly with the patient's perception of "obstruction." Therefore, a useful measurement of nasal obstruction is not easily obtained.

BIBLIOGRAPHY

1. Duchateau GSMJE, Graamaans K, Zuidema J, et al: Correlation between nasal ciliary beat frequency and mucus transport rate in volunteers. Laryngoscope 95:854–859, 1985.
2. Messerklinger W: Endoscopy of the Nose. Baltimore, Urban & Schwarzenberg, 1978.
3. Proctor DF, Andersen I (eds): The Nose: Upper Airway Physiology and the Atmospheric Environment. Amsterdam, Elsevier, 1982.
4. Rice DH, Schaefer SD: Endoscopic Paranasal Sinus Surgery. New York, Raven Press, 1988.

17. NASAL SEPTAL ABNORMALITIES

Abilio Muñoz, M.D., and Michael Leo Lepore, M.D.

1. Describe the anatomy of the nasal septum.

The nasal septum is made up anteriorly by the nasal septal cartilage (quadrangular septal cartilage), posteriorly by the vomer and the perpendicular plate of the ethmoid, and anteroinferiorly by the maxillary crest.

2. What is the most common deformity of the nasal septum resulting from trauma?

Caudal deformity involving the anterior cartilaginous septum. Usually, the cartilage is displaced off the maxillary crest, lying either in the left or right nasal cavity, depending of the direction of the force. The caudal septum (anterior-most part of the cartilaginous septum) projects into the nasal cavity, causing obstructive symptoms.

3. Which complications commonly result from trauma to the nasal septum?

Epistaxis, hematomas, and dislocations of the quadrangular septal cartilage are the most common complications. Nose bleeds usually involve the anterior septum at Kiesselbach's plexus (or Little's area). Hematomas result from disruption of the vascular supply within the perichondrial layer with subsequent bleeding into the soft tissue. This will appear as a fluctuant swelling of the septum covered by reddish-purple mucosa. Hematomas are uncommon in children, but when they occur spontaneously, a blood dyscrasia needs to be excluded. Dislocations of the cartilage cause nasal obstruction.

4. What characteristic deformity results from untreated septal hematomas?

Septal hematomas that are not surgically drained may become infected, leading to destruction of the cartilage. This destruction of cartilage causes a loss of nasal support with a resultant cosmetic deformity termed a **saddle-nose deformity**.

5. List the causes of a septal perforation.

Perforations of the anterior nasal septum may be caused by trauma, digital manipulation (nose-picking), and surgery (submucous resection). Chrome workers are susceptible to a septal perichondritis causing a perforation. Posterior perforations involving the vomer and perpendicular plate of the ethmoid bone may be the result of gumma formation secondary to tertiary syphilis.

6. What is the significance of granulation tissue attached to the nasal septum?

Granulation tissue is a response to nasal infections and a history of foreign body. The granulation tissue must be biopsied to rule out sarcoidosis, tuberculosis, malignant lethal midline granuloma (Wegener's disease), and neoplasms.

7. How is nasal biopsy used in detecting Wegener's granulomatosis?

Wegener's granulomatosis is a potentially lethal systemic disease that affects the upper respiratory tract, including the nasal mucosa and the kidneys. It is characterized histologically by granulomatous inflammation, focal necrosis, fibrinoid degeneration, and multinucleated giant cells. Nasal mucosal biopsy is a fairly innocuous method for obtaining histologic proof of Wegener's disease. It is essential to differentiate this disease from other nasal processes, such as infections, connective tissue disorders, Goodpasture's syndrome, and hypersensitive vasculitis. Biopsy specimens > 5 mm in diameter from ulcerated areas are recommended for better yield.

8. What are inverted papillomas?

Inverted nasal papilloma is a histologically benign but clinically malignant neoplasm. It primarily affects the lateral wall, with the most common site of occurrence in the area of the ethmoid sinus and the opening of the maxillary antrum. Occasionally, a biopsy of the nasal septum will reveal this entity. A nasal papilloma is usually unilateral and causes nasal obstruction. Physical exam reveals a fleshy papillary exophytic growth in either one or both nasal passages. Treatment involves complete resection since inverted nasal papilloma is associated with a 13% transformation into squamous cell carcinoma.

9. Describe the effects of cocaine inhalation on the septum.

Chronic cocaine inhalation can result in symptoms of nasal stuffiness, anosmia, rhinorrhea, sinusitis, and bleeding. In addition, its use results in crusting and nasal septum perforation. Furthermore, chronic obstruction might lead to abuse of internasal sprays, which further exacerbate the problem and contribute to the formation of a septal perforation. Vasoconstriction from cocaine leads to inflammation, infection, chondritis, and nasal septal perforations with chronic rhinitis.

10. How should you treat nasal septal defects?

Conservative treatment for mild symptoms includes saline irrigation, emollients (mineral oil), and ointments such as bacitracin. Some physicians recommend "nasal rest" by occluding the nasal airflow with an ointment-impregnated cotton for several hours a day. Surgical repair is usually considered in symptomatic patients who fail to respond to conservative care. Perforations > 2 cm in diameter are seldomly closed successfully, and repair is contraindicated in perforations caused by cocaine abuse, infection, neoplasm, granulomatous disease, or vascular diseases.

11. How does nasal septal deviation affect nasal physiology?

Nasal septal obstruction is the most common symptom of septal deviation. Where mucosa is closely approximated, dryness occurs secondary to a **Bernoulli effect** of airflow, causing mucus formation and impairing ciliary mobility. This, in time, may lead to inflammatory disease, termed **bacterial rhinitis**. Also, septal deviation may impair the normal flow of sinus secretions, producing symptoms and signs of sinusitis (infection, purulent drainage, pain, tenderness, fever).

12. Which organism is most commonly found in bacterial rhinitis? How is it treated?

Alterations of airflow cause an inflammatory response with associated mucosal drying, crusting with retained secretions, and bacterial rhinitis, which further aggravates the inflammatory response. Frequently, *Staphylococcus aureus* is found on nasal cultures. Treatment consists of the following:
• Saline douches—mix 1 cup of water with 1/2 tsp of salt and a pinch of baking soda
• Saline nasal sprays
• Topical applications of mupirocin (Bactroban) ointment twice daily for 1 week and once daily at bedtime for 2 weeks.

13. Describe the presentation and treatment of primary squamous cell carcinoma arising from the nasal septum.

These tumors are extremely rare. The usual presentation is nasal obstruction, bleeding, and crusting of the nasal septum. The clinical picture often depends on the direction of extension. Local and distant metastases are very rare, and the treatment of choice is wide surgical excision with postoperative radiation.

14. What are the otolaryngologic manifestations and diagnostic criteria for polychondritis?

Polychondritis is probably of autoimmune origin and is characterized by inflammation of cartilage with its consequent destruction. It is often associated with Hashimoto's thyroiditis, Sjögren's syndrome, scleroderma, and collagen III antibodies. Otolaryngologic manifestations are common, with 70–80% of cases exhibiting septal involvement, commonly presenting as rhinitis and epistaxis with progression to saddle-nose deformities. For diagnosis, patients must meet 3 out of 6 criteria:

1. Bilateral, recurrent ear chondritis
2. Noneroding polyarthritis
3. Nasal chondritis
4. Ocular inflammation
5. Laryngotracheal chondritis
6. Cochlear or vestibular lesions

15. Postoperative nasal adhesions can be seen following septal and/or turbinate surgery. How often do nasal adhesions occur, and how are they managed?

Studies cite an incidence of up to 14% following nasal surgery. Turbinate resection is associated with one of the highest complication rates for adhesions (up to 36%). Adhesions may lead to nasal obstruction requiring a second surgery, and up to 80% of patients who develop postoperative adhesions may require this second operation. A study by White and Murray in 1987 found that up to 49% of patients with postoperative adhesions require general anesthetic for correction, while 33% required local. Although nasal splints are recommended to prevent postoperative adhesions, their efficacy is questioned.

CONTROVERSIES

16. Intranasal splints have been recommended for prevention of postoperative nasal adhesions. What is their efficacy? Are they associated with comorbidity?

Although intranasal splints have been advocated (Gilchrist, 1974) as a preventive measure for postoperative nasal adhesion formation, recent studies have found that splints do not decrease the rate of adhesion formation. Many patients find them very uncomfortable and significantly painful. In addition, intranasal splints may contribute to septal perforations. Adequate nasal toilet has been proposed as an alternative strategy to reduce nasal adhesion formation.

17. Does surgery on the nasal septum affect midfacial growth in children?

This subject has been argued among otolaryngologists for quite some time. Some surgeons are conservative in their approach, only operating on children after their last growth spurt. Although controversial, recent literature suggests the following: "Although septal cartilage appears to be a factor in midfacial growth in the human fetus, it does not appear to be a factor in midfacial growth postnatally." Therefore, septoplasty and rhinoplasty in childhood failed to demonstrate any significant effect in retarding midfacial growth by anthropometric studies.

BIBLIOGRAPHY

1. Blaugrund SM: The nasal septum and concha bullosa. Otolaryngol Clin North Am 22:291–305, 1989.
2. Cook JA, Murrant NJ, Evans KL, Lavelle RT: Intranasal splints and their effects on internasal adhesions and septal stability. Clin Otolaryngol 17:24–27, 1992.
3. Del Buono EA, Flint A: Diagnostic usefulness of nasal biopsy in Wegener's granulomatosis. Hum Pathol 22:107–110, 1991.
4. Granados R, Constantine NM, Cibas ES: Nasal scrape cytology in the diagnosis of Wegener's granulomatosis. A case report. Acta Cytol 38:463–466, 1994.
5. Kpemissi E, Mathias A, Napo-Koura G, et al: Polychondrited chronique atrophiante: A propos d'une observation. Ann Oto-Laryngol Chir Cervicofac 111:411–414, 1994.

6. Kurloff DB: Nasal septal perforations and nasal obstruction. Otolaryngol Clin North Am 22:333–349, 1989.
7. Leeman DJ, Shuler K, Han K, Mirani N: Anaplastic transformation of primary squamous cell carcinoma arising from nasal septum [abstract]. In American Academy of Otolaryngology Meeting Abstracts, 1994.
8. Ortiz-Monasterio F, Olmedo A: Corrective rhinoplasty before puberty: A long-term follow-up. Plast Reconstr Surg 68: 381–390, 1981.
9. Stankiewicz JA, Girgist SJ: Endoscopic surgical treatment of nasal and paranasal sinus inverted papilloma. Otolaryngol Head Neck Surg 109:988–995, 1993.
10. White A, Murray JA: Intranasal adhesion formation surgery for chronic nasal obstruction. Clin Otolarynogol 13:139–143, 1988.

18. RHINITIS

Bruce Murrow, M.D., Ph.D.

1. Define rhinitis.
Rhinitis is nasal hyperfunction and tissue inflammation which leads to nasal congestion, rhinorrhea, nasal obstruction, pruritus, and sneezing. Although rhinitis is generally not life-threatening, it often leads to general annoyance and a decreased quality of life, prompting many to seek medical care.

2. How is rhinitis categorized?
Although very difficult to categorize, rhinitis can be divided into **allergic** and **nonallergic** types. Allergic rhinitis can be further subcategorized into **seasonal** and **perennial** types. Accurate classification and subsequent therapy require a careful history, physical exam, and appropriate laboratory studies.

3. What is the pathophysiology that underlies rhinitis?
Nasal congestion arises from engorgement of blood vessels due to the effects of vasoactive mediators and neural stimuli. Rhinorrhea is due to hypersecretion of the nasal glands, leading to tissue transudate. The autonomic nervous system mediates both vascular tone and secretions. Sympathetic innervation constricts the vessels, decreasing secretions, while the parasympathetic innervation vasodilates the vessels, enhancing nasal secretions. Pruritus occurs in association with histamine release from mast cells and basophils secondary to antigenic stimulation.

4. What are the most common causes of rhinitis?
Allergy is the most common cause of chronic rhinitis, while **infection** is the most common cause of acute rhinitis.

5. Allergic rhinitis is most often mediated by what Gell and Coombs' type of hypersensitivity?
Type I. Antigen binds to IgE on mast and basophilic cells, causing release of mediators (i.e., histamine) that produce the symptomatic response of allergy.

6. Which types of antigens cause allergic rhinitis?
In general, inhalants, foods, and chemicals cause allergic rhinitis. **Inhalants** usually produce an immediate response upon exposure and include pollens, animal dander, mold spores, and dust. Food allergies can be more difficult to diagnose. A **fixed food allergy** causes symptoms each time the food is ingested, while a **cyclic food allergy** is based on the amount and frequency of the allergen consumed.

7. **What are the etiologies of nonallergic rhinitis?**

Causes of Nonallergic Rhinitis

Pharmacologic (rhinitis medicamentosa)
Hormonal
Irritative
Atrophic
Structural
Infectious
Substance abuse (cocaine, alcohol, nicotine)
Emotions
Temperature
Exercise
Recumbency
Trauma
Foreign bodies
Decreased nasal airflow states (post-laryngectomy or tracheostomy)
Systemic diseases (Wegener's granulomatosis, sarcoid, superior vena cava syndrome, and Horner's syndrome)
Idiopathic (vasomotor rhinitis, eosinophilic or basophilic nonallergic rhinitis)

8. **Can laboratory tests aid in the diagnosis of rhinitis?**

Nasal smears and cytologic examination indicate the presence or absence of eosinophils or neutrophils. Large numbers of eosinophils suggest allergy or nonallergic rhinitis, whereas large numbers of neutrophils suggest infection. Blood work for serum IgE, total eosinophils, thyroid hormone, estrogen levels, and drug levels can point to the appropriate cause of rhinitis. Skin testing has become a mainstay for the diagnosis of allergic rhinitis.

9. **Describe the endocrine or hormonal causes of nonallergic rhinitis.**

Pregnancy, menstruation, and oral contraceptive use can all cause nasal congestion. The increased estrogen levels associated with these states inhibit acetylcholinesterase, leading to increased parasympathetic tone and tissue edema. Hypothyroidism is also associated with rhinitis. In this state, parasympathetic activity predominates over the hypoactive sympathetic state, causing vasodilation of the nasal mucosa.

10. **How does the effect of irritants in nonallergic rhinitis differ from an allergic response?**

Dust, gases (formaldehyde), chemicals, and air pollution (smoke, sulfur dioxide) can cause nasal congestion and rhinorrhea via direct irritative effects on the mucosa. In contrast, an allergic response is due to interaction with IgE antibodies and histamine-releasing cells.

11. **Name some common structural abnormalities that can cause rhinitis.**

Deviated nasal septums
Nasal valve collapse
Neoplasms (e.g., papilloma, angiofibroma, malignancy)
Polyps
Intranasal and extranasal deformities

12. **What is atrophic rhinitis?**

Atrophic rhinitis, or **ozena**, is associated with atrophy of the nasal mucosa and turbinates in association with excessive crusting and mucopurulent discharge. This socially debilitating condition is marked by an extremely foul odor which can be easily detected by others. Patients often complain of epistaxis, nasal obstruction, headaches, and the foul smell. Although the etiology is unknown, hereditary, infectious, developmental, nutritional, and endocrine factors have been implicated. Atrophic rhinitis may also be iatrogenic, as it may be associated with excessive turbinate resection. Although no cure exists, treatment revolves around frequent saline irrigation and topical antibiotics. Surgical options are aimed at narrowing the cavity and nostril.

13. What is vasomotor rhinitis?

Vasomotor rhinitis is idiopathic nasal congestion and rhinorrhea that is not associated with sneezing or pruritus. After other causes of the rhinitis are ruled out, it becomes a diagnosis of exclusion. In this disorder, autonomic imbalance with parasympathetic predominance causes vasodilation and hyperresponsive glands.

14. Describe the treatment of allergic rhinitis.

Treatment includes avoidance of the stimulus, pharmacologic agents, and immunotherapy. **Avoidance** of the offending antigen is most applicable with food allergies and chemical allergies. **Pharmacotherapy** includes antihistamines (to block the effects of histamine release), topical or systemic sympathomimetics (which decongest the nasal tissue), cromolyn sodium (to stabilize mast cell membranes), and topical or systemic corticosteroids (to reduce inflammation). **Immunotherapy** involves injecting the offending antigen into the patient. This therapy decreases the serum levels of IgE, increases IgG antibody ("blocking antibody"), decreases sensitivity of histamine-releasing cells, and decreases responsiveness of lymphocytes. However, the specific mechanism behind the relief of immunotherapy is unknown.

15. Describe the medical treatment of nonallergic rhinitis.

In general, treatment should be directed toward the specific etiology of the rhinitis (e.g., removal of the offending agent, correction of the hormonal problem, treatment of infection). Symptomatic treatment includes the use of antihistamines, sympathomimetic agents (topical or systemic), anticholinergics, and steroids.

16. How do antihistamines aid in the treatment of chronic rhinitis?

Antihistamines act by blocking H1 receptor sites, thereby interfering with basophil and mast cell histamine release. While the first-generation antihistamines are associated with drowsiness, the newer antihistamines are nonsedating.

17. How do sympathomimetics aid in the treatment of chronic rhinitis?

Sympathomimetics are decongestants that can be orally (e.g., ephedrine, pseudoephedrine, phenylpropanolamine) or topically (e.g., oxymetazoline, phenylephrine) administered. Side effects of oral decongestants include nervousness, insomnia, irritability, and difficulty urinating. They should be avoided in patients with hypertension, cardiac arrhythmias, or glaucoma. While topical decongestants are potent, their duration of use must be limited secondary to rebound decongestion.

18. What is rhinitis medicamentosa?

Rhinitis medicamentosa is drug-induced rhinitis that is due to rebound nasal congestion. It is most often associated with prolonged use of topical decongestants. It is thought that a semi-ischemic state is induced by the strong vasoconstrictive effect of topical decongestants. With time, this effect leads to the metabolic accumulation of vasodilators that are responsible for the rebound vasodilation. The condition can become irreversible with the development of vascular atony.

19. How long should topical decongestants be continuously used for symptomatic relief of rhinitis?

Because of the risk of rhinitis medicamentosa, topical decongestants should not be used for more than 3–5 days.

20. How is rhinitis medicamentosa treated?

Topical decongestants should be completely discontinued. Systemic decongestants and nasal saline spray can be substituted for symptomatic relief. The etiology of the nasal congestion should be specifically treated (i.e., allergy, structural problem, infection).

21. What is the role of ipratropium bromide in the treatment of rhinitis?

Ipratropium bromide is a topical anticholinergic agent that antagonizes the effect of acetylcholine at parasympathetically innervated submucosal glands. It is effective in reducing mucosal gland hypersecretion that causes rhinorrhea. Systemic side effects are limited because of poor absorption topically. Unlike topical vasoconstrictors, ipratropium bromide does not exhibit rebound on withdrawal.

22. How do steroids aid in treating chronic rhinitis?

Corticosteroids can be given topically or orally, but oral agents are limited by suppression of the hypothalamic-pituitary-adrenal axis. Topical steroids decrease local inflammation caused by vasoactive mediators, decrease rhinorrhea by reducing the reactivity of acetylcholine receptors, decrease basophil and eosinophil counts, and decrease sneezing by desensitizing irritant receptors. Allergic and nonallergic rhinitis (including vasomotor rhinitis, hypothyroid-related rhinitis, and polyposis) are effectively treated with topical corticosteroids. Short duration systemic steroids are useful as initial decongestants in cases of severe obstruction or polyposis.

23. What are the side effects of corticosteroids when they are used to treat rhinitis?

Systemic corticosteroids can suppress the hypothalamic-pituitary-adrenal axis. The newer topical steroids, in general, are thought to be free of this problem at their recommended dosages. However, nasal steroids can cause mucosal edema, mild erythema, burning, drying, and epistaxis.

24. If chronic rhinitis is refractory to the usual medical modalities, what disorders should be further considered in the differential diagnosis?

Uncommon chronic conditions are likely to be referred to an otolaryngologist. Chronic infectious processes, such as tuberculosis, syphilis, and fungal rhinosinusitis, may lead to granulomas, ulceration, masses, or necrosis. In these cases, it is important to rule out neoplasia histologically. Tissue should also be stained and cultured for mycobacteria and fungi.

CONTROVERSIES

25. What is the role of corticosteroid turbinate injections in the treatment of rhinitis?

Injection of the inferior turbinate with a small-size particle corticosteroid, such as triamcinolone (Kenalog), provides relief from chronic hypertrophy of the turbinates that is refractory to medical treatment. Opponents argue that turbinate injection, if intravascular, can lead to embolization/vasospasm of the orbital vessels and possible blindness. In addition, some patients do not experience long-term relief.

26. Is surgical management indicated for rhinitis?

Though controversial, surgical options exist for the management of rhinitis. Most surgical procedures are directed toward mechanical-obstructive issues. The options may decrease nasal congestion and improve the penetration of topically applied medication. Surgeries include septoplasty for the repair of deviated septums, polypectomies, out-fracture of the inferior turbinates, and total or partial inferior turbinectomies. The inferior turbinates may also be treated with electrical/chemical cautery or cryosurgery. Cryosurgery of the inferior turbinates with vidian nerve sectioning has also provided relief from the secretory aspect of vasomotor rhinitis.

27. Should an inferior turbinectomy be utilized for treatment of rhinitis?

Some advocate a **total inferior turbinectomy**, as this procedure may provide relief of nasal congestion. Others argue that the relief is often not permanent. In addition, normal humidification and warming of inspired air is compromised. Postoperative bleeding can be problematic. This group argues that most patients have extensive nasal crusting which is debilitating, and atrophic rhinitis can ensue. However, there are reports of minimal crusting complications and no atrophic rhinitis following **partial inferior turbinectomies** (anterior aspect).

28. What role does vidian neurectomy play in rhinitis?
The vidian nerve carries sympathetic and parasympathetic supply to the nasal mucosa. In medically refractory cases of vasomotor rhinitis, sectioning of this nerve can relieve hypersecretion in > 90% of cases. Others argue that serious risks of this procedure include ophthalmoplegia, decreased lacrimation, and paresthesias.

BIBLIOGRAPHY

1. Bailey BJ (ed): Head and Neck Surgery–Otolaryngology. Philadelphia, J.B. Lippincott, 1993.
2. Borts MR, Druce HM: The use of intranasal anticholinergic agents in the treatment of nonallergic perennial rhinitis. J Allergy Clin Immunol 90:1065–1070, 1992.
3. Cummings CW, et al (eds): Otolaryngology–Head and Neck Surgery, 2nd ed (vol 4). St. Louis, Mosby, 1993.
4. Hogan MB, Grammer LC, Patterson R: Rhinitis. Ann Allergy 72:293–302, 1994.
5. Jones NS: The place of surgery in the management of rhinosinusitis. Clin Exp Allergy 24:888–892, 1994.
6. Malm L: Pharmacological background to decongesting and anti-inflammatory treatment of rhinitis and sinusitis. Acta Otolaryngol (Stockh) 515:53–56, 19xx.
7. Paparella MM, Shumrick DA, Gluckman JL, Meyerhoff WL (eds): Otolaryngology, 3rd ed (vol 3). Philadelphia, W.B. Saunders, 1991.

19. SINUS ANATOMY AND FUNCTION
Kent E. Gardner, M.D.

1. Name the paranasal sinuses and describe their location.
There are four pairs of paranasal sinuses: the frontal, maxillary, ethmoid, and sphenoid sinuses.

1. The **frontal sinus** is located in the vertical portion of the frontal bone. It is pyramidal in shape with its base formed by the floor of the sinus. The apex of the sinus projects superiorly.

2. The **maxillary sinus** occupies the body of the maxilla. It is bound medially by the lateral nasal wall, superiorly by the orbital floor, anteriorly by the canine fossa, and inferiorly by the alveolar process of the maxilla.

3. The **ethmoid sinuses** are located in the superior half of the lateral nasal wall. They are bound superiorly by the skull base in the region of the cribriform plate and laterally by the lamina papyracea (medial wall of the orbit).

4. The **sphenoid sinus** lies in the body of the sphenoid bone. It is surrounded posteriorly, superiorly, and laterally by important structures. These important structures include the pons, pituitary gland, carotid artery, optic nerve, and cavernous sinus. Anteroinferiorly, the sinus wall is exposed to the choanae and nasal cavity.

2. What are the uncinate process, hiatus semilunaris, and ethmoid infundibulum?
The **uncinate process** is a small thin piece of bone, covered by mucoperiosteum, that runs parallel and medial to the lateral nasal wall in the anterior middle meatus. Anteriorly and inferiorly, the bone is attached to the lateral nasal wall. The posterosuperior margin ends freely without attachment to other structures. This posterior margin is concave in shape and runs parallel to the anterior surface of the ethmoid bulla. The two-dimensional trough formed by the gap between the

ethmoid bulla and uncinate is known as the **hiatus semilunaris**. The hiatus semilunaris is the opening to the three-dimensional space bound medially by the uncinate process and laterally by the lateral nasal wall. This three-dimensional space is known as the **ethmoid infundibulum**. The frontal, anterior ethmoid, and maxillary sinuses all usually drain into the infundibulum and then out through the hiatus semilunaris.

3. What is the osteomeatal complex?

The osteomeatal complex is a term used to describe the region of the uncinate process, maxillary ostium, middle turbinate, bulla ethmoidalis, and ethmoid infundibulum. It is important because the frontal, ethmoid, and maxillary sinuses all drain through this area, which contains very narrow clefts. Any mucosal thickening or congenital variation is likely to produce obstruction, stasis, and recurrent infection of the "upstream" sinuses. Functional endoscopic sinus surgery (FESS) is based on the concept that the osteomeatal complex, also known as the osteomeatal unit, must be cleaned to restore and enhance normal sinus drainage.

4. Where do each of the sinuses drain into the nasal cavity?

Each paranasal sinus communicates with the nasal cavity through an opening known as an ostium. The ostium of the frontal sinus opens into the frontal recess in the anterior portion of the middle meatus. It may drain directly into the ethmoid infundibulum lateral to the uncinate process, or medial to the uncinate if the uncinate process inserts into the lamina papyracea. The ostium of the maxillary sinus is located in the ethmoid infundibulum of the middle meatus. The ostia of the ethmoid sinuses are inconsistent in location. Anterior ethmoid cells generally drain into the ethmoid infundibulum or in the region of the ethmoid bulla. Posterior ethmoid cells drain into the superior meatus. The ostium of the sphenoid sinus opens into the sphenoethmoidal recess above the superior concha.

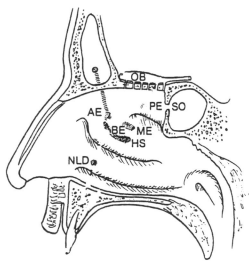

Sagittal section of the head illustrating position of ostia of paranasal sinuses. *OB*, olfactory bulb; *SO*, sphenoid ostium; *PE*, posterior ethmoidal ostium; *ME*, middle ethmoidal ostium; *BE*, ethmoidal bulla; *HS*, hiatus semilunaris; *AE*, anterior ethmoidal ostium; *NLD*, nasolacrimal duct (From Cummings CW, et al (eds): Otolaryngology–Head and Neck Surgery. St. Louis, Mosby, 1986, p 902, with permission.)

5. Describe the development of the maxillary sinuses.

The maxillary sinus is the first to develop in the human fetus. Initial pneumatization is seen during the 65–70th day of fetal life. At birth, this sinus is 4–7 mm in diameter. Further growth of the maxillary sinus is biphasic. The first growth spurt occurs from birth until 3 years of age. At the end of this growth spurt, the floor of the sinus lies approximately 4–5 mm above the nasal floor. The second spurt occurs from 7 years of age until adolescence. By adolescence, the sinus lies 3–4 mm below the level of the nasal floor. Later in adult life, the sinus floor may be 5 –10 mm below the nasal floor, and the roots of the second maxillary premolar and first and second maxillary molars may break through into the sinus cavity. The average volume of the adult maxillary sinus is 14.75 ml.

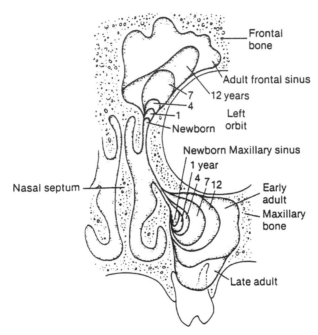

Developmental stages of maxillary frontal sinuses. (From Cummings CW, et al (eds): Otolaryngology–Head and Neck Surgery. St. Louis, Mosby, 1986, p 902, with permission).

6. Describe the development of the frontal sinuses.

Frontal sinus development begins during the fourth month of fetal life. Initially, it is only an upward extension in the region of the frontal recess. At birth, it is not clinically significant and cannot be distinguished from the anterior ethmoid cells. At about 2–4 years of age, the sinus begins to invade the vertical portion of the frontal bone. At 6 years of age, it is visible radiographically. At 12 years, the sinus is quite large. During the teens, the sinus becomes fully developed with a volume of 6–7 ml. Frontal sinus development is extremely variable, and approximately 5% of the population has at least one undeveloped frontal sinus.

7. Describe the development of the ethmoid sinuses.

Ethmoid sinus development begins during the third or fourth month of fetal development. Ethmoid cells are classified into anterior and posterior divisions based on the cells' location relative to the ground lamella of the middle turbinate. Anterior ethmoid cells develop from the lateral nasal wall in the region of the middle meatus. Posterior ethmoid cells begin as evaginations of the lateral nasal wall in the region of the superior meatus. At birth, there are usually 3 or 4 cells present. The ethmoid and maxillary sinuses are the only sinuses at birth which are large enough to be of clinical significance. Through childhood, the sinuses continue to grow, until age 12 when they reach adult size. An average adult ethmoid sinus has 10–15 cells with a total volume of 15 ml.

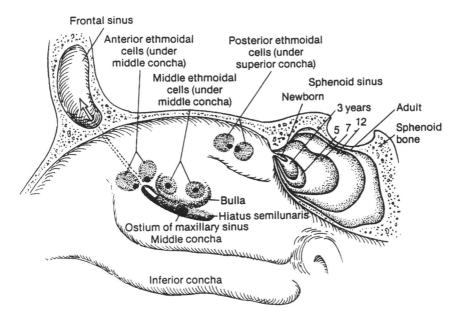

Developmental stages of the ethmiod and sphenoid sinuses. (From Cummings CW, et al (eds): Otolaryngology–Head and Neck Surgery. St. Louis, Mosby, 1986, p 904, with permission).

8. How does the sphenoid sinus develop?

Sphenoid sinus development begins in the fourth month of fetal development as an evagination of the nasal mucosa in the posterior nasal cavity. At birth, there is no clinically significant sphenoid sinus. Significant further development begins after the fifth year of life. By age 7, the sinus has extended posteriorly to the sella turcica. Its final volume of 7.5 ml is usually attained by 12–15 years of life.

9. Which arteries supply each of the paranasal sinuses?

The frontal sinus is supplied by the supraorbital and supratrochlear arteries. The maxillary sinus is supplied predominantly by branches of the maxillary artery, with some contribution from the facial artery. The ethmoid sinus receives contributions from the sphenopalatine artery and anterior and posterior ethmoid arteries. The sphenoid sinus receives input predominantly from the sphenopalatine and posterior ethmoid arteries.

10. Describe the course of the sphenopalatine artery.

The sphenopalatine artery is a branch of the internal maxillary artery. It enters the nasal cavity through the sphenopalatine foramen just posterior to the middle turbinate in the sphenoethmoidal recess. It then divides into two main branches. The first branch passes across the inferior aspect of the face of the sphenoid sinus to supply the septum. It can cause significant hemorrhage if violated during sphenoidotomy. The second branch supplies the lateral wall of the nose.

11. Where are the anterior and posterior ethmoid arteries located?

These arteries are branches off the ophthalmic artery in the orbital cavity. They leave the orbital cavity through the anterior and posterior ethmoid foramina. These foramina occur on the medial wall of the orbit at or just superior to the frontoethmoid suture line. The anterior ethmoid foramen is usually located 14–22 mm posterior to the maxillolacrimal suture line. The location of the posterior ethmoid foramen is more variable, but it is usually 3–13 mm posterior to the anterior ethmoid foramen. The anterior and posterior arteries lie at the level of the ethmoid sinus roof and are helpful landmarks during external ethmoidectomy.

12. What is the innervation of each of the paranasal sinuses?

The paranasal sinuses are predominantly innervated by the sensory branches of the trigeminal nerve. Sensory innervation of the frontal sinus mucosa is via the supraorbital and supratrochlear nerves. Sensory innervation of the maxillary sinus is via multiple branches of the maxillary nerve, including the greater palatine, posterolateral nasal, and superior alveolar branches of the infraorbital nerve. Postganglionic parasympathetic secretomotor fibers from the pterygopalatine ganglion also supply the mucosa of the maxillary sinus. The ethmoid sinuses receive innervation from both the ophthalmic and maxillary divisions of the trigeminal nerve. The anterior cells are supplied by the anterior ethmoid nerve. The posterior cells are supplied by the posterior ethmoid nerve and sphenopalatine nerve. The sphenoid sinus is supplied by the posterior ethmoid nerve and sphenopalatine nerve.

13. What is the functional significance of the sinuses?

The clinical significance of the sinuses can be appreciated by anyone who has had an acute or chronic sinus infection. Multiple theories exist about the possible functional significance of the sinuses, including humidification and warming of inspired air, lightening the weight of the skull, improving vocal resonance, absorption of shock to the face or skull, increasing the area of the olfactory membrane, regulation of intranasal pressure, and secretion of mucus to keep the nasal chambers moist. However, all of these theories have flaws. The real functional significance of the sinuses is unknown.

14. What type of cells form the lining of the paranasal sinuses?

The paranasal sinuses are lined with ciliated, pseudostratified, columnar epithelial cells. Also, numerous mucoserous glands and goblet cells produce the **mucous blanket** which lines the sinuses. This lining consists of two layers. The first layer is the inner serous layer, or **sol phase**, in which the cilia beat. The second layer is a more viscous layer, or **gel phase**. The gel phase is transported by the beat of the cilia toward the sinus ostia.

15. Discuss the pattern of mucous clearance or secretion from the maxillary sinus.

In the maxillary sinus, secretion transport starts from the floor of the sinus in a stellate pattern. The mucus is transported along the anterior, medial, posterior, and lateral walls of the sinuses as well as along the roof. All of the secretions converge at the natural ostium of the maxillary sinus. After secretions leave the sinus ostium, they flow out the middle meatus over the medial aspect of the posterior inferior turbinate and into the nasopharynx.

16. How is the mucus cleared or secreted from the frontal sinus?

The frontal sinus has a flow of secretions both into and out of the sinus. Inward flow begins on the medial aspect of the sinus ostium. This flow continues superiorly and then laterally along the roof of the frontal sinus. Next, secretions are transported back toward the ostium along the floor of the sinus as well as along the inferior aspect of the anterior and posterior sinus walls. Secretions then flow out the nasofrontal duct and into the ethmoid infundibulum. These secretions then merge with the secretions of the maxillary sinuses and are transported out through the nasopharynx.

17. What factors can lead to inadequate drainage of sinus secretions?

Normal clearance of sinus secretions requires normal secretion and transport mechanisms. The secretion mechanism involves the amount and consistency of the mucus produced. A normal transport mechanism requires normal mucosal cilia, normal ciliary beat, and a patent sinus ostia or drainage opening. Factors that influence the secretion and transport mechanisms include environmental pollution, humidity, other airborne external irritants, parasympathetic nerve fibers, and neuromediators.

18. Where do you find agger nasi cells? What is their significance?

Agger nasi cells are the most anterior of the anterior ethmoid cells. These cells are located at the agger ridge, just anterior to the anterosuperior attachment of the middle turbinate. They are in close proximity to the frontal recess. The agger nasi cells are often opened during endoscopic sinus surgery to get a better view of the nasofrontal duct. They also can occasionally obstruct outflow from the frontal sinus.

19. What are Haller cells?

Haller cells are ethmoid cells that have extended into the maxillary sinus and are adherent to the roof of the maxillary sinus in the region of the maxillary sinus ostium. Haller cells occur in 10% of the population. They can be asymptomatic or can have a negative influence on maxillary sinus ventilation and drainage, leading to recurrent or chronic sinusitis.

20. What is an Onodi cell? What structure can lie within an Onodi cell?

Onodi cells are posterior ethmoid cells that extend posteriorly, either laterally or superiorly, along the sphenoid sinus. Because of their location, the optic nerve can lie within an Onodi cell. These cells should be recognized prior to endoscopic sinus surgery to avoid injury to the optic nerve on posterior dissection of the ethmoids.

21. What is the clinical significance of a concha bullosa?

The term concha bullosa refers to the pneumatization of the middle turbinate. Approximately 30% of the population have concha bullosa, and in most circumstances, these are asymptomatic. If the drainage system of the concha bullosa itself becomes obstructed, it can become symptomatic and require surgical drainage. Also, the concha bullosa is associated with enlargement of the middle turbinate. This enlarged turbinate is felt to have a negative effect on paranasal sinus ventilation and mucociliary clearance in the osteomeatal complex. To relieve the obstruction, either one wall of the concha or the entire concha bullosa must be removed surgically.

22. Where is the grand (basal) lamella?

The grand lamella is the bony insertion of the middle turbinate into the skull base and lateral nasal wall. This landmark is used to differentiate anterior from posterior ethmoid cells. The grand lamella can be divided into thirds. The anterior third inserts directly into the lamina cribosa. The middle third inserts into the lamina papyracea and runs in an oblique anterosuperior to postcroinferior course. The posterior third inserts into the lateral nasal wall and runs in a horizontal direction.

23. What is the relationship of the face of the sphenoid sinus to the nasal sill?

The face of the sphenoid sinus lies 7 cm from the nasal sill at a 30° angle with the floor of the nasal cavity.

CONTROVERSIES

24. What is an accessory ostium? Is it an effective drain of the maxillary sinus?

In addition to the natural maxillary sinus ostium, one or more accessory sinus ostia can be located in the lateral nasal wall. There is some controversy as to whether these accessory ostia are effective drainage sites for sinus secretions. Accessory ostia may be quite large. However, studies have shown that the mucous blanket tends to bypass the accessory ostium and leave through the natural ostium. This is thought to occur secondary to the natural beat of all cilia in the maxillary sinus toward the natural ostium. For the same reason, nasoantral windows which are surgically placed in the inferior meatus tend to be less effective at improving sinus drainage than nasoantral windows made at the natural ostium.

25. Is the correct term "osteomeatal" or "ostiomeatal"?

Actually, either spelling is correct. Some use *osteo-*, referring to the bone. Others argue that *ostio-* is the proper prefix, referring to the ostium, or meatal opening.

BIBLIOGRAPHY

1. Anand FK, Panje WR: Practical Endoscopic Sinus Surgery. New York, McGraw-Hill, 1993.
2. Becker SP: Anatomy for endoscopic sinus surgery. Otolaryngol Clin North Am 22:677, 1989.
3. Becker SP: Applied anatomy of the paranasal sinuses with emphasis on endoscopic sinus surgery. Ann Otol Rhinol Laryngol 103:3, 1994.
4. Bolger WE, Butzin CA, Parson DS: Paranasal sinus bony anatomic variations and mucosal abnormalities: CT analysis for endoscopic sinus surgery. Laryngoscope 101:56, 1991.
5. Graney DO, Rice DH: Paranasal sinuses: Anatomy. In Cummings CW (ed): Otolaryngology—Head and Neck Surgery, 2nd ed. St. Louis, Mosby, 1993.
6. May M: The location of the maxillary os and its importance to the endoscopic sinus surgeon. Laryngoscope 100:1037, 1990.
7. Stammberger H: Functional Endoscopic Sinus Surgery. Philadelphia, Mosby, 1991.
8. Wolf G, Anderhuber W, Kuhn F: Development of the paranasal sinuses in children: Implications for paranasal sinus surgery. Ann Otol Rhinol Laryngol 120:705, 1993.

20. SINUSITIS

Tyler M. Lewark, M.D.

1. Define sinusitis.

In general terms, sinusitis is inflammation of the paranasal sinuses, the etiology of which includes both infectious agents and allergic mechanisms.

2. What are the major categories of sinusitis?

Sinusitis may be categorized in many ways, but the most common description is by duration of symptoms. Acute, subacute, and chronic sinusitis refers to symptoms lasting < 4 weeks, 4 weeks to 3 months, and > 3 months, respectively.

3. What pathogenic mechanisms are important in sinusitis?

Three major factors contribute to the development of sinusitis:

1. Patency of the sinus ostia is perhaps the most important factor. Obstruction of any sinus ostia may occur. Although this obstruction is most often due to mucosal edema, an anatomic abnormality interfering with drainage may be present. Bacterial growth is favored due to the resulting stagnation of secretions, lowered oxygen tension, and decreased pH.

2. Failure of the normal mucous transport mechanism of the paranasal sinus mucosa supports further bacterial colonization. Ciliary beat frequency, normally 700/minute, decreases to < 300 beats/minute. This slowing is usually in response to a virus, bacterium, or allergen. The transport mechanism is impaired by hypersecretion of mucus and inflammatory mediators released in response to one of these offending agents.

3. Finally, a change in the quality of sinus secretions occurs. Inspissated mucus cannot be cleared from the sinuses and becomes a culture medium for bacterial growth and a source of inflammation.

4. What are the predisposing factors of acute sinusitis?

The most common cause of acute **bacterial** sinusitis is recurrent viral upper respiratory tract infections (URI). Approximately 0.5% cases of viral URI are complicated by bacterial sinusitis.

Other predisposing factors include allergy, foreign body, dental procedures, and barotrauma. Iatrogenic factors have become increasingly important due to mechanical ventilation, nasogastric tubes, nasotracheal tubes, and nasal packing. Less common causes of sinusitis include trauma and mucosal edema associated with pregnancy. Factors predisposing to **fungal** sinusitis usually are related to immune deficiency. These opportunistic infections may be life-threatening.

5. What are the predisposing factors of chronic sinusitis?

Factors predisposing to chronic bacterial sinusitis include allergic rhinitis, nasal polyposis, anatomical disorders (e.g. nasal septal deviation), immunodeficiency disease, cystic fibrosis, and primary ciliary dysfunction such as seen in Kartagener's and Young's syndromes.

6. How do allergies predispose a patient to sinusitis?

No data confirm a direct causal relationship between allergies and sinusitis. However, it is rarely disputed that allergies predispose a patient to sinus disease. Hypersecretion caused by upper respiratory tract allergies is likely the causative factor. Studies implicating this mechanism have demonstrated hyperemia and increased metabolic activity of the paranasal sinuses after exposure to ragweed pollen.

7. How does the clinician recognize allergy-related sinusitis?

A complete history is vital when evaluating the sinusitis patient. The typical patient with allergy-associated sinusitis reports a history of inhalant allergies. Infectious sinusitis may develop in acute, subacute, or chronic forms. The patient may have known allergies, or this may be the first allergic presentation. The patient with full-blown sinusitis may be difficult to evaluate for allergic etiology, because purulent secretions and congestion often overshadow the symptoms that are characteristic of allergic rhinitis. In this case, evaluation of potential inciting allergens is conducted after appropriate treatment and resolution of symptoms.

8. What organisms are responsible for acute bacterial sinusitis?

Studies have shown that 70% of community-acquired acute sinusitis in adults is caused by *Streptococcus pneumoniae* and *Haemophilus influenzae*. In recent years, the prevalence of ß-lactamase-producing strains of these organisms has increased, with reports as high as 52% for *H. influenzae*. Usually associated with dental infections, anaerobic organisms including *Fusobacterium, Peptostreptococcus*, and *Bacteroides* account for about 6–10% of cases. In children, the pathogens responsible for acute bacterial sinusitis are similar to those in adults. *S. pneumoniae* and *H. influenzae* are responsible for the majority of cases, although *Moraxella catarrhalis* has been implicated in approximately 20% of acute sinusitis in children. Both *H. influenzae* and *M. catarrhalis* may be ß-lactamase producing.

9. Are these same organisms responsible for chronic bacterial sinusitis?

No. Anaerobic organisms have a significant role in the pathogenesis of chronic sinusitis in adults, mostly *Bacteroides* and anaerobic cocci. Aerobes may also play a role, with *Streptococcus* species and *Staphylococcus aureus* representing the majority. Although widely differing reports of the prevalence of anaerobes (*Bacteroides, Fusobacterium*, and anaerobic cocci) have been reported, it seems that in children with long-standing symptoms, both anaerobic and *Staphylococcus* species should be suspected.

10. What organisms are responsible for fungal sinusitis?

Fungi are normal commensals of the upper airway, but they can occasionally lead to the development of sinusitis. *Aspergillus* species are the most common cause of both noninvasive and invasive (seen in immunocompromised patients) fungal sinusitis. Other organisms implicated in noninvasive cases include *Pseudallescheria boydii, Schizophyllum commune*, and *Alternaria* species.

11. Describe the symptoms of acute bacterial sinusitis.

In the early phase of the illness, the symptoms of acute sinusitis may be difficult to distinguish from those of the common cold or allergic rhinitis. Certain symptoms, including headache or pain and elevation of temperature and pulse rate, are common to sinusitis affecting any of the sinuses. The location of facial pain will vary and is related to the sinus involved. Depending on the patency status of the ostium, purulent nasal discharge may or may not be present. Less frequent symptoms include postnasal drip with cough, vague headache, halitosis, and anosmia.

In children, symptoms may be less specific than in adults. Children are less likely to complain of facial pain or headache. Persistent nasal congestion and cough (> 7 days), high fever, purulent nasal discharge, and especially mild periorbital edema probably represent sinusitis.

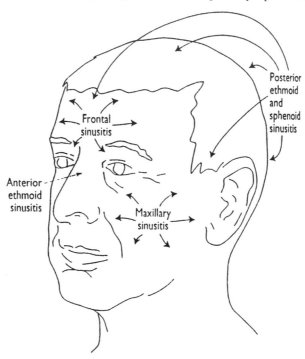

Sites of referred pain from the sinuses. (From Evans KL: Diagnosis and management of sinusitis. BMJ 309:1416, 1994, with permission.)

12. How do the symptoms of chronic bacterial sinusitis differ?

In adults, the symptoms of chronic sinusitis are similar to those for acute sinusitis. However, nasal congestion and purulent nasal discharge are prolonged. Chronic sinusitis in children is usually manifest as purulent rhinorrhea that may be associated with postnasal drip, cough, and wheezing. Many children also have an associated chronic or recurrent otitis media.

13. What are the signs of acute bacterial sinusitis?

Tenderness to palpation may be present over the affected sinus. In sinusitis secondary to dental infection, the offending tooth is usually tender to percussion. On examination of the nose, the mucous membranes are red and edematous. If an associated acute rhinitis is present, the nose will be congested and reveal little information as to the affected sinus. If one or more of the anterior sinuses (frontal, maxillary, or anterior ethmoid) are affected, the middle turbinate may be red and swollen, and the uncinate process may be prominent. The middle meatus may be closed or have pus emanating from it. If one of the posterior sinuses (posterior ethmoid and sphenoid) is affected, the abnormal appearance of the mucous membrane will be confined to the upper posterior portion of the nose. Pus may be seen above the posterior end of the middle turbinate or descending from the sphenoethmoid recess.

14. Discuss the differential diagnosis of sinusitis.
- The association of **rhinitis** with sinusitis is complex. Many patients with a dripping nose assume they have sinusitis when they actually have simple rhinitis. Rhinitis may cause sinusitis by blocking the sinus ostium.
- The symptoms of **dental disease** may mimic those of sinusitis due to the proximity of the apical dentition to the sinuses.
- Pain which is associated with **migraine** and **intracranial causes** can usually be distinguished on clinical grounds. In the elderly, atypical pain which is localized to the face or head may be due to **temporal arteritis**.
- Symptoms that are associated with **stress** or **tension**, such as "eye strain," may be clinically indistinguishable from mild pain due to chronic sinusitis.

15. When diagnosing a patient as having "sinusitis," do you risk missing the diagnosis of sinonasal malignancy?
Compared with sinusitis, malignancy in the paranasal sinuses is very rare. It is seldom picked up at an early stage, and symptoms and signs relate to expansion of the sinus wall or local extension. Local symptoms include epistaxis, proptosis, trismus, fullness of the cheek or palate, cranial nerve palsy, facial numbness, and loosening of the upper teeth. Nodal metastases are rare and usually indicate a poor prognosis.

16. Can any maneuvers aid the clinician in diagnosing sinusitis?
- **Transillumination** of the frontal and maxillary sinuses involves placing a light on the palate and observing the amount of transmitted light through the sinuses. This technique has been mostly abandoned due to concern about its clinical significance.
- **Nasal culture** is not recommended due to frequent contamination by nonoffending organisms.
- **Nasal endoscopy** affords the thorough evaluation of nasal anatomy with visualization of the accessible components of the osteomeatal complex and is easily performed in the clinic setting with topical anesthetics.
- **Maxillary sinus aspiration** (for microscopy, culture, and antimicrobial sensitivities) is suggested for immunocompromised patients and cases refractory to medical therapy.

17. Are plain film radiographs helpful in evaluating sinusitis?
Traditionally, obtaining plain films of the sinuses has facilitated evaluation of the patient with suspected sinusitis. These films provide a noninvasive evaluation of the sinuses and the lower one-third of the nasal cavity. However, the anterior ethmoid sinuses and osteomeatal complex are poorly visualized. Studies have also shown that a significant number of patients with radiographic abnormalities do not have sinusitis. Plain films are diagnostically useful with certain findings. Air-fluid levels and sinus opacification are highly suggestive of sinus involvement, and a clear radiograph makes sinus pathology unlikely.

18. You are evaluating a patient with symptoms suggestive of acute sinusitis. Your attending asks you if sinus x-rays are indicated. How do you respond? When indicated, what radiologic views should be ordered?
Sinus x-rays are most likely not indicated when evaluating the patient with uncomplicated acute sinusitis. The findings of air-fluid levels and sinus opacification rarely lead to a change in management. When indicated, the most commonly obtained films include the occipitomental (Waters), occipitofrontal (Caldwell), and lateral views.

19. What is the best imaging technique for evaluating sinus disease?

Computed tomography (CT). Thin coronal sections effectively allow visualization of the osteomeatal complex and ethmoid sinuses. Contrast injection is not necessary when evaluating sinusitis but may be valuable if malignancy is suspected.

20. When is obtaining a CT indicated in the evaluation of sinusitis?

In the evaluation of chronic refractory sinusitis, complications of sinusitis, and suspected malignancy. In addition, it is helpful for the evaluation of anatomy prior to endoscopic or conventional sinus surgery.

21. Compare the advantages and disadvantages of magnetic resonance imaging for evaluating sinusitis.

Advantages: MRI is emerging as a valuable tool for evaluating certain disease processes of the paranasal sinuses. MRI has superior soft-tissue resolution compared with CT and can better distinguish fungal sinusitis, sinus neoplasia, and intracranial extension of sinus disease. MRI avoids the use of ionizing radiation, which is particularly important for children.

Limitations: The ethmoid sinus mucosa and nasal cavity have a natural cycle of mucosal edema followed by mucosal shrinkage. During the edematous phase, the signal intensity of normal mucosa is largely indistinguishable from that of inflammatory disease, which may yield a false-positive result on imaging. In addition, MRI resolution of bony landmarks is poor, providing little information when planning endoscopic sinus surgery. The small size of the machine portal, high cost, and need for sedation of most young children due to long imaging time are other limitations.

22. You are evaluating an HIV-positive patient in the clinic. Is this patient predisposed to developing sinusitis? What percentage of AIDS patients develop sinusitis?

Patients who are HIV-positive have deficits in cell-mediated and humoral immunity. Therefore, they are more susceptible to bacterial infection. Sinusitis occurs in approximately 75% of AIDS patients and is often extensive and difficult to treat. Causative pathogens are similar to those for immunocompetent patients. In addition, *Cryptococcus neoformans*, cytomegalovirus, and *Pseudomonas aeruginosa* may be implicated.

23. Should your evaluation of the immunocompromised patient with possible sinusitis differ from that for the immunocompetent patient?

The clinician needs to have a high index of suspicion when evaluating the immunocompromised patient with possible sinusitis. Headache, facial pain, fever of unknown origin, and nasal crusting should prompt urgent CT evaluation of the sinuses. In addition, hospital admission with prompt initiation of treatment is indicated for the patient with suspected sinusitis.

24. You are evaluating a patient with persistent sinusitis. On oral exam, you discover the patient has very poor dentition. What should be considered?

Sinusitis may be related to periapical or periodontal disease. An oroantral fistula, usually occurring after extraction of molar teeth, may also cause sinusitis. Adults are at greater risk than children because of continued expansion of the sinus into alveolar bone after secondary dentition eruption. Symptoms of dental sinusitis include facial pain, swelling, tenderness, and nasal or oral fistula discharge. The maxillary sinus may appear opaque on plain films or CT. Offending organisms are predominantly anaerobic, and treatment should be adjusted accordingly.

25. In broad terms, what are the complications of sinusitis? Which is most common?

In general, complications may affect the orbit or intracranial structures. Sinusitis may also lead to osteomyelitis or a mucocele. Complications of the orbit occur most commonly. Approximately 75% of all orbital infections in patients are a direct result of sinusitis.

26. How are orbital complications classified?

Inflammatory Orbital Involvement by Sinusitis

Group 1	Inflammatory edema	Most common type. Upper eyelid is swollen without evidence of orbital infection. No visual acuity loss or limitation of extraocular movement.
Group 2	Orbital cellulitis	Inflammatory cells and bacteria diffusely invade orbit without forming abscess. Proptosis of globe results from inflammatory edema. Extraocular movement impaired. Chemosis present.
Group 3	Subperiosteal abscess	Pus collection at medial aspect of orbit between periorbital and bone. Globe displaced downward and laterally. Extraocular movement impaired. Visual acuity may be affected.
Group 4	Orbital abscess	Abscess formation within orbit. Severe proptosis and complete ophthalmoplegia. Visual acuity usually impaired, leading to possible irreversible blindness.
Group 5	Cavernous sinus thrombosis	Sepsis, chemosis, proptosis, orbital pain, ophthalmoplegia. Opposite eye may be affected through spread of infection through cavernous sinus.

27. What are the intracranial complications of sinusitis?

Meningitis is usually regarded as the most common intracranial complication of sinusitis. The source of infection is most often the sphenoid and/or ethmoid sinuses. Lumbar puncture should be performed with CSF culture. Almost always occurring in relation to the frontal sinus, an **epidural abscess** is often found along with frontal bone osteomyelitis. Although the frontal sinuses may be locally painful or tender, symptoms are often mild and neurologic deficits are usually absent. The frontal sinus is also the most common offender in a **subdural abscess**, which today is a rare complication of sinusitis. The route of spread is thought to be by thrombophlebitis. Fever and meningeal signs may be present with associated tenderness and swelling of the frontal sinus. A **brain abscess** carries a high mortality rate (20–30%). When it is due to sinusitis (approximately 15%), the frontal and ethmoid sinuses are the most often implicated sources. Most abscesses occur in the frontal lobe, and symptoms include headache and behavioral changes (which may be mild). Clinical suspicion should prompt CT or MRI scan for confirmation. A **venous sinus thrombosis** may involve the cavernous sinus or the superior sagittal sinus. Thrombosis of the superior sagittal sinus may occur from meningitis or a sinus infection. If it is due to sinusitis, usually only one-third of the superior sagittal sinus is affected and patients may recover with appropriate treatment. In advanced cases, however, the outcome is almost always fatal.

28. What is a mucocele?

A mucocele is an expanding mass of mucoid secretions lined by cuboidal epithelium. As a complication of chronic sinusitis, mucoceles usually occur due to obstruction of the sinus ostia secondary to inflammation and scarring. Mucoceles associated with sinusitis are classified as secondary, whereas mucous retention cysts are considered primary. They are potentially dangerous if they invade surrounding structures, including the orbit and brain. A secondary infection, or mucopyocele, facilitates the expansion and extension of these lesions. They can rupture intracranially with catastrophic results. The most commonly affected sinuses are the posterior ethmoid, sphenoid, and frontal. CT scan or MRI will aid in the diagnosis.

29. What is a Pott's puffy tumor?

Originally described by Sir Percivall Pott in 1760, Pott's puffy tumor is a doughy swelling on the forehead caused by erosion of the anterior sinus wall secondary to frontal sinus osteomyelitis.

Infection of the bone can occur via direct extension or, more commonly, by thrombophlebitis of the diploic veins, leading to infection of the marrow. The frontal bone is most frequently involved. The complication is seen most often in adolescents and young adults, possibly due to the more extensive system of diploic veins in this group. The most common offending organism is *Staphylococcus aureus*. The characteristic radiographic pattern is a "moth-eaten" pattern of the bone. Early in the course of the infection, however, plain films and CT scan are notoriously normal.

CONTROVERY

30. How common is sinusitis in the intensive care unit (ICU) population?
Hospitalization with ICU stay has been shown to be a risk factor for the development of sinusitis. The relationship between sinusitis and nasal cannulation is well-established. The condition is thought to occur from direct mechanical obstruction of the sinus ostia, occlusion of the ostia from mucosal edema, and disruption of the normal nasal cyclic airflow with secondary changes in sinus outflow. Early studies indicated that sinusitis occurs in 2–17% of nasally cannulated ICU patients. More recent investigations show that sinusitis may occur in 100% of nasaotracheally intubated patients and in as many as 80% of patients with nasogastric tubes.

BIBLIOGRAPHY

1. Borman KR, Brown PM, Mezera KK, Jhaveri H: Occult fever in surgical intensive care unit patients is seldom caused by sinusitis. Am J Surg 164:412–416, 1992.
2. Calhoun K: Diagnosis and management of sinusitis in the allergic patient. Otolaryngol Head Neck Surg 107:850–854, 1992.
3. Colman BH: Sinusitis. In Hall & Colman's Diseases of the Nose, Throat and Ear, Head and Neck. Edinburgh, Churchill Livingstone, 1992, pp 49–54.
4. Evans KL: Diagnosis and management of sinusitis. BMJ 309:1415–1422, 1994.
5. Gluckman JL, Righi PD, Rice DH: Sinusitis. In Donald PJ, Gluckman JL, Rice DH (eds): The Sinuses. New York, Raven Press, 1995, pp 161–171.
6. Lebeda MD, Haller JR, Graham SM, Hoffman HT: Evaluation of maxillary sinus aspiration in patients with fever of unknown origin. Laryngoscope 105:683–685, 1995.
7. Stankiewicz JA, Newell DJ, Park AH: Complications of inflammatory disease of the sinuses. Otolaryngol Clin North Am 26:639–655, 1993.
8. Wagenmann M, Naclerio RM: Complications of sinusitis. J Allergy Clin Immunol 90:552–554, 1992.
9. Wilson J: Current approaches to sinusitis. Practitioner 238:467–472, 1994.

21. MEDICAL MANAGEMENT OF SINUSITIS

Tyler M. Lewark, M.D.

1. What therapeutic agents can be used to manage sinusitis?
There are many therapeutic agents available to the clinician for the management of sinusitis. However, to treat this condition properly, one must understand and treat all the contributory factors in each individual case (*see* chapter 20). Therapeutic agents include antibiotics, decongestants, mucolytics, nasal sprays or irrigation, and corticosteroids.

2. What percentage of cases of acute bacterial sinusitis spontaneously resolve? Should antibiotics still be used?
An estimated 40% of cases of acute bacterial sinusitis will spontaneously resolve. Antibiotics should still be used, as they are felt to facilitate recovery from the acute episode, prevent complications, and prevent progressive mucosal changes that may result in chronic sinusitis.

3. What factors should be considered when choosing an antibiotic?

History of drug allergies, cost, prior antibiotic failures, and incidence of ß-lactamase-producing strains of bacteria.

4. Which antibiotics should be used in adults with acute sinusitis?

Many clinicians employ ampicillin or amoxicillin as first-line antimicrobials in the treatment of sinusitis. Other antibiotics proven clinically effective include trimethoprim-sulfamethoxazole, cefaclor, cefuroxime axetil, and azithromycin. Although appropriate antibiotic therapy can be chosen on the basis of culture and sensitivity results, usually the choice is empiric. If the patient presents with continued evidence of purulent sinusitis despite prior adequate treatment with ampicillin or amoxicillin, a ß-lactamase-resistant antibiotic may be necessary. Amoxicillin with clavulanate (ß-lactamase inhibitor), trimethoprim-sulfamethoxazole, and cefuroxime axetil all appear to be effective in eradicating most ß-lactamase producing strains of bacteria.

5. Which antibiotics should be used in children with acute sinusitis?

As for adults, one must consider the patient's drug allergy history, previous antibiotic failures, potential side effects, and prevalence of ß-lactamase-producing bacteria in the population. Coverage of likely pathogens varies and is provided by a variety of antimicrobials, including amoxicillin, erythromycin, trimethoprim-sulfamethoxazole, cefaclor, and amoxicillin-clavulanic acid.

6. How long is antimicrobial therapy continued in uncomplicated acute sinusitis?

In uncomplicated maxillary sinusitis, treatment with ampicillin or amoxicillin for 10–14 days is usually adequate. Clinical improvement usually occurs within 48–72 hours of initiation of antimicrobial therapy. However, antibiotic therapy should be continued for a minimum 7 days after the disappearance of symptoms. Because of the increased prevalence of ß-lactamase-producing bacteria in the pediatric population, lack of clinical improvement after 48–72 hours should prompt an antibiotic change to cover these pathogens. Lack of symptom resolution after 10–14 days requires that antibiotics be continued until all symptoms are resolved.

7. What factor must be addressed for the successful treatment of recurrent or chronic sinusitis?

The most important factor contributing to the development of sinusitis is obstruction of the sinus ostia. Accordingly, the key to effective management of recurrent or chronic sinusitis is early correction of osteomeatal complex obstruction. Medical management of this condition is necessary if the obstruction is due to, or affected by, physiologic abnormalities. If the obstruction is anatomic, surgery may be necessary (*see* chapter 22).

8. Does antimicrobial treatment differ in chronic sinusitis?

When compared to that for acute sinusitis, medical management in chronic sinusitis treatment has a limited role. Antibiotic therapy differs both in choice of agent and duration of treatment. Because anaerobes or a combination of aerobes and anaerobes are often implicated in chronic cases, antibiotic choice should include anaerobic coverage. Penicillin VK is useful, but as many as 44% of anaerobic isolates may be ß-lactamase-positive, and so amoxicillin–clavulanic acid or clindamycin may be necessary. Antibiotic therapy should be administered for a minimum of 4 weeks. Treatment of chronic sinusitis in children is similar to that for the adult. Special care should be given to the choice of antibiotic due to the increased prevalence of ß-lactamase-producing bacteria in this population.

9. What is rhinitis medicamentosa? What therapeutic agent causes it?

Rhinitis medicamentosa is **rebound rhinitis** that occurs with the use of topical **decongestants**, usually after 5 days of treatment. In addition to antibiotics, decongestants are used in the treatment of most cases of sinusitis to diminish local mucosal edema, improving access for air and egress of secretions via the sinus ostia. Topical and systemic agents are available and produce vasoconstriction via their α-adrenergic effect. Use of topical agents should be limited to 5 days, although systemic decongestants (e.g., pseudoephedrine, phenylpropanolamine) may be continued longer. Patients taking systemic agents should be monitored for potential side effects, including nervousness, insomnia, tachycardia, and hypertension.

10. What is the Mecca position? When is it used?

Topical nasal decongestants are more effective when given in the Mecca position. It should be maintained for 2–3 minutes after decongestants are administered.

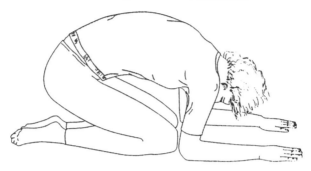

The Mecca position for receiving topical nasal decongestion. (From Evans KL: Diagnosis and management of sinusitis. BMJ 309:1418, 1994, with permission.)

11. Describe the role of mucolytics in the treatment of sinusitis.

Mucolytic agents are used in sinusitis to decrease the tenacity of mucus. Home remedies include horseradish, chicken soup, and increased fluid intake. Although less well established in cases of sinusitis, organic iodide preparations have been shown to be effective in treating patients with bronchitis. The most widely used mucolytic agent in the treatment of sinusitis is **guaifenesin**. Because effective doses approach levels that cause emesis, guaifenesin may cause gastrointestinal side effects.

12. Should corticosteroids be used in the treatment of sinusitis? When? What type?

Because of the significant potential for undesirable side effects on multiple organ systems, systemic corticosteroids have largely been supplanted by topical preparations. Nasal steroids reduce edema of the osteomeatal complex. Because they may decrease inflammation necessary for combating infection, appropriate antibiotic therapy should be initiated prior to topical steroids. Thus, they may be helpful when treating chronic sinusitis or when used prophylactically in recurrent sinusitis.

To be beneficial, the medication must contact the affected mucosa. Topical steroids are less effective if the airway is obstructed by septal deviation, turbinate hypertrophy, polyps, or anterior nasal edema. Maximal benefit will not be seen for 1–2 weeks, and further therapy depends on therapeutic response and other treatment employed. Potential side effects of topical preparations include nasal irritation, crusting, bleeding, and even septal perforation. Local candidiasis and significant systemic absorption may result from prolonged use.

13. Are any nonpharmacologic treatments effective in sinusitis?

Great benefit is derived from **regular saline nasal irrigations** in many patients with sinusitis. Delivered with a bulb syringe or nasal irrigator, this treatment helps to move secretions through the nasal cavity. Saline solutions of roughly physiologic proportions can be prepared by patients or may be purchased as a commercially prepared, sterile physiologic solution. Self-prepared solutions are easily delivered with the use of an empty conventional squeeze-spray or pump-spray bottle. Irrigations must be thorough and performed several times a day. For patients with bothersome thick postnasal secretions, powered, pulsating devices that deliver warm saline into the nasal cavity are available. Moist heat to the face and the inhalation of steam may give some relief to the patient with facial pressure. This can be accomplished with a hot shower, sauna, or hot towel.

14. How is fungal sinusitis treated? Is medical management effective?

Fungal sinusitis may be invasive or noninvasive, and medical management alone rarely eradicates the disease. Acute noninvasive fungal sinusitis most commonly involves the maxillary sinus and is treated surgically. Antifungal therapy is usually not indicated. Invasive fungal sinusitis can be life-threatening and requires surgical debridement and prompt fungal chemotherapy, usually with intravenous amphotericin B.

15. Does the medical management of sinusitis differ for the patient with allergy?

Repeated or severe allergic reactions lead to osteomeatal complex obstruction and stasis of secretions within the sinus. Therefore, it is important either to prevent or to rapidly and effectively treat acute reactions. If possible, the patient should avoid inciting allergens. Antibiotics, decongestants, mucolytics, corticosteroids, and nasal irrigation should be employed as for acute and chronic sinusitis. Because histamine is the major product released during an anaphylactic or immediate allergic reaction, **antihistamines** are usually employed in the treatment of allergy-associated sinusitis. Potential side effects of antihistamines include sedation and excessive dryness and crusting within the nose. The newer second-generation antihistamines (e.g., terfenadine, loratadine) are less sedating because they are lipophobic and do not cross the blood-brain barrier. Unlike first-generation antihistamines, these newer agents do not cause dryness and crusting. **Cromolyn sodium**, a mast cell stabilizer, may also be administered to the allergic patient with sinusitis. Because this agent acts on acute and late-phase allergic reactions, its use is limited to prevention and treatment of sinusitis cause by allergic flares.

16. When is immunotherapy indicated in the treatment of sinusitis?

Immunotherapy is the administration of carefully determined allergen doses over a period of years. IgG-blocking antibodies prevent the allergic event by disrupting the IgE–allergen–mast cell interaction. This therapy should be considered in patients with allergen-induced sinusitis whose symptoms are not controlled by simple pharmacologic measures. It should also be used when the offending allergens are unavoidable.

17. How does the medical management of sinusitis differ for the immunocompromised patient?

Fungal infections are prevalent in the immunocompromised population, especially in those patients with lymphoproliferative neoplasms. The clinician's threshold for administration of antibacterial and antifungal agents in this population should be quite low. Because AIDS patients have deficits in both cell-mediated and humoral immunity, they are more susceptible to bacterial infection. Treatment is often very difficult, especially when the patient's CD4 count is $< 200 \times 10^6$/liter. Antral aspiration may be necessary for organism identification and antibiotic sensitivity determination. Uncomplicated cases may respond to oral antibiotics. However, when patients appear systemically affected, hospital admission may be required for antral lavage (*see* chapter 22) and intravenous therapy.

18. How are orbital complications of sinusitis managed?

Early preseptal infections may be managed on an outpatient basis with oral antibiotics active against ß-lactamase-producing strains of bacteria. However, the clinician must have a low threshold for hospital admission and aggressive treatment because unrecognized orbital infection may have catastrophic consequences. Advanced cases of orbital infection require intravenous antibiotics. Strict visual acuity monitoring, CT scan evaluation, and ophthalmology consultation are also necessary. Surgical intervention is indicated if the patient experiences visual loss, progression of symptoms over 24 hours, or no improvement after 48–72 hours.

19. How are the intracranial complications of sinusitis treated?

Despite the reduced frequency of these complications, they are life-threatening and require immediate attention. In all cases, the underlying sinus disease should be treated. High-dose intravenous antibiotic therapy is the primary medical treatment. Sinusitis-induced meningitis requires antibiotics with good cerebrospinal penetration. Surgery may be indicated if symptoms persist. Surgery is required for the treatment of epidural, subdural, and brain abscesses and for venous sinus thrombosis. Concurrent high-dose intravenous antibiotics should be administered. Some clinicians advocate the use of heparin for the treatment of cavernous venous thrombosis. In cases of superior sagittal sinus thrombosis, aggressive medical management may be lifesaving.

20. Can sinusitis-induced mucocele be treated medically?

If infection is suspected, broad-spectrum antibiotics should be instituted. Otherwise, mucoceles are primarily treated surgically (*see* chapter 22).

21. How is sinusitis-induced osteomyelitis managed? How long should you follow the patient after resolution of the infection?

The mainstay of treatment of sinusitis-induced osteomyelitis is prolonged antibiotic therapy with wide surgical debridement of necrotic bone. Although ineffective when used alone, antibiotics should be continued for at least 6 weeks. The patient should be followed on a long-term basis due to the tendency for the condition to recur many years after resolution of the infection.

22. When should the primary care physician refer a patient with sinusitis to an otolaryngologist?

1. If there is no response to a first-line course of antibiotics, a course of a second-line medication may be administered. If there is no response to the second course, the patient should be referred to an otolaryngologist.

2. Any symptom suggestive of incipient complications should prompt immediate referral.

3. Patients who have at least three attacks/year for 2 years or four or more attacks in 1 year warrant referral. Specialist care is necessary to investigate a possible correctable local anatomic factor or predisposing systemic condition, such as immunosuppression.

CONTROVERSIES

23. When is a case considered a medical failure? When is surgical management indicated?

This question has both medical and financial considerations. Although some third-party payers have guidelines for the management of sinusitis, no set criteria are generally accepted. Some clinicians do not easily abandon medical therapy and favor long-term antimicrobial treatment. Some argue that surgery is only indicated in cases of proven mechanical obstruction. Others argue that surgery is indicated with either evidence of mechanical obstruction or residual infection following adequate medical management. Further concerns revolve around medical and surgical management in the pediatric patient. Cost-effectiveness of the various modalities is also disputed. Consideration should be given to the cost of sinus surgery versus the cost of long-term second-line antimicrobial treatment.

24. The ICU team consults you on a patient who is intubated, obtunded, and has a fever of unknown origin. CT scan of the patient's sinuses indicate the patient has sinusitis. Should maxillary sinus aspiration be performed to identify possible sinus pathogens contributing to the patient's fever?

The controversy concerns how often sinusitis causes a fever of unknown origin in the ICU patient. Some investigators have found sinusitis to be an often overlooked cause of occult fever and sepsis in the ICU patient. These authors advocate more aggressive search for and treatment of sinusitis in these patients, including maxillary sinus aspiration. In contrast, others argue that although radiographic evidence of sinusitis is very common in the nasally cannulated ICU patient, this condition is rarely the cause of occult fever. These authors also argue that maxillary sinus aspiration for identification of possible inciting pathogens is often not necessary and that medical management, including decongestants and antibiotics, often eliminates the need for this procedure.

BIBLIOGRAPHY

1. Borman KR, Brown PM, Mezera KK, Jhaveri H: Occult fever in surgical intensive care unit patients is seldom caused by sinusitis. Am J Surg 164:412–416, 1992.
2. Calhoun K: Diagnosis and management of sinusitis in the allergic patient. Otolaryngol Head Neck Surg 107:850–854, 1992.
3. Colman BH: Sinusitis. In Hall & Colman's Diseases of the Nose, Throat and Ear, Head and Neck. Edinburgh, Churchill Livingstone, 1992, pp 55–57
4. Evans KL: Diagnosis and management of sinusitis. BMJ 309:1415–1422, 1994.
5. Gluckman JL, Righi, PD, Rice DH: Sinusitis. In Donald PJ, Gluckman JL, Rice DH (eds): The Sinuses. New York, Raven Press, 1995, pp 166–171.
6. Mabry RL: Therapeutic agents in the medical management of sinusitis. Otolaryngol Clin North Am 26(4):561–570, 1993.
7. Stankiewicz J, Osguthorpe JD: Medical treatment of sinusitis. Otolaryngol Head Neck Surg 110:361-362, 1994.
8. Stankiewicz JA, Newell DJ, Park AH: Complications of inflammatory disease of the sinuses. Otolaryngol Clin North Am 26(4):639–655, 1993.
9. Wilson J: Current approaches to sinusitis. Practitioner 238:467–472, 1994.

22. SURGICAL MANAGEMENT OF SINUSITIS

Nicolas G. Slenkovich, M.D.

1. What is the aim of surgical intervention for sinus infections?

The goal for any treatment of sinusitis is to clear infection rapidly and to prevent serious complications from orbital or intracranial spread. The aim of surgery is to establish effective sinus drainage, cither through minimal techniques to restore physiologic mucociliary drainage or through more aggressive techniques involving wide sinus opening, sinus removal, or sinus obliteration. Except in the case of sinus obliteration, these techniques are said to be *mucosa-sparing*, where removal of diseased mucosa facilitates re-establishment of a healthy mucosal blanket.

2. What preexisting knowledge is needed to understand the surgical management of sinusitis?

Sinus anatomy and physiology. Observing an endoscopic sinus procedure can be a humbling experience to the neophyte. Surgical landmarks such as the uncinate process, ethmoid bulla, and ground lamella are foreign concepts. How they relate to the pathology may not be initially understood from the endoscopic view. Before attempting to decipher the complex surgical anatomy, it is important to study the relatively simple anatomic and physiologic basis of sinusitis.

3. Describe the details of sinus drainage into the osteomeatal complex via the infundibulum and semilunar hiatus.

Endoscopic sinus surgery is based on the fact that the anterior sinuses drain to the middle meatus. The **osteomeatal complex** defines a region of sinus drainage into the middle meatus. The posterior ethmoids drain via small ostia directly into the middle meatus. The frontal, anterior cthmoid, and maxillary sinuses all drain through the osteomeatal complex into the middle meatus via anatomic spaces referred to as the infundibulum and semilunar hiatus. The **infundibulum,**

which is Latin for *funnel*, refers to an inverted funnel that originates at the frontonasal duct superiorly and receives small anterior ethmoid ostia and the maxillary ostium through its lateral wall.
The **semilunar hiatus**, which translates as "a curved aperture," refers to a slot-like aperture in the
lateral nasal wall that curves from the frontonasal duct inferiorly and posteriorly to just below the
maxillary ostium.

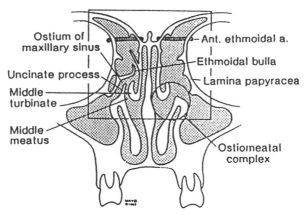

Anatomy of the midportion of the nasal cavity. The box identifies the boundaries of ethmoid bone, and the
circle identifies the osteomeatal complex. (From McCaffrey TV: Functional endoscopic sinus surgery: An
overview. Mayo Clin Proc 68:572, 1993, with permission.)

4. What is a "FESS"?

FESS is an acronym for **functional endoscopic sinus surgery**, a term that describes endoscopic techniques that have revolutionized the approach to sinus disease. These techniques were
initially developed in Europe by Messerklinger and Stammberger and were popularized in the
United States in the mid-1980s. The procedure is aimed at restoring the **functional** physiology of
sinus aeration and drainage via the osteomeatal complex while minimizing surgical intervention.
Accurate coronal CT images, together with advances in endoscopic instrumentation and techniques, led to the development of FESS.

5. What are the principles behind FESS?

Detailed CT scans led to our current understanding that anterior ethmoid sinusitis plays a
predominant role in initiating widespread sinus disease. FESS allows the surgeon to initiate dissection in the anterior ethmoids and limit surgical intervention to the diseased anatomy. FESS
techniques have reduced the length of hospitalization and discomfort associated with traditional
sinus surgery. Also, in the past, many patients with anterior ethmoidal disease may have escaped
diagnosis and can now be diagnosed accurately and treated successfully.

6. How are patients selected for endoscopic sinus surgery?

Surgery is reserved for patients with refractory sinusitis or complicated cases of sinusitis.
The highest success rates have been achieved in patients with chronic or recurrent acute episodes
of sinusitis despite maximal medical therapy. Patients with recurrent polyps, severe allergies, a
history of previous external procedures, or an immunocompromised state may undergo endoscopic sinus surgery, but with lower success rates.

7. Describe the physical exam and surgical workup performed in evaluating patients for
sinus surgery.

In addition to the complete head and neck exam, nasal endoscopy using rigid or flexible scopes
is performed to evaluate for mucosal inflammation and a source of purulence. Nasal cultures are
not routinely indicated unless a source of purulence is visualized, as results correlate poorly with

cultures of sinus aspirates. With the price of CT scans decreasing, CT is increasingly being utilized to image the sinuses due to its superior definition of bone as well as mucosal changes.

8. Which FESS techniques are used to gain access to the anterior ethmoid area?

Coronal sinus CT scans are consulted both preoperatively and in the operating room to assist in identifying landmarks and diseased areas. Following inward fracturing of the middle turbinate, an incision is made in the infundibulum to allow for removal of the uncinate process and to provide access to the anterior ethmoid area. Many surgeons will perform a middle turbinate reduction together with FESS techniques to provide additional anatomic relief. Generally, the anterior two-thirds of the inferior portion of the middle turbinate is removed, taking care to avoid a major sphenopalatine artery branch posteriorly.

9. Describe the FESS techniques used for anterior ethmoid sinus removal and frontal duct identification.

The anterior ethmoids are removed laterally by entering the sinuses via the semilunar hiatus. Working posteriorly, the middle ethmoids are entered through the ethmoid bulla, taking care to identify the roof of the ethmoid, the lamina papyracea, and the anterior ethmoid artery. From the anterior ethmoid area, a 120° endoscope allows one to look backward up into the infundibulum and view the frontal recess and frontonasal duct anterosuperiorly. The frontonasal duct may be probed to ensure its patency, but this is controversial, as some feel it may lead to scarring and stenosis.

10. How is FESS used to reestablish maxillary sinus drainage?

The maxillary ostium is identified using the 30° endoscope or by palpating the area. If the ostium is small or obstructed, it can be enlarged anteriorly and inferiorly, taking care not to damage the nasolacrimal duct anteriorly. If needed, instruments can be used to remove diseased mucosa by entering the anterior maxillary wall from an oral approach (above the superior gumline at the canine fossa). In this situation, mucosa can be removed via the anterior puncture under direct endoscopic visualization through the maxillary ostium. Some surgeons feel that creating an additional nasoantral window under the inferior turbinate may improve maxillary drainage and ventilation by more favorably utilizing gravity as well as the "beer-can" effect of creating two patent openings.

11. Describe FESS techniques for dissection of the posterior sinuses.

Surgery proceeds posteriorly as needed to address disease. To enter the posterior ethmoids, the basal lamella is taken down. The basal lamella is somewhat thicker than the rest of the eggshell septae in the ethmoids and represents the intersinus lateral projection of the middle turbinate. If necessary, the sphenoid sinus can be identified posteriorly and opened under direct vision.

12. What postoperative care is needed in patients having endoscopic sinus surgery?

Endoscopic sinus surgery is commonly performed on an outpatient basis. Nasal packing, if placed, is usually removed before discharge. Prophylactic oral antibiotics are commonly given. Careful postoperative care and nasal hygiene with rinses are important in preventing recurrence and adhesions. Some advocate early nasal steroids to decrease inflammation and the potential for adhesions.

13. What types of complications result from endoscopic sinus surgery?

Recurrence of disease is a frustrating complication that tends to occur more readily in immunocompromised patients and patients with severe allergies or polyps. Other complications are generally either orbital or intracranial and have decreased in frequency with improvements in technique and experience. A large retrospective comparison study of endoscopic versus traditional nonendoscopic intranasal sinus surgery found no statistical difference in the overall incidence of complications. Major complications occurred in < 1% of patients and minor complications in < 7% of patients.

14. What are the major complications of endoscopic sinus surgery?

Major complications include CSF leak, orbital hematoma, hemorrhage requiring transfusion, and symptomatic lacrimal duct obstruction requiring surgical intervention. Rarer major complications include diplopia, loss of vision, meningitis, brain abscess, intracranial hemorrhage, stroke, carotid artery injury, and death.

15. What minor complications may result from endoscopic sinus surgery?

Minor complications most commonly result from middle turbinate adhesions or orbital penetration. Other minor complications include sinus infection, periorbital edema or ecchymosis, epistaxis, bronchospasm, and loss of smell. Retrobulbar orbital hematomas tend to occur more often in traditional intranasal techniques, probably owing to a lack of direct visualization. Middle turbinate adhesions occur in endoscopic surgery and not in traditional techniques, as the middle turbinate is routinely removed in the latter. Even with turbinate reduction in conjunction with endoscopic techniques, some authors still report a similar rate of adhesions.

16. How can you minimize complications of endoscopic sinus surgery and manage complications when they occur?

Orbital complications generally occur from penetration of the lamina papyracea along the lateral wall of the ethmoids. Orbital fat may be visible through the lamina papyracea and will float if placed in a specimen cup filled with water. Pressing on the eye may reveal transmitted movement of the suspected area. Retrobulbar accumulation of blood in the orbit is suspected in the presence of proptosis, pupillary dilation with decreased light reactivity, and pain around the eye. When visual impairment is present, it is imperative to decompress the orbit within 60–90 minutes, as blindness can result. Traumatic injury of the optic nerve, medial rectus, or superior oblique muscle is often irreversible and requires immediate ophthalmologic consultation. CSF leaks and other intracranial complications are minimized by meticulous attention to detail. In particular, all instruments should be placed under direct vision, and the mucosa along the roof of the ethmoid should be left intact. The procedure should be terminated if landmarks or surgical relationships are unclear.

17. Do residency training programs experience increased complications in endoscopic sinus surgery?

This is a question that goes to the heart of the American surgical educational system. Surgeons report that there is a learning curve in developing expertise in endoscopic sinus procedures and that formal training should be mandatory for the sinus endoscopist. However, a recent study reported some increase in minor complications but concluded that endoscopic sinus surgery can be safely performed by residents in carefully structured and supervised training programs.

18. What is the traditional approach to chronic maxillary sinusitis?

With the proliferation of endoscopic sinus surgery, traditional techniques are less commonly employed, in part due to our current understanding that ethmoiditis typically serves as the impetus for maxillary sinusitis. The traditional approach to refractory chronic sinusitis begins with weekly puncture and lavage of the maxillary sinus. If three or more antral lavages fail to clear maxillary sinusitis, a large antrostomy is created to remove diseased mucosa.

19. What is a Caldwell-Luc procedure?

The **Caldwell-Luc procedure** is an external approach to the anterior maxillary wall through the canine fossa above the gumline. Alternatively, an intranasal approach may be used to create an inferior meatal antrostomy. The Caldwell-Luc procedure provides excellent sinus visualization and subsequent creation of a large nasoantral window in the inferior meatus for permanent sinus drainage. The Caldwell-Luc procedure has the potential for more complications, and care must be taken to protect the infraorbital nerve superiorly and the tooth roots inferiorly. When performing an inferior meatal antrostomy, care must be taken to avoid damage to the nasolacrimal duct anteriorly and the greater palatine artery and branches of the sphenopalatine artery posteriorly.

20. Are there traditional surgical approaches that address ethmoid sinusitis?
Yes. External ethmoidectomy, transantral ethmoidectomy, and intranasal ethmoidectomy without direct endoscopic visualization all predate current endoscopic techniques. In cases of sinusitis complications, sinus mucoceles, or sinus neoplasms, the external and transantral approaches are commonly employed.

21. How are external ethmoidectomy and transantral ethmoidectomy performed?
External ethmoidectomy provides exposure of the orbit and excellent visualization of the ethmoid labyrinth. From the Lynch incision at the medial orbital rim, external ethmoidectomy proceeds posteriorly with exposure of the ethmoids via removal of the medial orbital wall (the lamina papyracea). This approach also provides access to the frontal sinuses superiorly and sphenoid posteriorly. Important landmarks include the suture line between the frontal bone and lamina papyracea, which identifies the plane of the cribriform plate, and the anterior and posterior ethmoid arteries. The optic nerve lies 0.5 cm behind the posterior ethmoid artery. Transantral ethmoidectomy is performed through a large Caldwell-Luc antrostomy and allows an inferior approach to the ethmoids. The procedure can be combined with intranasal ethmoidectomy, allowing nasal instrumentation under direct vision through the maxillary sinus.

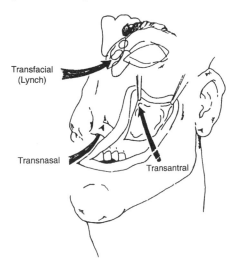

Three approaches to ethmoidectomy: transfacial (Lynch), transantral, and transnasal. (From Osguthorpe DJ, Hochman M: Inflammatory sinus diseases affecting the orbit. Otolaryngol Clin North Am 26:657–671, 1993, with permission.)

Transfacial
(Lynch)

Transnasal

Transantral

22. What are the surgical approaches to the frontal sinus?
The internal approach to the frontal sinus in FESS allows identification of the frontal recess and cannulation of the frontonasal duct. However, removal of diseased frontal mucosa is better accomplished via external approaches. The frontal sinus can be approached externally from the Lynch incision as used in external ethmoidectomy or by elevating a large bicoronal tissue flap forward from within the hairline to the orbital rims.

23. Compare the Lynch approach to the bicoronal osteoplastic approach to the frontal sinuses.
A Lynch incision at the medial orbital rim provides access to the anterior table of the frontal sinus and can be used in combination with ethmoidectomy, allowing a combined frontoethmoidectomy with removal of the frontal sinus floor and establishment of a widely patent frontonasal duct. The Lynch incision can also be used to perform a frontal trephination, where the frontal sinus is entered and drained externally, without dissection to the nasal passage. In either case, external frontal sinus approaches permit access to the intersinus septum, which can be taken down to facilitate drainage of both sinuses through either frontonasal duct.

The bicoronal flap is used in osteoplastic frontal sinus obliteration for chronic recurrent frontal sinusitis. A scalp flap is raised in the subperiosteal plane and elevated anteriorly to expose the frontal bone over the sinuses. Using a template made from a cutout of a plain film radiograph, bone incisions are planned and created, raising the anterior table of the frontal sinuses in a single bony flap. Sinus mucosa is removed, and the sinus is obliterated using a fat graft and packing of the frontal ducts with bone and muscle.

24. What are the surgical approaches to the sphenoid sinus?
The sphenoid sinus is approached through its anterior wall. This can be accomplished alone or in combination with external ethmoidectomy or intranasal ethmoidectomy. Resection of the pituitary is commonly performed using a transsphenoidal approach.

CONTROVERSY

25. When should pediatric sinusitis be treated surgically?
Although a technically feasible procedure, endoscopic sinus surgery in young children is controversial. There is general agreement that surgical techniques can be indicated in children with orbital or intracranial complications of sinusitis or in patients with mucoceles or nasal polyps. However, some authors argue against pediatric sinus surgery in all but extreme refractory cases. This group argues that pediatric sinusitis is generally a self-limited disease, rarely persisting past age 7–8 years, and complications are rare. Minimum criteria for consideration of surgery should include:
1. Persistent or recurrent symptoms, most often unabated rhinorrhea
2. Failure of maximal medical therapy
3. Abnormal mucosal changes on CT scan

BIBLIOGRAPHY

1. Feldman BA, Feldman DE: The nose and sinuses. In Lee KJ (ed): Essential Otolaryngology, 6th ed. Norwalk, CT, Appleton & Lange, 1995, pp 715–756.
2. Kinsella JB, Calhoun KH, Bradfield JJ, et al: Complications of endoscopic sinus surgery in a residency training program. Laryngoscope 105:1029–1032, 1995.
3. May M, Levine HL, Mester SJ, Schaitkin B: Complications of endoscopic sinus surgery: Analysis of 2108 patients—incidence and prevention. Laryngoscope 104:1080–1083, 1994.
4. McCaffrey TV: Functional endoscopic sinus surgery: An overview. Mayo Clin Proc 68:571–577, 1993.
5. Netter FH: Atlas of Human Anatomy. Summit, NJ, Ciba-Geigy, 1989.
6. Poole MD: Pediatric sinusitis is not a surgical disease. ENT J 71:622–623, 1992.
7. Rice DH (ed): Inflammatory diseases of the sinuses. Otolaryngol Clin North Am 26(4):509–704, 1993.
8. Rice DH: Endoscopic sinus surgery. Otolaryngol Head Neck Surg 111:100–110, 1994.
9. Weymuller EA Jr, Rice DH: Surgical management of infectious and inflammatory disease. In Cummings CW, et al (eds): Otolaryngology–Head and Neck Surgery, 2nd ed. St. Louis, Mosby, 1993, pp 955–964.

IV. General Otolaryngology

23. TEMPOROMANDIBULAR JOINT DISEASE

Steven B. Aragon, M.D., D.D.S.

1. Are the terms temporomandibular disorder and temporomandibular joint disease synonymous?

No. Temporomandibular disorders (TMD), also called craniomandibular disorders, encompass a variety of disorders affecting not only the temporomandibular joint (TMJ) but also areas extrinsic to the joint. TMD has traditionally been described as a constellation of related pathologic changes that produce musculoskeletal symptoms. These may present as pain associated with jaw function, limited range of mandibular motion, masticatory muscle tenderness, and TMJ tenderness. TMD has a very broad interpretation and describes a general population of patients suffering from abnormal and usually painful function of the jaw muscle and joints. This is not a homogeneous group of patients, as many different etiologies and mechanisms of pain are responsible for similar presentations. It is imperative to definitively diagnose the specific causal factor in order to treat the patient effectively.

2. Describe the anatomy of the TMJ.

The TMJ is a diarthrodial (freely movable) joint with articulation between the condyle of the mandible and the glenoid fossa of the temporal bone. It is a true synovial joint with gliding and hinging motions. Avascular fibrocartilage lines both the condyle and glenoid fossa. A meniscus made of fibrocartilage lies between the condyle and temporal bone, producing a superior and inferior joint space.

3. Describe the normal relationship of the disc within the TMJ.

The disc is composed of a posterior band, an intermediate zone, and an anterior band. The posterior band is usually thicker (about 3 mm) than both the anterior band (about 2 mm) and the central zone (about 1 mm thick). The upper band conforms to the depth of the glenoid fossa, while the central and anterior bands conform to the articular eminence anteriorly. The inferior surface adapts to the contour of the mandibular condyle. Posteriorly, the disc is contiguous with the posterior attachment tissue, which is attached to the tympanic plate of the temporal bone superiorly and the neck of the condyle inferiorly. Anteriorly, the disc is contiguous with the superior head of the lateral pterygoid muscle.

4. What are the common signs and symptoms of TMD?

Preauricular (TMJ) pain	Deviation in mandibular motion
Limited mandibular range of motion	Pain in the muscles of mastication
Clicking and/or crepitus within the TMJ	Locking of the jaw in open or closed position

5. What is the differential diagnosis in these disorders?

TMJ disorders
    Arthralgia (capsulitis)
    Disc displacement
    Disc dysfunction
    Disc perforation

Masticatory muscle disorders (myogenic disorders)
  Muscle trismus or splinting
Chronic mandibular hypomobilities
  Fibrosis of muscular tissue (contracture)
  Capsular fibrosis
  Ankylosis (bony ankylosis, bony fusion)
  Adhesions (intracapsular fibrosis, fibrous ankylosis)
  Coronoid process elongation
Chronic mandibular hypermobilities
  Subluxation
  Dislocation
Fractures
  Mandible
  Maxilla
Inflammatory disorders
  Synovitis, capsulitis
  Traumatic arthritis
  Degenerative arthritis
  Infectious arthritis
  Rheumatoid arthritis
  Hyperuricemia
Disorders of maxillomandibular growth
  Masticatory muscle hypertrophy or atrophy
  Maxillomandibular or condylar hypoplasia or hyperplasia
  Neoplasia

6. Explain the etiology of myogenic disorders.

Myogenic disorders were previously classified as myofunctional pain dysfunction (MPD), but this term is outdated and not generally used today. Most patients with myogenic pain have normal TMJs. They present with limitation of the normal mandibular movement secondary to muscle pain and stiffness. Pain usually develops without a specific history of significant trauma.

Myogenic pain is usually considered to be the result of hyperactivity or hyperfunction. Many of these patients will have a history of nocturnal or diurnal bruxism (grinding or clenching), which may become more exaggerated during periods of physical or emotional stress. This stress results in hyperactivity, which leads to muscle fatigue and spasm, resulting in pain and limitation. This disorder is usually classified as a strain due to overuse or improper use and is treated as such. This category of disorders includes myalgias (myofascial pain, fibrositis), muscle splinting (trismus), spasm, myositis (muscle swelling), contracture, hypertrophy, dyskinesia, and bruxism.

7. How are muscle disorders diagnosed?

The most common sign of myogenic disorders is **diffuse facial pain**. The pain of muscular origin is poorly localized and diffuse, as opposed to the well-localized pain associated with internal derangement of the TMJ. While muscle disorders may occur with true internal derangement of the TMJ, this entity must be diagnosed separately from internal derangement. There is usually no clinical or radiographic evidence of internal derangement.

8. Which muscles are usually affected?

1. The **masseter muscle** is the most common muscle involved, producing what is described as "jaw pain."
2. The **temporalis muscle** is the second most common site, producing "headache."
3. Involvement of the **lateral pterygoid muscle** produces otalgia or retrobulbar pain.
4. The **medial pterygoid** may result in odynophagia or the sensation of a painful swollen gland beneath the angle of the mandible.

9. How is myogenic pain treated?

Muscle hyperactivity is treated as most strains—by reducing the functional load and stress. Patients are placed on a soft diet and utilize heat or ice to reduce the pain and inflammation. The most commonly prescribed medications include nonsteroidal anti-inflammatory drugs (NSAIDs) and muscle relaxants. Other useful medications include anxiolytics, antidepressants, and, less commonly, narcotics such as codeine or hydrocodone. Orthotic (splint) therapy may be useful to prevent or alter excessive muscle contraction and tight intercuspation (wearing of the dentition). Physical therapy, behavioral training, and stress management are also effective modalities of treatment.

10. What is internal derangement of the TMJ?

Internal derangement has been traditionally accepted to be synonymous with disc displacement. However, the strict orthopedic use of the term includes all abnormal processes that occur in the confines of the TMJ, including not only disc displacements, but also osteoarthrosis, inflammatory arthritides, congenital deformities, and traumatic, neoplastic, and developmental abnormalities. With the use of newer technologies such as arthroscopy, other abnormalities such as adhesions are also considered to be part of this diagnostic nomenclature. Disc displacement is no longer the only diagnosis considered when discussing internal derangement.

11. Explain the pathophysiology of disc displacement.

Disc displacement is usually in the anteromedial direction, probably due to the orientation of the lateral pterygoid muscle and its attachment to the capsule of the TMJ. Disruption of the ligamentous attachment of the disc to the condyle and subsequent pull by the lateral pterygoid muscle result in such displacement. While it is easy to understand how a significant external force may result in such a derangement, the exact cause often remains a mystery. Any cause of ligamentous rupture or tear can lead to displacement. This trauma may be due to a purely structural weakness or to hyperextension due to prolonged dental visits or forceful extraction of teeth, difficult anesthetic intubation, or use of retraction during a tonsillectomy.

12. What is the significance of meniscal displacement?

While osteoarthritis has been documented in > 50% of patients with disc displacement, it is unclear if disc displacement is a cause or result of osteoarthritis. Several animal studies have shown osteoarthritis after producing disc displacement, but osteoarthritis has been seen in joints with normal disc–condyle relationships. Pain is often associated with disc displacement. As the disc becomes displaced, the condyle may function on the innervated posterior attachment, resulting in marked discomfort. However, not all disc displacements lead to pain—as much as 20% of the random population may have some form of disc displacement without pain.

13. Describe the nonsurgical treatment of disc displacement of the TMJ.

Initial therapy includes **NSAIDs** to reduce inflammation and provide analgesia. Limitation of function with **restricted opening** and **soft diet** help reduce painful loads on the inflamed joint. **Hyaluronate injection** has shown some promise as a therapy for the painful, persistent clicking disorder. Often a concomitant muscular disorder is present which requires simultaneous treatment. **Splint therapy** may reduce the symptoms of both TMJ and muscular pain. **Physical therapy** may provide relief of symptoms. If painful symptoms persist despite therapy, surgical correction is indicated.

14. What imaging studies are available for the TMJ?

Plain films, such as the **panoramic view**, are capable of screening gross disease, destruction, and general joint configuration. Panoramic films may be useful for bony alterations, such as degenerative joint disease, ankylosis, or other gross deformities. However, if fine detail is required, **computed tomography** (CT) is far superior to the panoramic or plain films for fine osseous or fibrous evaluation.

Disc position can be evaluated by **arthrography**. A contrast material is placed into the superior and inferior joint space and outlines the disc and its position. Although this modality is an effective tool for evaluating disc position and even perforation, it is an invasive study and may have a fair amount of discomfort associated with its use. **Magnetic resonance imaging** (MRI) is an excellent technique for evaluating disc morphology and position and is also a sensitive indicator of early degenerative bone changes. It is also a noninvasive technique and requires no injection of a contrast material.

15. When is a bite appliance used?

An appliance is a device worn on the teeth to relieve acute muscle and TMJ pain. The bite appliance is also known as an interocclusal appliance, orthopedic appliance, night guard, orthotic, and occlusal appliance. Many types of splints are available with different purposes. These appliances are used to stabilize an occlusion when a bruxing disorder is present. They may also decrease the load on a compromised joint when it is acutely inflamed. These devices are considered conservative and reversible. However, close follow-up is in order when these splints are worn for long periods to prevent permanent occlusal changes from occurring.

16. Are narcotics useful in the management of TMD?

Because TMD is often a prolonged or recurrent problem, long-term use of narcotics is to be avoided to prevent chemical dependence. The other often-utilized medications include NSAIDs, muscle relaxants, benzodiazepines, antidepressants, and local anesthetics.

17. What is the role of nonsteroidal anti-inflammatory drugs (NSAIDs) in the treatment of TMD?

NSAIDs inhibit cyclo-oxygenase and the production of prostaglandins. Recent evidence suggests they may also have a central analgesic effect. Individual response to NSAIDs is highly variable, and when response to a particular NSAID is poor, a different one should be prescribed rather than turning to narcotics.

NSAIDs and TMD

GENERIC NAME	BRAND NAME	DOSE
Ibuprofen	Motrin	900–2400 mg/day in divided doses
Naproxen	Anaprox	275–550 mg twice daily
Meclofenamate	Meclomen	50 mg every 4–6 hrs
Etodolac	Lodine	200–400 mg every 8 hrs
Piroxicam	Feldene	20 mg/day

18. What is the role of muscle relaxants in the treatment of TMD?

Muscle relaxants can be divided into centrally-acting or peripherally-acting agents. The centrally-acting agents relax skeletal muscle via their generally sedating effect on the CNS and are more commonly prescribed.

Commonly Used Muscle Relaxants

GENERIC NAME	BRAND NAME	DOSE
Carisoprodol	Soma	100–1400 mg/day in divided doses
Methocarbamol	Robaxin	1500–3000 mg/day in divided doses
Cyclobenzaprine	Flexeril	5–30 mg/day in divided doses

19. Benzodiazepines?

Benzodiazepines bind to gamma-aminobutyric acid (GABA) type A receptors in the CNS. These are indicated for reduction of anxiety and muscle hyperactivity. Sedation is the most common side effect.

Commonly Used Benzodiazepines

GENERIC NAME	BRAND NAME	USUAL DOSE
Diazepam	Valium	2–10 mg 1–4 times a day
Clonazepam	Clonopin	0.5–1 mg 1–4 times a day
Alprazolam	Xanax	0.5 mg 1–3 times a day

20. And antidepressants?

Recent evidence suggests that antidepressant medication is often useful for chronic pain management in patients without symptoms of depression. Antidepressants have been used to manage chronic pain, headaches, sleep disorders, panic disorders, and neurologic and sympathetically mediated pain. Tricyclic and serotonin-reuptake inhibitors are most commonly used.

Commonly Used Antidepressants

GENERIC NAME	BRAND NAME	INITIAL DOSE
Amitriptyline	Elavil	10–25 mg/day
Imipramine	Tofranil	10–25 mg/day
Nortriptyline	Pamelor	10–25 mg/day
Fluoxetine	Prozac	5 mg/day
Sertraline	Zoloft	50 mg/day

21. When is surgery indicated for TMD?

When nonsurgical therapy has been ineffective and when pain and/or dysfunction is moderate to severe in nature. Surgery is not indicated for asymptomatic or minimally symptomatic patients. It is not indicated for masticatory muscle disorders without internal derangement. Surgery also is not indicated for preventive reasons in patients without pain and with satisfactory function. **Arthroscopy** and **arthrotomy** are the two general techniques employed by most TMJ surgeons.

22. Describe TMJ arthroscopy and its usefulness.

TMJ arthroscopy enables the surgeon to treat the TMJ via a closed technique. An arthroscope is placed into the superior joint space. The articular surfaces are evaluated for synovitis, osteoarthritis, and articular dysfunction. Adhesions can be lysed to achieve improved mobility and function. Small shavers are now available to remove degenerated fibrocartilage, create smooth articulating surfaces, and remove fibrillated cartilage. It is believed that this procedure will restore more normal function and hopefully halt the progression of degeneration.

Arthroscopy is accomplished in an outpatient setting with minimal morbidity. Patients enjoy a faster recovery following arthroscopy than arthrotomy. Arthroscopy has greatly enhanced the treatment of patients with internal derangement.

23. When is an arthrotomy indicated?

Arthrotomy is the more traditional surgical approach to the TMJ. It is an external approach utilizing a preauricular incision for access. Arthrotomy is indicated when the surgical treatment is beyond the scope of arthroscopy. The internal derangement may be so severe as to require a menisectomy or even joint reconstruction. Disc repositioning, disc replacement, and grafting can be accomplished with the greater access of open joint surgery. Furthermore, TMJ reconstruction with autologous or alloplastic materials can be achieved with the open technique.

CONTROVERSY

24. How is occlusion related to TMDs?

Dental occlusion has been a central theme in the etiology and treatment of TMD for decades. Proponents argued that malocclusion leads to abnormal function and proprioceptive alterations in occlusal function, resulting in clenching and grinding, inappropriate muscle use, and myogenic pain. Others believed that occlusion has little to do with malocclusion and that these parafunctional habits are the result of stress, leading to clenching, grinding, muscle hyperactivity, and eventually myogenic pain. Today, a multifactorial etiology is believed to be responsible, which may include portions of both theories.

BIBLIOGRAPHY

1. Bell WE: Temporomandibular Disorders: Classification, Diagnosis, Management, 3rd ed. Chicago, Year Book Medical Publishers, 1990.
2. Bertolami CN, Gay T, Clark GT, et al: Use of sodium hyaluronate in treating temporomandibular joint disorders: A randomized, double-blind, placebo-controlled clinical trial. J Oral Maxillofac Surg 51:232–242, 1993.
3. Clark GT, Kim YJ: A logical approach to the treatment of temporomandibular disorders. Oral Maxillofac Surg Clin North Am 7:149–166, 1995.
4. Dolwick MF: Intra-articular disc displacement: Part 1. Its questionable role in temporomandibular joint pathology. J Oral Maxillofac Surg 53:1069–1072, 1995.
5. Hall HD: Intra-articular disc displacement: Part II. Its significant role in temporomandibular joint pathology. J Oral Maxillofac Surg 53:1073–1079, 1995.
6. Helfrick JF, Kelly JF, Carberry A (eds): Parameters of Care for Oral and Maxillofacial Surgery. J Am Assoc Oral Maxillofac Surg 53(suppl 5), 1995.
7. Laskin DM, Greene CS: Technological methods in the diagnosis and treatment of temporomandibular disorders. Quintessence Int 23:95, 1992.
8. Montgomery MT, Van Sickels JE, Harms SE, et al: Effects on signs, symptoms, and disc position. J Oral Maxillofac Surg 47:1263–1271, 1989.
9. Mosby EL: Efficacy of temporomandibular joint arthroscopy: A retrospective study. J Oral Maxillofac Surg 51:17–21, 1993.
10. Truelove E, Sommers E, LeResche L, et al: Clinical diagnostic criteria for TMD. J Am Dent Assoc 123:47–54, 1992.
11. Zoppi M, Zamponi A: Anti-inflammatory drugs. In Lipton S, Tunks E, Zoppi M (eds): Advances in Pain Research and Therapy: The Pain Clinic, vol. 13. New York, Raven Press, 1990, pp 329–337.

24. ORAL LESIONS

Thomas D. MacKenzie, M.D., and Michael L. Lepore, M.D.

1. What is the most common cause of xerostomia?
Medications are the most common cause of oral dryness, especially in older persons. In fact, increased medication use in the geriatric population may explain the widely believed myth that salivary gland dysfunction is a part of the normal aging process.

2. How do medications cause xerostomia?
Numerous mechanisms are responsible for the xerostomia: salivary gland hypofunction, mucosal dehydration, total body dehydration, altered sensory function, and cognitive disorders. Medications that frequently cause decreased salivary flow rates by blocking cholinergic activity include tricyclic antidepressants, antipsychotics, centrally acting antihypertensives such as clonidine, diphenhydramine, and the belladonna alkaloids such as atropine, scopolamine, and hyoscyamine.

3. Which medical conditions are commonly associated with xerostomia?
Two of the most common are Sjögren's syndrome and radiation-induced salivary gland dysfunction. The vast majority of patients with radiation-induced salivary gland dysfunction have received ionizing radiation for head and neck carcinoma. Several other disorders also can lead to dysfunction of one or more of the major salivary glands (parotid, submandibular, and sublingual),

but patients are rarely symptomatic because salivary flow must decrease by approximately 50% before xerostomia develops.

4. Are there complications of salivary gland hypofunction?
Saliva contains a variety of polypeptides and glycoproteins that have antimicrobial activity. In the absence of these elements, the most common complications are recurrent **oral candidiasis** and **dental caries**.

5. A 27-year-old woman comes to your office with painful mouth sores that began 24 hours ago. On exam, she has several white lesions on her pharynx, soft palate, and tongue. She had similar lesions 3 years ago, which resolved over 2 weeks. What is the most likely diagnosis?
Most likely, recurrent aphthous stomatitis. Aphthous ulcers are the most common type of nontraumatic ulcers. In the general population, the incidence is 10–20%. The incidence in professionals and upper socioeconomic groups is higher.

6. What causes aphthous ulcers?
The cause of these lesions is still unknown. However, the following have been implicated:
1. Viral agents (herpes simplex virus)
2. Bacteria (*Streptococcus sanguis*)
3. Nutritional deficiencies (B_{12}, folate, iron)
4. Hormonal alterations
5. Stress
6. Trauma
7. Food allergies (nuts, chocolate, gluten)
8. Immunologic abnormalities

7. Name the three types of aphthous ulcers.
Minor, major, and herpetiform.

8. How do the various types of aphthous ulcers differ?
Minor: A tingling or burning sensation is usually noticed by the patient prior to the appearance of the ulceration. The ulcerations usually measure < 1.0 cm and are localized to the freely moveable keratinized gingiva. They are white in the center surrounded by a red border. They are extremely painful and usually resolve in approximately 7–10 days.

Major: These can occur on the moveable mucosa, soft palate, tongue, and tonsillar pillars. They are much more painful than the minor ulcers and are also much larger, measuring 1–3 cm. Anywhere from 1–10 ulcers may be present.

Herpetiform: These ulcers are similar to herpetic lesions. There are usually 10–100 ulcers present, measuring 1–3 mm in diameter. These small ulcers may coalesce to form larger ulcers.

The minor and major types generally do not leave a scar, whereas the herpetiform variety may leave a scar if the ulcerations coalesce.

9. What is the current treatment for aphthous stomatitis?
Treatment includes both medical management and cauterization. Cauterization of the ulcer bed can be done either chemically or electrically. Silver nitrate is commonly used for chemical cauterization. After the application of silver nitrate, the area should be swabbed with a cotton-tip applicator impregnated with sodium chloride. This agent converts the silver nitrate to silver chloride, preventing a deep burn. When using electrical cauterization, care must be taken not to produce a deep burn.

Medical treatment includes oral antibiotics, anti-inflammatory agents, or immunosuppressants. Treatment with yogurt, cultured buttermilk, and *Lactobacillus* capsules has also been recommended. Local measures include the use of an oral suspension of tetracycline or topical steroids, such as 0.5% fluocinonide ointment or betamethasone solution.

10. A 30-year-old otherwise healthy man presents with small, creamy white, curdlike lesions on his tongue and buccal mucosa of several weeks' duration. What is your diagnosis?

This presentation is consistent with the diagnosis of thrush, or **oral candidiasis**. *Candida* species are present in normal oral flora in 40–60% of the population. In certain immunocompromised states, overgrowth of the candida can occur, leading to thrush. The lesions represent patches of *Candida albicans* with leukocytes and desquamated epithelial cells.

11. How is the diagnosis of thrush made?

The diagnosis can easily be made by scraping the lesions (they are easy to remove and have an erythematous base) and then examining the scrapings in potassium hydroxide under the microscope. Characteristic hyphae and blastospores are easily recognized.

12. When thrush is suspected, what should your diagnostic workup include?

Common conditions that lead to thrush include inhaled corticosteroid use for reactive airways disease, debilitating systemic illnesses such as cancer, and other immunocompromised states such as AIDS and neutropenia. Less common etiologies include diabetes, pregnancy, adrenal insufficiency, systemic antibiotic and systemic steroid use, nutritional deficiencies, and poor oral hygiene. The differential diagnosis includes leukoplakia and hyperkeratosis. Patients who have thrush for no obvious reason, such as the patient presented above, should be evaluated for HIV disease.

13. A 60-year-old woman seen in your office complains of ulcerations involving the free and attached gingiva. She noted some raised areas and a diffuse redness and peeling of the mucous membrane prior to the appearance of the ulcerations. What is the most likely diagnosis?

Desquamative gingivitis affects females after the age of 30. It is characterized by a diffuse erythematous desquamation, ulceration, and, at times, bullae formation involving the free and attached gingiva. Associated conditions include lichen planus, cicatricial pemphigoid, bullous pemphigoid, pemphigus vulgaris, dermatitis herpetiformis, and drug reactions. Incisional biopsy is frequently necessary for diagnosis. Immunofluorescent studies may aid in differentiating the various entities.

14. How often are white oral lesions malignant?

Acutely, lesions of the oral cavity may be erythematous. However, during the course of the disease, white elements may appear and predominate. White lesions of the mouth are often benign. However, 5–10% of oral malignancies present as white lesions. Thus, the examining physician must always be concerned that the lesion in question is a possible malignancy.

15. What are the two broad clinical categories of white lesions?

Keratotic and nonkeratotic. The most important clinical feature distinguishing the two groups is the lesion's ability to adhere to the surface epithelium. The more common lesions can therefore be categorized into one of these two groups. In some cases, the pathologic process causing the oral lesions also involves the skin. If a diagnosis cannot be made clinically by observation or association with a cutaneous counterpart, a biopsy with immunofluorescent staining will be of value in establishing a diagnosis.

Keratotic	Nonkeratotic
Firmly adherent	Removed relatively easily
Usually of long duration	Usually of short duration
Usually change slowly	Frequently change rapidly
Surface is usually elevated and may be smooth, roughened, or even verrucous	Usually erosive or ulcerative

16. Which disease states can lead to keratotic and nonkeratotic white lesions?

Keratotic

Clinical leukoplakia

Stomatitis nicotina of the palate

Carcinoma in situ

Squamous cell carcinoma

Florid oral pappilomatosis

Verruca

Squamous papilloma

Chronic candidiasis

Interstitial glossitis (tertiary syphilis)

Hereditary and nevoid white lesions

Primary skin lesions

Lichen planus

Lupus erythematosus

Psoriasis

Nonkeratotic

Acute candidiasis

Aphthous stomatitis

Vesiculobulbous diseases

Viral infection

Contact dermatitis

Drug reaction

Pemphigus vulgaris

Benign mucous-membrane pemphigus

Bullous pemphigoid

Erythema multiforme

Trauma

  Mechanical

  Chemical

  Thermal

Desquamative gingivitis

Acute lupus erythematosus

Secondary syphilis

Psoriasis

17. A 45-year-old man who drinks and smokes heavily has a white plaque lesion on the undersurface of his tongue. He noticed the area when brushing his teeth and could not rub it off with the brush. What is the most likely diagnosis?

Clinical **leukoplakia** is the most likely diagnosis. Leukoplakia refers to a white patch or plaque of the mouth that cannot be removed by rubbing and cannot be ascribed to other diseases (such as lichen planus). Because 30% of these lesions are malignant, a biopsy is necessary. Asymptomatic, velvety red lesions of the mouth may be even more suspect for carcinoma in situ and should be biopsied.

18. What is a "geographic" tongue?

Loss and regrowth of papillae lead to red patches on the tongue. This map-like appearance is asymptomatic and results from an idiopathic inflammatory condition.

19. Where does squamous cell carcinoma most often occur in the mouth?

The lower lip, floor of the mouth, and tongue. Painless ulcers that do not heal in 1–2 weeks are highly suspect and should be biopsied.

20. What is the differential diagnosis of an oral pigmented lesion?

The most worrisome diagnosis is malignant melanoma, but other possibilities include nevi and benign macules, lesions of Peutz-Jeghers disease, or Addison's disease. Any new suspicious lesion should by followed and biopsied early.

21. Who develops hairy leukoplakia?

White painless lesions that appear "hairy" are often found in patients with AIDS, usually on the lateral aspects of the tongue. These lesions are caused by the Epstein-Barr virus and may temporarily respond to high-dose acyclovir.

22. What is torus mandibulae? Torus palatinus?

Both torus mandibulae and torus palatinus are usually an incidental finding on routine examination of the oral cavity. **Torus mandibulae** consists of an enlargement of bone, usually on the lingual surface of the mandible. The enlargement is found above the insertion of the mylohyoid muscle. It is covered by normal mucosa of the oral cavity. The mass may consist of one single bony formation or multiple bony ridges. These bony abnormalities are thought to be autosomal dominantly inherited with variable penetration.

Torus palatinus is a slow-growing enlargement located on the hard palate at its midportion. It may be single or multiple and is covered by normal-appearing oral mucosa. This bony growth is more frequent in females, although in the American Indian population, males predominate. It is thought to be inherited in an autosomal dominant pattern, but X-linked dominance may be a factor.

23. How is torus mandibulae managed? Torus palatinus?

Neither of these lesions should be surgically removed unless they interfere with denture placement or normal function. However, a torus palatinus may become excessively large, altering speech and thus necessitating its removal. Occasionally, they ulcerate, causing persistent discomfort and pain and again necessitating surgical removal.

24. What is trench mouth?

Acute necrotizing ulcerative gingivitis (ANUG), or Vincent's gingivitis, is a synergistic infection involving multiple oral anaerobic bacteria that is found in adolescents and young adults. Numerous factors increase the susceptibility to bacterial destruction and include debilitating disease, nutritional deficiencies, psychogenic factors, and degenerative disease. ANUG spares the edentulous patient.

Patients usually complain of ulcerations on the gingival margin. On physical examination, the typical lesions are punched-out, crater-like depressions in the interdental papillae and along the gingival margins. The lesions are covered by a gray pseudomembrane containing a meshwork of fibrin, necrotic epithelial cells, and various bacterial organisms. During the acute phase, the patient may have malaise, fever, regional lymphadenitis, fetid oris, increased salivation, and spontaneous gingival hemorrhage. Treatment consists of local measures (vigorous oral hygiene and removal of callus formation) and antibiotics to cover predominantly anaerobic organisms.

25. What are Fordyce spots?

Fordyce spots are very small, yellowish, granular lesions consistent with sebaceous glands on histologic examination. They are normally located in the mucosa lateral to the anterior pillar but also can be found in the upper lip, along the distal portion of the lower lip, and on the buccal mucosa at the angle of the mouth. To see them, one must spread the oral mucosa by placing it under tension. Removal of these structures is unnecessary unless the lesions are increasing in size, denoting an underlying pathologic condition.

26. What is a mucocele?

A mucous retention cyst, or mucocele, is a lesion of the lower lip or buccal mucosa. Chiefly of cosmetic concern, this benign nodule is either translucent or bluish in color and ranges from 1–2 cm in diameter. These cysts result from the retention of salivary gland contents and are commonly caused by trauma to the lower lip. The lesions are usually superficial and very thin-walled, transparent in nature, and true cysts. If a thin wall is not present with mucoid material, this type of lesion is commonly referred to as a mucous retention cyst. Mucoceles located deep in the lip tissue may appear as ill-defined discrete masses. These lesions may be surgically excised in their entirety or they may be marsupialized (the lining is incised and the mucoid material allowed to drain). Because there are numerous minor salivary glands present in the lip and other areas of the oral mucosa, the recurrence rate after removal of these lesions is high. Treatment may also involve repeated needle aspiration.

BIBLIOGRAPHY

1. Allen CM, Blozis GG: Oral mucosal lesions. In Cummings CW, et al (eds): Otolaryngology–Head and Neck Surgery, 2nd ed, St. Louis, Mosby, 1993.
2. Aragon SB, Jafek BW: Stomatitis. In Bailey BJ, et al (eds): Head & Neck Surgery–Otolaryngology. Philadelphia, J.B. Lippincott, 1993, p. 531.

3. Atkinson JC, Fox PC: Salivary gland dysfunction. Clin Geriatr Med 8:499–508, 1992.
4. Barker RL, Burton JR, Zieve PD (eds): Principles of Ambulatory Medicine. Baltimore, Williams & Wilkins, 1991.
5. Epstein JB: The painful mouth: Mucositis, gingivitis, stomatitis. Infect Dis Clin North Am 2:183-200, 1988.
6. Krull EA, Fellman AC, Fabian LA: White lesions of the mouth. Ciba Clin Symp 25(2):1–32, 1973.
7. Lucente FE: Otolaryngologic aspects of acquired immunodeficiency syndrome. Med Clin North Am 75:1389–1398, 1991.
8. Mandell GL, Bennett JE, Dolin R (eds): Principles and Practice of Infectious Disease. New York, Churchill Livingstone, 1995.

25. FACIAL NERVE DISORDERS

Shawna Harris Abbey

1. Name the five segments of the facial nerve. What are their course and length?

1. **Meatal:** from brainstem to internal auditory canal (IAC); 23–24 mm

2. **Labyrinthine:** from fundus of IAC to facial hiatus, where the fallopian is the narrowest; 3–5 mm

3. **Tympanic:** from geniculate ganglion to pyramidal eminence; 8–11 mm

4. **Mastoid:** from pyramidal process to stylomastoid foramen; 10–14 mm

5. **Extratemporal:** from the stylomastoid foramen to the muscles of facial expression and posterior belly of digastric, stylohyoid, and postauricular; 15–20 mm

2. Name the five major branches of the extratemporal segment of cranial nerve VII. What do they innervate?

1. **Cervical:** platysma

2. **Ramus mandibularis:** lower orbicularis oris, depressor anguli oris, depressor labii inferioris, and mentalis; it travels superficial to the facial vein at the inferior border of the mandible

3. **Buccal:** zygomaticus major and minor, levator anguli oris, buccinator, and upper orbicularis oris; it courses in close relation to the parotid duct

4. **Zygomatic:** lower orbicularis oculi; it anastomoses with the buccal branch

5. **Temporal:** frontalis, corrugator supercilii, procerus, and upper orbicularis oculi

3. What is the blood supply to the VIIth nerve?

Labyrinthine branches of the anterior inferior cerebellar artery (AICA) supply the meatal segment within the IAC. The petrosal branch of the middle meningeal artery supplies the nerve in the perigeniculate region. The stylomastoid branch of the postauricular artery feeds the mastoid and tympanic segments.

4. During surgery, what are the landmarks for identifying the facial nerve?

First, follow the sternocleidomastoid muscle to its insertion on the mastoid process. Now, identify the tragal pointer, a triangular extension of the tragal cartilage which points toward the main trunk. The nerve usually lies 10 mm inferior and 10 mm deep to the tragal pointer. Next, follow the posterior belly of the digastric muscle. At this point, find the styloid process. The nerve courses posterior and lateral to this process. Now, identify the tympanomastoid fissure. Find the marginal mandibular nerve as it crosses the posterior facial vein, following it proximally. Next, identify branches distally as they exit the parotid, also following them proximally. Lastly, find the nerve in the mastoid and follow it distally to the extratemporal portion.

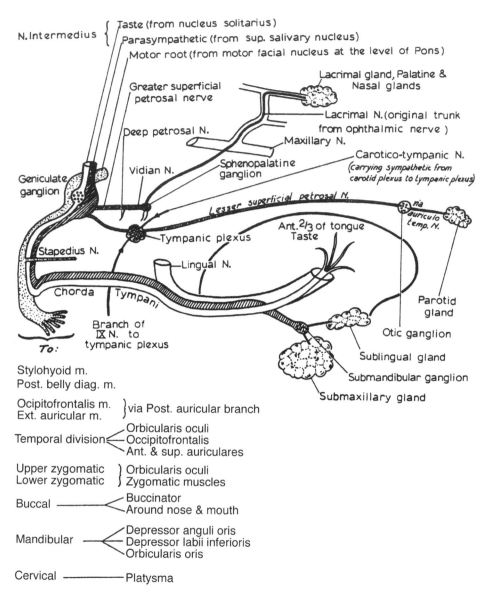

The facial nerve. (From Lee KJ: The vestibular system and its disorders. In Lee KJ (ed): Essential Otolaryngology–Head and Neck Surgery. Norwalk, CT, Appleton & Lange, 1995, p 194, with permission.)

5. Discuss the pathophysiology of nerve injury.

Nerve injury is classically described in terms of neuropraxia, axonotmesis, or neurotmesis.

Neurapraxia results when a lesion compresses the flow of axoplasm from the somata to the distal axons. In this case, the nerve is viable and returns to normal function when the blockade is corrected. Electrophysiologic testing reveals normal function, except that EMG fails to show voluntary motor action potentials because they are not conducted across the blockade.

Axonotmesis is a state of wallerian degeneration distal to the lesion with preservation of the motor axon endoneural sheaths. Electrically, the nerve shows rapid and complete degeneration, with loss of voluntary motor units. Regeneration to the motor end plates will occur, as long as the endoneural tubules are intact.

The lesion in **neurotmesis** is characterized by both wallerian degeneration and loss of endoneural tubules. Electrophysiologic studies yield evidence of complete nerve degeneration. Regeneration is dependent on many factors, including the integrity of the endoneurium, perineurium, and epineurium and the extent of ischemia and scarring around the lesion.

6. List the most common causes of facial paralysis.

Causes of Facial Paralysis

Idiopathic	**Neoplasia**
Bell's palsy	Cholesteatoma
Recurrent facial palsy	Glomus jugulare or tympanicum
Melkersson-Rosenthal syndrome	Carcinoma (primary or metastatic)
	Facial neuroma
Trauma	Schwannoma of lower cranial nerves
Temporal bone fractures*	Meningioma
Birth trauma	Leukemia
Facial contusions/lacerations	Histiocytosis
Penetrating wounds to face and temporal bone	Rhabdomyosarcoma
Iatrogenic injury	
	Congenital
Infection	Compression injury
Herpes zoster oticus (Ramsay Hunt syndrome)	Möbius syndrome*
Otitis media with effusion	Lower lip paralysis
Acute suppurative otitis media	
Coalescent mastoiditis	**Metabolic and systemic**
Chronic otitis media	Pregnancy
Malignant otitis externa (*Pseudomonas* osteomyelitis)	Diabetes mellitus
Tuberculosis	Sarcoidosis*
Lyme disease*	Guillain-Barré syndrome*
AIDS	Autoimmune disorders
Infectious mononucleosis	

* May present with bilateral palsy.
Adapted from Coker NJ: Acute paralysis of the facial nerve. In Bailey BJ, et al (eds): Head and Neck Surgery–Otolaryngology. Philadelphia, J.B. Lippincott, 1993, p 1715.

7. What elements of the history and physical examination are important in evaluating a facial paralysis?

Evaluation of Facial Paralysis

History	**Physical examination**
Onset	Complete head and neck evaluation
Duration	Microscopic otoscopy
Rate of progression	Upper aerodigestive tract examination
Recurrent or familial	Cranial nerve assessment (III–XII)
Associated symptoms	Palpation of parotid gland and neck
Major medical illness or previous surgery	
Trauma	**Facial palsy**
	Complete vs. incomplete (paresis)
Neurologic evaluation	Segmental vs. uniform involvement
Cerebellar signs	Unilateral vs. bilateral
Motor	Schirmer
Evidence of trauma	

Modified from Coker NJ: Acute paralysis of the facial nerve. In Bailey BJ, et al (eds): Head and Neck Surgery–Otolaryngology. Philadelphia, J.B. Lippincott, 1993, p 1714.

8. How can you evaluate the five branches of the extratemporal segment of the facial nerve during physical examination?

It is important to test each of the five branches of the nerve in order to exclude isolated branch paralysis or central lesions. To ensure that contraction of the masseter or temporalis muscle is not mistaken for facial nerve function, you should make each of the following assessments while jaw movements are minimized.

Cervical—contract the neck muscles
Ramus mandibularis—whistle or pucker the lips
Buccal—smile or show teeth
Zygomatic—squeeze eyes shut tightly
Temporal—raise eyebrows

9. What is Schirmer's test?

Schirmer's test is a method to assess parasympathetic innervation to the lacrimal gland via the greater superficial petrosal nerve. The procedure entails placing 5-mm × 35-mm paper strips in the conjunctival fornix of each eye and measuring lacrimation by comparing the length of paper moistened by tear flow over a 5-minute period. An abnormal Schirmer's test involves a 25% reduction of the ipsilateral eye as compared to normal lacrimation, a 30% reduction of the involved side versus total lacrimation, or < 25 mm bilateral lacrimation.

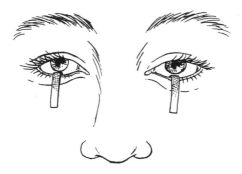

Schirmer's test. (From Pender DJ: Practical Otology. Philadelphia, J.B. Lippincott, 1992, p 118, with permission.)

10. Which radiologic studies should be part of the diagnostic workup for a patient with a facial paralysis?

Radiologic tests are not indicated for the assessment of every patient presenting with a facial nerve paralysis. The need for such studies is based on both the clinical history and course of the paralysis (i.e., if a neoplasm is suspected). If radiologic imaging is deemed necessary, high-resolution CT or MRI is the study of choice. MR scans are superior to CT in imaging the nerve at the cerebellopontine angle and internal auditory canal. Gadolinium-enhanced MRI is the test of choice for facial nerve paralysis secondary to inflammatory and other nontraumatic etiologies. CT, on the other hand, is preferred for the evaluation of traumatic VII nerve paralysis.

11. Which electrophysiologic tests are important in evaluating a patient with a facial paralysis?

Nerve Excitability Test (NET): In this study, a 1/sec^2 wave pulse which is 1 msec in duration is applied over both the affected and unaffected facial nerves. Thresholds for minimal facial muscle response are recorded and compared. A 3–4-mA or greater difference is considered significant, suggesting denervation. Limitations to this test include the requirement that the patient must be 3 days after the onset of symptoms and the patient must not have had the paralysis for > 3 months.

Maximal Stimulation Test (MST): A variation of the NET, the MST stimulates the ipsilateral and contralateral facial muscles at a level sufficient to depolarize all motor axons underlying the stimulator. Therefore, it utilizes maximal as opposed to minimal stimulation to evaluate muscular response. The results of the test are recorded as a subjective account of the difference in facial muscle movement between the normal and involved sides. Generally, it is thought that the MST becomes abnormal before the NET and is therefore a better prognostic indicator. However, the MST is limited by its lack of objectivity.

Electroneuronography (ENoG): ENoG measures and compares the amplitudes of the summation potentials that are elicited when a supramaximal level of current is applied over the main trunk of the facial nerve on the affected and unaffected sides. The peak-to-peak amplitude is directly proportional to the number of intact motor axons, thus providing a gauge to assess neuronal degeneration. An evoked summation potential of ≤ 10% indicates 90% degeneration, and surgical decompression is warranted. ENoG is limited by a short window of opportunity, and it must be done within 2 weeks of the onset of paralysis.

Electromyography (EMG): EMG is complementary in the evaluation of acute facial paralysis, helping to eliminate false-positive results obtained by NET, MST, and ENoG. The EMG determines the activity of the muscle rather than the activity of the nerve. This test can (1) provide information regarding intact motor units in the acute phase and (2) confirm the integrity of intact axons in the recovery phase, detecting reinnervation potentials 6–12 weeks before the return of facial muscle function is clinically evident. However, unlike NET, MST, and ENoG, an EMG cannot assess the degree of degeneration or prognosis for recovery.

Audiometry: Audiometry should be performed to evaluate the potential for conductive and sensorineural hearing losses which can be coexistent in patients with facial nerve palsies. Conductive hearing losses are most consistent with middle ear tumors, cholesteatomas, and other middle ear processes involving the horizontal segment of the facial nerve. Sensorineural deficits, on the other hand, indicate conditions such as acoustic neuroma, meningioma, congenital cholesteatoma, and dermoid and facial nerve neuromas which affect the nerve in the cerebellopontine angle or internal auditory canal.

12. What is Bell's palsy?

Bell's palsy is an idiopathic demyelinating inflammatory disease characterized by:
1. An acute onset usually preceded by a viral prodrome
2. 3–5 day duration with a peak in symptoms at 48 hours
3. Unilateral loss of facial expression

The patient may have a widened palpebral fissure, diminished taste, difficulty chewing, hypesthesia in one or more branches of the fifth cranial nerve, and hyperacusis. In 10% of patients with Bell's palsy, family history will be positive. Some 12% of patients may have recurrent facial paralysis, either ipsilateral or contralateral.

13. How common is Bell's palsy?

Bell's palsy accounts for over 50% of acute facial palsies. However, it is important to realize that this is a diagnosis of exclusion. A diagnosis of Bell's palsy is less probable if any of the following signs and symptoms are present:

History of known trauma along the course of the nerve
Multiple cranial nerve involvement
Bilateral paralysis
Slowly progressive paresis evolving for > 3 weeks
Signs of neoplasia
Vesicles on the head or neck
Evidence of a temporal bone infection
Palsy at birth
Signs of a CNS lesion
Failure to have onset of recovery within 6 months after onset

14. What is the most common complication following the onset of facial paralysis?

Corneal desiccation secondary to (1) paralysis with inability to close the eyelid completely, (2) diminished tearing, and (3) loss of corneal sensitivity with trigeminal nerve involvement. Evidence for corneal irritation includes redness, itching, foreign-body sensation, and visual blurring. Treatment involves using artificial tears 4–5 times /day. Ophthalmic lubricant should be followed by patching or taping the eye shut at night. The eye should be protected from wind, foreign bodies, and drying with glasses and/or moisture chambers.

15. What are crocodile tears?

Injuries to the facial nerve may be associated with nerve regeneration. Fibers that normally innervate the submaxillary gland may regenerate to innervate the lacrimal gland. This leads to "crying" when the patient eats.

16. How do you treat facial nerve paralysis medically?

The medical management of facial nerve paralysis employs several philosophies:

1. If infectious processes are ascertained, appropriate treatment with antimicrobial and/or antiviral agents, in addition to eradication of the infectious nidus (i.e., mastoidectomy/myringotomy), should be instituted.

2. Though controversial, a 7–10 day course of oral steroids, if initiated within the first 48 hours after onset of symptoms, may improve recovery via decreased inflammation.

3. Electrophysiologic assessment of the extent of nerve damage provides valuable information, particularly in cases where surgical decompression may be a treatment option.

4. Finally, prophylactic eye care to protect against corneal desiccation should be initiated in all patients with a facial nerve paralysis.

However, if paralysis is incomplete, many clinicians hold the belief that no treatment is necessary, especially with idiopathic facial palsy.

17. When is surgical treatment indicated?

Clinical Scenario	Surgical Intervention
Facial paralysis due to trauma	Nerve decompression, anastomosis
Paralysis secondary to acute OM	Myringotomy
Nerve paralysis due to chronic OM	Decompression, mastoidectomy
Iatrogenic injury to facial nerve	Decompression, anastomosis
Complete idiopathic paralysis	Decompression

OM—otitis media.

18. If the nerve is cut during surgery, can it be fixed?

Yes. A nerve that is cut during surgery can be repaired by using the same techniques that are employed in the surgical management of traumatic facial nerve lacerations. Nerve anastamosis via epineural or perineural repair is performed by exact end-to-end approximation under the illumination and magnification of the operating microscope. A 9.0 or 10.0 monofilament suture is then used to tie the nerve ends together without putting tension on the anastomosis. Interpositional grafts, most often from the greater auricular or sural nerves, can enhance nerve-end apposition if the anastomosis creates tension.

19. What is the Möbius syndrome?

This congenital condition is characterized by facial paralysis that can be either unilateral or bilateral, complete or incomplete, in association with bilateral abducens nerve palsies. Concomitant findings include tongue weakness and talipes equinovarus (clubfoot) in one-third of patients. Abnormal development of the VIIth nerve itself, of the facial musculature, or of the facial motor nucleus has been postulated as a cause of the syndrome, although the etiology may also be a destructive process secondary to in utero hypoxia.

20. What is the association between facial nerve paralysis and otitis media? Mastoiditis? Cholesteatoma?

In **otitis media** (OM), facial palsy can present as a complication of acute suppurative OM, OM with effusion, and chronic OM. The palsy results from an inflammatory reaction within the narrow fallopian canal to the inciting infectious agent. In both **mastoiditis** and **cholesteatoma**, direct mass compression, in addition to the inflammatory response, results in a facial nerve palsy. The mainstay of treatment, particularly if the palsy is a complication of OM, is to eradicate the infection with a combination of aggressive antibiotic therapy and, if necessary, surgical decompression via myringotomy and drainage or tympanomastoid surgery. Facial palsy secondary to coalescent mastoiditis may be managed surgically with myringotomy followed by a mastoidectomy. Surgical excision is necessary in patients with cholesteatomas.

21. Describe the most common traumatic injuries to the facial nerve.

Traumatic injuries to the facial nerve generally fall within two categories, penetrating wounds and temporal bone fractures.

Penetrating wounds of the cheek, face, or parotid gland may lacerate the facial nerve trunk or one of its branches. VII nerve lacerations such as these are repaired surgically by approximating the two ends of the cut nerve using 10.0 monofilament nylon suture. Generally, the results of facial nerve repairs are excellent. However, if the main facial nerve trunk has been divided by the laceration, synkinesis results during the regenerative process.

Temporal bone fractures involve the facial nerve nearly 50% of the time via laceration or contusion of the nerve within its bony fallopian canal. The mechanism of immediate traumatic facial paralysis is most often complete severance of the nerve within the bony canal. In these instances, surgical repair is indicated, but the surgery is not performed until 3 weeks after injury. This delay optimizes the results by taking advantage of the physiologic processes occurring within the nerve. If, following a closed head injury, a delayed facial paralysis develops over a period of 1–7 days, medical management with steroidal anti-inflammatory agents and electrophysiologic monitoring to map the course of recovery is instituted.

22. What conditions suggest the possibility of a neoplastic etiology for facial paralysis?

Paresis evolving slowly over a period exceeding 3 weeks
Coexistence of facial twitching with an evolving paresis
Development of chronic eustachian tube dysfunction in a patient with no prior history of chronic middle ear disease
Presence of multiple cranial nerve deficits
No return of facial function when the process has had an opportunity for regeneration
Recurrent palsy on the same side
Presence of neck or parotid mass
History of cancer

23. A patient presents to the ENT clinic complaining of involuntary, annoying facial movements. What are the most common types of facial "tics"?

Essential blepharospasm is a neurologic disease of unknown origin that results in rapid blinking of the eyes bilaterally, indicating that the lesion is central rather than peripheral. Some patients suffering from essential blepharospasm are declared legally blind because their eyelids close so frequently and so tightly. Medical treatment consists of injections of modified botulinum toxin into the orbicularis oris muscle. Surgically, the nerve branches and/or the orbicularis oculi muscle can be resected.

Hemifacial spasm, a spastic disease that is most often unilateral, is thought to be the result of an idiopathic demyelination of the peripheral facial nerve. It is characterized by severe, grotesque contraction of the muscles of facial expression. While treatment with botulinum toxin injections often provides effective relief, some patients benefit from surgical intervention in the form of a posterior fossa craniotomy with isolation of the nerve from a compressing artery.

Facial myokymia, usually associated with multiple sclerosis or a malignant neoplasm of the brainstem, is a peculiar wormlike motion in the midfacial muscles.

Segmental fasciculation, consisting of barely perceptible twitches of one or two facial muscles, is often a precursor to a facial nerve neuroma. Clinically, this disorder begins with slight twitches around the eye or in the cheek, followed by enlargement of the involved area with concomitant paralysis. Surgical removal is the only treatment.

24. What are herpes zoster oticus and Ramsay Hunt syndrome?

Herpes zoster oticus, in its simplest form, is characterized by intense ear pain and vesicles on the external auditory canal and concha, thus indicating that the dormant herpes zoster (chickenpox) virus has reactivated to affect sensory afferent neurons. If viral involvement progresses to involve the efferent motor axons of the facial nerve, then Ramsay Hunt syndrome has developed. This syndrome is characterized by the coexistence of (1) a facial nerve palsy and (2) vesicular eruptions on the head and neck in the distribution of the affected cranial nerve or cervical plexus. Treatment includes narcotic analgesics for pain relief, tapering doses of oral steroids to decrease inflammation, and acyclovir to inhibit viral DNA replication. If a secondary bacterial otitis externa develops, a topical otic antibiotic-hydrocortisone solution may be employed.

CONTROVERSIES

25. If the facial nerve is surgically removed (i.e., secondary to a parotid tumor), can facial function spontaneously return?

Yes. Although the exact mechanism behind this rare occurrence remains obscure, it is a phenomenon that has been extensively documented. Martin and Helsper consider the most likely mechanism to be fifth-nerve takeover. However, regrowth of facial nerve fibers has also been hypothesized.

26. What role do corticosteroids play in the treatment of Bell's palsy?

The use of corticosteroids in the treatment of idiopathic facial nerve paralysis is indeed an area of controversy. While some protocols recommend steroids to treat all patients with Bell's palsy, others indicate steroid therapy only in cases with total facial palsy. Still others advocate no role whatsoever for corticosteroid treatment. A 1993 study by Austin and colleagues strongly advocates the use of prednisone therapy, citing that patients given prednisone early in their disease course benefited significantly. These patients had less denervation and improvement in facial grade at recovery. Various other studies have shown less than promising results with steroid therapy.

BIBLIOGRAPHY

1. Austin JR, Peskind SP, Austin S, Rice DH: Idiopathic facial nerve paralysis: A randomized double blind controlled study of placebo versus prednisone. Laryngoscope 103:1326–1333, 1993.
2. Brownlee RE, Lee KJ, Drake AF: Facial nerve paralysis. In Lee KJ (ed): Essential Otolaryngology–Head and Neck Surgery, 6th ed. New York, Elsevier Science Publ., 1991, pp 181–196.
3. Coker NJ: Acute paralysis of the facial nerve. In Bailey BJ, et al (eds): Head and Neck Surgery–Otolaryngology. Philadelphia, J.B. Lippincott, 1993, pp 1711–1728.
4. Crumley RL: Facial nerve disorders. In American Academy of Otolaryngology–Head and Neck Surgery Foundation: Common Problems of the Head and Neck Region. Philadelphia, W.B. Saunders, 1992, pp 187–194.
5. Harker LA, Pignatari SS: Facial nerve paralysis secondary to chronic otitis media without cholesteatoma. Am J Otol 13:372–374, 1992.
6. Martin H, Helsper JT: Spontaneous return of function following surgical section or excision of the seventh cranial nerve in the surgery of parotid tumors. Ann Surg 151:538, 1960.
7. Shafshak TS, Essa AY, Bakey FA: The possible contributing factors for the success of steroid therapy in Bell's palsy: A clinical and electrophysiological study. J Laryngol Otol 108:940–943, 1994.

26. ESOPHAGEAL DISORDERS

Michael F. Spafford, M.D.

1. Where are most esophageal foreign bodies found?

95% of esophageal foreign bodies are located just inferior to the cricopharyngeus muscle. The force of this powerful sphincter muscle and the pharyngeal constrictors can transmit objects into the esophagus but they cannot be transported further by the esophageal musculature. The remaining 5% of foreign bodies are normally found in regions of anatomic narrowing of the esophagus: the gastroesophageal junction and the indentations of the esophagus caused by the arch of the aorta and left mainstem bronchus.

2. Where is Killian's triangle?

Killian's triangle is an area of weakness in the posterior esophagus. Specifically, it is located in the midline pharyngoesophageal segment, above the cricopharyngeus muscle and below the midline raphe of the inferior constrictor. This is the location of Zenker's diverticulum, a mucosal sac that protrudes between the oblique and transverse fibers of the cricopharyngeus muscle. This sac is thought to be formed by the repeated pulsion forces created by the contracting pharyngeal constrictors.

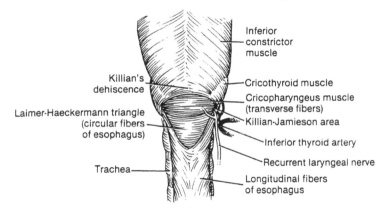

Pharyngoesophageal segment. (From Cummings CW, et. al (eds): Otolaryngology–Head and Neck Surgery, 2nd ed. St. Louis, Mosby, 1993, p 2370, with permission.)

3. How is a Zenker's diverticulum diagnosed and treated?

A Zenker's diverticulum is diagnosed primarily by history. About 70% of patients with a Zenker's diverticulum are over 60 years old. They typically report gradual-onset dysphagia of long duration, with food "sticking" at the level of the suprasternal notch. Another typical feature is regurgitation of the undigested food from the pouch with a foul odor and taste. Physical exam may show a palpable mass in the left neck, posteroinferior to the sternocleidomastoid muscle. Barium swallow is diagnostic and shows a pouch with multiple radiographic lucencies from retained food. Treatment usually consists of cricopharyngeal myotomy alone, although large diverticula should be resected.

4. In the complex neuromuscular sequence of swallowing, which step is most important for airway protection?

Laryngeal elevation. As the swallowing reflex begins, the suprahyoid muscles contract, as well as the thyrohyoid muscle. The resulting elevation brings the laryngeal inlet into a protected position under the tongue base. It also passively deflects the epiglottis to a position 60° below the horizontal, shielding the airway and directing food laterally. Finally, laryngeal elevation serves to dilate the upper esophageal sphincter, allowing food passage into the esophagus.

5. **Which type of caustic ingestion causes more severe esophageal injury, acid or alkaline?**

Acid causes coagulation necrosis, which creates a barrier to deeper penetration. **Alkaline** agents, however, cause a liquefaction necrosis and therefore tend to penetrate more quickly and deeply through tissue layers. Nevertheless, strong acids may produce severe burns and strictures.

6. **Where are the three anatomic narrowings of the esophagus?**

The upper esophageal sphincter, or **cricopharyngeus**, is at the level of the cricoid cartilage. The anterior compression by the **aortic arch and left mainstem bronchus** is approximately 20–25 cm from the upper incisors in the adult. The **gastroesophageal junction** is 40–45 cm away. These locations are significant because they are common sites for foreign bodies to lodge, and swallowed corrosive liquids may produce more damage in these areas.

7. **A child has ingested a caustic substance, but physical exam reveals no oral or pharyngeal burns. Is there cause for concern?**

Yes. After caustic ingestion, there is little correlation between the presence of burns on the lips, oral cavity, and pharynx and the presence of burns in the esophagus. If the substance is crystalline (i.e. detergent), there is a greater chance of proximal burning, because these substances are harder to swallow and the immediate pain prevents further ingestion. Liquid substances, on the other hand, are more likely to produce distal burns. Nevertheless, observation is indicated based on history alone.

8. **What intervention is required after a caustic ingestion?**

If the airway is compromised on presentation, it should be controlled with intubation or tracheotomy if the supraglottic structures are severely burned. All patients should be kept NPO, supported with intravenous fluids, and observed for acute complications. These include laryngeal edema with airway obstruction, esophageal perforation with mediastinitis, gastric perforation with peritonitis, and tracheoesophageal fistula with pneumonia. Esophagoscopy under general anesthesia is performed approximately 24 hours after ingestion. It is used to determine if a burn is present and the extent of the burn. A feeding tube may be placed carefully if severe or circumferential burns are encountered, although this is controversial. If burns are encountered, antibiotics and steroids are initiated. Antibiotics are shown to prevent intramural spread of infection and mediastinitis, and steroids have been found to help prevent formation of strictures if given in the first 24–48 hours. A contrast esophagogram is performed at 6 weeks to evaluate for stricture.

9. **What is globus pharyngeus?**

Globus pharyngeus is a foreign-body sensation, or "lump," in the throat. First described by Hippocrates, the sensation is familiar to many. This sensation localizes in the midline between the suprasternal notch and thyroid cartilage and occurs during strong emotion. The persistent sensation is estimated to account for 3–4% of otolaryngology referrals, and a workup is indicated to exclude serious underlying disease. Globus pharyngeus is considered a diagnosis of exclusion. Although controversial, several authors have recently reported a high incidence of gastroesophageal reflux disease (GERD) in patients with globus pharyngeus.

10. **What are the most common otolaryngologic manifestations of gastroesophageal reflux disease?**

Koufman recently studied 225 patients with GERD using 24-hour pH monitoring and found that the most common symptoms were hoarseness (71%), cough (51%), globus pharyngeus (47%), throat–clearing (42%), and difficulty swallowing (35%). Only 43% of patients had

GI symptoms such as heartburn or acid regurgitation. On physical exam, these patients often have laryngoscopic findings of chronic laryngitis, including vocal cord granulomas. The inflammation may be localized to the posterior larynx.

11. What are the most common causes of GERD?

The most common causes of GERD are factors that decrease lower esophageal sphincter pressure and include hiatal hernia and a variety of substances such as dietary fat, chocolate, mints, tobacco, ethanol, and many drugs. Other less common etiologies include abnormal esophageal motility, delayed gastric emptying, increased intra–abdominal pressure, and gastric hypersecretion.

12. How is GERD treated?

Treatment has three phases:

1. Lifestyle modification, including raising the head of the bed 6–8 inches, losing weight, and avoiding overeating and eating before bedtime. Tobacco, alcohol, and caffeine should be eliminated.

2. Pharmacologic therapy, including H2 blockers (i.e., ranitidine) or proton–pump inhibitors (i.e., omeprazole).

3. If these therapies fail, surgery may be considered (Nissen fundoplication).

13. Where do you find a Schatzki's ring?

Schatzki's ring is a concentric or weblike narrowing that appears at the junction of the esophageal and gastric mucosa in 6–14% of barium swallows. It is symptomatic only one–third of the time, when the esophageal lumen is reduced to < 13 mm. Intermittent solid food dysphagia is the most common symptom.

14. Are the terms "esophageal web" and "esophageal ring" interchangeable?

No. An **esophageal web** is a thin membrane that projects into the esophageal lumen and is covered with squamous epithelium. Webs can occur anywhere in the esophagus and may be single or multiple, concentric or eccentric. **Esophageal rings**, on the other hand, occur at the gastroesophageal junction and are covered with squamous epithelium on the upper surface and columnar epithelium on the lower surface.

15. What is Plummer-Vinson syndrome?

This syndrome typically occurs in patients of Scandinavian descent between the ages of 20 and 50; 90% of these patients are female. Manifestations include iron-deficiency anemia, dysphagia, hiatal hernia, atrophic gastritis, and achlorhydria. Upper esophageal webs occur in 86% of cases. There is an increased incidence of postcricoid and cervical esophageal carcinoma. Although the etiology is unclear, iron-deficiency anemia generally precedes the esophageal presentation, and iron therapy alone often improves the dysphagia.

16. Are any systemic diseases associated with esophageal motility disorders?

Polymyositis, characterized by systemic degenerative and inflammatory changes of the skin and striated muscle, is associated with esophageal dysmotility in 30% of cases. The affected portion is the pharynx and striated upper one-third of the esophageal musculature.

Scleroderma and other **connective tissue disorders** such as systemic lupus erythematosus, dermatomyositis, and Raynaud's disease produce a distinct pattern of esophageal dysmotility. Scleroderma, the most common of these disorders, produces a 52% rate of dysphagia and a 74% rate of histologic involvement. Small vessel arteritis and collagen deposition in the region of esophageal smooth muscle produce a dilated and aperistaltic lower two-thirds of the esophagus. This, combined with decreased function of the lower esophageal sphincter, leads to unremitting reflux with a high rate of esophagitis. This may lead to dysphagia, bleeding, and stricture.

Other systemic diseases that can affect esophageal motility include **diabetes mellitus** and **alcoholism**, causing a peripheral neuropathy. The degenerative and demyelinating **CNS diseases** also can decrease motility. **Chagas' disease** is a systemic parasitic infection that destroys the ganglion cells of Auerbach's plexus and produces a picture similar to achalasia.

17. Name the types of hiatal hernia.
  • **Type I**, or **sliding hiatal hernia**, features a phrenoesophageal membrane that is intact. Although a portion of the stomach can "slide" into the thorax, its size is limited, and no peritoneum actually enters the thorax.
  • In **type II hiatal hernia**, the membrane is defective, allowing a peritoneal sac to enter the thorax, which can progressively increase in size.

18. Describe the characteristic radiographic finding associated with diffuse esophageal spasm.
The barium esophagogram in this condition has been described to demonstrate a **corkscrew esophagus**, with curling or beading of the barium column. This curling develops because non-peristaltic simultaneous contraction of the lower two-thirds of the esophagus occurs. The symptoms are intermittent and consist of dysphagia, odynophagia, and chest pain that often forces a cardiac evaluation. Treatment includes reassurance and pharmacologic relaxation of the smooth muscle with nitrates, calcium channel blockers, and anticholinergic agents. Underlying GERD is also treated. Dilatation and myotomy are reserved for incapacitating cases.

19. What is dysphagia lusoria?
Dysphagia lusoria is caused by extrinsic esophageal compression by an anomalous right subclavian artery. Arising from the descending aorta, it must cross posteriorly behind the esophagus to reach the right arm. In 15% of cases, it passes between the trachea and esophagus. It is a fourth branchial arch anomaly.

20. How is a tracheoesophageal fistula diagnosed?
Esophageal atresia (EA) is the most common congenital anomaly affecting the esophagus, with an incidence of 1 in 3000. Variations are classified anatomically by whether a fistula is present and by its location relative to the atresia. The most common variation (86%) is esophageal atresia with a distal tracheoesophageal fistula (TEF), followed by isolated EA (7.7%), and then isolated TEF or H-type anomaly (4.2%). When esophageal atresia is present, fluids will be quickly regurgitated during and after feeding. A small **isolated TEF** (H-type anomaly) may remain asymptomatic until recurrent or refractory pneumonia presents. When a **distal TEF** is present, the stomach becomes distended with inspired air. Repeated aspiration of stomach contents will manifest itself as recurrent pneumonia. With a **proximal TEF**, feeding results in immediate choking and gagging, and if the distal segment is not connected to the airway, no gas will appear in the GI tract. Diagnosis can be made by the inability to pass a soft rubber catheter into the stomach or by the absence of gas on abdominal plain film, and is confirmed with a barium contrast study.

21. What is the embryologic etiology of TEF?
TEF results from a developmental failure of the tracheoesophageal septum between weeks 4–8 and/or failure of recannulation of the esophagus between weeks 3–8.

22. What sort of swallowing complaints can be expected in the elderly population?
Presbyesophagus is a term for the abnormalities of esophageal motility seen in the elderly. Histologically, partial denervation (a decrease in the number of ganglion cells in Auerbach's plexus) has been documented with aging. Although some degree of reduced peristalsis and occasional failure of lower esophageal relaxation can be seen in the elderly, most of these patients remain asymptomatic. When dysphasia does occur in this group, its location is most often oropharyngeal or hypopharyngeal, and its etiology is neuropathologic.

23. How do you approach dysphagia or odynophagia in the immunocompromised patient?

In the immunocompromised patient, one must have a high index of suspicion for esophageal infection. In HIV-infected patients, candida esophagitis is the most common etiology of new-onset esophageal symptoms. Initial empiric treatment with oral antifungal therapy (fluconazole or ketaconazole) is indicated. In contrast, esophageal symptoms in non–HIV-infected immuno-compromised patients, such as transplant recipients, are likely to represent infection with viral disease such as herpes or cytomegalovirus, and, less often, candida and fungal diseases. Therefore, these patients are more commonly taken initially for endoscopy and biopsy to help establish a diagnosis.

24. What are the three manometric findings in achalasia?

The three manometric findings that distinguish achalasia from other esophageal motility disorders are:
1. Increase in lower esophageal sphincter (LES) pressure
2. Absence of LES relaxation
3. Absence of esophageal peristalsis.

In its primary form, achalasia is associated with an idiopathic degeneration of the ganglion cells of Auerbach's plexus. The above forces produce esophageal dilatation or "megaesophagus."

25. How can cardiac pain be distinguished from esophageal pain?

It is thought that Galen (130–200 AD) coined the term *cardia* for the gastroesophageal region because pain arising there can closely mimic cardiac pain. Esophageal spasm can present with substernal chest pain which radiates to the arms and back. An esophageal spasm can be exacerbated by emotion and stress and can be relieved by nitroglycerin. The absence of an exertional component, temporal relationship to swallowing, and concomitant complaints of dysphagia or odynophagia may help identify an esophageal source of pain, but the more common and serious cardiac etiology must always be first ruled out.

26. What is nutcracker esophagus?

Nutcracker esophagus is the most common esophageal motility disorder in patients evaluated for noncardiac chest pain. It resembles diffuse esophageal spasm with substernal chest pain and dysphagia; however, the esophageal contractions remain peristaltic. Its etiology is also unknown. Calcium-channel blockers are the initial medical therapy.

BIBLIOGRAPHY

1. Couturier D, Samama J: Clinical aspects and manometric criteria in achalasia. Hepato-Gastroenterology. 38:481–487, 1991.
2. Ergon GA, Miskovitz PF: Aging and the esophagus: Common pathologic conditions and their effect upon swallowing in the geriatric population. Dysphagia 7(2):58–63, 1992.
3. Jones KR: The esophagus. In Lee KJ (ed): Essential Otolaryngology, 6th ed. Norwalk, CT, Appleton & Lange, 1995, pp 481–497.
4. Koufman JA: Gastroesophageal reflux disease. In Cummings CW, et al (eds): Otolaryngology–Head and Neck Surgery, 2nd ed. St. Louis, Mosby, 1993, pp 2349–2367.
5. Koufman JA: The otolaryngologic manifestations of gastroesophageal reflux disease (GERD): A clinical investigation of 225 patients using ambulatory 24-hour pH monitoring and an experimental investigation of the role of acid and pepsin in the development of laryngeal injury. Laryngoscope 101(4 pt 2/suppl 53):1–78, 1991.
6. Seiden AM: Esophageal Disorders. In Paparella MM, et. al (eds): Otolaryngology, 3rd ed. Philadelphia, W.B. Saunders Co., 1991, pp 2439–2481.
7. Snow JB: Esophagology. In Ballenger JJ (ed): Diseases of the Nose, Throat, Ear, Head and Neck, 14th ed. Malvern, PA, Lea & Febiger, 1991, pp 1297–1321.
8. Timon C, O'Dwyer T, Cagney D, Walsh M: Globus pharyngeus: Long-term follow-up and prognostic factors. Ann Otol Rhinol Laryngol 100(5 pt 1):351–354, 1991.
9. Wilcox CM, Karowe MW: Esophageal infections: Etiology, diagnosis, and management. Gastroenterologist 2(3):188–206, 1994.

27. THE THYROID AND PARATHYROID GLANDS

Catherine Winslow, M.D.

1. What does thyroid hormone do?

Thyroxine (T4) and triiodothyronine (T3) increase cellular metabolism, influence genomic expression, and alter the transcellular flux of substrates. The production is dependent on iodine, of which the normal adult requires 80 μg/day.

2. What is the embryologic origin of the thyroid gland? How is the origin important clinically?

In the fourth week of gestation, the thyroid appears as an invagination of the foramen cecum at the base of the tongue. The gland migrates inferiorly over the next 3 weeks to rest anterior to the larynx. It remains attached to the foramen cecum by the thyroglossal duct, a structure which later atrophies. Alteration in this process results in ectopic thyroid tissue, which may occur anywhere from the base of the tongue (**lingual thyroid**) along the persistent thyroglossal duct. A cyst along this duct is evident as a midline mass which moves with swallowing and protrusion of the tongue.

3. A patient presents with a mass at the base of his tongue, which you suspect is a lingual thyroid. How should you evaluate this patient?

If the thyroid gland fails to descend during development, lingual thyroid tissue may persist. A mass at the base of the tongue may be such a remnant or it may be an oral cancer. First, a good history and physical exam are of utmost importance. Evaluate the patient for oral cancer risk factors, such as smoking and alcohol intake. Feel the mass for irregularities, and palpate the neck for a normally located thyroid gland. If there is doubt, a thyroid scan which includes the base of the tongue should be done.

4. Does the lingual thyroid function normally in patients with no other thyroid tissue?

Most lingual thyroids are asymptomatic, and they may exist in up to 10% of the population. They are the only functioning thyroid tissue in 70–80% of patients with lingual thyroids. About 15% of these patients are hypothyroid. Intervention is warranted if the mass is symptomatic, as evidenced by airway obstruction, dysphagia, or dysphonia. Excision should be performed if the symptoms are refractory to suppression therapy.

5. What is the most common cause of hyperthyroidism?

Grave's disease, or diffuse toxic goiter, is the most common cause of hyperthyroidism. Usually affecting women aged 20–50, this autoimmune disease leads to enlargement of the thyroid gland. **Plummer's disease**, or nodular toxic goiter, is a less common cause of hyperthyroidism and affects elderly individuals. Rarer causes of hyperthyroidism include subacute thyroiditis, pituitary tumors, and struma ovarii.

6. Are there options to thyroidectomy in Grave's disease?

For hyperfunctioning thyroid tissue, antithyroid medications, radioactive iodine ablation of the gland, or surgical excision are all options. Radioactive iodine is contraindicated in women of childbearing age, and recurrence of hyperthyroidism is common after antithyroid medications. Hypothyroidism requiring lifelong replacement is common following surgery or iodine ablation.

7. What is the blood supply to the parathyroids?

The inferior thyroid artery, a branch of the thyrocervical trunk, supplies the parathyroids. The superior parathyroid artery, a branch of the external carotid, may also give branches. With vascular compromise, the parathyroids darken from tan to black.

8. Where do the parathyroids originate? Where are they anatomically located?
The superior parathyroids originate from the fourth branchial pouch, and the inferior parathyroids originate from the third branchial pouch. The superior glands lie between the upper and middle third of the thyroid gland. They may lie in the tracheoesophageal groove or on the posterior surface of the thyroid gland. Occasionally, they may be found within the thyroid gland itself. As a general rule, the superior parathyroid glands lie posteriorly to the recurrent laryngeal nerve, while the inferior parathyroid glands lie anterior to the nerve. The inferior parathyroids can occasionally be found in the thymus.

9. What is the most common cause of hyperparathyroidism?
Adenoma is the etiology in 80% of hyperparathyroidism cases. **Diffuse hyperplasia** is the etiology in 20% of cases. Carcinoma is rare (1–3%).

10. How often is hypercalcemia associated with hyperparathyroidism?
Hyperparathyroidism accounts for 20% of hypercalcemia cases. Over half of cases of hypercalcemia are due to bone metastases.

11. What are the predisposing factors associated with hyperparathyroidism?
Although most cases arise spontaneously without a known cause, > 10% of patients have a history of **radiation** to the neck. Familial parathyroid hyperplasia and multiple endocrine neoplasia syndromes suggest that **genetic factors** also may play an important role.

BIBLIOGRAPHY

1. Ackerstrom G, Malmaeus J, Bergstrom R: Surgical anatomy of human parathyroid glands. Surgery 95:14, 1984.
2. Cope O: Hyperparathyroidism: Diagnosis and management. Am J Surg 99:394, 1960.
3. Fish J, Moore R: Ectopic thyroid tissue and ectopic thyroid carcinoma. Ann Surg 157:212, 1963.
4. Hempleman L, ct al: Neoplasms in persons treated with x-rays in infancy for thymic enlargement. J Natl Cancer Inst 38:317, 1967.
5. Lore JM: An Atlas of Head and Neck Surgery. Philadelphia, W.B. Saunders, 1988, pp 726–810.
6. Noyek A, Friedberg J: Thyroglossal duct and ectopic thyroid disorders. Otolaryngol Clin North Am 14:187, 1981.
7. Walling A: Ectopic thyroid tissue. Am Fam Physician 36:147, 1987.

28. SALIVARY GLAND DISORDERS

Bruce W. Jafek, M.D.

1. What is the origin of the salivary glands?
The salivary glands arise as epithelial outpouchings from the primitive oral cavity (stomodeum), beginning in the 4th week. The parotids usually arise first (4th week), followed by the submandibular glands (6th week), and the sublingual glands (9th week).

2. What is Stenson's duct?
The mature **parotid gland** is the largest of the salivary glands and lies on the side of the face, just anterior and inferior to the ear, and is in contact with the posterior surface of the ascending ramus of the mandible. **Stenson's duct** arises at the anterior border of the gland, travels forward over the masseter muscle, and passes through the buccinator muscle to enter the oral cavity in proximity to the second upper molar.

do you find Wharton's duct?

 submandibular gland lies under the horizontal ramus of the mandible just superficial oglossus muscle. Its duct, called **Wharton's duct**, opens anteriorly in the floor of the mou. just lateral to the base of the frenulum of the tongue.

4. What is the plica sublingualis?

The smallest named salivary glands are the sublingual glands, which lie along a fold under the tongue called the plica sublingualis. This fold originates anteriorly at the frenulum of the tongue, and travels posteriorly and laterally toward the angle of the mandible. The sublingual glands have 8–15 excretory ducts with their minute orifices along the plica.

5. How do the submandibular and submaxillary glands differ?

These two terms are interchangeable. Both are descriptive terms, based on the location of the gland. The gland, after all, lies beneath both the maxilla and mandible. Because the gland lies closer to the mandible, many authors prefer the term "submandibular."

6. What are the superficial and deep lobes of the parotid gland?

Although not having true "lobes," the parotid gland does have superficial and deep portions. The facial nerve (CN VIII) runs between these portions of the gland. This nerve exits the skull via the stylomastoid foramen, enters the substance of the parotid gland between its superficial and deep "lobes," and divides into five terminal branches. These branches leave the gland anteriorly to supply the mimetic musculature of the face.

7. Describe the branches of the facial nerve.

Following its exit from the stylomastoid foramen, the facial nerve divides into an upper and lower division at the pes anserinus (foot of the goose). The upper division divides into the **temporal branch**, which supplies the frontalis and orbicularis oculi, and the **zygomatic branch**, which also supplies the orbicularis oculi. The lower division divides into the **mandibular branch**, which supplies the muscles of the lower lip and chin, and the **cervical branch**, which supplies the platysma. A middle branch, the **buccal branch**, supplies the buccinator. The buccal branch may receive contributions from the upper and lower divisions, or it may arise separately at the pes. Other variations occur, making careful identification of the facial nerve and its branches critical.

8. Which nerves are at risk when the submandibular gland is resected?

During removal of the submandibular gland, for any reason, the lingual, marginal mandibular, and hypoglossal nerves are at risk. The marginal mandibular nerve is superior to the gland, while the hypoglossal nerve is inferior and deep to the gland. The lingual nerve is deep to the gland in the resection bed. These branches should be identified and preserved.

9. What common problems, besides tumors, cause salivary gland enlargement?
Parotitis
Salivary calculi or duct stricture
Benign lymphoepithelial disease (e.g., Sjögren's syndrome, Mikulicz' disease, Heerfordt's syndrome, Melkersson's syndrome)
Granulomatous parotitis (e.g., tuberculosis)
Bulimia
Lead or mercury intoxication
Chronic fatty infiltration (e.g., secondary to alcoholism, hypovitaminoses)

10. What causes viral parotitis?

Inflammation of the parotid gland, or parotitis, may be nonsuppurative or suppurative. The most common example of nonsuppurative viral parotitis is **mumps**, a once-common childhood disease. Mumps, caused by a paramyxovirus, is associated with bilateral painful parotid swelling, malaise, and trismus. Treatment is conservative (e.g., bedrest, heat, fluids, pain medications), as the condition is usually self-limited.

11. How is recurrent, nonsuppurative sialadenitis treated?

Recurrent, nonsuppurative enlargement of the submandibular or parotid salivary gland may occur due to obstruction of the draining duct by mucous plugs or stones. Mucolytic agents, massage, hydration, and secretagogues (e.g., lemon wedges) may be helpful.

12. Discuss suppurative sialadenitis.

Suppurative sialadenitis may be acute or chronic. **Acute** suppurative sialadenitis is characterized by swelling of the involved gland, pain, fever, and purulent discharge which may be expressed from the affected duct. It is often a complication of chronic dehydration in a debilitated patient such as a diabetic. Acute suppurative sialadenitis may also follow immunosuppression, radiation therapy, or chemotherapy. Classically, *Staphylococcus* is involved. Treatment revolves around hydration and antibiotics, but surgical drainage may be required in unresponsive cases. **Chronic** or **recurrent** suppurative sialadenitis may also require removal of the gland. Removal of these glands is more surgically complex than removal of a tumor because extensive fibrosis and bleeding are often present.

13. Which gland is most commonly affected by sialolithiasis?

The submandibular gland is affected in about 80% of cases. The stones are most commonly composed of hydroxyapatite. Sialolithiasis is characterized by pain and swelling of the affected gland, and symptoms may worsen when the patient eats.

14. How are salivary gland calculi managed?

Calculi are usually apparent on intraoral inspection or bimanual palpation. Sometimes they can be expressed bimanually. If this is impossible, an intraoral incision made over the stones facilitates their removal. Often, the duct eventually fistulizes into the oral cavity in this area, relieving the retrograde obstruction. If a stricture of the duct results, the duct can be reconstructed with a procedure termed sialodochoplasty. It may be necessary to remove the involved gland if the stones are recurrent and symptomatic or if the two described maneuvers are unsuccessful.

15. What is benign lymphoepithelial disease of the salivary glands?

Benign lymphoepithelial disease is an autoimmune disease commonly known as **Sjögren's syndrome**. The main salivary manifestations are xerostomia, recurrent infections, and glandular hypertrophy. Sialectasis of the ducts may be demonstrated on sialography. The diagnosis is confirmed with a minor salivary gland biopsy from the lip. Cholinergic drugs tend to produce significant side effects, and artificial saliva is poorly tolerated. Therefore, these patient often must carry a small bottle of water at all times. Infections are managed as necessary. Steroids are inconstant in effect. A parotidectomy may be indicated for cosmetic reasons.

16. How are parotid cysts managed? Why are special precautions needed?

Prior to the HIV era, cystic lesions of the parotid were thought to occur rarely. However, over the past decade, the reported incidence of these lesions has increased substantially. The classic management for any parotid mass includes a superficial parotidectomy as well as biopsy. However, because elective surgery on HIV patients poses additional risks for patients and health-care workers, and because surgical management does not affect the underlying disease, nonsurgical management of parotid cysts in these patients is now gaining favor.

Huang et al., in a recent review, recommend CT scanning to confirm the cystic nature and a fine needle aspiration (FNA) of all parotid tumors in patients at high risk for HIV infection. If the lesion is cystic on CT and benign on FNA, then watchful waiting and a nonsurgical approach are recommended, with repeat FNA for palliation. Although patients may request surgery for cosmetic or other unpleasant symptoms, Huang et al. do not recommend this procedure. Surgery should be reserved for suspicious solid lesions, especially with findings such as abnormal cells or a uniform lymphoid population on cytologic exam. In these cases, further pathologic diagnosis is warranted. Huang et al. also feel that an elevated amylase level in the parotid FNA specimen is suggestive of benign cystic disease. Finally, they suggest that any patient who presents with a parotid cyst should be investigated for possible HIV infection. Injection of the cyst with a sclerosing agent, such as tetracycline, has recently been shown to be helpful in treating these cysts.

17. What is a ranula?

Ranula is a nonspecific term for a cystic mass in the floor of the mouth. A localized form is limited to the oral cavity and is usually cured by excision or by marsupialization. A "plunging" form, characterized histologically by extravasated mucus, is more extensive and extends along muscle planes. It requires a more extensive procedure, often including excision of the submandibular gland.

18. How is drooling managed?

A normal person produces 1–1.5 pints of saliva a day. This saliva is important in initiating digestion, lubricating the teeth, etc. In neuromuscular problems such as cerebral palsy, drooling may occur, even though the production is normal. Treatment with anticholinergics is rarely successful, but salivary duct re-routing is often curative. In this procedure, the duct is mobilized and the orifice is sutured to a new, more posterior location in the mouth. This surgery facilitates swallowing and eliminates drooling.

19. How is trauma to the salivary glands managed?

For practical purposes, significant trauma to the salivary glands most commonly affects the parotid and submandibular glands, primarily the former. For **submandibular gland trauma**, the wound can be closed and observed, or the gland can be removed. A superficial salivary fistula is exceedingly rare in these cases; the gland usually undergoes atrophy if the saliva is unable to enter the oral cavity, either via the duct or via a new fistula. Where the duct is identified, it can be stented over a small silastic cannula. Trauma to the adjacent nerves (marginal mandibular, lingual, or hypoglossal) is managed by microsurgical approximation of the divided segments, with sharp freshening of the edges if necessary.

With **parotid trauma**, the facial nerve is managed similarly. After presurgical evaluation, the divided ends are microscopically approximated with 8-0 to 10-0 monofilament sutures. The duct is stented, if possible, or ligated. Subsequent external salivary fistulas can be managed by observation, elimination of parotid function (e.g., denervation or radiation therapy), or re-establishment of flow to the oral cavity. A sialocele can be managed by eliminating parotid function or re-establishing flow to the oral cavity, possibly by an intraoral incision and placement of a long-term drain.

BIBLIOGRAPHY

1. Cummings CW, et al (eds): Otolaryngology–Head and Neck Surgery. St. Louis, Mosby, 1993, pp 56–58, 997–1028.
2. Huang RD, Pearlman S, Friedman WH, Loree T: Benign cystic vs solid lesions of the parotid gland in HIV patients. Head Neck 13:522–526, 1991.
3. Norman, JE DeBurgh, McGurk M: Color Atlas & Text of the Salivary Glands: Diseases, Disorders & Surgery. London, Mosby-Wolfe/Times Mirror International Publishers Ltd., 1995.

29. DEEP SPACE NECK INFECTIONS

Ethan Lazarus, M.D.

1. How is the cervical fascia important in deep space neck infections?

The cervical fascia dictates the presentation, spread, and treatment of deep space neck infections (DSNIs). Enveloping structures and separating the neck into potential spaces, this fibrous connective tissue is composed of two main components, the **superficial** and **deep** cervical fascia. The deep cervical fascia is further divided into the superficial, middle, and deep layers.

2. Name the main deep neck spaces.

The hyoid bone is a critical landmark that divides the neck into 3 different general areas and limits the spread of infection.

Above the hyoid bone
   Submandibular (sublingual, submaxillary)
   Pharyngomaxillary (lateral pharyngeal)
   Peritonsillar
   Masticator
   Parotid
Below the hyoid bone
   Anterior visceral (pretracheal)
Spaces involving the entire length of the neck
   Vascular (involvement of carotid sheath)
   Prevertebral (can spread to coccyx)
   Danger space (spreads to superior mediastinum)
   Retropharyngeal (spreads to danger space)

3. What organisms typically cause DSNIs?

Most DSNIs contain mixed flora. Aerobic organisms include *Streptococcus* and *Staphylococcus*. Aerobic organisms tend to be associated with intravenous drug abuse. Infections of dental origin generally involve anaerobes, especially *Bacteroides*. In > 50% of cases, the specific pathogen is not identified.

4. Where do most DSNIs originate?

Before the era of antibiotics, most DSNIs were the result of pharyngeal and tonsillar infections which spread to the pharyngomaxillary space. Today, the most common origin is **odontogenic**. In addition, **salivary gland** infections are a common source and spread to involve the submaxillary space. **Intravenous drug abusers** are particularly prone to DSNI of the vascular region, as they may inject this area. In the pediatric population, acute **tonsillitis** can lead to infection of the peritonsillar space.

5. How do you diagnose a DSNI?

Fever, pain, and neck swelling are the most common presenting symptoms. Other findings may include trismus, fluctuance, dysphagia, and dental abnormalities. If a DSNI is suspected, a CT should be ordered. It helps to differentiate cellulitis from abscess and to delineate which structures are involved. MRI can also provide excellent visualization. Ultrasound is useful for guiding needle aspiration.

6. What is the initial step in managing a DSNI?

A stands for airway. Most patients require only humidified oxygen. If an airway is needed, endotracheal intubation is often difficult, and tracheotomy or cricothyrotomy may be necessary.

7. In addition to airway compromise, what other emergencies are associated with DSNI?
Septic shock, carotid blowout, internal jugular vein thrombosis.

8. Why is the danger space dangerous?
Infections of the retropharyngeal space can readily spread through the alar fascia to the superior mediastinum, or danger space, and from there into the posterior mediastinum to the level of the diaphragm. Treatment consists of drainage and intravenous antibiotics.

9. If a DSNI spreads to the coccyx, which space did it spread in?
The **prevertebral space** extends the length of the vertebral column to the level of the coccyx. Such infection is a relatively rare condition but can lead to vertebral osteomyelitis.

10. What three critical structures are contained in the vascular space?
The carotid artery, internal jugular vein, and vagus nerve. These structures are contained in the carotid sheath, a structure formed by all three layers of the deep cervical fascia.

11. A patient has suffered a stab wound to the face and develops a DSNI. What are you most concerned about?
The parotid space has the potential to become infected. In cases of parotitis, you should be concerned of spread to the pharyngomaxillary space and subsequent spread to the danger space.

12. Who is most prone to develop an infection in the spaces involving the entire length of the neck?
Patients who have sustained esophageal trauma, have a foreign body that pierces the posterior esophageal wall, or have vertebral fractures. In addition, infections of the ears, nose, and throat can lead to infections of this area. The characteristic infection of this space is the **midline retropharyngeal abscess**, which is most common in infants and young children. The onset can be slow, often following an upper respiratory tract infection. Frequently, a feverish child will have difficulty swallowing or breathing. Trismus is generally not present. On inspection, the posterior pharyngeal wall is bulging. Mediastinal extension is characterized by its widening on chest x-ray, chest pain, dyspnea, and fever.

13. A patient presents with trismus, dysphagia, drooling, and a fever. What diagnosis should you consider?
Peritonsillar abscess. This infection can also be associated with fever, a "hot potato" voice, deviation of the uvula, and bulging of the soft palate. Intraoral drainage is indicated, which can generally be performed in the clinic or emergency department with local anesthesia. Treatment options range from drainage and needle aspiration to primary tonsillectomy.

14. What is Ludwig's angina?
Ludwig's angina is an emergent condition that presents with firmness of the tissues in the floor of the mouth due to an infection of the submandibular space. The patient may have a swollen tongue, sometimes so swollen that it causes breathing difficulties. The patient may experience severe pain, difficulty swallowing, drooling, and trismus. Typically, the sublingual and both submaxillary spaces are involved.

In general, there is no abscess and little or no frank pus. Ludwig's angina is a bilateral cellulitis, involving connective tissue, fascia, and muscle. The infection can spread via the styloglossus muscle back into the pharyngomaxillary space, resulting in possible seeding of the retropharyngeal space and superior mediastinum. Intravenous antibiotics may be curative if started early. However, rapid surgical intervention is crucial because of potential airway compromise. The goals of surgery are drainage and release of tension.

15. An immunocompromised patient develops rhinosinusitis while in the hospital. What diagnosis should you consider?

In the hospitalized immunocompromised patient with rhinosinusitis, fungal infections should be high on your differential. Diagnosis can be confirmed with biopsy. Treatment generally consists of surgical debridement and antifungal chemotherapy.

16. A patient with a DSNI presents with severe dyspnea, chest pain, and fever. What is the diagnosis, and how is it confirmed?

This picture is characteristic of **mediastinitis**. This diagnosis can be confirmed with a chest radiograph that shows characteristic mediastinal widening.

17. A patient with a suspected DSNI develops bleeding from the external auditory canal. What is the cause?

Inadequate treatment of DSNI is associated with serious complications. In this case, the infection has likely spread to the carotid area, eroding the carotid artery and resulting in major hemorrhage.

18. Which antibiotics are most appropriate in DSNIs?

Since infections of these spaces are frequently spread from odontogenic origin, providing good anaerobic coverage is essential. Clindamycin or metronidazole is appropriate. In addition, potential staphylococcal pathogens should be covered with oxacillin or cefoxitin.

19. An infection appears to be confined to a single potential neck space. What is the appropriate treatment?

It is crucial to identify and drain the space properly. Appropriate antibiotics should be initiated. The primary space and its secondary compartments to which the infection may have spread should be opened. The incision must be large enough to expose the entire abscess cavity.

20. Where should the incision be made?

Frequently, the anatomy of the neck can become very distorted due to a DSNI. The hyoid bone, cricoid cartilage, and styloid process are useful landmarks for orientation. It is important to provide drainage as near as possible to the portal of entrance. It is generally felt that a wide incision that exposes the entire space is necessary. However, such an incision can result in a poor cosmetic outcome, and more desirable approaches have been described for most neck spaces.

21. If a drain is placed into a DSNI, how long should it remain in place?

Generally, closed suction drainage is employed to prevent fluid collection. Depending on the presentation, the drain is left in place for 2–7 days, for at least 24 hours after it ceases to drain fluid. If the drain is removed too early, you risk reaccumulation of fluid in the abscess cavity. Another option is delayed primary closure. With this approach, the space is exposed and packed with gauze for approximately 5 days, at which time the number of phagocytic cells at the wound margins peaks.

CONTROVERSY

22. Must all cervical esophageal lacerations be explored to avoid DSNI?

Perforation of the esophagus remains a diagnostic and therapeutic challenge. Reinforced primary repair of the perforation is the most frequently employed and preferable approach to the surgical management of esophageal laceration. However, nonoperative management consisting of antibiotics and parenteral nutrition is particularly successful for certain types of limited esophageal injuries. One recent study had good results treating iatrogenic esophageal perforation with antibiotics, a stomach catheter, enteric or parenteral nutrition, and suction drainage. Early evaluation and treatment are critical to ensure a good outcome.

BIBLIOGRAPHY

1. Harada T, Sakakura Y: Recent intractable bacterial infections in otolaryngology. Nippon Rinsho 55:502–506, 1994.
2. Herr RD: Serious soft tissue infections of the head and neck. Am Fam Physician 44:878–888, 1991.
3. Johnson JT: Abscesses and deep space infections of the head and neck. Infect Dis Clin North Am 6:705–717, 1992.
4. Kaplan HT, Eichel BS: Deep neck infections. In English GM (ed): Otolaryngology. Philadelphia, J. B. Lippincott, 3(30):1–35, 1991.
5. Levitt GW: Cervical fascia and deep neck infections. Otolaryngol Clin North Am 9:703–728, 1976.
6. Scott BA, Stiernberg CM: Deep neck space infections. In Bailey BJ (ed): Head and Neck Surgery–Otolaryngology. Philadelphia, J. B. Lippincott, 1993, pp 738–753.

30. SLEEP APNEA AND SNORING

Abilio Muñoz, M.D.

1. What is sleep apnea?

Sleep apnea is a disorder of intermittent cessation of air flow during sleep that lasts 10 seconds or longer. This cessation in air flow is usually measured at the nose and lips. Sleep apnea consists of three classes: central, obstructive, and mixed.

2. How do central, obstructive, and mixed sleep apnea differ?

Central sleep apnea—The cessation in air flow is due to a transient lack of respiratory effort. The phrenic nerve and diaphragm are temporarily inactive due to intermittent failure in the respiratory drive centers of the CNS.

Obstructive sleep apnea (OSA)—There is normal respiratory effort, but temporary upper airway obstruction causes intermittent cessation of air flow.

Mixed sleep apnea—Exhibits components of both central and obstructive apnea but is considered a variant of OSA.

OSA is the most common type of apnea and often involves the otolaryngologist's care. Treatment of mixed sleep apnea is similar to that for OSA. Central apnea is generally treated by neurologists and sleep specialists.

3. What are the symptoms of OSA?

Typical symptoms include snoring, daytime somnolence, morning headache, and restless sleep. The spouse may witness periods of apnea, and the patient may complain of frequent arousals at night. Impotence and hypertension have also been associated with OSA. However, none of these signs and symptoms is pathognomonic of OSA, and even spousal reports of apneas have been found to be unreliable in predicting the presence or severity of OSA. A formal sleep study is the only means to make the diagnosis.

4. Define the term "pickwickian."

Pickwickian syndrome is characterized by obesity and hypersomnolence. These features were described by Charles Dickens in *The Pickwick Papers*. Obesity definitely contributes to OSA due to the weight of the neck, redundancy in the soft palate, and fullness in the base of the tongue.

5. What questions should you ask when evaluating a patient with suspected OSA?

1. Does your snoring ever awaken you from sleep?
2. Do you ever awaken suddenly, gasping for air?
3. Do family members complain about your snoring?

4. Does your spouse notice periods in which breathing temporarily stops?
5. Do you feel rested after a night's sleep?
6. Do you feel drowsy at work, or do you fall asleep at inappropriate times (such as at work, while driving, or while on the telephone)?
7. Do you have morning headaches?

6. What should you look for on the physical examination of a patient with suspected OSA?

A complete head and neck examination should be performed, as well as further exams if problems such as cor pulmonale or hypertension are suspected. The nose should be examined for signs of obstruction due to a deviated septum, hypertrophic turbinates, allergic rhinitis, etc. Examination of the oral cavity may reveal potential obstruction due to large tonsils, redundant soft palate and uvula, redundant lateral pharyngeal walls, and/or a full base of the tongue. Retrognathia and/or macroglossia can also contribute to OSA. Full, thick necks may also predispose patients to OSA, especially in the setting of an overall "pickwickian" patient. Laryngeal examination should be performed to rule out any obstructing lesion.

7. What is Müller's maneuver?

Müller's maneuver is performed by passing the flexible fiberoptic scope into the hypopharynx to obtain a view of the entire hypopharynx and larynx. The examiner then pinches the nostrils closed, and the patient closes his or her lips while attempting to inhale. If the hypopharynx and/or larynx collapse, then the test is positive. A positive test means that the site of upper airway obstruction is very likely below the level of the soft palate, and the patient will probably not benefit from a uvulopalatopharyngoplasty (see Question 19). These patients will probably benefit only from a tracheostomy.

8. Which diagnostic tests are useful in the workup of OSA?

Polysomnography is the most sensitive and specific test in the evaluation of OSA. This test measures brain activity (EEG), leg muscle movements (EMG), cardiac rhythm (EKG), eye movements (EOG), pulse oximetry, respiratory effort, and air movement at the nose and mouth. Polysomnography can differentiate between snoring without OSA, pure OSA, and central sleep apnea and can characterize the severity of the apnea. This test, however, is very expensive and requires the patient to spend a night in a formal sleep lab.

Home sleep studies have recently been implemented in an effort to reduce cost. These studies range from simple continuous pulse oximetry recordings to multichannel recording devices similar to those used in a formal sleep lab. Although these tests are gaining popularity, none is as sensitive or specific as a formal sleep lab study.

The **multiple sleep latency test** (MSLT) is also performed in a sleep lab, but it is done during the day. The subject is given the chance to take several naps, and this test assesses the time it takes for the subject to fall asleep. An average sleep onset of < 5 minutes is generally considered pathologic and suggests excessive daytime sleepiness.

9. How are mild, moderate, and severe OSA defined?

Several parameters can be used to classify the severity of OSA, the most common of which is the respiratory disturbance index (RDI). This is the sum of the number of apneas (cessation of air flow for > 10 sec) and hypopneas (reduction of airflow by 50%) per hour. The degree of oxyhemoglobin desaturation can also be useful.

	RDI	SaO_2
Mild OSA	10–30	—
Moderate OSA	30–50	< 85%
Severe OSA	> 50	< 60%

10. What is the pathophysiology of OSA?

OSA can be due to an obstruction at any level of the upper airway (i.e., above the true vocal cords or glottis). Respiratory physiology dictates that during inspiration, there is a *negative pressure* within the upper airway. Sleep physiology reveals that during the deeper stages of sleep (stages III, IV, and REM), there is *muscle relaxation* of the entire body, including the muscles of the upper airway. Most patients with OSA have redundant tissue or an abnormally small air passage. In the presence of these anatomic variants, these two physiologic events combine to result in collapse of the upper airway, with resulting obstruction to air flow. Oxyhemoglobin desaturation eventually leads to an arousal to a lighter level of sleep, and the airway is re-established with the characteristic loud snoring respiration. Any factor that adds to upper airway obstruction can cause or exacerbate OSA, including adenotonsillar hypertrophy, obstructive laryngeal masses, bulky soft palate or uvula, fullness in the base of the tongue, a low-lying hyoid bone, or nasal obstruction.

11. During which stage of sleep do most obstructive events occur?

Most obstructive events occur during the deeper stages of sleep, including stages III, IV, and REM sleep. It is during these stages that muscles are most relaxed, and thus pharyngeal wall collapse is most likely. OSA patients are therefore being deprived of deep sleep. This explains the restless sleep patterns and daytime somnolence. In fact, the hallmark of successful treatment of OSA is REM rebound, or a significant increase in REM sleep due to previous sleep deprivation.

12. Describe the classic sleep pattern seen in OSA.

Typically, OSA patients exhibit a quick onset of sleep and multiple arousals. The patient maintains relatively more stage I and II sleep and less stage III, IV, and REM sleep. This lack of deep sleep results in the symptoms of sleep deprivation.

13. What exacerbates OSA?

Alcohol and sedatives are known to exacerbate OSA. A physician should be aware that even mild sedatives, such as cough suppressants, may be dangerous if administered to a patient with OSA. Allergic rhinitis, upper respiratory infections, and other causes of nasal obstruction may also exacerbate the problem. Weight gain is known to cause or exacerbate OSA. If this factor is reversed, the patient's OSA may be alleviated, obviating the need for devices or surgeries.

14. Are children with OSA more likely to exhibit a specific etiology?

Yes. OSA in children is usually due to tonsil and adenoid hypertrophy. Other causes include nasopharyngeal cysts, encephaloceles, choanal atresia, a deviated nasal septum, and craniofacial or orthodontic malformations.

15. Do all people who snore loudly have OSA?

No. About 1 in 4 adult males snore, with the prevalence rising with increasing age until it reaches about 60% in males over age 60 years. However, although snoring does indicate some degree of obstructed breathing, and although patients who have OSA are typically loud snorers, not all people who snore have OSA. Most snoring is not pathologic and may be prevented by lifestyle changes, such as weight loss, alcohol abstinence, or change in sleep position.

16. Should everyone who snores have a sleep study?

When the snoring is accompanied by symptoms of OSA, such as hypersomnolence, morning headache, and restless sleep, a thorough examination and sleep study are probably indicated. When snoring is socially disruptive but not accompanied by symptoms of sleep apnea, the picture is not so clear. Unfortunately, even "apneas" witnessed by the spouse are not predictive of OSA. The only reasonably accurate method of detecting OSA remains the formal sleep study. Therefore, current recommendations suggest obtaining a sleep study prior to any surgery for sleep apnea or snoring.

17. What are the complications of OSA?

Left untreated, chronic OSA is definitely associated with significant morbidity and mortality. An increased rate of nocturnal death has been reported, presumably due to lethal cardiac arrhythmias. Cor pulmonale and chronic heart failure have also been well documented and improve dramatically after successful treatment. Idiopathic hypertension has also been associated with OSA, although the precise mechanism has not yet been elucidated. Again, this hypertension often reverses after successful treatment of the apnea, reducing the need for antihypertensive medication. There is also a higher rate of mortality in OSA patients due to automobile accidents, presumably due to excessive daytime somnolence. The physician who recognizes OSA should also recognize the dangers associated with excessive somnolence and driving or operating dangerous equipment. It appears that the natural history of OSA tends to worsen with age and with weight gain. Often, a vicious cycle develops in which daytime somnolence leads to less exercise, more weight gain, and more severe sleep apnea. Therefore, once it is identified, OSA should be treated promptly and aggressively.

18. Are there nonsurgical treatments for OSA?

Nasal continuous positive airway pressure (CPAP) is the most effective nonsurgical treatment of OSA. An air-tight mask is held over the nose by a strap wrapped around the patient's head. CPAP is maintained by a machine that is similar to a ventilator. Although nasal CPAP is nearly 100% effective in relieving OSA, it is very poorly tolerated. Even when it is initially successful, many (30% or more) patients eventually stop using it due to discomfort.

Tongue-retaining devices and **mandibular positioning devices** also may be implemented. These devices open the airway by holding the tongue and/or mandible forward during sleep. As with CPAP, discomfort and poor compliance are major problems.

Behavioral modifications, such as weight loss and avoidance of alcohol and sedatives, may also reduce OSA. Again, patient compliance is a major stumbling block.

Finally, attempts have been made at altering the **patient's sleeping position** (e.g., sewing a tennis ball into the back of a patient's pajamas to discourage sleeping on the back); in general, these approaches have been unsuccessful.

19. What is a "U-triple-P"?

Uvulopalatopharyngoplasty (UPPP) is the most common procedure performed for OSA. In this procedure, the tonsils are removed (if they have not been removed previously), along with the posterior edge of the soft palate, including the uvula. The tonsillar pillars are then sewed together, and the mucosa on the nasal side and oral side of the cut edge of the soft palate arc sewed together. This procedure enlarges the oropharyngeal airway in an anterior-superior and lateral dimension. UPPP is a not a technically difficult operation, but it generally requires a 1- or 2-day stay in the hospital.

20. Can other surgeries be used to treat OSA?

Several procedures have been devised to advance the base of the tongue. These procedures are based on the premise that fullness in the base of the tongue contributes to upper airway collapse.

1. A partial midline **glossectomy**, using either a laser or Bovie cautery, can be performed, although this procedure has not gained wide acceptance.

2. A more popular method is an **advancement genioplasty** combined with a **hyoid suspension**. In this procedure, the genial tubercle of the mandible, which attaches to the genioglossus muscle, is advanced anteriorly, and the hyoid bone is suspended from the mandible by permanent sutures or wires. This results in an enlarged airway at the level of the base of tongue.

3. A third procedure involves mandibular and maxillary advancements via **sagittal split** and **LeFort I osteotomies**, respectively. These are much larger operations than the UPPP, but they do successfully alter the anatomic anomalies that appear to cause OSA. They also appear to be very effective and long-lasting treatments.

4. Nasal obstruction may contribute to or worsen OSA, but rarely is it the sole cause. Thus, **nasal surgery**, including septoplasty and/or surgery on the turbinates, may be performed in combination with some of the other procedures, if it is indicated.

5. **Tracheostomy** bypasses the upper airway entirely and is thus highly effective in the treatment of OSA. However, the patient must live with and care for the tracheostomy on a daily basis, which is undesirable to most patients.

21. Which is the most effective treatment for OSA?

Tracheostomy remains the gold standard in the treatment of OSA. It is effective in almost all patients, including those with severe disease. In patients with very severe disease or those who are markedly obese or debilitated, it is probably the initial procedure of choice. The other methods that have been described realistically have little chance of benefit.

22. What are the surgical options for treatment of snoring without OSA?

An outpatient procedure has been devised in which a Bovie or laser (usually CO_2) is used to amputate the uvula and to create 1-cm trenches in the soft palate on either side of the uvula. The laser procedure is termed **laser-assisted uvulopalatoplasty** (LAUP), and the Bovie procedure is termed **Bovie-assisted uvulopalatoplasty** (BAUP). As healing occurs, the soft palate elevates and stiffens, reducing the tendency to vibrate. This procedure is usually performed in a doctor's office or in an outpatient setting under local anesthesia. It is also performed in stages, titrating the resection to resolve the snoring without causing velopharyngeal insufficiency. Two to four treatments are usually required, each separated by about 1 month. The superiority of the laser over the Bovie has not been established, although both appear to be effective treatments for snoring. The Bovie is less expensive and more widely available, but the laser may prevent deep tissue damage.

23. How effective is using UPPP to treat OSA or snoring without OSA?

UPPP is very successful in treating snoring alone but is not as successful in treating OSA. Approximately 90% of patients stop snoring after a UPPP, regardless of whether or not they have sleep apnea. However, significant improvement in OSA occurs in only about 50% of patients. In addition, significant improvement may mean a reduction in the RDI of 50% or more, but the patient still may have significant OSA, especially if their RDI was very high at the start. Overall, studies have not shown a reduction in the mortality of OSA following UPPP alone. Studies, however, have shown dramatically improved mortality rates following treatment with tracheostomy or CPAP. Therefore, the decision to proceed with UPPP must be individualized to each patient, and the patient must be aware of the possible need for additional procedures if the UPPP fails.

24. Describe the potential complications of a UPPP.

UPPP has been described as a "radical tonsillectomy," and therefore the potential complications are similar to those of a tonsillectomy. Bleeding is by far the most common postoperative complication, occasionally requiring another visit to the operating room for control. Transient velopharyngeal insufficiency occurs in 5–10% of patients but is rarely permanent. Nasopharyngeal stenosis is a very rare but devastating complication in which the nasopharynx scars down completely. Patients may complain of a dry mouth, tightness in the throat, an increased gag reflex, and/or a change in taste; however, these are usually transient.

CONTROVERSY

25. What is the role of laser-assisted uvulopalatoplasty (LAUP) in OSA and snoring?

LAUP is highly effective in the treatment of snoring, with resolution of snoring occurring in 85–90% of patients. However, the effectiveness of LAUP in the treatment of OSA has not been established. Snoring and OSA probably represent a continuum of a similar pathology, but along this continuum, it is hard to differentiate where LAUP is effective and where it is not effective. In addition, a patient's symptoms, including snoring or daytime somnolence, cannot be used as predictors of OSA nor as indicators for successful treatment of OSA. Therefore, the current recommendation is that all patients undergo a sleep study prior to surgery for snoring or OSA and that OSA of any degree is a contraindication to LAUP. It should be noted, however, that there is ongoing research in this area, and LAUP may well prove to be effective for the treatment of mild or moderate OSA.

BIBLIOGRAPHY

1. Braver HM: Treatment for snoring: Combined weight loss, sleeping on side, and nasal spray. Chest 107:1283–1288, 1995.
2. Fairbanks DN: Uvulopalatopharyngoplasty: Strategies for success and safety. Ear Nose Throat J 72:46–47, 50–51, 1993.
3. Hausfeld JN: Snoring and sleep apnea syndrome. In American Academy of Otolaryngology–Head and Neck Surgery Foundation: Common Problems of the Head and Neck. Philadelphia, W.B. Saunders, 1992, pp 85–96.
4. Koopman CF, Moran WB: Sleep apnea—A historical perspective. Otolaryngol Clin North Am 23:571–573, 1990.
5. Poole MD: Obstructive sleep apnea. In Bailey BJ (ed): Head and Neck Surgery–Otolaryngology. Philadelphia, J.B. Lippincott, 1993, pp 598–611.
6. Riley RW, Powell NB, Guilleminault C: Maxillofacial surgery and obstructive sleep apnea: A review of 80 patients. Otolaryngol Head Neck Surg 101:353, 1989.
7. Sher AE: Obstructive sleep apnea syndrome: A complex disorder of the upper airway. Otolaryngol Clin North Am 23:593–605, 1990.
8. Schlesinger AE, Hernandez RJ: Radiographic imaging of airway obstruction in pediatrics. Otolaryngol Clin North Am 23:609–633, 1990.

31. THE HOARSE PATIENT

Abilio Muñoz, M.D.

1. What is hoarseness?

Hoarseness is a vague term that patients often use to describe a change in voice quality, ranging from voice harshness to voice weakness. However, the term can reflect abnormalities anywhere along the vocal tract, from the oral cavity to lungs. Ideally, the term *hoarseness* refers to laryngeal dysfunction caused by abnormal vocal cord vibration.

2. How is speech produced?

There are three phases in speech: pulmonary, laryngeal, and oral. The **pulmonary** phase creates the energy flow with inflation and expulsion of air. This activity provides the larynx with a column of air for the laryngeal phase. In the **laryngeal** phase, vocal cords vibrate at certain frequencies to create sound that is unique to the individual. The **oral** phase occurs in the oral cavity where sound is modified. Words are formed by the action of the pharynx, tongue, lips, and teeth. Dysfunction in any of these stages can lead to voice changes which may be interpreted as hoarseness by the patient.

3. What clinical signs in voice quality and frequency may help to localize the speech abnormality?

When the speech abnormality is limited to the lungs or tracheobronchial tree, the patient exhibits a weak, damped voice. The lungs may be restricted in movement, making the voice barely perceptible. On the other hand, if the patient has difficulty articulating words or if the voice resonates as if coming from the nose, the problem probably originates in the oral stage. Oral-stage abnormalities may also lead to a muffled or "hot potato" voice. Abnormalities originating in either the lung or oral cavity are not considered to be true hoarseness. True hoarseness from a laryngeal origin usually results in a rough, raspy voice.

4. Where is frequency produced?

Different frequencies are produced by expiratory pulmonary force in conjunction with changes in the length, breadth, elasticity, and extension of the vocal cords. The adductor laryngeal muscle modifies length of the vocal cords. Vocal cords are approximated, and the pressure of moving air causes vibration of the elastic cord. It is important to note that vocal cord vibration is not an active process caused by laryngeal muscles.

5. What terms are useful in characterizing hoarseness or voice change?

Dysphonia—describes a general alteration in voice quality.

Diplophonia—describes a sound made by vibrating cords at two different frequencies. It indicates that the vocal cords are being affected differently.

Aphonia—occurs when no sound is emanated from the vocal cords. It often occurs secondary to a lack of air passing through the vocal cords or a deficiency in vocal cord approximation.

Stridor—indicates noise emanating from the upper airway during inspiration due to an obstruction. Stridor is a medical emergency; it is not considered hoarseness. It may coexist with hoarseness when the obstruction occurs at the level of the vocal cords.

6. How is hoarseness categorized?

Hoarseness can be broken down into two broad categories, acute onset and chronic onset. **Acute onset** is more common and is often caused by local inflammation of the larynx, such as seen with acute laryngitis. It may be secondary to viral infection, voice abuse, or smoking. **Chronic hoarseness**, on the other hand, may be caused by benign polyps, vocal cord nodules, laryngeal papillomatosis, tumor, functional dysphonia, neurologic involvement, or chronic inflammation secondary to smoking or voice abuse. Note that acute hoarseness is unlikely to have a malignant etiology. A malignant process should always be considered if hoarseness has been progressive and present for several months.

7. What are the most common problems associated with hoarseness?

Acute viral laryngitis	Laryngeal cancer
Vocal cord nodules	Postnasal drip
Vocal cord paralysis	Gastroesophageal reflux

8. Which chronic benign lesions cause hoarseness?

Chronic laryngitis	Recurrent benign lesions
Vocal cord nodules	Altered laryngeal architecture
Single benign lesions of the larynx	Laryngeal papillomatosis

9. How is chronic laryngitis treated?

Chronic laryngitis is general inflammation of the larynx often caused by smoking, voice abuse, or gastroesophageal reflux. The voice usually improves if the irritating factors are discontinued. This may involve smoking cessation or voice rest. Antacid medication often relieves hoarseness due to reflux. In addition, patients with reflux may benefit from resting their voice, sleeping with the head of their bed elevated, and waiting 3–4 hours after eating before going to bed.

10. How are vocal cord nodules treated?

Vocal cord nodules often arise as a result of excessive laryngeal use. Voice therapy often can correct hoarseness in many patients. If voice therapy is not effective, surgical removal of nodules may improve the voice. Generally, surgery will not resolve the hoarseness completely, and it is rarely indicated since vocal coaching usually solves the problem.

11. How is a laryngeal polyp treated?

A laryngeal polyp is a single benign lesion of the larynx. A polyp is usually removed with a CO_2 laser or cryotherapy. Normal voice usually returns after treatment.

12. How are laryngeal papillomas treated?

Laryngeal papillomas are recurrent benign lesions caused by infection with human papillomavirus. They tend to recur despite surgery. Multiple surgical resection, often with a laser, is required. Normal baseline voice does not usually return.

13. Which infections are likely to cause hoarseness?

Viral infections are most commonly responsible for laryngitis, causing diffuse erythema of the vocal cords and an increase in vocal cord mass. In children, **subglottic edema** also may cause croup (barking cough). In contrast, epiglottitis does not typically present with hoarseness but instead causes a muffled "hot potato" voice due to supraglottic swelling. **Bacterial infections** of the endolarynx are not common, but they can occur. **Laryngeal papillomatosis** is a relatively common infectious cause of hoarseness. It results from human papillomavirus infection, inducing wart-like growths on the vocal cords. Because laryngeal papillomatosis is more common in children, examination of the larynx with a flexible laryngoscope should be considered if this disorder is suspected.

14. What questions should be included in the history when evaluating a patient with hoarseness?

1. What is the duration of symptoms, and is there any progression? Such questions determine whether the process is acute or chronic.

2. Is there a coexistent sore throat or otalgia?

3. Is there dysphagia or odynophagia? If present, these symptoms may indicate a problem with the pharynx, esophagus, or larynx.

4. Is there a cough? Although cough may be associated with an infection, cancer of the lung with vocal cord paralysis (secondary to recurrent laryngeal nerve impingement) often presents with hoarseness and cough.

5. Is there hemoptysis? This potentially serious symptom may indicate malignancy.

6. What are the occupation and habits of patient? Singers, sports fanatics (shouting), and people who eat spicy foods are more likely to suffer from benign hoarseness.

15. Which parts of the physical exam are vital when evaluating a patient with hoarseness?

The physical exam is very helpful in separating a malignant process from a benign one. In the head and neck exam, pneumatic otoscopy, nasal exam, oral exam, and neck palpation are extremely important. If the history and exam fail to provide a clear picture, visual examination of glottis with a laryngoscope is necessary.

16. What innervates voice production?

The motor neurons that innervate the larynx are found in the nucleus ambiguous of the medulla. Fibers travel from the nucleus ambiguous with the vagus nerve to exit through the jugular foramen within the carotid sheath. Superiorly, the vagus nerve gives rise to the superior laryngeal nerve which innervates the cricothyroid muscle of the larynx and provides sensory innervation to the endolarynx. The vagus continues traveling inferiorly. In the thorax, it gives rise to the recurrent laryngeal nerve. The recurrent laryngeal nerve loops around the arch of the aorta on the left and around the subclavian artery on the right to innervate the larynx inferiorly.

17. Which neurologic abnormalities may cause hoarseness?

If a neoplasm is present, **nerve compression** may lead to hoarseness. This compression can occur anywhere from the brainstem to the larynx. For example, vocal cord paralysis can be secondary to tumors of the jugular foramen (glomus jugulare), neck, thyroid, bronchus, or esophagus.

Thyroid tumors are the most common cause of bilateral vocal cord paralysis, while malignant esophageal and pulmonary tumors are common causes of unilateral vocal cord paralysis. **Nerve injury** should also be suspected if a patient is hoarse after any neck procedure. Injury may be due to transection, cricothyroid joint injury, or compression from an overinflated endotracheal cuff.

18. What are the neoplastic disorders of the vocal cords?

The true vocal cords are most commonly affected by squamous cell carcinoma. Such a malignancy is exophytic in appearance and, if treated early, has a high cure rate and excellent possibility of voice preservation. Therefore, laryngeal examination of the hoarse patient is vital for early diagnosis and intervention.

19. Can nonorganic disorders present as hoarseness?

A **conversion disorder**, a psychiatric condition, may present as hoarseness. One of the most common nonorganic causes of hoarseness is **hysterical aphonia**. Patients exhibit paradoxical motion of the vocal cords during speech. During quiet respiration or sleep, the vocal cords work normally. During speech, the vocal cords abduct and fail to vibrate adequately to produce sound. The diagnosis can be made if a normal cough is present. The laryngoscope exam will reveal normal-appearing vocal cords in the face of dramatic voice manifestations.

20. Voice abuse may result in benign vocal cord polyps, nodules, or contact granulomas. How are these lesions differentiated?

Polyps are asymmetrical and appear soft and smooth. Polyps may occur on one or both cords. In contrast, **vocal nodules** are easily identified because they are usually paired. Nodules are small and discrete and are located in the middle of the membranous vocal cord. Finally, **contact granulomas** are not actually found on the vocal cord itself. Contact granulomas are found on the vocal processes of the arytenoid cartilage.

21. What is the differential diagnosis of laryngeal edema?

Laryngeal edema is usually related to trauma or infection. Some systemic diseases cause laryngeal swelling with concomitant hoarseness, including:
- Obstruction of venous drainage at the heart, great veins, or internal jugular veins
- Dilated pulmonary artery or aortic arch (left recurrent laryngeal nerve compression)
- Obstruction of lymphatic drainage, as in postradiation
- Hypoproteinemia with decreased plasma oncotic pressure
- Increased capillary permeability to protein, seen in diseases such as rheumatoid arthritis, lupus, polyarteritis, diabetes, and leukemia
- Hypothyrodism with myxedema

It is important to recognize these conditions, because they can cause rapid inflammation with potential airway obstruction.

BIBLIOGRAPHY

1. Chan P: Cardiovocal (Ortner's) syndrome left recurrent laryngeal nerve palsy associated with cardiovascular disease. Eur J Med 1:492–495, 1992.
2. Davidson TM: Clinical Manual of Otolaryngology, 2nd ed. New York, McGraw-Hill, 1992.
3. Dettelbach M, Eibling DE, Johnson JT: Hoarseness: From viral laryngitis to glottic cancer. Postgrad Med 95:143, 1994.
4. Lyons BM: "Doctor, my voice seems husky." Austr Fam Physician 23:2111–2119, 1994.
5. MacKenzie K: Diagnosis and treatment of hoarseness. Practitioner 238(1539):474–478,1994.
6. Passy V: Hoarseness: Evaluation and Treatment: Common Problems of the Head and Neck Region: A Manual and Guide for Management of Diseases and Injuries in Otolaryngology–Head and Neck Surgery. Alexandria, VA, American Academy of Otolaryngology–Neck and Head Surgery Foundation, 1992.
7. Waring JP, Lacayo L, Hunter J, et al: Chronic cough and hoarseness in patients with severe gastroesophageal reflux disease: Diagnosis and response to therapy. Dig Dis Sci 40:1093–1097, 1995.

32. OTOLARYNGOLOGIC MANIFESTATIONS OF AIDS

Daniel W. Watson, M.D.

1. What is the primary mode of transmission of HIV?

Sexual intercourse, especially receptive anal intercourse. Other modes of transmission include transfusion of infected blood products, needle-sharing in intravenous drug abuse, and perinatal transmission. In the United States, 64% of patients have been homosexual or bisexual men, while 25% have been intravenous drug abusers. In 1992, 6% of AIDS cases were classified as due to heterosexual contact. About 3% of cases are due to receipt of contaminated blood or blood products.

2. What is the risk of acquiring HIV infection from a "six pack" of platelets? From 3 units of packed red blood cells?

Estimates are 1:11,000 for a six-pack platelet transfusion and 1:23,000 for 3 units of packed red cells.

3. What are the three potential modes of HIV transmission from mother to child?

Transplacental, perinatal (during the birth process), and postnatal (during breastfeeding).

4. What is the chance of transmitting HIV from an infected mother to her infant?

Approximately 25%. Vertical transmission in the United States occurs in 15–35% of HIV-positive pregnancies. This rate is influenced by stage of maternal disease, type of delivery, birth order, and concurrent sexually transmitted diseases (especially syphilis). Pediatric cases account for 1.7% of the approximately 200,000 infected individuals. AIDS is the leading cause of childhood immunodeficiency and ranks among the top 10 causes of death in children.

5. Following HIV infection, what percentage of seropositive patients will develop AIDS within 10 years?

Data from the San Francisco City Clinic Cohort Study suggest that 50% of seropositive patients will develop AIDS within 10 years. Remember, the CDC has developed a list of specific indicator diseases for the diagnosis of AIDS in the presence of HIV seropositivity.

AIDS Indicator Diseases

Infectious diseases	Neoplastic diseases
Pneumocystis carinii pneumonia	Kaposi's sarcoma
Cytomegalovirus retinitis	Primary lymphoma of the brain
Esophageal candidiasis	Non-Hodgkin's lymphoma of B-cell or
Cryptococcosis, extrapulmonary	unknown immunologic phenotype
Cryptosporidiosis with diarrhea persisting > 1 mo	if small noncleaved or immunoblastic
Coccidioidomycosis, disseminated	sarcoma
Toxoplasmosis of the brain	
Disseminated histoplasmosis	**Others**
Disseminated mycobacterial disease (other than	HIV encephalopathy (AIDS dementia)
by *M. tuberculosis*)	HIV wasting syndrome
Extrapulmonary disease caused by	CD4 count < 200
M. tuberculosis	
Recurrent nontyphoid *Salmonella*	
Isosporiasis with diarrhea persisting > 1 mo	

From Tami T, Lee K: AIDS and the otolaryngologist. SIPAC from AAOHNS, 1993, p 23, with permission.

6. Once the diagnosis of AIDS is made, how long does the patient usually live?

The median survival is about 15 months, with an estimated 5-year survival rate of approximately 6%.

7. Which is the most common index disease for the diagnosis of AIDS?

Pneumocystis carinii pneumonia. More than 60% of reported cases of AIDS have *P. carinii* pneumonia as the index for diagnosis.

8. The CD4 count is a serum marker currently used to measure progression of AIDS. What is considered a normal value? What level is associated with progression to AIDS?

The CD4 count, normally at about 1,000 cells/mm³, represents the absolute helper T-lymphocyte count. This test is widely available, and its levels correlate directly with disease stage. At levels below 200 cells/mm³, there is a higher incidence of progression to AIDS. Many prophylactic regimens are initiated at this level.

9. Name the most common cause of focal intracerebral lesions in patients with AIDS.

The protozoan *Toxoplasma gondii*. The general population harbors latent infection with *Toxoplasma*, depending on the geographic area and the person's dietary habits (consuming raw, infected meat). In AIDS patients, toxoplasmosis results from reactivation of the latent infection. Patients subsequently develop toxoplasmic encephalitis with a characteristic hypodense, ring-enhancing CNS lesion on computed tomographic scan.

10. Name the most common viral opportunistic pathogen seen with HIV infection.

Cytomegalovirus (CMV). Infection can lead to chorioretinitis, pneumonia, esophagitis, colitis, encephalitis, and hepatitis.

11. What are the common dermatologic manifestations of HIV infection?

Several dermatologic manifestations of HIV infection are due to fungal and viral infections—e.g., candidiasis, tinea versicolor, and molluscum contagiosum. *Staphylococcus aureus* is the most common bacterial pathogen causing cutaneous infections in HIV patients. These cutaneous manifestations may all present in the head and neck region.

12. An HIV-positive patient presents with pinkish purple, slightly raised lesions over the face, neck, upper trunk, and oral mucosa. What is your diagnosis?

Besides the usual skin infections, do not forget neoplasia. This patient may have **Kaposi's sarcoma**, the most common malignant manifestation of AIDS. Not all AIDS patients are equally affected, as homosexual or bisexual AIDS patients are disproportionately affected. Treatment for AIDS-associated Kaposi's sarcoma is primarily palliative. In most patients, ultimate survival is determined by the infectious complications of AIDS and not by this neoplasm.

13. An HIV-positive patient presents with chronic otitis externa. Should you be concerned?

Probably not, since otitis externa is relatively common. Keep in mind, however, that skin conditions such as Kaposi's sarcoma of the auricle and seborrheic dermatitis in the external ear canal, are commonly seen in HIV-infected patients. These skin infections can become secondarily infected. Aural polyps due to *Pneumocystis carinii* have been reported to cause canal obstruction.

14. What is the most common otologic condition seen in HIV-infected patients?

Serous and **acute otitis media**. In pediatric patients, eustachian tube dysfunction in association with depressed cell-mediated immunity creates a high risk for middle ear infection. In adults, eustachian tube dysfunction may be secondary to nasopharyngeal (adenoid) lymphoid hypertrophy. The otolaryngologist must carefully examine the nasopharynx in an HIV patient with eustachian tube dysfunction, since neoplastic processes, such as Kaposi's sarcoma or non-Hodgkin's lymphoma, may be present.

15. What is the most common middle ear pathogen in an HIV-infected patient with otitis media?

Pneumococcus. The usual middle ear pathogens apply to both HIV- and non-HIV-infected patients (*Streptococcus pneumoniae, Haemophilus influenzae, Moraxella catarrhalis*), but otitis media due to *Staphylococcus* and *Pseudomonas* is seen with greater frequency in HIV patients than in the normal population. Unusual organisms, such as *Norcardia asteroides* and *Mycobacterium*, can occur. *Pneumocystis carinii* otitis media and mastoiditis is an opportunistic otologic infection unique to AIDS.

16. What is Ramsay Hunt syndrome?

Ramsay Hunt syndrome, or herpes zoster oticus, is a vesicular eruption of the ear and face with ipsilateral facial paralysis. It is thought to be caused by reactivation of a latent varicella-zoster virus. Patients may have intense otalgia, vesicular eruptions (occasionally extending onto the tympanic membrane), sensorineural hearing loss (in up to 40%), tinnitus, and vertigo. Herpes zoster infections have been reported in up to 16% of AIDS patients.

17. HIV-infected patients often present with acute and chronic sinus problems. What are the indications to perform sinus lavage in an HIV patient with sinusitis?

1. Failure to respond to initial medical therapy
2. Complication of sinusitis
3. Severe systemic toxicity from sinusitis

These are not absolute indications but merely guidelines. As AIDS patients become more immunocompromised, unusual pathogens are seen in sinusitis, including *Legionella, Alternaria, Cryptococcus, Candida,* and *Acanthamoeba.*

18. An AIDS patient presents with tender, white, pseudomembranous lesions on the mucosal surfaces of the oral cavity. What is your diagnosis?

It is probably **oral candidiasis**, or thrush, which is the most common oral manifestation of AIDS. If the patient also complains of severe odynophagia, then esophageal candidiasis must be considered. Herpetic infections of the oral mucosa are also quite common, but these usually are vesicular, extremely painful, and may coalesce to form large ulcers up to several centimeters. Kaposi's sarcoma lesions may also occur in the oral cavity, where they may ulcerate and become secondarily infected.

19. Which oral cavity lesion is seen almost exclusively in HIV patients?

Hairy leukoplakia. This white, vertically corrugated lesion occurs along the anterior lateral border of the tongue. It is a reliable prognostic indicator of AIDS, as 50% of HIV-infected patients with this lesion will develop AIDS in 16 months. Electron microscopy has revealed Epstein-Barr virus and papillomavirus in these lesions.

20. An AIDS patient presents with tender, bleeding gums and erythema at the gumline. Explain the concerns you might have with this presentation.

HIV-associated **periodontitis** and **gingivitis** are much more severe in the immunocompromised patient. The process of HIV gingivitis, HIV periodontitis, ANUG (acute necrotizing ulcerative gingivitis), and necrotizing stomatitis represent a continuum of disease from moderate to severe. In ANUG, the gingiva appear red and swollen, then subsequently undergo necrosis, turning yellow-gray. There is often significant destruction of periodontal soft tissue.

21. An HIV-infected patient has had asymptomatic bilateral parotid swelling for 3–4 months. What is the most likely diagnosis?

Salivary gland disease is not uncommon in HIV patients. In particular, **lymphoepithelial cysts** are fairly common, usually involving the tail of the parotid. The cysts are often bilateral, multiloculated, and contained within the parotid fascia. The etiology is unknown, although these lesions exhibit reactive lymphocytes which infiltrate parotid tissue. However, salivary flow is usually preserved, and amylase is normal.

In children with HIV infection, the lymphocytic response implies a strong anti-HIV response, and survival is much longer in children with parotid enlargement. Other diagnoses to consider include parotid neoplasms, such as **Kaposi's sarcoma** or **non-Hodgkin's lymphoma**.

22. What is the risk of seroconversion after needlestick exposure from an HIV-positive patient?

Estimates range from 0.31–0.50%. Presently, many institutions recommend zidovudine prophylaxis, 200 mg every 4 hours for 6 weeks, if exposure occurs.

23. An AIDS patient presents with fever, night sweats, and weight loss in addition to a nontender, rapidly enlarging neck mass. Which neoplasm might this represent?

Non-Hodgkin's lymphoma (NHL). NHL is the second most common AIDS-associated malignancy. It is very aggressive in HIV patients, involving extranodal sites in 89% of cases and the CNS in 42%. NHL appears late in the spectrum of HIV disease. Most lymphomas in this patient population are classified as high-grade. Chemotherapy and radiation therapy often yield poor control.

24. Baseline, palpable adenopathy is common in HIV patients. When should you do a cervical lymph node biopsy?

Lymph node biopsy often reveals follicular hyperplasia. **Malignant** etiologies, such as Kaposi's sarcoma and non-Hodgkin's lymphoma, and **infectious** etiologies, such as tuberculosis, atypical tuberculosis, histoplasmosis, toxoplasmosis, and cat-scratch disease, should be considered. Indications for cervical lymph node biopsy are as follows:

1. Marked constitutional symptoms with an otherwise negative evaluation
2. Localized, enlarging adenopathy
3. Single, disproportionately large node in a patient with persistent generalized lymphadenopathy
4. Cytopenia or an elevated erythrocyte sedimentation rate, or both, in a patient with an otherwise negative evaluation
5. Patient (or physician) reassurance of an ambiguous tissue diagnosis

Often a fine-needle aspirate can provide valuable information, thus eliminating the need for a formal open biopsy.

25. After performing fiberoptic nasopharyngoscopy on an HIV-infected patient, how should you clean the scope for future use?

After each use, the endoscope should be wiped with an alcohol sponge to remove secretions and any organic matter. The scope should then be immersed in 2% glutaraldehyde for 10 minutes. The instrument is then rinsed with water and air-dried. To prevent corrosion on the endoscope's coating, it is important to rinse the glutaraldehyde thoroughly. In addition, glutaraldehyde residue may be irritating to future patients' nasal mucosa.

CONTROVERSIES

26. How should sinusitis be managed in an HIV-infected patient?

Often AIDS patients are referred for sinusitis refractory to antibiotic therapy. In addition to temporarily relieving pressure symptoms, a sinus lavage will sometimes yield an organism. These benefits must be weighed against the risks of antral puncture, a risk not only to the immunocompromised patient but also to the physician who is performing the procedure. Special consideration needs to be given to AIDS patients with thrombocytopenia or other coagulopathy.

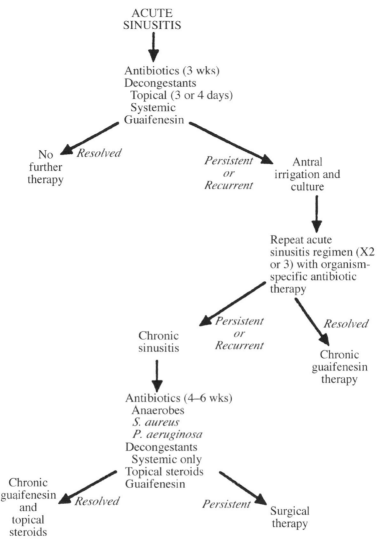

Sinusitis management in the HIV-infected patient. (From Tami T, Wawrose S: Diseases of the nose and paranasal sinuses in the HIV-infected population. Otolaryngol Clin North Am 25:1208, 1992, with permission.)

27. How should benign lymphoepithelial cysts be managed?
    Some advocate parotidectomy with facial nerve dissection, while others advocate needle aspiration. Recurrence is common. Therapeutic attempts have included intralesional tetracycline sclerosis and low-dose radiation. Further study is needed.

BIBLIOGRAPHY

 1. Barzan L, Tavio M, Tirelli U, et al: Head and neck manifestations during HIV infection. J Laryngol Otol
    107(2):133–136, 1993.
 2. Burton F, Patete ML, Goodwin WJ: Indications for open cervical node biopsy in HIV-positive patients.
    Otolaryngol–Head Neck Surg 107:367–369, 1992.
 3. Casiano R, Cooper J, Gould E, et al: Value of needle biopsy in directing management of parotid lesions
    in HIV-positive patients. Head Neck 13:411–414, 1991.

4. Eversole LR: Viral infections of the head and neck among HIV-seropositive patients. Oral Surg Oral Med Oral Pathol 73:155–63, 1992.
5. Gates G: Current Therapy in Otolaryngology–Head and Neck Surgery, 5th ed. St. Louis, Mosby, 1994.
6. Greenspan D, Greenspan JS, Hearst NG, et al: Relation of oral hairy leukoplakia to infection with the human immunodeficiency virus and the risk of developing AIDS. J Infect Dis 155:475, 1987.
7. Lucente F: Impact of the acquired immune deficiency syndrome epidemic on the practice of laryngology. Ann Otol Rhinol Laryngol 102(8):3–21, 1993.
8. Mayer M, Haddad J: Human immunodeficiency virus infection presenting with lymphoepithelial cysts in a six-year-old child. Ann Otol Rhinol Laryngol 105:242–244, 1996.
9. Principi N, Marchisio P, Tornaghi R, et al: Acute otitis media in human immunodeficiency virus-infected children. Pediatrics 88:556–571, 1991.
10. Tami T, Lee K: AIDS and the otolaryngologist. Self-Instructional Packet from American Academy of Otolaryngology–Head and Neck Surgery, 1993.
11. Tami T, Wawrose S: Diseases of the nose and paranasal sinuses in the HIV-infected population. Otolaryngol Clin North Am 25:6, 1992.
12. Tucci F, Castelli G, Bottero S, et al: Parotid swelling in children with HIV infection [abstract PB0462]. Int Conf AIDS 10:258, 1994.
13. Wenig BM, Kuruvilla A, Goldrich MS, et al: Pathologic manifestations of acquired immunodeficiency syndrome in the head and neck. Ear Nose Throat J 69:406–415, 1990.

33. ANTIMICROBIAL THERAPY IN OTOLARYNGOLOGY

Tyler M. Lewark, M.D.

1. What factors need to be considered when choosing an antibiotic?

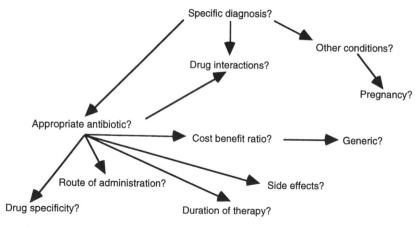

Decision-making process in pharmacotherapy. (Adapted from Mabry RL: Principles of pharmacology and medical therapy. In Bailey BJ (ed): Head and Neck Surgery–Otolaryngology. Philadelphia, J.B. Lippincott, 1993, pp 44–51.)

1. Specific diagnosis —antibiotics may be administered for a proven infection, suspected infection, or prophylaxis against a possible infection.
2. Antibiotic specificity—may be determined with laboratory testing.
3. Route of administration—depends on type and severity of infection.
4. Duration of therapy—depends on type and severity of infection.

5. Concurrent medical conditions—including physical ailments and pregnancy.
6. Other medications—possible drug interactions.
7. Previously identified drug allergy.
8. Potential side effects— must be discussed with the patient.
9. Cost

2. What determines whether an antibiotic should be given orally or parenterally?

The mode of administration depends primarily on the specific infection that is being treated. Parenteral therapy should be considered when topical or oral therapy would be ineffective—e.g., otitis externa is readily treated with topical preparations. In addition, the severity of the infection may dictate that parenteral therapy is necessary.

3. When should cost play a role in choosing an antibiotic?

The physician must consider cost when choosing an antibiotic. However, a less expensive medication that is *ineffective* should not be substituted for the more expensive but *effective* treatment. If there are good indications for using the more expensive antibiotic, then it should be chosen. In addition, the patient should be informed as to why a particular choice is made. The use of generic formulations, when available, can dramatically decrease the cost of an antibiotic course.

4. What is the clinical spectrum of the penicillins? What are their side effects?

Penicillins are bactericidal and penetrate well into the CSF in the presence of inflammation.

Activities of the Penicillins

ANTIBIOTIC	ACTIVE AGAINST	SIDE EFFECTS
Penicillin V or K	*Streptococcus pyogenes* Most *Streptococcus pneumoniae* Many oral anaerobes	Hypersensitivity: rash (5%), anaphylaxis (1/10,000)

Antistaphylococcals
  Methicillin
  Oxacillin
  Dicloxicillin
	Staphylococcus aureus
	Pneumococcus species
	Streptococcus species
	Many anaerobes
		Hypersensitivity

Aminopenicillins
  Ampicillin
  Amoxicillin
	Many *Haemophilus influenzae*
	Escherichia coli
	Proteus species
	Streptococcus pyogenes
	Most *Streptococcus pneumoniae*
	Most anaerobes
		Hypersensitivity

Augmented penicillins (with
  β-lactamase inhibitor)
  Amoxicillin/clavulanate
  Ampicillin/sulbactam
	Haemophilus influenzae
	Moraxella catarrhalis
	Staphylococcus aureus
	Most *Streptococcus pneumoniae*
	Most anaerobes
		Hypersensitivity

Antipseudomonals
  Ticarcillin
  Carbenicillin
  Piperacillin
	Pseudomonas aeruginosa
	Most gram-negatives
		Hypersensitivity

Adapted from Fairbanks DNF: Antimicrobial therapy in otolaryngology–head and neck surgery. In Lee KJ (ed): Essential Otolaryngology–Head and Neck Surgery. Norwalk, CT, Appleton & Lange, 1995, pp 427–436.

5. How are cephalosporins categorized? What is their clinical spectrum?

The cephalosporins are categorized into first-, second-, and third-generation agents. The first-generation agents are most active against gram-positive cocci. *Staphylococcus aureus*, streptococci, and most pneumococci. They are also active against a few gram-negative organisms. The second-generation agents are active against the gram-positive cocci but also against *Haemophilus influenzae* and *Moraxella catarrhalis*. The third-generation agents are more active against gram-negative bacteria, including *Haemophilus influenzae, Moraxella catarrhalis,* and *Neisseria gonorrhoeae*. In addition, the third-generation cephalosporin ceftazidine is highly active against *Pseudomonas aeruginosa*.

6. Should cephalosporins be avoided in the penicillin-hypersensitive patient?

Cephalosporins have a similar structure to penicillin's and are also categorized as β-lactam antibiotics. This chemical relationship dictates that patients with a history of penicillin anaphylaxis should probably avoid cephalosporins. However, cephalosporins are often used safely in patients with a history of penicillin rashes.

7. What other β-lactam antibiotics may be used for head and neck infections?

Imipenem and aztreonam. These antibiotics are administered parenterally and are widely bactericidal. **Imipenem** exerts the broadest spectrum of activity of any antimicrobial agent, which includes *Staphylococcus aureus, Streptococcus pyogenes, Streptococcus pneumoniae, Neisseria gonorrhoeae,* and most gram-negatives and anaerobes. Penicillin-allergic patients may also be hypersensitive to imipenem. **Aztreonam** is effective in penicillin-hypersensitive patients against aerobic gram-negative pathogens.

8. What are the macrolides? What is their clinical spectrum?

The macrolides are bacteriostatic agents that are used for respiratory tract infections. They include erythromycin, azithromycin, and clarithromycin. Erythromycin is active against most streptococci, *Staphylococcus aureus, Haemophilus influenzae* (with a sulfa preparation), *Mycoplasma, Legionella, Chlamydia, Corynebacterium diphtheriae, Bordetella pertussis,* and *Clostridium tetani* (tetanus). Side effects include nausea, cramps, vomiting, and reversible jaundice. Azithromycin and clarithromycin have similar activity, except that they are active against *Haemophilus* species as a single agent. In addition, they cause less nausea, and clarithromycin may be taken with meals.

9. What is the clinical spectrum of clindamycin? What are its side effects?

Clindamycin is a bacteriostatic agent that concentrates in bone. It is highly effective against anaerobic infections of the aerodigestive tract, including *Bacteroides fragilis*. It is also effective against *Staphylococcus aureus, Streptococcus pyogenes,* and *S. pneumoniae*. Its side effects include nausea, cramps, and diarrhea. In addition, it can cause pseudomembranous colitis due to overgrowth of *Clostridium difficile*.

10. What are the limitations of the tetracyclines? When should they be used?

The tetracyclines are inexpensive bacteriostastic agents to which most streptococcal, staphylococcal, and *Haemophilus influenzae* infections have become resistant. They are effective against *Mycoplasma* and *Legionella* infections. They should only be used in respiratory infections when they are proven sensitive by culture. Side effects include the staining of enamel, and they should thus be avoided in children under age 10 and in pregnant women.

11. When should chloramphenicol be used for head and neck infections?

Chloramphenicol has broad-spectrum activity against all gram-positive cocci and most gram-negative bacteria. However, *Pseudomonas aeruginosa* is resistant. Chloramphenicol penetrates the CSF more effectively than any other antibiotic. Because of potentially fatal bone marrow suppression, occurring in 1 of 24,000 patients, it should be used only in life-threatening infections when other effective agents are unavailable.

12. Which oral agents are available for treatment of pseudomonal infections of the head and neck?

The only agents available for the treatment of head and neck infections by *Pseudomonas* are the fluoroquinolones, including ciprofloxacin and ofloxacin. These antibiotics are bactericidal and also active against *Haemophilus influenzae, Moraxella catarrhalis,* and *Neisseria gonorrhoeae.* However, because other ordinary antibiotics are available for treatment of these three infections, the fluoroquinolones should only be used for pseudomonal infections. They may be used only in adults and are not primary agents for common respiratory or pharyngeal infections.

13. How should the aminoglycosides be administered? What is their clinical spectrum?
The aminoglycosides are not effective orally and are thus available only for parenteral use. They are effective against hospital-acquired infections, including *Escherichia coli, Serratia, Klebsiella, Proteus,* and *Enterobacter.* When combined with β-lactam agents, they are particularly effective against *Pseudomonas aeruginosa.* Anaerobic infections are almost universally resistant to the aminoglycosides.

14. In addition to β-lactams and clindamycin, which agent has activity against anaerobes?
Metronidazole is highly active against anaerobic infections, including *Bacteroides fragilis* and *Clostridium difficile.* It penetrates the CSF well. However, metronidazole is inactive against all aerobic infections. When this drug is administered, alcohol must be avoided.

15. What agent is most commonly used for methicillin-resistant strains of *Staphylococcus aureus*?
Vancomycin is unrelated to other antimicrobial groups and is often used for treatment of infections caused by methicillin-resistant *S. aureus.* It is also active against the streptococci. Vancomycin is only available in parenteral form, but when it is given orally, it is active against pseudomembranous colitis caused by *Clostridium difficile.*

16. When are sulfonamides effective for the treatment of bacterial infections?
The sulfonamides are bacteriostatic agents that are active only when combined with erythromycin or trimethoprim. They are effective in the treatment of infections caused by *Haemophilus influenzae, Moraxella catarrhalis,* and some streptococci.

17. How should a carrier of a nasopharyngeal infection be treated?
Rifampin is useful for prophylaxis and treatment of patients who carry *Haemophilus influenzae* and meningococcus. When combined with other antistaphylococcal agents, it is useful against resistant *Staphylococcus aureus.* It is also active against streptococci, *Legionella,* and anaerobes.

18. An asthmatic patient who is currently taking theophylline has pharyngitis, and you want to prescribe an antibiotic. Which should you avoid?
Erythromycin. The hepatic clearance of theophylline may be decreased by erythromycin, leading to high serum theophylline levels and toxicity within 1 week.

19. Which agents should be used to treat acute and chronic otitis media?
The first-line antibiotic for treating **acute otitis media** is often amoxicillin. Of the most common pathogens implicated in this infection, amoxicillin effectively treats *Streptococcus pneumoniae,* but 20% of *Haemophilus influenzae* strains and 80% of *Moraxella catarrhalis* strains are resistant. These pathogens are covered by the inexpensive trimethoprim-sulfamethoxazole preparations, but pneumococcal coverage is less effective. Although more expensive, erythromycin plus sulfonamide, amoxicillin plus clavulanic acid, cefixime, and cefuroxime combat all of these organisms. These should be considered second-line antibiotics. **Chronic otitis media** with effusion usually harbors the same pathogens as the acute form and is treated with the same agents.

20. How does the treatment of sinusitis differ from that of otitis media?
Acute sinusitis is caused by the same organisms that cause otitis media, and drug choices are similar. Intracranial and orbital complications of acute sinusitis require agents that penetrate the

blood-brain barrier, which include ceftriaxone, cefuroxime, ampicillin plus chloramphenicol, and vancomycin plus aztreonam. Chronic sinusitis is caused by anaerobic organisms and often *Staphylococcus aureus*. Effective agents include amoxicillin plus clavulanic acid, clindamycin, cephalexin, and dicloxacillin. Fungal infections should be treated with ketoconazole. Pseudomonal infections are often associated with extensive nasal polyposis and are treated with ciprofloxacin.

21. Which agents are useful for treating tonsillitis?

Bacterial tonsillitis is most often caused by *Streptococcus pyogenes*. However, a number of anaerobic organisms may be present in a mixed infection. Penicillin is often ineffective due to the production of β-lactamase by these organisms. Effective alternatives include clindamycin, amoxicillin plus clavulanic acid, dicloxacillin, and cephalexin. If the infection is mononucleosis, the amoxicillin will cause a severe rash in 50% of cases.

22. When should pharyngitis be treated with antibiotics? Which antibiotic should be used?

Antibiotics should be given to the sore throat patient when bacterial infection is suspected. Bacterial infection is favored when there is a history of contact with a bacterially infected individual, prolonged or severe sore throat, severe erythema or exudate, and lymphadenopathy. Penicillin's effectiveness is limited by β-lactamase-producing bacterial strains but may be administered. Effective alternatives include a macrolide or cephalexin.

23. When should antibiotic therapy be administered to the patient with epiglottitis? Which antibiotic?

Airway management takes priority in these patients. Antibiotics should be administered once the airway is secured. *Haemophilus influenzae* is often implicated in this infection. Antibiotics should be administered parenterally and may include ampicillin plus sulbactam, ampicillin plus chloramphenicol, or a second- or third-generation cephalosporin.

24. When should croup be treated with antibiotics?

Croup is usually caused by a virus but may become secondarily infected with *Staphylococcus aureus* or *Haemophilus influenzae*. Antibiotics should be administered when thick yellow secretions are encountered. Croup is treated with the same antibiotics that are used to treat epiglottitis.

25. Should laryngitis be treated with antibiotics?

Laryngitis is usually a viral infection that recovers with a few days of voice rest. Antibiotics may be necessary if the viral infection becomes secondarily infected with bacteria. Prolonged hoarseness suggests such a secondary infection and is effectively covered with erythromycin plus sulfonamide or amoxicillin plus clavulanic acid.

26. Which organisms predominate in deep neck abscesses? How should they be covered?

Deep neck abscesses and chronic intracranial infections spreading from the ears or sinuses are usually caused by mixed bacteria with a predominance of anaerobes. Clindamycin is a good antibiotic choice, covering anaerobic organisms and all cocci. If a pseudomonal infection is suspected, gentamicin should be added. If CNS penetration is required, nafcillin plus metronidazole should be utilized.

27. What agents should be used when treating mastoiditis?

Acute mastoiditis with a subperiosteal abscess is usually caused by the same organisms that cause acute otitis media, and therefore antibiotic choices are similar. Ceftriaxone is a good initial choice as the pneumococci and *Haemophilus influenzae* may extend intracranially. Chronic suppurative otomastoiditis requires additional coverage for *Staphylococcus aureus, Proteus* species, anaerobes, and possibly *Pseudomonas*.

28. What therapy is necessary for acute otitis externa?

Combination topical antibiotic therapy is necessary for the draining ear of acute otitis externa. Pseudomonal infections are covered by polymyxin, and *Staphylococcus aureus, Proteus* species, and others are covered by neomycin. Cortisporin includes both of these preparations.

29. What are the polyenes? When are they used by otolaryngologists?

The polyenes are antifungal agents and include nystatin and amphotericin B. Nystatin is available only in topical and oral preparations and is useful only for oral candidiasis. It is not absorbed systemically. An oral suspension is swished around in the mouth and swallowed. Amphotericin B is also poorly absorbed from the gastrointestinal tract and is thus limited to intravenous use. Lower doses that are administered for 1–2 weeks are used to treat esophageal candidiasis. High doses are required for treating documented infections due to *Aspergillus* species or zygomycosis. Therapy duration is determined by total cumulative dose, which should be from 2–3 gm.

30. Can any additional agents be used for treating candidiasis?

The azoles, including cotrimazole, ketoconazole, fluconazole, and itraconazole, may be used in candidiasis. In addition, fluconazole may be used when treating histoplasmosis, coccidioidomycosis, and paracoccidioidomycosis. Itraconazole is approved for the treatment of pulmonary and extrapulmonary blastomycosis and histoplasmosis.

31. Which antiviral agents are used by the otolaryngologist?

The number of effective antiviral agents is sharply limited. Acyclovir may be used for prophylaxis or treatment of herpes infections. Amantadine is effective against influenza type A and is used primarily for severe infections, especially in the immunocompromised patient. Zidovudine and didanosine are used in patients infected with HIV.

CONTROVERSIES

32. When should prophylactic antibiotics be administered to patients undergoing surgery of the head and neck?

This question has received much attention, and an abundance of clinical research has revolved around it. Overall, a decreased wound infection rate has been shown for patients undergoing surgery when appropriate short-term antibiotic prophylaxis has been implemented. Cost analysis data suggest that antibiotics should not be withheld to reduce hospital costs in head and neck surgery. Prophylactic antibiotic therapy has been shown clearly to be of benefit in patients undergoing **clean** operations with a foreign-body implant. This is also evident for **clean-contaminated** wounds, which are sterile initially but have a mucosal barrier crossed or a hollow viscus entered during the operation. The **contaminated** wound results from a major lapse in sterile technique or exposure to acute nonpurulent inflammation. The **dirty** wound is the infected traumatic wound that is contaminated with bacteria or environmental debris. These wounds clearly benefit from the administration of prophylactic antibiotics.

33. What is the appropriate timing for administration of surgical prophylactic antibiotics?

The effective use of prophylactic antibiotics depends on the appropriate timing of their administration. Although most head and neck surgeons agree that prophylactic antibiotics are necessary, many disagree as to the dosing schedule. The current recommendation is that parenteral antibiotics be administered within 30 minutes of the initial incision. If they are given 3–4 hours before the initiation of surgery, levels of the antibiotic in serum and tissues may be low or absent during the procedure. Although some surgeons have advocated continuation of antibiotics for 2–5 days after a procedure, many argue that a single day of administration is adequate.

34. What determines which antibiotics should be given to the patient who is undergoing head and neck surgery?

The agent should be chosen depending on its efficacy against the microorganisms that are known to cause infectious complications in each particular clinical setting. In addition, safety profile and cost should be considered. For example, parenteral administration of a first-generation cephalosporin is appropriate for clean procedures in which common infecting organisms include *Staphylococcus aureus* and *S. epidermidis*. Procedures that frequently involve contamination with anaerobic organisms require appropriate coverage with an antibiotic such as clindamycin.

BIBLIOGRAPHY

1. Blair EA, Johnson JT, Wagner RL, et al: Cost analysis of antibiotic prophylaxis in clean head and neck surgery. Arch Otol Head Neck Surg 121:269–271, 1995.
2. Brook I: Diagnosis and management of anaerobic infections of the head and neck. Ann Otol Rhinol Laryngol 101:9–15, 1992.
3. Fairbanks DNF: Bacteriology and antibiotics. Otolaryngol Clin North Am 26:549–559, 1993.
4. Fairbanks DNF: Microbiology, infections, and antibiotic therapy. In Bailey BJ (ed): Head and Neck Surgery–Otolaryngology. Philadelphia, J.B. Lippincott, 1993, pp 52–61.
5. Fairbanks DNF: Antimicrobial therapy in otolaryngology–head and neck surgery. In Lee KJ (ed): Essential Otolaryngology–Head and Neck Surgery. Norwalk, CT, Appleton & Lange, 1995, pp 427–436.
6. Medoff G: Antimicrobial use in otolaryngeal infections: General considerations: Ann Otol Rhinol Laryngol 101:5–8, 1992.
7. Neibart E, Gumprecht J: Antifungal agents and the treatment of fungal infections of the head and neck. Otolaryngol Clin North Am 26:1123–1131, 1993.
8. Nichols RL: Surgical antibiotic prophylaxis. Med Clin North Am 79:509–522, 1995.
9. Velanovich V: A meta-analysis of prophylactic antibiotics in head and neck surgery. Plastic Reconst Surg 87:429–434, 1991.
10. Weber RS, Callender DL: Antibiotic prophylaxis in clean-contaminated head and neck oncologic surgery. Ann Otol Rhinol Laryngol 101:16–20, 1992.

34. PHARMACOLOGY OF OTOLARYNGOLOGY

Erik Vinge and Stephen Batuello, M.D.

1. What are the pharmacological treatments for xerostomia?

Xerostomia is a dry mouth due to salivary gland dysfunction. It is associated with many diseases and is often a pharmacologic side effect. Among the many complications associated with a chronic dry mouth are dental caries, infection, discomfort, dysphagia, and halitosis. For some patients, a cholinergic agonist such as pilocarpine may be effective in alleviating the symptoms. Others may find saliva substitutes, containing either carboxymethyl-cellulose or hydroxyethyl-cellulose, to be the best treatment.

2. For what conditions are intranasal corticosteroids utilized?

Hayfever	Chronic sinusitis
Perennial noninfectious rhinitis	Nasal polyposis

3. How long must nasal corticosteroids be used before they demonstrate their desired effects?

Some people experience relief of symptoms as quickly as a few hours after beginning use. However, the vast majority of people who use nasal corticosteroids must use the drugs for several weeks before achieving maximum relief of symptoms. Therefore, patients should be instructed to use the inhalers continuously for a few weeks before they decide whether the drug is helpful.

4. What are the common side effects of intranasal corticosteroids?

Some of the most common side effects are transient irritation, burning, and sneezing. Long-term use of these steroids may cause capillary fragility, predisposing the patient to epistaxis. Side effects associated with chronic use of systemic steroids, such as adrenal suppression and a cushingoid body morph, have not been observed.

5. Which drugs are associated with increased serum theophylline levels?

Erythromycin, ciprofloxacin, cimetidine, propranolol, and high-dose allopurinol may significantly raise serum theophylline levels. This relationship is important to remember because of the many asthmatics who receive long-term theophylline therapy. Signs and symptoms of theophylline toxicity include nausea, restlessness, ventricular arrhythmias, convulsions, and even death. The more serious presentations are not necessarily preceded by the milder symptoms.

6. How do antihistamines work?

Antihistamines are competitive antagonists that occupy histamine receptor sites on histamine-releasing cells. The two subclasses of histamine receptors are denoted as H_1 and H_2. The H_1 receptors are primarily involved in bronchial and gastrointestinal smooth muscle contraction, vasodilation of arteries and veins, and stimulation of sensory nerve endings. Conversely, H_2 receptors predominantly affect gastric acid secretion. Unfortunately, because many other types of chemical mediators are released during an anaphylactic reaction, antihistamines are ineffective in treating of the profound vasodilation and bronchospasm associated with anaphylactic shock.

7. What is the most common side effect of H_1 antihistamines?

Sedation. Other less common ones include vision changes, fatigue, and incoordination.

8. What are the stimulatory side effects of H_1 antagonists?

The stimulatory side effects of antihistamines include euphoria, restlessness, nervousness, insomnia, and tremor. Patients with underlying neuropathology may be prone to seizures. Whether a person experiences stimulatory or depressive side effects varies from person to person. This response also varies with the dose of the drug.

9. Define rhinitis medicamentosa.

Rhinitis medicamentosa develops when over-the-counter preparations of topical antihistamine and decongestant sprays (e.g., Afrin) are used for prolonged periods. Rebound nasal congestion results with discontinued use of the spray. Patients become dependent on the medication and are often reluctant to accept that the medicine is the source of, not the solution to, their problem.

10. How should a patient using potentially ototoxic drugs be evaluated for ototoxicity?

Patients should be questioned regarding the development of tinnitus, hearing loss, imbalance, and vertigo. They should be instructed to report the development of any such symptoms while they are taking these medications.

11. What drugs are commonly associated with ototoxicity?

Streptomycin	Minocycline
Neomycin	Quinine (more marked than usually appreciated)
Kanamycin	Quinidine
Tobramycin	Salicylates (often reversible on drug withdrawal)
Amikacin	Cisplatin
Netilmicin	Ethacrynic acid
Vancomycin	Furosemide
Erythromycin	

12. Why is an ototoxic agent such as streptomycin used in the treatment of Meniere's disease?

Because streptomycin sulfate has a strong toxic affinity for the vestibular system, it can be used to treat intractable, bilateral Meniere's disease. The toxic effect of the drug is dose-related. Generally, a patient is given 2 gm/day until he or she no longer has a caloric response.

13. What are some special considerations regarding the ototoxicity of quinine?

Tinnitus and hearing loss are side effects associated with quinine use. Both are considered to be reversible. However, in pregnant women, therapeutic doses may not cause hearing loss in the mother but may cause bilateral sensorineural hearing loss in the child.

14. Why are sinus infections often difficult to treat pharmacologically?

It is thought that sinus infections result from stasis of pooled secretions. This stasis may be secondary to obstruction or inadequate function in the sinuses. Once secretions are infected, antibiotics may be less effective because of the absence of blood supply to the infected reservoirs. Antibiotic therapy for sinusitis may require prolonged courses and high doses. Antibiotic therapy may also be prescribed in combination with treatments aimed at increasing sinus drainage.

15. What is the mechanism of action of cromolyn sodium?

Cromolyn sodium indirectly blocks the uptake of calcium by the mast cell, thereby preventing degranulation when the cell is exposed to an allergen. Without the release of the chemical mediators contained in the granules, the allergic hypersensitivity reaction cannot occur.

16. Should cromolyn sodium be used in the acute setting?

Because cromolyn sodium must be given prior to allergen presentation to the mast cell, the drug is not administered in acute hypersensitivity reactions. Four weeks may be required before the desired effects of the drug are observed. For example, a patient should begin treatment 1 month before the onset of hayfever season and continue taking the drug for the duration that symptoms are present.

17. Should intravenous corticosteroids be used in place of epinephrine in the treatment of severe allergic hypersensitivity reactions?

The effective use of IV corticosteroids requires at least 60–120 minutes following administration before desired effects are observed. Therefore, IV corticosteroids are not a good substitute for epinephrine.

18. What are some possible treatments of motion sickness?

Most treatments for motion sickness belong to either the anticholinergic or antihistamine class of drugs. Scopolamine, an anticholinergic, is considered the most effective. Other anticholinergics include atropine and glycopyrrolate (Robinul). Dimenhydrinate, diphenhydramine, promethazine, and piperazine derivatives are H_1 blockers also known to provide effective treatments for motion sickness.

19. How should drugs for motion sickness be administered?

Motion sickness medications are much more effective when given prophylactically. Once severe nausea or vomiting has commenced, the effectiveness of these agents is significantly reduced.

20. A patient regularly takes birth control pills. Should ampicillin be prescribed for otitis media?

Some antibiotics, when given for > 10–14 days, interact with oral contraceptives and reduce their effectiveness. Ampicillin, bacampicillin, penicillin V, sulfonamides, and tetracyclines have all been shown to have such an effect. Patients should be advised of this increased risk, and other methods of contraception should be employed for at least one cycle after the drug has been discontinued.

21. When are antibacterial/anti-inflammatory drops indicated?

Preparations of neomycin combined with hydrocortisone and polymyxin B are used to treat superficial infections of the external auditory canal.

22. Of what use is the diluent in otic drops?

In otic preparations, the diluent promotes an acidic pH, inhibiting bacterial growth. Therefore, the diluent is just as important as the preparation's antibiotic or steroid.

23. How are antibacterial/anti-inflammatory drops used?

The dosing varies with the severity of the disease. A severe infection might require one-half of a dropper four times daily. As the patient improves, the dosing schedule and amount can both be decreased.

24. Should ear drops be used prophylactically?

As long as the tympanic membrane is intact, it is safe for someone to use ear drops a couple of times every week for prolonged periods of time.

25. Why is cocaine sometimes used in ENT procedures?

Cocaine is used primarily because it has both anesthetic and vasoconstrictive effects that are rapid in onset. Although topical cocaine is useful in the clinic, emergency department, and operating room, it should not be prescribed.

26. How does cocaine promote vasoconstriction?

Cocaine is a catecholamine re-uptake inhibitor. Therefore, topical administration should precede injection of epinephrine preparations.

27. Describe the pharmacology of lidocaine.

Lidocaine is an ester that inhibits action potentials by interrupting ion transfer across cell membranes.

28. What are the maximum recommended doses of lidocaine, lidocaine with epinephrine, and cocaine?

In the normal-hearing adult, lidocaine should not be given in excess of 4.5 mg/kg, not to exceed 300 mg. Lidocaine with epinephrine is more slowly absorbed and is given in a dosage not greater than 7.0 mg/kg or 500 mg. The maximum dosage of cocaine is 3.0 mg/kg or 200 mg.

29. When is the peak anesthetic effect and what is the duration of action of topical cocaine and lidocaine?

Peak anesthetic effect occurs within 2–5 minutes and lasts for 30–45 minutes.

30. What is the first-line antibiotic for acute otitis media in a child?

In children, the most frequent pathogens associated with otitis media are *Streptococcus pneumoniae* and *Haemophilus influenzae*. In uncomplicated episodes of acute otitis media, amoxicillin is active against all *S. pneumoniae* and most strains of *H. influenzae*. If the patient is allergic to penicillins, erythromycin with sulfisoxazole preparations may be used.

31. When is botulinum-A toxin indicated?

Botulinum-A toxin may be used to treat facial dystonias (blepharospasm, torticollis, hemifacial spasm) and spastic dysphonia. This therapy may be an alternative or adjunct to surgery.

32. Which drugs are part of the first-line therapy for gastroesophageal reflux?

Liquid antacids are considered an integral part of treatment for gastroesophageal reflux. Sucralfate and Gaviscon are examples. Anatacids may be used along with postural and dietary changes.

33. Aggressive therapy has been shown to increase survival in patients with mucormycosis. What does this entail?

Mucormycosis is a fungal infection that tends to affect people with diabetic ketoacidosis, neutropenia, malnutrition, or iron overload. Survival appears to be improved by aggressive measures such as surgical debridement and intravenous amphotericin B.

BIBLIOGRAPHY

1. Blakely BW, Swanson RW: ENT Formulary: Otolaryngology for the House Officer. Baltimore, Williams & Wilkins, 1989, pp 187–201.
2. Lee KJ: Pharmacology and therapeutics. In Lee KJ (ed): Essential Otolaryngology–Head and Neck Surgery. Norwalk, CT, Appleton & Lange, 1995, pp 1069–1085.
3. Physicians Desk Reference, 49th ed. Oradell, NJ, Medical Economics, 1995.
4. Principato JJ: Chronic rhinitis. In Gates GA (ed): Current Therapy in Otolaryngology–Head and Neck Surgery—4. Toronto, B.C. Decker, 1990, pp 280–283.
5. Sugar AM: Mucormycosis. Clin Infect Dis 14(suppl 1):S126–S129, 1992.
6. Willett JM, Lee KJ: Pharmacology and Therapeutics. Otolaryngology–Head and NeckSurgery—630 Questions and Answers. Norwalk, CT, Appleton & Lange, 1995, pp 287–291.

V. Endoscopy

35. LARYNGOSCOPY

Bruce W. Jafek, M.D.

1. What is laryngoscopy used for?
To visualize the larynx, or "voicebox."

2. How is "indirect" laryngoscopy done?
Actually, you should have done indirect laryngoscopy during your initial examination of the head and neck region. This is done with a mirror and is termed "indirect" because you do not visualize the larynx "directly" but only see it in the mirror. If additional evaluation of the larynx is necessary, then a more direct method may be indicated.

3. What are the indications for direct laryngoscopy?
  1. Additional evaluation of suspected or actual pathology within the larynx (e.g., hoarseness, laryngeal tumor)
  2. Therapy within the larynx (e.g., removal of vocal cord polyp, subglottic dilatation)
  3. Preliminary step to intubation (the anesthesiologist usually uses a scope with a curved blade and visualizes only the posterior larynx)
  4. Preliminary step to the insertion of a rigid bronchoscope (rarely required)

4. Direct laryngoscopy is considered a "surgical procedure," even though it does not require an external incision. Is there another way to evaluate the larynx before proceeding with direct laryngoscopy?
Additional visualization of the larynx may be required in the outpatient setting. If the larynx cannot be visualized with the mirror—for example, due to arthritic changes in the patient's neck or a vigorous gag reflex—fiberoptic laryngoscopy may be performed.

5. How is fiberoptic laryngoscopy performed?
This procedure is performed through the patient's nose. It avoids the problems associated with the deep pressor receptors of the tongue base and prevents the uncooperative patient from biting your expensive fiberoptic laryngoscope! The nose is first sprayed with a vasoconstrictor (e.g., 0.5% ephedrine) and then with a local anesthetic (e.g., 1% lidocaine). Alternatively, 1% cocaine may be used, accomplishing both anesthesia and vasoconstriction. The flexible scope is then inserted through the nose and down through the pharynx to visualize the larynx.

6. Fiberoptic laryngoscopy seems much simpler. What are its advantages and disadvantages over direct laryngoscopy?
The primary advantage is, indeed, simplicity and patient comfort. The procedure is easily accomplished in the office and provides a good view of the larynx. This procedure is disadvantageous because a fiberoptic viewing cable is used, and the view of the larynx is not as good as with a Hopkins rod telescope or direct visualization with or without the microscope. Although not impossible, biopsy or vocal cord injection are more complex via fiberoptic laryngoscopy, and other surgical manipulation (e.g., dilatation) is nearly impossible.

7. Can vocal cord biopsies and injections be performed without direct laryngoscopy?

Yes. Biopsies can be obtained using a curved biopsy forceps and a mirror or a fiberoptic laryngoscope. However, this procedure requires an extremely skilled otolaryngologist and cooperative patient. Similarly, injections can be made directly into the vocal cord (e.g., Teflon or fat injection for vocal cord medialization) with this technique. Botulinum injections into the vocal cords can either be performed with this technique or via the cricothyroid membrane.

8. How is anesthesia obtained for manipulation of the larynx?

Cocaine or lidocaine/ephedrine can be used in the nose if the fiberoptic laryngoscope is utilized. These agents are not necessary if the mirror rests on the soft palate, as in indirect laryngoscopy. Anesthesia of the larynx can then be achieved by either dripping 1% cocaine through a curved cannula or by anesthetizing the superior laryngeal nerve.

9. What is superior laryngeal nerve anesthesia?

The superior laryngeal nerve (SLN) provides sensory innervation to the epiglottis, aryepiglottic folds, and upper larynx. In addition, this nerve provides parasympathetic secretomotor fibers to the associated glands in the mucous membrane of these structures. Passing downward, the SLN parallels the carotid artery, until a branch (internal branch) swings anteriorly to cross and then pierce the superior aspect of the thyrohyoid membrane. It is here that the nerve is accessible to infiltration of anesthesia.

The otolaryngologist's left (nondominant) index finger is placed in the trough between the hyoid, superiorly, and thyroid cartilage, inferiorly (over the thyrohyoid membrane). This finger is advanced posteriorly until the pulsations of the carotid artery are palpable. The common carotid artery lies posteriorly and is avoided and protected with the index finger. Through a #25 needle, 2% lidocaine without epinephrine is injected approximately 1 cm deep into the tissues, just off the tip of the palpating index finger. This injection is just anterior to the posterior edge of the hyoid bone or superior cornua of the thyroid cartilage. Usually an injection of 2 ml/side provides excellent anesthesia. Alternatively, the needle is inserted until the patient complains of pain in the ear (via Arnold's nerve), but this is usually unnecessary. The area of injection is then massaged briefly to promote spread through the tissues. A similar injection is then carried out on the other side.

10. Why is lidocaine *without* epinephrine preferred?

Lidocaine spreads through the tissues easily, obviating the need to inject the SLN directly. This spread is inhibited by epinephrine because of the associated vasoconstriction.

11. What other endoscopic procedures are used to evaluate the larynx?

Two of the most important recent methods of evaluating the larynx prior to manipulation are **videolaryngoscopy** and **videolaryngostroboscopy**. These examinations are best done with the transoral rigid telescope with a rigid-rod quartz lens system (e.g., Ward-Berci scope) but can be done with the flexible laryngoscope. They are the best ways to assess the dynamic function of the larynx, as observation during both quiet breathing and during a variety of tasks is possible. The addition of a **video camera** (videolaryngoscopy) produces an enlarged image that may be recorded for detailed evaluation or saved for comparison with future examinations. Videolaryngoscopy also allows accurate evaluation of the closing and opening pattern of the larynx.

The addition of the **stroboscope** provides a flashing light to simulate a slowed vocal cord vibration and further facilitates evaluation of dynamic laryngeal function, particularly the mucosal wave of the vocal folds. The stroboscope has a microphone to sense the fundamental frequency of the vibrations and coordinates the flashing light to the same frequency. If the light flashes at the fundamental frequency, the stroboscope will freeze one image in the vibratory cycle. The slowed motion allows the most accurate assessment of the mucosal wave. This wave may be impaired by scarring, edema, or subtle defects in the mucosa. With stroboscopy, lesions such as very early carcinoma may be best seen as an adynamic segment of the vocal cord.

12. Name the other ancillary tests used for the evaluation of laryngeal function.
- **Acoustic analysis** measures fundamental frequency, spectral analysis, and perturbation (shimmer = loudness and jitter = pitch).
- **Aerodynamic ability** is an aerodynamic assessment of flow and pressure.
- **Photoglottography** and **electroglottography**
- **Electromyography** provides information about the nerves and muscles of the larynx.
- **Cineradiography** is used to evaluate laryngeal closure and other functions.
- **Aspiration tests**

13. How is direct laryngoscopy performed?
If general anesthesia is employed, the patient is placed supine and intubated. The neck is then extended and the scope inserted. With insertion, it is important to avoid injury to the lips, tongue, or teeth. The initial landmark is the uvula, followed by the epiglottis. The epiglottis is lifted superiorly into the patient's anterior neck, allowing visualization of the larynx. At this point, the operator can stabilize the patient's head by holding the scope with the palm of the non-dominant hand on the patient's forehead. Alternatively, the patient can be "suspended" with various devices (e.g., Lewy, Benjamin). This arrangement allows the microscope to be positioned so that the surgeon may proceed with both hands.

14. Are there any other tricks to direct laryngoscopy?
The larynx is usually cocainized prior to manipulation (4% cocaine-soaked neurosurgical patties are placed on the laryngeal mucosa).

15. Why use cocaine, since the patient is already under general anesthesia?
The cocaine serves three purposes:
  1. It is a vasoconstrictor and therefore minimizes bleeding if biopsies are to be obtained.
  2. It is an anesthetic and minimizes the potential for laryngospasm upon extubation, a problem due to irritation from bleeding.
  3. Cocaine decreases the laryngocardiac reflex.

16. Why does laryngospasm occur?
During recovery, especially during stage II anesthesia, the glottis occasionally "clamps" closed. This action is probably a primitive defense mechanism in response to an irritant and acts to protect the lower respiratory tree. It usually "breaks up" as the patient starts breathing spontaneously. However, reanesthetizing the patient, especially with paralytic agents, is occasionally required.

17. What is the laryngocardiac reflex?
Observers have noted that pressure on the larynx occasionally produces bradycardia or cardiac arrest. This response is believed to be due to reflexive laryngocardiac innervation, although the neural pathways are not precisely defined. Anesthetizing the larynx prior to manipulation avoids this problem.

18. How do the various types of laryngoscopes differ?
Each type of laryngoscope is designed to deal with a certain type of problem encountered during laryngoscopy. One has an "anterior flare" (anterior commissure scope) and allows for improved visualization of the anterior commissure of the larynx. Another is "wasp-waisted" (constricted in the middle) and minimizes pressure on the teeth. Another has a broad viewing port and facilitates the use of the microscope. Another has a "double bill" which allows the larynx to be spread somewhat, facilitating the use of a laser for a transoral supraglottic laryngectomy.

19. What are the special postoperative considerations with direct laryngoscopy?
This procedure is usually performed on an outpatient basis. Voice rest is indicated for 7–10 days if a biopsy has been obtained, especially if the lesion involved most of a vocal cord. One or

two doses of 8 mg dexamethasone IV (4 hours apart) minimizes postoperative edema. Cool mist is also soothing if the cord has been "stripped."

20. What are the potential complications associated with direct laryngoscopy?
The most common is inadvertent injury to the lips, tongue, or teeth. This should be avoided by watching these areas carefully during the procedure. A tooth guard minimizes pressure on the teeth. Laryngospasm and the laryngocardiac reflex are discussed earlier (see Questions 16 and 17). If a cord is stripped (deepithelialized), care should be taken to protect the anterior commissure mucosa on the opposite side to avoid anterior laryngeal webbing.

CONTROVERSIES

21. Is laryngoscopy best done under local or general anesthesia?
Direct laryngoscopy is usually done under general anesthesia, but in the cooperative, preferably sedated patient, direct laryngoscopy can easily be done under local anesthesia. However, the real decision as to local or general anesthesia relates to the purpose. A detailed examination of the larynx can easily be accomplished under local anesthesia in the office. Manipulation, on the other hand, may require general anesthesia, depending on the skill of the operator, specific procedure to be performed, and patient preference.

22. Should the laryngoscope be hand-held, or is suspension best?
Again, the best means depends on the procedure. For simple examination of the larynx or minimal biopsying, holding the laryngoscope shortens the procedure and minimizes tooth injury. For prolonged procedures (e.g., use of the laser or microscope), suspension is indicated.

BIBLIOGRAPHY

1. Hanson DG, Gerratt BR, Ward PH: Glottographic measurements of vocal cord dysfunction: A preliminary report. Ann Otol Rhinol Laryngol 92:413, 1983.
2. Hirano M: Stroboscopic examination of the normal larynx. In Blitzer, et al (eds): Neurologic Disorders of the Larynx. New York, Thieme, 1992.
3. Ward PH, Hanson DG, Berci G: Observations on central neurologic etiology for laryngeal dysfunction. Ann Otol Rhinol Laryngol 90:430, 1990.
4. Woodson GE, et al: Use of flexible laryngoscopy to classify patients with spasmodic dysphonia. J Voice 5:85, 1991.
5. Woodson GE, Blitzer A: Neurologic evaluation of the larynx and pharynx. In Cummings CW, et al (eds): Otolaryngology–Head and Neck Surgery, 2nd. ed. St. Louis, Mosby, 1995, pp 61–71.

36. ESOPHAGOSCOPY

Stephen G. Batuello, M.D.

1. Describe the embryology of the esophagus.
The esophagus is derived from the embryonic foregut of the primitive gut tube. The foregut is separated by the tracheoesophageal septum into the dorsal esophagus and the more ventral trachea. The shortened esophagus lengthens as it descends with the heart and lungs to reach its full length in the 7th embryonic week. The stratified squamous epithelium and glands of the esophagus are derived from endoderm, whereas the striated and smooth muscle are derived from mesenchyme. During development, epithelial proliferation obliterates the lumen of the esophagus, which re-canalizes by the 8th week.

2. How do congenital esophageal atresia, esophageal stenosis, and tracheoesophageal fistula occur?

Esophageal atresia occurs as a result of dorsal deviation of the tracheoesophageal septum and subsequent blind closure of the esophagus. Because the fetus is then unable to swallow amniotic fluid, this condition is frequently associated with polyhydramnios.

Esophageal stenosis, or congenital webbing, usually occurs in the distal third of the esophagus and results from incomplete recanalization of the lumen after epithelial proliferation.

Tracheoesophageal fistula, usually associated with esophageal atresia, occurs in about 1 in 2,500 births. As the name implies, this disorder is an abnormal communication between the trachea and esophagus which results from a defective tracheoesophageal septum.

3. What are the four major types of tracheoesophageal fistula?

1. Most commonly, the superior portion of the esophagus ends blindly, and the inferior portion joins the trachea directly.

2. The inferior portion of the esophagus ends blindly, and the superior portion joins the esophagus directly.

3. Both superior and inferior portions join the trachea directly without joining each other.

4. The esophagus is a continuous tube with a side-to-side communication with the trachea.

4. Describe the anatomy of the esophagus.

The esophagus is a 25-cm neuromuscular tube extending from the mouth to the stomach. The outer musculature layer is composed of outer longitudinal and inner circular fibers of striated muscle in the upper third of the esophagus and nonstriated muscle in the lower third of the esophagus. Between the two muscle layers is the myenteric (Auerbach's) parasympathetic plexus and the submucous (Meissner's) plexus. An intervening submucosa contains mucous glands, blood vessels, and lymphatics. The esophageal mucosa is lined by stratified squamous epithelium. The arterial supply and venous drainage systems of the esophagus are segmental. The lymphatic drainage of the cervical esophagus is via paraesophageal cervical and lower jugular nodes. The thoracic esophagus drains via mediastinal, hilar, and paraesophageal nodes, and the abdominal portion of the esophagus drains into gastric and celiac nodes. The esophagus receives both sympathetic and parasympathetic innervation from cranial nerves IX and X.

5. What are the three points of anatomic narrowing of the esophagus?

1. Cricopharyngeus muscle
2. Point at which the aorta and left mainstem bronchus cross anteriorly
3. Lower esophageal sphincter

6. At what distances from the incisor teeth are major esophageal landmarks encountered in the adult? In the 3-year-old? In the 1-year-old?

	Adult	*3-year-old*	*1-year-old*
Cricopharyngeus	12–16	9–11	8–10
Aorta	20–24	13–15	12–14
Esophageal hiatus	35–38	20–23	18–20
Cardia	38–42	25–27	21–22

Distances are in cm.

7. What is the function of the esophagus? How is this evaluated?

The esophagus transports nutrients from the mouth to the stomach and prevents regurgitation. The former is accomplished by involuntary peristalsis initiated by delivery of a food bolus from the oropharynx. The latter is accomplished by tonic closure of the lower esophageal sphincter. The tone and transport functions of the esophagus may be evaluated by cinepharyngography (tailored barium swallow).

8. Define esophagoscopy.

The term esophagoscopy is derived form the Greek word *oisophagos*, meaning gullet, and *skopos*, meaning to aim or inspect. Esophagoscopy is a procedure involving direct examination of the interior of the esophagus.

9. Who performed the first esophagoscopy?

The first rigid esophagoscopy was performed by Kussmaul in 1868. Interestingly, early esophagoscopes contained a bend to accommodate the oropharynx. Kussmaul studied the techniques of sword swallowers and adapted these techniques to his practice. This obviated the need for curved esophagoscopes and optimized direct examination with straight instruments.

10. What are the indications for esophagoscopy?

Esophagoscopy has both diagnostic and therapeutic indications.

Diagnostic uses: dysphagia, odynophagia, atypical chest pain, hematemesis, suspected gastroesophageal reflux, webs, strictures, and neoplasia.

Therapeutic uses: removal of foreign bodies, sclerotherapy, myotomy, dilation, and coagulation of bleeding.

11. When is esophagoscopy contraindicated?

• Aneurysm of the thoracic aorta
• Severe deformities of the cervical or thoracic spine
• Uncooperative or combative patient
• Severe erosive burns to the esophagus
• Chronic administration of high-dose steroids
• Laryngeal edema

12. What are the potential complications of esophagoscopy?

Esophageal perforation	Hypotension
Trauma to the lips, tongue, or oral mucosa	Arrhythmias
Fracturing or dislocation of the teeth	Pneumothorax
Aspiration pneumonia	Bleeding
Respiratory depression	

The most common complication of esophagoscopy, esophageal perforation, occurs in 1–2 % of cases.

13. Why does the esophagus have a greater propensity to rupture than other sites in the alimentary tract?

The esophagus has no serosal layer. This anatomic fact, combined with the presence of negative intrathoracic pressure, makes the esophagus more susceptible to perforation.

14. What are the symptoms of esophageal perforations?

Pain, followed by fever, hematemesis, tachycardia, hypotension, and shock.

15. How is an esophageal perforation diagnosed?

The patient with fever after esophagoscopy should be presumed to have a perforation until proved otherwise. Chest radiography and Gastrograffin contrast studies should be performed immediately. The white blood cell count is usually elevated. An electrocardiogram is obtained to rule out possible myocardial ischemia.

16. How do you treat an esophageal perforation?

The patient should receive nothing by mouth and be placed on broad-spectrum antibiotics initially. The patient's vital signs and white blood cell count are followed closely. Oral suctioning of saliva, rather than swallowing, is helpful. If symptoms resolve and there is no evidence of infection in 7–10 days, the Gastrograffin contrast is repeated to reassess the perforation. If there is no evidence of leakage, the diet may be advanced slowly and the patient closely observed. Antibiotics are discontinued if there is no evidence of recurrent infection. Should symptoms persist or recur, surgical exploration with drainage is indicated.

17. Describe the technique of rigid esophagoscopy.

In general, esophagoscopy should not be performed without a preoperative esophagogram viewable during the procedure. Rigid esophagoscopy is best tolerated by the patient under general anesthesia. The patient is positioned with the shoulders at the free end of the operating table, the head in the neutral position, and the neck flexed initially. The lubricated esophagoscope is introduced laterally in the region of the premolars and advanced to the level of the epiglottis. The epiglottis is retracted, and the esophagoscope is then brought into the midline. The esophagoscope then is carefully advanced to the level of the cricopharyngeus muscle, the most dangerous location of the procedure. The lumen is maintained in the center of the visual field as the instrument is advanced toward the stomach, and the esophagus is carefully examined to and through the gastroesophageal junction. The esophagoscope is never advanced unless it moves easily and the lumen is visible at all times. The esophagus may be re-inspected during careful removal of the instrument.

18. Describe the technique of flexible esophagoscopy.

Flexible endoscopes are more easily passed from the oropharynx into the esophagus and may be used with local or topical anesthesia. With the patient in the sitting or decubitus position (to minimize aspiration), the endoscope is introduced past the cricopharyngeus muscle as the patient swallows. The esophagus and stomach are then inspected during cautious advancement of the instrument.

CONTROVERSIES

19. Which is better, rigid or flexible esophagoscopy?

Because each procedure has advantages and disadvantages, many endoscopists consider them as adjunctive rather than mutually exclusive techniques. In general, rigid esophagoscopy provides better visualization of the pharynx and upper esophageal sphincter, more controlled foreign-body removal, direct visualization during dilation, easier debulking of tumor, and easier securing of biopsies. Flexible esophagoscopy obviates the need for general anesthesia, allows inspection of the stomach and duodenum, and can be used to maneuver through tortuous anatomy.

20. Should esophagoscopy be performed in cases of caustic ingestion?

Some authors have identified caustic ingestion as an absolute contraindication to endoscopy, but others report the necessity to evaluate the esophagus so that appropriate treatment may be instituted. However, it is generally agreed that esophagoscopy is contraindicated in cases of severe burns or evidence of laryngeal edema. Most also agree that it is contraindicated for patients on high-dose steroids.

BIBLIOGRAPHY

1. Hollinshead WH: Anatomy for Surgeons: vol 1. The Head and Neck, 3rd ed. Philadelphia, J.B. Lippincott, 1982.
2. Huizinga E: On esophagoscopy and sword swallowing. Ann Otol Rhinol Laryngol 78:32–39, 1969.
3. Krepsi YP: Complication in Head and Neck Surgery. Philadelphia, W.B. Saunders, 1993. pp 292–295.
4. Lee KJ: The chest. In Essential Otolaryngology–Head and Neck Surgery. Norwalk, CT, Appleton & Lange, 1995, p 335.
5. Moore KL: The Developing Human, 4th ed. Philadelphia, W.B. Saunders., 1988.
6. Orringer MC: Esophagoscopy. In Sabiston DC (ed): Textbook of Surgery: The Biological Basis of Modern Surgical Practice, 14th ed. Philadelphia, W.B. Saunders, 1991.
7. Shockley WW: Esophageal disorders. In Bailey BJ (ed): Head and Neck Surgery–Otolaryngology, Philadelphia, W.B. Saunders, 1993, pp 292–295.

37. BRONCHOSCOPY

Bruce W. *Jafek*, M.D.

1. Describe the embryologic development of the trachea and bronchi.

A median tracheobronchial groove appears in the ventral wall of the embryonic pharynx during the third week of development. As this groove deepens, the lateral septae grow together and fuse to divide the esophagus from the trachea. Superiorly, the fusion is incomplete, forming the laryngeal inlet. The caudal end of the embryonic trachea elongates and divides into two lateral outgrowths, the right and left lung bud. These buds grow out into the coelom, which forms the primitive pleural cavity. The buds are enveloped in splanchnic mesoderm from which the connective tissues of the lungs and bronchi develop. Subsequent divisions of the lung buds form the lobes of the lungs and progressively smaller divisions of the tracheobronchial tree (e.g., bronchopulmonary segments down to alveolar sacs).

2. What are the functions of the trachea and bronchi?

The trachea and bronchi conduct air from the upper aerodigestive cavity. The larynx serves to protect these airways. While air is being conducted, it is being conditioned by the ciliated tracheobronchial epithelium. This specialized epithelium traps and expels small foreign bodies (e.g., 1–5-μm particles), propelling them back up to the pharynx where they are swallowed. Larger foreign bodies may trigger the cough reflex. The air is warmed and humidified by exposure to the tracheobronchial epithelium and mucus, although most of this activity occurs in the nose. In addition to these respiratory functions, the trachea and bronchi have a lesser role in vocal resonation. These structures provide a column of air from the lung to the vocal cords.

3. Describe the structure of the trachea and bronchi.

The trachea is composed of horseshoe-shaped cartilages with membranous connections. The trachea extends from the larynx to the carina. At approximately the level of the fifth thoracic vertebra, the trachea divides into the right and left main bronchi. Posteriorly, the trachea is closed by fibrous tissue. Interspersed in the fibrous membranes are smooth and voluntary (trachealis) muscle fibers. As the bronchi divide and become progressively smaller, the cartilages become less complete, until the alveoli are formed. At this point, there is no cartilage present. The tracheobronchial tree is lined by a ciliated respiratory epithelium.

4. What biomechanical characteristics of the trachea must be considered for reconstructive surgery?

The trachea is a dynamic organ that expands and contracts longitudinally in response to the demands of deglutition, respiration, and gravity. Following tracheal resection, reconstruction should allow the trachea to resume its dynamic functions. The upper tracheal segments assume a larger stress load than the lower tracheal segments following tracheal resection. By severing the suprahyoid musculature from the hyoid, the trachea may be loosened superiorly, and by severing intrathoracic connective tissue, the trachea may be loosened inferiorly. This allows maximal tracheal resection of 5 or more rings and subsequent reconstruction without tension.

5. What is bronchoscopy?

The word *bronchoscopy* is derived from the Greek word *bronchios*, meaning windpipe, and *skopos*, meaning to aim or inspect. In practice, bronchoscopy refers to the endoscopic examination of the trachea and tracheobronchial tree.

6. What is "open" bronchoscopy? When is it indicated?

Open or rigid bronchoscopy was the first type of bronchoscopy developed. During this procedure, a rigid hollow tube measuring 6–8 mm in its inside diameter is inserted through the larynx into the tracheobronchial tree. Specialized telescopes, such as the Hopkins rod telescope, and other specialized magnification devices may be inserted into the bronchoscope to facilitate observation of the tracheobronchial tree.

This procedure is indicated for the evaluation of actual or suspected tracheobronchial pathology (e.g., hemoptysis, neoplasm) and tracheobronchial therapy (e.g., foreign-body removal, dilatation). It is especially useful for the establishment of an emergency airway via the peroral route. Open bronchoscopy is limited by two major disadvantages: (1) it is technically difficult to visualize tissue beyond the second order of bronchi, even with mirrors; and (2) this procedure is associated with significant discomfort, and the patient may need general anesthesia.

7. What is the Hopkins rod?

Optical telescopes, used to magnify the tracheobronchial tree, initially used a lens or series of lenses separated by air. Hopkins, an ingenious British inventor, reversed the traditional design, replacing the former air spaces with a series of glass rods and then replacing the former lens with small air spaces. As a result, this system allows a much larger viewing angle with greatly increased illumination and resolution. The use of this viewing telescope through the rigid endoscope has revolutionized the field of endoscopy.

8. What is "closed" bronchoscopy, and when is it indicated?

Closed or flexible bronchoscopy was popularized by Ikeda in 1971. In this technique, a flexible bronchoscope is inserted through the larynx and into the lungs. This instrument is approximately 5 mm in diameter and carries a viewing channel via light-bearing, flexible, coherently arranged glass fibers. One or two noncoherent glass fiber bundles carry the light. Another open channel permits suctioning or biopsy. Closed bronchoscopy is indicated to inspect the second- to fifth-order bronchi for peripheral or upper lobe lesions, to evaluate x-ray-negative hemoptysis, and to evaluate patients whose lung spaces are inaccessible with rigid bronchoscopes (e.g., kyphosis). It is also used to retrieve small foreign bodies and to evaluate occult carcinoma (x-ray-negative, sputum-positive). Unfortunately, closed bronchoscopic images are not as sharp as the images that are obtained with a rigid bronchoscope and telescope.

9. Which type of anesthesia is used for bronchoscopy?

For flexible bronchoscopy, topical local anesthesia usually suffices. Rigid bronchoscopy can also be performed under local anesthesia with sedation. This includes glossopharyngeal and superior laryngeal nerve blocks, supplemented by spraying local anesthesia through the scope as it is advanced. However, general anesthesia is more commonly used for rigid bronchoscopy.

10. Describe the landmarks seen as the bronchoscope is introduced and advanced.

The **flexible** scope is commonly inserted through the nose. This provides a straight path to the larynx and avoids the contamination of the tongue. (More importantly, this route prevents the patient from biting your several-thousand-dollar instrument in half!) With advancement, landmarks include the posterior choana, pharynx, larynx, and vocal cords. Insertion of the **rigid** bronchoscope is facilitated by remaining close to the midline. The landmarks in sequence are the uvula, epiglottis, and larynx. The patient's head is retroflexed upon the occiput to recreate the "sniffing position." To expose the larynx, the tongue is placed anteriorly.

11. What is the first endobronchial landmark?

Once the scope traverses the larynx, you should see the cartilaginous rings of the trachea and the carina. If you err posteriorly, you enter the esophagus, which lacks the rings and carina.

12. How many divisions does the lung have?

The bronchoscopist should regard the lungs as being divided according to bronchial distribution, rather than by fissures. Starting at the carina, there is a left and right lung. The right lung has three major divisions exiting from the right main, or mainstem, bronchus. These divisions are the upper, middle, and lower lobes. The left lung has two divisions, the upper and lower lobe. A third division on the left, corresponding to the middle lobe on the right, is called the lingula. The lingula shares its initial bronchus with the upper lobe.

13. How many bronchopulmonary segments are there in the right lung? In the left?

In American nomenclature, there are 10 segments on the right and 8 on the left. Variations in anatomy include an occasional subapical division. Each bronchopulmonary segment has its own bronchus and blood supply.

Right Lung	Left Lung
Upper lobe	Upper lobe
Apical (bronchopulmonary segment)	Apical-posterior
Posterior	Anterior
Anterior	Lingula
Middle lobe	Lateral
Superior	Inferior
Medial	Lower Lobe
Lower lobe	Superior
Superior	Anteromedial basal
Lateral basal	Lateral basal
Medial basal	Posterior basal
Posterior basal	
Anterior basal	

14. Beyond the bronchopulmonary segments, how do you indicate location of findings?

Examination of this area requires an extended anatomic nomenclature to describe the site of the findings. One system correlates closely with the endobronchial system. An *a* represents the more anterior and a *b* the more posterior segments as the endoscopist views the patient internally and progresses to the more peripheral bronchopulmonary tree. Using this system, a lesion in a sub-sub-subsegmental (fifth-order) bronchus in the right lung could be designated RB1b1ß, and the location is described reliably to another endoscopist.

15. What is the eparterial bronchus, and why is this important?

The right upper lobe bronchus is the eparterial (above the artery) bronchus. This bronchus passes over the right pulmonary artery. The left upper lobe bronchus passes under the left pulmonary artery. This difference is important to remember when obtaining biopsies. If a deep biopsy (e.g., with a 5-mm cup forceps) is taken from the right upper lobe spur, or secondary carina, the pulmonary artery may be violated with obviously disastrous results.

16. If you encounter major bleeding when performing a bronchoscopy, how is it managed?

The only treatment for major bleeding, such as with a pulmonary artery biopsy, is the immediate placement of the rigid bronchoscope down the opposite main bronchus. This allows ventilation of the "good" lung until the thoracic surgeon can open the chest and control the bleeding. Any attempt at suctioning or local endobronchial control is disastrous, as both lungs fill rapidly with blood. Once this blood clots, it is impossible to extract. Because ventilation is impossible, the patient suffocates. Immediate action is the only life-saving measure.

17. What non-neoplastic lung conditions are commonly evaluated with bronchoscopy?

Bronchoscopy is indicated for nearly all patients with prolonged respiratory disease. Specific non-neoplastic indications include unexplained chronic cough, stridor, wheezing, hemoptysis, noncardiac shortness of breath, suspected foreign body, stenosis, vocal cord paralysis, neck mass, obstructive emphysema, atelectasis, and radiographic abnormalities. Of course, each of these indications may result in the finding of a neoplasm. The differential diagnosis is dependent on specimens gathered for microbiology, cytology, or pathology at the time of bronchoscopy. Therapeutic aspiration of secretions or foreign-body retrieval may also be performed.

18. How are endobronchial foreign bodies removed?

Smaller foreign bodies may be removed with a cup forceps via the fiberoptic bronchoscope. Removal of larger foreign bodies may require the use of intricate foreign-body forceps and complex maneuvers. Organic foreign bodies may be especially tricky, because they tend to swell (e.g., bean), cause inflammatory responses (e.g., peanut), and break up. This prevents their complete removal, and the fragment may be lodged further down the tracheobronchial tree. If all else fails, open removal with a thoracotomy or partial lobectomy may be required.

19. How does tuberculosis appear on bronchoscopy in the lung?

The incidence of tuberculosis is again increasing. Characteristically, it appears as a "cottage cheese" exudate. It is associated with surprisingly little inflammatory response in the epithelium. When this diagnosis is suspected, special stains for acid-fast bacilli may help with the early diagnosis. This facilitates early therapy, as the organisms are often fastidious and difficult to culture. It is important to protect the endoscopist, anesthesiologist, and other staff from accidental inoculation. Protection can be facilitated by interposing a glass or Plexiglas shield over the viewing channel. This step is, of course, an important routine precaution in the age of HIV and antibiotic-resistant organisms. Special precautions are also indicated when cleaning the operating room after the case.

20. What kinds of samples should you obtain by bronchoscopy?

Depending on the evaluated condition, biopsies, brushings, washings, or specimens for culture are obtained.

21. How are these samples obtained?

1. **Biopsies** are generally obtained with the cup forceps through the open bronchoscope or with the flexible-cup forceps through the closed scope. Often, the flexible forceps are not withdrawn through the small biopsy channel; instead, they are withdrawn to the opening, and the scope and biopsy are withdrawn together, which avoids dislodging the biopsy in the channel.

2. **Brushings** are obtained with a tiny stiff-bristled brush. The brush can be withdrawn through the biopsy channel, but it should be irrigated into a trap at the conclusion of the procedure to retrieve all cells for cytologic examination. Alternatively, a sheathed brush can be used to retain all possible cells.

3. **Washings** are obtained by flushing the suspicious segment with physiologic saline and retrieving the washings into a sterile trap.

4. **Materials for culture** can be obtained in the same fashion.

22. How does cancer appear in the lung?

The most common cancer of the lung is squamous cell carcinoma. Since this is an epithelial lesion, it presents as an irregularity of epithelial lining. Some adjacent blood vessels may be somewhat tortuous, and the lesion is usually raised. In more advanced cases, the lumen may be completely occluded.

23. How is a "sputum cytology" obtained?

Because neoplastic cells commonly exfoliate, they may be found in the sputum. Because early-morning specimens are the most concentrated with these cells, the patient is asked to cough deeply and produce samples when they awaken. The samples are examined by the trained pathologist, usually using Papanicolaou or other stains. They are examined for the usual malignancy criteria (pleomorphism, increased nuclear/cytoplasmic ratios, etc.). Newer technology uses lasers to identify suspicious cells, which are then visually evaluated by the pathologist.

24. Why are translobar lung biopsies performed? How are they performed?

If the lung is diffusely involved (e.g., *Pneumocystis carinii* pneumonia or metastatic disease), the fiberoptic bronchoscope is advanced to the periphery, and the biopsy forceps are advanced blindly until gentle resistance is encountered. The patient is advised to "take a deep breath," and the biopsy cups are advanced further. The patient is then requested to exhale. This maneuver brings lung tissue into the biopsy cups. The biopsy is removed along with the scope. This procedure carries the associated danger of creating a pneumothorax if the biopsy is performed too peripherally.

CONTROVERSIES

25. Is a bronchial adenoma benign?

Bronchial adenomas were formerly classified as benign neoplasms, but this is now known to be incorrect. Histologically, two types of adenoma are recognized, a **carcinoid** type with uniform, benign-appearing, cuboidal cells, and a **cylindromatous** type, with equally benign-appearing cells. Both tend to present with hemoptysis and appear at endoscopy as a reddish mass. Both tend to bleed vigorously on biopsy. Both also tend to cause problems because of distal obstruction. Here the similarities cease. Metastases are occasionally seen with the carcinoid variant, and endobronchial resection is often helpful. In contrast, the cylindroma is clearly malignant, and resection is indicated.

26. Which is better, rigid or flexible bronchoscopy?

Although some may advocate one method over the other, each has specific limitations and indications as discussed above. Depending on the problem, the bronchoscopist should be able to perform either technique.

BIBLIOGRAPHY

1. Arroliga AC, Matthay RA: The role of bronchoscopy in lung cancer. Clin Chest Med 14:87–98, 1993.
2. Baselski VS, Wunderlink RG: Bronchoscopic diagnosis of pneumonia. Clin Microbiol Rev 7:533–538, 1994.
3. Carter DR, Jafek BW: Endoscopic anatomy for bronchopulmonary anatomy. Otol Head Neck Surg 87:815–817, 1979.
4. Ikeda S: Flexible bronchofiberscope. Ann Otol Rhinol Laryngol 79:916–925, 1970.
5. Jackson C, Huber JF: Correlated applied anatomy of the bronchial tree and lungs with a system of nomenclature. Dis Chest 9:319, 1970.
6. Jackson C, Jackson CL: Bronchoesophagology. Philadelphia, W.B. Saunders, 1950.
7. Jafek BW, Sasaki C: Head and Neck Surgery: vol III. In Lee, KJ (ed): Comprehensive and Comparative Atlases in Otolaryngology. New York, Grune & Stratton, 1983.
8. Meyers AD, Bishop HE: Biomechanical characteristics of the canine trachea. Ann Otol Rhinol Laryngol 87:538–543, 1978.
9. Norris CM, Norris CM Jr: Bronchology. In English GM (ed): Otolaryngology: Vol 3. Diseases of the Larynx, Pharynx, and Upper Respiratory Tract. Philadelphia, J.B. Lippincott, 1994.
10. O'Neil KM, Lazarus AA: Hemoptysis: Indications for bronchoscopy. Arch Intern Med 151:171–174, 1991.
11. Rowe LD, Jafek BW: Bronchial adenoma, a malignant misnomer. Laryngoscope 89:1991–1999, 1979.
12. Stradling P: Diagnostic Bronchoscopy: A Teaching Manual, 6th ed. New York, Churchill Livingstone, 1991.

38. MEDIASTINOSCOPY

Bruce W. Jafek, M.D., and Marv Pomerantz, M.D.

1. What is mediastinoscopy used for?

Mediastinoscopy is a method used to explore and biopsy the superior mediastinum. It can be used to define the resectability of bronchogenic cancer, determine cancer spread prior to thoracotomy, and provide pathologic confirmation of mediastinal masses. Mediastinoscopy assists in the accurate staging of lung cancer. It helps to identify patients who will gain little benefit from a thoracotomy, therefore sparing them the risks of a major surgical procedure.

2. Who is the "father of mediastinoscopy"?

Eric Carlens, who described the endoscopic technique in 1959.

3. What are the indications for mediastinoscopy?

Absolute and Relative Indications for Mediastinoscopy

Absolute indications
  1. Presence of enlarged mediastinal lymph nodes (> 1.5 cm) on CT scan

Relative indications
  1. Presence of T2 or T3 primary lesion
  2. Presence of lesions located within the inner third of the lung field
  3. Presence of adenocarcinoma or large-cell undifferentiated tumors on preoperative biopsy
  4. Presence of small-cell cytology on preoperative biopsy with apparently resectable stage 1 lesions
  5. Suspected presence of multiple primary lesions or synchronous lung tumors
  6. Presence of vocal cord paralysis in the setting of left upper lobe primary lesion
  7. Intent to use neoadjuvant therapy

From Sugarbaker DS, Strauss GM: Advances in surgical staging and therapy of non-small-cell lung cancer. Semin Oncol 20:163–172, 1993, with permission.

4. How is the dissection made in preparation for mediastinoscopy?

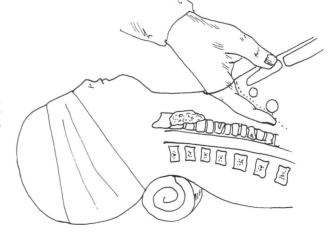

Dissection into the mediastinum. (From Jepsen O: Mediastinoscopy. Copenhagen, Munksgaard, 1966, with permission.)

The patient is placed on the back with a roll under the shoulders. A 2–3-cm curvilinear incision is made just above the suprasternal notch and is carried deeper until the pretracheal fascia is reached. The fascia is then incised to confirm the presence of tracheal rings. Blunt finger dissection is carried down into the superior mediastinum, with careful palpation anteriorly for the innominate artery. The dissection must be performed beneath the innominate to avoid injury to this vessel. Usually, the tip of the surgeon's finger can reach the carina and may feel the pulsation of the aortic arch deep in the superior mediastinum. The mediastinoscope is then inserted, and the necessary diagnostic or therapeutic measures are performed.

5. What are the divisions of the mediastinum? Why are these important?

The mediastinum is systematically divided into superior and inferior halves. The inferior portion is further divided into anterior, middle, and posterior portions. Ordinarily, only lesions which occupy the superior mediastinum are accessible to mediastinoscopy. Intrathoracic metastases are commonly found in the superior mediastinum, as are primary mediastinal tumors such as lymphoma and germ cell tumors. The heart occupies the middle mediastinum. Neurogenic neoplasms commonly are found in the posterior mediastinum.

6. Where is the innominate artery in the mediastinum?

The innominate artery is usually in the anterior mediastinum. Mediastinoscopy occurs deep and inferior to this vessel. In approximately 25% of cases, the innominate may rise above the suprasternal notch, where it may be subject to injury.

7. How far down in the thorax can you reach with mediastinoscopy?

Mast and Jafek reported a fairly constant distance of 11 cm from the cricoid cartilage to the carina in adults. The mediastinoscopist should find this well within the range of the 14.5-cm mediastinoscope. This gives access to an average of 31 mediastinal lymph nodes.

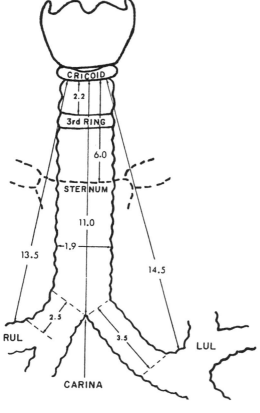

Distances between major cervical and mediastinal landmarks (in cm). RUL = right upper lobe, LUL = left upper lobe. (From Mast WR, Jafek BW: Mediastinal anatomy for the mediastinoscopist. Arch Otol 101:596–599, 1975, with permission.)

8. Where are you unable to reach (and shouldn't try to)?

Lymph nodes which are extremely anterior and those in the aortopulmonary window are difficult to reach by standard mediastinoscopy. Lymph nodes in the posterior mediastinum (posterior subcarinal and paraesophageal nodes) are inaccessible.

9. How does the lymphatic drainage of the lungs relate to tumor spread?

A number of lymph node groups are identified within the chest, and there are many anatomic variations in normal lymphatic drainage of the lungs and adjacent esophagus. Under pathologic conditions, blockage of lymph nodes may lead to collateral and retrograde lymph flow, resulting in deviations from predicted lymphatic spread patterns in bronchogenic carcinoma. Generally, sidedness (e.g., right lung to right nodes) and position (e.g., superior lung field to superior lymph nodes) are maintained. However, a major part of the left lung lymphatics may drain into the inferior tracheobronchial nodes and subsequently into the right paratracheal nodes. Therefore, the site of the primary tumor helps to guide the mediastinoscopist to the proper node chain.

X   **Supraclavicular nodes.**

2R   **Right upper paratracheal nodes.** Nodes to the right of the midline of the trachea, between the intersection of the caudal margin of the brachiocephalic artery with the trachea and the apex of the lung or above the level of the aortic arch.

2L   **Left upper paratracheal nodes.** Nodes to the left of the midline of the trachea, between the top of the aortic arch and the apex of the lung.

4R   **Right lower paratracheal nodes.** Nodes to the right of the midline of the trachea, between the cephalic border of the azygos vein and the intersection of the caudal margin of the brachiocephalic artery with the right side of the trachea or the top of the aortic arch.

4L   **Left lower paratracheal nodes.** Nodes to the left of the midline of the trachea, between the top of the aortic arch and the level of the carina, medial to the ligamentum arteriosum.

5   **Aortopulmonary nodes.** Subaortic and paraaortic nodes, lateral to the ligamentum arteriosum or the aorta or left pulmonary artery, proximal to the first branch of the left pulmonary artery.

6   **Anterior mediastinal nodes.** Nodes anterior to the ascending aorta or the innominate artery.

7   **Subcarinal nodes.** Nodes arising caudal to the carina of the trachea but not associated with the lower lobe bronchi or arteries within the lung.

8   **Paraesophageal nodes.** Nodes dorsal to the posterior wall of the trachea and to the right or the left of the midline of the esophagus below the level of the subcarinal region. (Nodes around the descending aorta should also be included.)

9   **Right or left pulmonary ligament nodes.** Nodes within the right or left pulmonary ligament.

10R   **Right tracheobronchial nodes.** Nodes to the right of the midline of the trachea, from the level of the cephalic border of the azygos vein to the origin of the right upper lobe bronchus.

10L   **Left peribronchial nodes.** Nodes to the left of the midline of the trachea, between the carina and the left upper lobe bronchus, medial to ligamentum arteriosum.

11   **Intrapulmonary nodes.** Nodes removed in the right or left lung specimen, plus those distal to the mainstem bronchi or secondary carina (includes interlobar, lobar, and segmental nodes)

14   **Superior diaphragmatic nodes.** Nodes adjacent to the pericardium within 2 cm of the diaphragm.

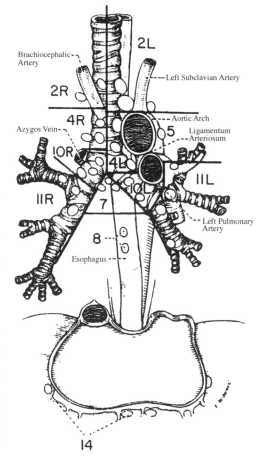

American Thoracic Society: definitions of regional nodal stations and lymph node mapping scheme. (From Am Rev Respir Dis 147:17–20 1986, with permission.)

10. Why do you aspirate lesions or lymph nodes prior to biopsy?

When a mass is encountered, you may not be able to palpate it directly to evaluate for pulsation. Therefore, before biopsying any mass, it should be aspirated to ensure that it is not a vascular structure. As carefully as possible, lesions should be bluntly dissected to inspect the lesion for consistency. This may be difficult and time-consuming if a lymph node exhibits extracapsular spread and adherence to adjacent tissue. Blind biopsies should never be performed during mediastinoscopy.

11. What if you enter the aortic arch or innominate artery?

Major vascular injury is the most dangerous complication of this procedure. Direct pressure should be placed on the area, optimally by a finger, and an immediate sternotomy should be performed to control the bleeding. However, this may not be possible, and the patient may exsanguinate. The superior vena cava, azygos vein, and other vessels are also at risk, but injury to these structures is less likely to lead to patient death.

12. What are some common complications that occur with mediastinoscopy?

In addition to major vascular injury, which is the most hazardous complication, other vital structures in the immediate vicinity of the operative field also pose potential hazards. If the surgeon has a thorough knowledge of the relevant anatomy and follows a gentle, meticulous approach, the risk of complications should be very low. Described complications include pleural damage leading to pneumothorax or hemothorax, left recurrent laryngeal nerve damage, tracheal or esophageal trauma, mediastinitis, wound infection, and tumor seeding. In patients with superior vena caval syndrome, special care is necessary due to venous engorgement.

13. Should tests be performed prior to mediastinoscopy to evaluate resectability of lung cancer?

A number of preoperative studies may be helpful in determining resectability, including x-rays, full-chest CT, bronchoscopy, and cardiac and pulmonary function tests. By means of these examinations, as many as 50% of all diagnosed patients may be found to have unresectable tumors.

14. What are the absolute contraindications to thoracotomy?

Absolute contraindications to thoracotomy, therefore unresectability, are **invasive growth** into the mediastinum and **advanced small-cell carcinoma**. While most thoracic surgeons feel that a single distal lymph node does not exclude the possibility of resection, **contralateral spread** or **fixation** is also an absolute contraindication to thoracotomy.

15. How is lung cancer staged?

Staging of Lung Cancer: TNM Classification

Primary Tumor (T)

Tx	Tumor proven by the presence of malignant cells in bronchopulmonary secretions but not visualized roentgenographically or bronchoscopically, or any tumor that cannot be assessed (as in retreatment staging).
T0	No evidence of primary tumor.
Tis	Carcinoma *in situ*
T1	A tumor that is ≤ 3.0 cm in greatest dimension, surrounded by lung of visceral pleura, and without evidence of invasion proximal to a lobar bronchus at bronchoscopy.
T2	A tumor > 3.0 cm in greatest diameter or a tumor of any size that either invades the visceral pleura or has associated atelectasis or obstructive pneumonitis extending to the hilar region. At bronchoscopy, the proximal extent of demonstrable tumor must be within a lobar bronchus or at least 2.0 cm distal to the carina. Any associated atelectasis or obstructive pneumonitis must involve less than an entire lung.
T3	A tumor of any size with direct extension into the chest wall (including superior sulcus tumors), diaphragm, or mediastinal pleura or pericardium without involving the heart, great vessels, trachea, esophagus, or vertebral body, or a tumor in the main bronchus within 2 cm of the carina without involving the carina.
T4	A tumor of any size with invasion of the mediastinum or involving heart, great vessels, trachea, esophagus, vertebral body, or carina, or presence of malignant pleural effusion.

(Continued on next page)

Staging of Lung Cancer: TNM Classification (cont'd)

Nodal Involvement (N)

N0   No demonstrable metastasis to regional lymph nodes.

N1   Metastasis to lymph nodes in the peribronchial or ipsilateral hilar region, or both, including direct expansion

N2   Metastasis to ipsilateral mediastinal lymph nodes and subcarinal lymph nodes

N3   Metastasis to contralateral mediastinal lymph nodes, contralateral hilar lymph nodes, and ipsilateral or contralateral scalene or supraclavicular lymph nodes.

Distant Metastasis (M)

M0   No (known) distant metastasis

M1   Distant metastasis present—Specify site(s)

From Miller JD, Gorenstein LA, Patterson GA: Staging: The key to rational management of lung cancer. Ann Thorac Surg 53:170–178, 1992, with permission.

Stage Groupings for Lung Cancer

Occult carcinoma	Tx	N0		M0
Stage 0	Tis		Carcinoma in situ	
Stage I	T1	N0		M0
	T2	N0		M0
Stage II	T1	N1		M0
	T2	N1		M0
Stage IIIa	T3	N0		M0
	T3	N1		M0
	T1–3	N2		M0
Stage IIIb	Any T	N3		M0
	T4	Any N		M0
Stage IV	Any T	Any N		M1

From Shields TW: General Thoracic Surgery, 3rd ed. Philadelphia, Lea & Febiger, 1989, with permission.

16. How does sarcoid appear upon mediastinoscopy?

Classically, mediastinal lymph nodes that have been affected by sarcoid are described as symmetrically enlarged, nonadherent, and somewhat purplish in color. A biopsy of a clinically involved lymph node should yield a positive diagnosis 80–90% of the time. In cross-section, affected nodes appear to possess microscopic noncaseous granulomas, leading to a "pebbly, salt crystal" gross description.

17. What is a "pawn broker" sign?

Historically, pawn brokers suspended three brass balls in front of their shops. On x-ray, the marked, symmetrical, and enlarged mediastinal lymph nodes characteristic of sarcoid resemble this symbol. At mediastinoscopy, biopsies of these lymph nodes provide a very reliable method of diagnosis.

18. Does a positive tuberculosis isolate from the mediastinum indicate active tuberculosis?

Bronchogenic carcinoma and tuberculosis may be difficult to distinguish because they generate similar clinical pictures. Mediastinal lymph nodes may harbor healed, childhood tuberculosis and may yield positive histology. However, this does not necessarily indicate that the identified intrathoracic disease process is caused by tuberculosis. In addition, attempts to make a diagnosis of tuberculosis by means of mediastinal biopsies are generally not rewarding.

19. How is the diagnosis of silicosis made?

The diagnosis of pulmonary silicosis may be difficult, especially when minimal changes are present on x-ray. Also, silicosis may coexist with tuberculosis, bronchogenic carcinoma, or other intrathoracic pathology. When mediastinal nodes are biopsied in a patient with silicosis, they are often densely fibrotic and adherent to surrounding structures. Polarized light microscopy showing birefringent crystals is diagnostic for silicosis.

20. What other lesions do you encounter during mediastinoscopy?

While mediastinoscopy is most commonly used to evaluate the resectability of primary lung tumors, other lesions may be evaluated. Sarcoidosis, metastatic tumors, tuberculosis, mediastinal cysts, lymphoma, Hodgkin's disease, malignant liposarcoma, silicosis, histoplasmosis, thymoma, germ cell tumors, neurogenic tumors, substernal thyroids, and parathyroid adenomas are not rare. Ward even described the removal of a foreign body, a bullet, from the mediastinum. Therefore, the mediastinoscopist must be prepared to evaluate a number of possibilities at surgery.

21. What vascular anomalies can occur in the superior mediastinum?

Knowledge of vascular anomalies of the mediastinum is essential to the mediastinoscopist. The embryologic development of the aortic system is complex, and a number of anomalies may be present. These anomalies include a double aortic arch, anomalous innominate artery, anomalous left common carotid artery, and aberrant right subclavian artery. A right aortic arch with a right recurrent laryngeal nerve and left ligamentum arteriosum may also be present. Aneurysms may be found in any vessel, most frequently the aorta, and should be diagnosed prior to biopsy.

22. Do other uses exist for mediastinoscopy?

Surgeons have described using the mediastinoscope to assist in the application of heart electrodes for atrial-triggered pacemakers. The mediastinoscope has also been considered for evaluating the resectability of esophageal neoplasms. Approaches to any intrathoracic region are theoretically possible, depending on the length of scope employed. The mediastinoscope has even been used to assist in removing thrombus from pulmonary arteries.

23. How accurate is the standard chest x-ray in evaluating mediastinal metastases?

Mediastinal nodes are apparent on standard chest x-rays when they are large enough to distort the normal mediastinal silhouette or cause widening of the carina. The standard chest x-ray is hardly sensitive, however, as 72% of patients with positive mediastinoscopy had a normal chest x-ray.

24. What is the diagnostic sensitivity and specificity of mediastinoscopy?

> 90%.

CONTROVERSIES

25. Instead of a diagnostic mediastinoscopy, wouldn't it be simpler and safer to do a supraclavicular fat pad biopsy?

Simpler and safer, yes, but a supraclavicular fat pad biopsy has a much smaller positive yield for intrathoracic disease. Therefore, this technique is now largely of historical interest, except where there is clinical adenopathy in the supraclavicular region or when it is used as a preliminary step in the diagnosis of tuberculosis.

26. A patient with lung cancer has radiologic lymph nodes < 1 cm. Is mediastinoscopy indicated?

Although some would say that mediastinoscopy is indicated, most would argue that it is probably not beneficial, as the positive yield in this situation is only 10–15%.

27. What contrast studies are helpful in the preoperative evaluation of a patient with lung cancer?

Although some advocate preoperative contrast studies, Miller et al. pointed out that routine radionuclide scans of brain, liver, and bone have no useful role in patients who do not have clinical or laboratory evidence of metastases to these sites. CT studies of the head and abdomen and nuclear bone scans are therefore reserved for patients with (1) signs or symptoms of metastatic disease at any site, (2) a histologic diagnosis of small cell cancer, (3) a previous history of malignancy, and (4) a high risk for resection.

28. Are patients with positive mediastinal lymph nodes candidates for resection?

Attitudes vary from one extreme to the other. Some surgeons consider the presence of malignant mediastinal nodes as a contraindication to thoracotomy and lung resection because the survival rates in these situations are extremely low. At the other extreme, some surgeons recommend lung resection and mediastinal node dissection even when contralateral nodes are involved. This group hopes to improve the salvage rate in a class of patients who have an otherwise dismal prognosis. The most reasonable approach utilizes neoadjuvant therapy for positive N2 nodes. The appropriate therapy for tumors with positive N3 nodes is still unclear.

BIBLIOGRAPHY

1. Carlens E: Mediastinoscopy: A method for inspection and tissue biopsy in the superior mediastinum Dis Chest 36:343–352, 1959.
2. Funatsu T, Matsubara Y, Hatakenaka R, et al: The role of mediastinoscopic biopsy in preoperative assessment of lung cancer. J Thorac Cardiovasc Surg 104:1688–1695, 1992.
3. Jepsen O: Mediastinoscopy. Copenhagen, Munksgaard, 1966.
4. Jahangiri M, Goldstraw P: The role of mediastinoscopy in superior venal caval obstruction. Ann Thorac Surg 59:449–455, 1995.
5. Kinzler DL, Jafek, BW: Techniques of mediastinoscopy. Ear Nose Throat J 60:63–70, 1981.
6. Kreutser EW, Jafek, BW: The mediastinum: Introduction. Ear Nose Throat J 60:5, 1981.
7. Kreutser EW, Jafek BW: Vistas of mediastinoscopy. Ear Nose Throat J 60:88, 1981.
8. Luke WP, Pearson FG, Todd TRJ, et al: Prospective evaluation of mediastinoscopy for assessment of carcinoma of the lung. J Thorac Cardiovasc Surg 91:53–56, 1986.
9. Mast WR, Jafek BW: Mediastinal anatomy for the mediastinoscopist. Arch Otol 101:596–599, 1975.
10. Merav AD: The role of mediastinoscopy and anterior mediastinoscopy in determining operability of lung cancer: A review of published questions and answers. Cancer Invest 9:439–442, 1991.
11. Miller JD, Gorenstein LA, Patterson GA: Staging: The key to rational management of lung cancer. Ann Thorac Surg 53:170–178, 1992.
12. Mountain CF: A new international staging system for lung cancer. Chest 89:225s–233s, 1986.
13. Sugarbaker DS, Strauss GM: Advances in surgical staging and therapy of non-small-cell lung cancer. Semin Oncol 20:163–172, 1993.
14. Ward PH, Jafek BW, Harris P: Interesting and unusual lesions encountered during mediastinoscopy. Ann Otol Rhinol Laryngol 80:487–491, 1971.

VI. Tumors

39. SALIVARY GLAND TUMORS

Bruce W. Jafek, M.D.

1. Name the most common benign tumors of the salivary glands.

Pleomorphic adenoma	Benign cyst
Monomorphic adenoma	Lymphoepithelial lesions
Warthin's tumor	Oncocytoma

2. What are the most common malignant tumors of the salivary gland?

Mucoepidermoid carcinoma	Adenocarcinoma
Malignant mixed	Adenoid cystic carcinoma
Acinic cell carcinoma	Epidermoid carcinoma

Some of these malignancies are low-grade, some are intermediate, and some are high-grade.

3. How does a tumor of the salivary gland typically present?

Patients usually have a clinical history of a slowly enlarging, painless mass in the area of the involved salivary gland (e.g., below the ear for the parotid). Any mass of this type should be considered a tumor until proved otherwise.

4. How is salivary gland disease evaluated?

Salivary gland disease is strongly suspected on the basis of the **history** and **physical examination**. Bimanual **palpation** of the involved gland is helpful in evaluating enlargement of the gland or presence of a mass. Palpation of the gland may also express pus or dislodge a stone, assisting in the diagnosis. **Sialography**, cannulation of the duct with instillation of contrast material to facilitate x-ray studies, is uncommon except when it is used to confirm benign lymphoepithelial disease. **CT**, **MRI**, or other techniques (e.g., technetium-99 scanning) help to visualize actual or suspected neoplasms but may not be indicated unless deep extension is suspected. Most of these studies only confirm the presence of a mass.

5. What are the important aspects of the history and physical exam in a patient with a suspected salivary gland tumor?

Historical information should include the rate of growth and presence or absence of pain. Other related history (e.g., keratoconjunctivitis, arthritis) might direct you toward a nonneoplastic etiology of salivary gland enlargement. Other conditions that might produce salivary gland enlargement include bulimia, actinomycosis, tuberculosis, parotitis, mumps, Sjögren's syndrome, and parotid lymphadenitis.

Physical examination should be directed toward determining the size of the mass, skin fixation, cervical adenopathy, and function of all branches of the facial nerve. A complete otolaryngologic exam is obviously in order, focusing on the exclusion of surface neoplasms of the upper aerodigestive tract which might have metastasized to the preparotid lymph nodes.

6. Why is a facial nerve palsy in association with a parotid mass significant?

A facial nerve palsy suggests that the underlying mass is malignant. Coexisting palsy or paresis is uncommon with benign neoplasms.

7. Why not biopsy the mass directly?

A direct biopsy of the mass is contraindicated for two reasons:

1. Risk is to the facial nerve. The tumor may have displaced the facial nerve to an abnormal location, and the surgeon may inadvertently injure the nerve because of its unexpected position.

2. Risk of tumor spillage. Tumor spillage increases the incidence of recurrence, even for benign lesions.

A fine-needle aspiration is 95% sensitive, and therefore, many surgeons regard it as a very appropriate diagnostic tool. Other surgeons may prefer to do a superficial parotidectomy primarily, as this procedure is therapeutic as well as diagnostic.

8. How do the major salivary glands differ histologically?

The parotid gland is made up of basophilic **serous cells**, which are arranged in acini, or grapelike clusters. The submandibular gland is a **mixed gland**, containing both serous and mucinous cells. The sublingual gland contains primarily **mucinous cells**.

9. How do low-grade and high-grade salivary gland malignancies differ in clinical behavior?

Of the malignant salivary gland tumors, some behave in a relatively benign fashion, while others are relatively aggressive. The relatively benign or low-grade tumors include acinic cell carcinoma, low-grade mucoepidermoid carcinoma, and "malignant" oncocytoma. The relatively aggressive or high-grade tumors include adenoid cystic carcinoma, squamous cell carcinoma, adenocarcinoma, carcinoma ex pleomorphic adenoma, and high-grade mucoepidermoid carcinoma.

10. Describe the staging system for salivary gland tumors.

Tumor

T0 No evidence of primary tumor
T1 Tumor ≤ 2 cm in greatest diameter
T2 Tumor > 2 cm but < 4 cm in greatest diameter
T3 Tumor > 4 cm but < 6 cm in greatest diameter
T4 Tumor > 6 cm in greatest diameter
All categories are subdivided:
   a. No local extension
   b. Local extension, defined as clinical evidence of skin, soft tissue, bone, or nerve invasion

Lymph nodes

N0   No regional lymph node metastasis
N1   Metastasis in a single ipsilateral lymph node, ≤ 3 cm in greatest diameter
N2a Metastasis in a single ipsilateral lymph node > 3 cm but < 6 cm in greatest diameter
N2b Metastases in multiple ipsilateral lymph nodes, none > 6 cm in greatest diameter
N2c Metastases in bilateral or contralateral lymph nodes, none > 6 cm in greatest diameter
N3   Metastasis in a lymph node > 6 cm in greatest diameter

Distant metastasis

M0   No distant metastasis
M1   Distant metastasis

11. How are parotid malignancies of the various grades managed?

Group 1: This group includes T1 and T2N0 low-grade malignancies (mucoepidermoid low-grade and acinous). Excision of the tumor with a cuff of normal tissue is recommended. Regional lymph nodes should be evaluated at the time of surgery. The facial nerve is preserved.

Group 2: This group includes T1 and T2N0 high-grade malignancies (adenocarcinoma, malignant mixed, undifferentiated, and squamous). Total parotidectomy with excision of digastric nodes and preservation of the facial nerve is recommended. If the nerve is involved, it is resected back to clear margins on frozen section and immediately grafted. All patients receive wide-field radiation to include the upper-echelon nodes.

Group 3: This group includes T3N0 or any N+ high-grade cancers and recurrent cancers. Radical parotidectomy with sacrifice of the facial nerve and modified neck dissection is recommended for N0 tumors. Radical neck dissection is recommended for N+ tumors. If there is evidence of facial nerve involvement into the mastoid, the nerve must be followed until negative margins are obtained. Primary nerve grafting is recommended. Postoperative radiation therapy is given to a wide field, from skull base to clavicle.

Group 4: This group includes all T4 tumors. In addition to radical parotidectomy and neck dissection, surgery may sometimes include resection of the masseter muscle, buccal fat pad, skin, mandible, ear canal, mastoid, or other involved structures as necessary. Postoperative radiotherapy is routine, and the facial nerve is grafted.

12. How is a parotid tumor removed?

Previously, tumors were "shelled out," which resulted in frequent recurrence. Current technique dictates excision of the tumor with a surrounding cuff of normal parotid tissue. This procedure is usually accomplished with a superficial lobectomy. The facial nerve must be carefully identified and spared.

13. During an operation on the parotid, where do you find the facial nerve?

The facial nerve is most often located just inferior to the external auditory canal, where it exits the stylomastoid foramen, approximately 6 mm medial to the tympanomastoid suture. The surgeon must know other ways to find the nerve in difficult cases. The facial nerve is just deep to the retrofacial vein at the inferior portion of the gland. The marginal mandibular branch passes over the facial artery at the anterior border of the masseter. The nerve lies just superficial to the styloid process. It crosses the zygomatic arch two-thirds of the way from the tragus to the lateral canthus of the eye. If all else fails, the otolaryngologist can drill out the mastoid process to identify the nerve.

14. What if the tumor is in the deep "lobe" of the parotid?

Fortunately, deep lobe tumors are uncommon, as they necessitate a complex surgery. The facial nerve is identified, and a superficial lobectomy is performed. The nerve is then carefully freed from the underlying tumor, and the tumor is removed with a cuff of normal gland.

15. What constitutes an "adequate operation" for a benign mixed tumor?

The pressure of an expanding benign mixed tumor compresses the surrounding salivary parenchyma, resulting in fibrosis and creating what is referred to as a **false capsule**. The false capsule is frequently incomplete, and tumor may project through the dehiscences and contact surrounding gland tissue. The lack of a complete capsule is a compelling reason for removing these tumors with wide margins. Once, these tumors were treated with enucleation, but this surgery resulted in an unacceptably high rate of recurrence, often as high as 40% over a 30-year period. Enucleation has now been largely abandoned in favor of superficial parotidectomies.

16. If a benign mixed tumor recurs, what's next?

A recurrent mixed tumor is to be feared. It represents not a discrete mass, but a multiplicity of nodules. A recurrence may appear in the previous scar, subcutaneous tissue, superficial or deep parotid parenchyma, facial nerve sheath, or perichondrium of the external meatus. Further attempts at surgery may be fruitless given the widespread nature of this condition, and further surgery may cause damage to the facial nerve. An eventual malignancy is seen in 2–5% of cases.

17. Is radiotherapy indicated in the treatment of a parotid tumor?
Indications for postoperative radiation therapy include:

High-grade tumors	Documented lymph node metastasis
Gross or microscopic residual disease	Extraparotid extension
Tumors involving or close to the facial nerve	Deep lobe cancers
Recurrent disease	All T3 and T4 cancers

18. Discuss the potential complications following parotid surgery.
Common complications include skin flap necrosis, hematoma, infection, and salivary fistula. **Hematoma** is generally related to inadequate hemostasis at the time of surgery. Treatment involves evacuation of the hematoma and hemostasis. **Salivary fistula** is a rare complication and usually responds to treatment with pressure dressings. It usually presents as an opening in the suture line below the lobule of the ear. A **temporary facial paresis** may occur in 10% of patients. It is seen more commonly in older patients, those with circulatory compromise (diabetes), and patients with deep lobe tumors. Permanent facial nerve dysfunction is uncommon (< 2% of patients). **Frey's syndrome** may occur in as many as 40% of parotid surgeries.

19. What is Frey's syndrome?
Frey's syndrome, also called **gustatory sweating**, is flushing and sweating of the skin overlying the surgical site. It occurs because of the postoperative growth of the interrupted preganglionic parasympathetic nerve branches to the parotid into the more superficial sweat glands. It may also occur following submandibular gland excision. The diagnosis is usually made from the history but can be confirmed by the starch-iodine test.

20. How is the starch-iodine test done?
Paint the affected skin with iodine, allow it to dry, dust the skin with starch, and feed the patient. The appearance of a bluish discoloration on the overlying skin is diagnostic. It is due to a reaction of the starch and iodine in the presence of moisture (sweat).

21. How do you treat Frey's syndrome?
Although Frey's syndrome is usually a very minor problem, it may require treatment. A **Jacobsen's neurectomy** involves surgically interrupting the preganglionic parasympathetic nerves in the ear which run to the parotid. Frey's syndrome may also be treated by re-elevating the skin flap and placing tissue, such as fascia, under the flap to prevent re-innervation. Parasympatholytic creams such as 1% glycopyrrolate lotion may also be applied to the skin.

22. Which parotid masses occur in children?
Parotid masses in children are very unusual, with only 3% of all parotid neoplasms occurring in the first 16 years of life.

Mixed tumors are by far the most common benign epithelial neoplasm in children. The peak incidence occurs at 10 years of age. The tumor behavior and treatment do not differ from those of similar tumors in adults.

Hemangiomas are the next most common, accounting for nearly 10% of all childhood parotid swellings. These tumors are usually present at birth and are located at the angle of the mandible. They are most common in white females. Whether these are true neoplasms or vascular malformations is an unresolved controversy.

Well-differentiated mucoepidermoid carcinoma is the most common malignant tumor in children.

CONTROVERSIES

23. Do benign parotid tumors ever undergo malignant degeneration?
Yes, but rarely. Carcinoma ex pleomorphic adenoma has been described. On the other hand, some pathologists argue that the tumor was malignant from the beginning. These masses have

been known to grow at an extremely slow rate over many years and then suddenly grow very rapidly. Because the rate changes so rapidly, it appears that some sort of malignant transformation has occurred.

24. Are diagnoses based on frozen sections of salivary tumors reliable?

This remains an area of controversy. It is often difficult for the pathologist to make a definitive diagnosis of a salivary gland neoplasm with frozen sections. The pathologist may require a second opinion and may need to send the specimen to an outside center before a definitive diagnosis can be reached. Many otolaryngologists are reluctant to proceed with a major, destructive operation, risking permanent facial nerve damage, given a frozen section diagnosis that may or may not be correct. Therefore, these otolaryngologists may perform a superficial parotidectomy and close, with the intention of performing a definitive operation later, should the final pathology require this.

25. Is a neck dissection indicated in the treatment of salivary malignancies?

This is only an issue in the case of selected high-grade salivary malignancies. Most otolaryngologists feel that it is indicated only when there is palpable, preoperative adenopathy or when a positive fine-needle aspirate of the involved mass has been obtained. The risk of occult metastasis to the cervical nodes is < 25%.

BIBLIOGRAPHY

1. Byun YS, Fayos JU, Kim YH: Management of malignant salivary gland tumors. Laryngoscope 90:1052–1060, 1980.
2. Cummings CW, et al (eds): Otolaryngology–Head and Neck Surgery, 2nd ed. St. Louis, Mosby, 1993.
3. Dawson AK, Orr JA: Long-term results of local extension and radiotherapy in pleomorphic adenoma of the parotid. Int J. Radiat Oncol Biol Phys 11:451–455, 1985.
4. English GM (ed): Otolaryngology, vol 5 [ch 30–31]. Philadelphia, J.B. Lippincott, 1990.
5. Huang RD, Pearlman S, Friedman WH, Loree T: Benign cystic vs solid lesions of the parotid gland in HIV patients. Head Neck 13:522–527, 1991.
6. Preston-Martin S: Brain and salivary gland tumors related to prior dental radiography. J Am Dent Assoc 120:151–157, 1990.
7. Seifert G: Diseases of the Salivary Glands. Stuttgart, Thieme, 1986.
8. Spiro RH: Diagnosis and pitfalls in the treatment of parotid tumors. Semin Surg Oncol 7:20–24, 1991.

40. TUMORS OF THE ORAL CAVITY AND PHARYNX

Vincent D. Eusterman, M.D., D.D.S.

1. Name the anatomic structures making up the oral cavity.

The oral cavity, extending from the vermilion border of the lips to the circumvallate papillae and the junction of the hard and soft palate, is composed of eight areas.

1. Lips
2. Buccal mucosa
3. Lower alveolar ridge
4. Upper alveolar ridge
5. Retromolar gingiva
6. Floor of the mouth
7. Hard palate
8. Oral tongue (anterior two-thirds of tongue)

2. What are the anatomic subdivisions of the pharynx?

The human pharynx is divided into three anatomic areas: the **nasopharynx** between the skull base and hard palate, **the oral pharynx** between the hard palate and hyoid bone, and the

hypopharynx between the hyoid bone and lower portion of the cricoid cartilage. Each of these three areas is divided into subunits which are beneficial for cancer staging. The larynx is not considered part of the pharynx but is significant for tumor staging when involved in the spread of pharyngeal cancer.

- **Nasopharynx**
  Posterior superior wall (skull base to the hard palate)
  Lateral wall (including the fossa of Rosenmüller and eustachian tube torus and orifice)
  Inferior wall (superior surface of the soft palate)
- **Oropharynx**
  Tongue base (posterior one-third of tongue)
  Vallecula
  Tonsils
  Tonsillar fossa
  Faucial pillars
  Inferior surface of the soft palate
  Pharyngeal wall
- **Hypopharynx**
  Pharyngoesophageal junction (postcricoid area)
  Pyriform fossa
  Posterior pharyngeal wall

3. What is the most common benign tumor of the oral cavity and pharynx?

Squamous papilloma. Unlike its nasal and laryngeal counterparts, oral papillomas are not locally invasive, and malignant degeneration is rare. Human papillomavirus (HPV) has been implicated as the etiology; however, polymerase chain reaction (PCR) studies of oral papilloma DNA show no evidence of HPV types 6a or 11a, suggesting that HPV may influence oral tumor development differently.

4. Which are the most common odontogenic neoplasms?

Odontogenic neoplasms arise from dental lamina (early ectoderm invagination into the jaw) or any of its derivatives. The **dentigerous cyst** is the most common follicular odontogenic neoplasm, constituting 95% of follicular cysts and 34% of odontogenic cysts. Multiple cysts can be seen in basal cell nevus syndrome and cleidocranial dysostosis. Aggressive neoplasms such as **odontogenic keratocysts** and **ameloblastoma** develop from the epithelial wall of a dentigerous cyst.

5. Which genetic disease is related to multiple osteomas of the jaw?

Osteomas are benign tumors in the oral cavity that may be related to **Gardner's syndrome**. This autosomal dominant hereditary defect of connective tissue consists of polyposis of the large bowel, epidermoid cysts of the skin, and multiple osteomas of the facial bones. The large bowel polyps appear late and lead to a 40% incidence of malignant degeneration.

6. What hard palate lesion appears as a painless ulcer and is often confused with malignancy?

Uninformed physicians often mistake **necrotizing sialometaplasia** for carcinoma and may treat it as such without an appropriate biopsy to confirm its benign nature. Histologic features include coagulative necrosis of minor salivary glands along with prominent squamous metaplasia of acini and ducts and pseudoepitheliomatous hyperplasia.

7. List some etiologic factors associated with cancer of the oral cavity and pharynx.

Tobacco smoking (cigarettes, cigars, pipes)   Sunlight exposure (carcinoma of the lower lip)
Smokeless tobacco use   Epstein-Barr virus (nasopharyngeal carcinoma)
Use of betel nut   Plummer-Vinson syndrome (cancer of the
Heavy alcohol consumption   tongue and hypopharynx)

Those who use tobacco and alcohol have a 15-fold increase for oral cancer when compared to those who abstain from both.

8. Describe the premalignant lesions of the oral cavity and pharynx.
All white or red patches should be viewed with suspicion:
- **Leukoplakia**, or white lesions, demonstrate invasive squamous cell carcinoma in 8% of cases, while the remainder represent a spectrum of epithelial hyperplasia (80%), dysplasia (30%), and carcinoma in situ (2%).
- **Lichen planus** appears as a white lace pattern on the buccal mucosa and has a squamous cell transformation rate of about 4%.
- **Erythroplakia**, or red velvety plaques on the floor of mouth or gingiva, carry a much higher risk of malignancy than leukoplakia.

9. What is the most common malignancy of the oral cavity?
About 90% of all carcinomas of the oral cavity and pharynx are **squamous cell carcinomas**. Other tumor types include minor salivary gland tumors, sarcomas, lymphomas, and melanoma.

10. Why do oral and pharyngeal neoplasms cause ear pain?
Cancers in the oropharyngeal region, which is supplied by cranial nerves IX and X, may cause **referred otalgia**, as the ear also receives sensory innervation along branches of the same nerves and sensory nuclei. A patient complaining of otalgia may be erroneously diagnosed with otitis or temporomandibular joint disease and may be treated with bite splints, antibiotics, or analgesics, while a throat cancer goes undiagnosed.

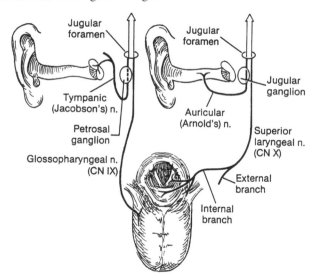

Pathways for referred pain from the oropharynx to the ear. (From Thawley SE, O'Leary MO: Malignant neoplasms of the oropharynx. In Cummings CW, et al (eds): Otolaryngology–Head and Neck Surgery, 2nd ed. St. Louis, Mosby, 1993, p 1315, with permission.)

11. What is the most common oral minor salivary gland cancer? Where is it likely to occur?
Adenoid cystic carcinoma is the most common, comprising 40% of all minor salivary gland malignancies. Adenocarcinoma (30%) and mucoepidermoid carcinoma (20%) are second and third, respectively. In the oral cavity, most salivary gland cancers occur in the posterior aspect of the hard palate near the greater palatine foramen.

12. The triad of nasal obstruction, nasopharyngeal mass, and recurrent epistaxis in a young male usually represents what nasopharyngeal neoplasm?

Angiofibromas (juvenile nasopharyngeal angiofibromas) are the most common benign tumors of the nasopharynx. Accounting for < 0.05 % of head and neck tumors, they are vascular neoplasms that occur only in males, usually during pubescence. This triad of symptoms indicates the presence of an aggressive and destructive neoplasm. If the patient is from China, **nasopharyngeal carcinoma** should also be in the differential diagnosis.

13. What is the etiology of nasopharyngeal carcinoma?

Nasopharyngeal carcinoma (NPC) accounts for 0.25% of all cancers among North American whites, but it accounts for approximately 18% of all malignant tumors among North American Chinese. In southern China, this rate is even higher, where it is the most common cancer in males and the third most common cancer in females. There is a significant increase in HLA-A2 and HLA-B-SIN2 in Chinese patients with NPC, but this association is not absolute. Other potential etiologic factors include the Epstein-Barr virus, polycyclic hydrocarbons, nitrosamine ingestion, and chronic rhinosinusitis, although the etiology is probably multifactorial.

14. What is the differential for a neck mass?

Remember the mnemonic **KITTENS**:

K   Congenital-developmental (sebaceous cysts, branchial cleft cysts, thyroglossal duct cysts, lymphangioma/hemangioma, dermoid cysts, ectopic thyroid tissue, laryngocele, pharyngeal diverticulum, thymic cysts)
I   Infectious-inflammatory (lymphadenitis: bacterial, viral, granulomatous, tuberculous, cat-scratch, actinomycosis, fungal)
T   Toxin (unlikely)
T   Traumatic (hematoma)
E   Endocrine (thyroid, parathyroid, carotid body, tumor, MEN)
N   Neoplastic (*metastatic:* unknown primary, epidermoid carcinoma, melanoma, adenocarcinoma, breast, lung, kidney, GI tract; *primary:* thyroid, lymphoma, salivary, lipoma, angioma, carotid body tumor, rhabdomyosarcoma)
S   Systemic, psychiatric

15. How do you evaluate a solitary neck mass?

The first step is a thorough **history** and **head and neck examination**, including flexible nasopharyngoscopy. A negative exam and low suspicion for malignancy may indicate an inflammatory node, which can be observed over 2–4 weeks with or without antibiotics. If the lesion persists or enlarges or if the clinical exam is suspicious for neoplasm, **fine-needle aspiration** for cytology and culture should be performed. A negative aspirate should not be accepted if the clinical suspicion for malignancy is high. **Imaging studies** of the neck (MRI, CT), chest x-ray, and **GI workup** (if indicated by fine-needle aspiration) should be done before the lesion is biopsied. An open biopsy should be preceded by **panendoscopy** (pharyngoscopy, laryngoscopy, esophagoscopy, and bronchoscopy) for an occult primary tumor. Multiple random **biopsies** of the most common occult sites (nasopharynx, tonsil, tongue base and valleculae, and pyriform sinus) should follow a negative panendoscopy. If an open biopsy of the neck mass is to be performed during the panendoscopy, the patient and surgeon should be prepared for a neck dissection if metastatic squamous cell carcinoma is found.

16. Why is lymphatic drainage of the oral cavity and pharynx a consideration in treating malignancy?

Carcinoma of the oral cavity and pharynx metastasize at different rates and in different directions. Pharyngeal tissues have abundant lymphatics, and tumors often metastasize earlier and to a greater extent. Also, "silent areas" exist in the pharynx, where lesions of the valleculae or pyriform sinus will remain asymptomatic for a longer time, resulting in great metastatic potential. Tongue-based lesions have extensive bilateral drainage and produce regional metastasis in as high as 70% of cases. Soft palate and other midline tumors spread to bilateral nodes approximately 30–40% of the time. Oral cancers, especially gingival cancers, rarely metastasize. Therefore, the location of the primary tumor and its lymphatic drainage must be taken into consideration when planning treatment of metastatic spread to the neck and other distant sites.

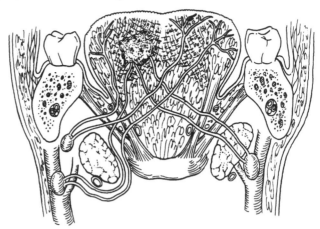

Bilateral lymphatic drainage of the base of the tongue. (From Thawley SE, O'Leary MO: Malignant neoplasms of the oropharynx. In Cummings CW, et al (eds): Otolaryngology– Head and Neck Surgery, 2nd ed. St. Louis, Mosby, 1993, p 1316, with permission.)

17. How do the rates of occult neck metastasis differ with respect to anatomic site in oral cavity and pharyngeal cancers?
The incidence of occult metastasis increases with the size of the primary tumor and the site. Oral cavity sites such as the tongue (34%) and floor of the mouth (30%) tend to have a high incidence of occult metastasis. In contrast, the lower alveolar ridge (19%) and buccal mucosa (9%) fare much better. Pharyngeal sites such as the pyriform sinus (38%) and tongue base (22%) also have a high incidence of occult metastasis, while the posterior pharynx (0%) is associated with virtually none. With this information, the management of an N0 neck should include surgical or radiation therapy to the nodes which drain the primary tumor.

18. How is cancer of the oral cavity and pharynx staged?
Primary tumors of the oral cavity and oropharynx are predominantly staged according to tumor size. In contrast, tumors of the nasopharynx and hypopharynx are staged by the involvement of subsites.

Oral Cavity and Oropharynx
T1   Tumor ≤ 2cm
T2   Tumor > 2 but ≤ 4 cm
T3   Tumor > 4 cm
T4   Tumor invades adjacent structures, such as cortical bone, tongue, skin, maxillary sinus, or soft tissues of neck.

Nasopharynx
T1   Tumor limited to 1 nasopharyngeal subsite
T2   Involvement of > 1 nasopharyngeal subsite
T3   Invasion of nasal cavity and/or oropharynx
T4   Invasion of skull and/or cranial nerves

Hypopharynx
T1   Tumor limited to 1 hypopharyngeal subsite
T2   Involvement of > 1 hypopharyngeal subsite or adjacent area without fixation of the hemilarynx
T3   Involvement of > 1 hypopharyngeal subsite or adjacent area with fixation of the hemilarynx
T4   Tumor of adjacent structures (neck soft tissue, etc.)

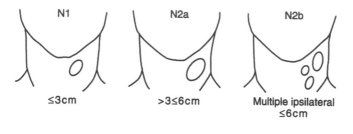

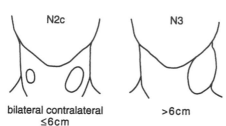

Neck node staging. (From Lee KJ: The vestibular system and its disorders. In Lee KJ (ed): Essential Otolaryngology–Head and Neck Surgery. Norwalk, CT, Appleton & Lange, 1995, p 539, with permission.)

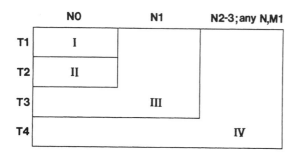

TNM staging of cancers of the oral cavity and pharynx. (From Lee KJ: The vestibular system and its disorders. In Lee KJ (ed): Essential Otolaryngology– Head and Neck Surgery. Norwalk, CT, Appleton & Lange, 1995, p 540, with permission.)

19. A 3.5-cm cancerous-appearing lesion is observed in the tonsillar fossa. It spreads down onto the tongue base, into the vallecula, and to the midline. The patient's neck has a large 3-cm matted node at the angle of the jaw. The remaining examination is incomplete. How is this tumor staged?

T2 N2b Mx. This lesion is contained entirely within the oral pharynx and is therefore staged similarly to oral cancers, with the T stage being determined by size, not by subunit involvement. Because the tumor is between 2–4 cm, it is considered a T2 lesion. The jugulodigastric node is matted, representing multiple nodes. Therefore, instead of a single node of 3 cm or less (N1), the nodal status increases to N2b. The presence of the matted nodes also moves the patient from stage III disease to stage IV disease. The x means that the staging category cannot be assessed; therefore, Mx designates that distant metastases are unaddressed.

20. What is the treatment of carcinoma of the oral cavity?

Radiation therapy and surgery have proved to be equally efficacious when used to treat stage I and II tumors of the oral cavity. Stage III and IV tumors are treated with combination therapy which consists of surgery with either preoperative or postoperative radiation. As the location of the tumor proceeds anatomically from the front of the lips to the hypopharynx, prognosis becomes poorer.

21. Is chemotherapy effective for the treatment of regionally advanced carcinoma of the oral cavity and pharynx?

Three methods of chemotherapy in local and regional sites in the head and neck have been utilized. **Neoadjuvant chemotherapy**, or induction chemotherapy, is given prior to surgery or irradiation. **Conventional adjuvant chemotherapy** is given after surgery and irradiation. Neither of these methods has improved disease control and survival when compared to regional treatment alone. In contrast, randomized studies looking at **combined modality therapy** (chemotherapy concomitantly with radiation therapy), using 5-fluorouracil or cisplatin in addition to radiation therapy, have found improved disease control and survival over irradiation alone.

22. What is a "commando" procedure?

The term commando, or **composite resection**, in head and neck surgery refers to the resection of the primary lesion (usually tonsil and lateral pharyngeal wall) in continuity with a partial mandibulectomy and a radical neck dissection with primary closure. This technique was described by Hayes Martin in the 1930s and is considered radical therapy today. Less radical and more functional approaches are currently used, including mandible preservation (mandibulotomy) with graft or flap reconstruction. When the cancer has involved the pterygoid musculature and directly invaded the mandible, consideration for more radical surgery is indicated. Commando procedures with primary closure are found to leave significant cosmetic and functional handicaps, including facial deformity, malocclusion, nasal regurgitation, aspiration, speech, and deglutition difficulties.

23. How do you reconstruct the pharynx following pharyngectomy for cancer?

Oral and pharyngeal tissue following ablative therapy were initially reconstructed with **free skin grafting, local skin flaps,** and **skin muscle flaps**. Due to the hypovascular effect following radiation therapy, reconstructions often failed because of wound breakdown, fistula formation, and stenosis. **Regional muscle-skin flaps** (pectoralis, trapezius, and latissimus dorsi) had improved outcomes due to the fact that the transferred tissue was vascularized and nonirradiated. These flaps are the current workhorses in head and neck reconstruction. Although time-consuming and expensive, **free vascularized flaps** have been highly successful. Free vascularized flaps are useful in replacing missing tissue with similar tissue and, in most cases, restore sensation, contour, and function.

CONTROVERSY

24. What is an N0 neck, and why is it controversial?

If there is no clinical or radiographic evidence of nodal spread from a primary oral or pharyngeal cancer, the neck is considered to have an N0 cervical node status. Treatment of the N0 neck is controversial because it can range from close observation with clinical and radiographic exams to surgery or radiation. Because of the high risk of occult metastases, N0 necks are uncommon with tongue base lesions, tonsillar fossa lesions, T3 or T4 oral tumors, and T3 or T4 pharyngeal tumors. Observation of the clinically negative neck under these circumstances is not recommended. Surgical treatment of suspected unilateral neck disease should be done with a **functional neck dissection**. For primary tumors with a higher incidence of occult bilateral cervical metastases, bilateral neck irradiation or neck dissections are performed. Patients with advanced cancer and clinically negative necks have no significant differences in neck cancer recurrence rates when the different treatment modalities, elective neck irradiation, neck dissection, and combined treatment, are compared.

BIBLIOGRAPHY

1. Baker SR: Malignant neoplasms of the oral cavity. In Cummings CW, et al (eds): Otolaryngology–Head and Neck Surgery, 2nd ed. St. Louis, Mosby, 1993.
2. Bhaskar SN: Synopsis of Oral Pathology, 7th ed. St. Louis, Mosby, 1986.
3. Eisele DW, Johns ME: Carcinoma of the oral cavity and pharynx. In Lee KJ (ed): Essential Otolaryngology–Head and Neck Surgery, 5th ed. New York, Elsevier Science Publishing Company, Inc., 1991.
4. Gustafson RO, Neel HB: Cysts and tumors of the nasopharynx. In Paparella MM, et al (eds): Otolaryngology, 3rd ed. Philadelphia, W.B. Saunders, 1991.

5. McGuirt WF: Differential diagnosis of neck masses. In Cummings CW, et al (eds): Otolaryngology–Head and Neck Surgery, 2nd ed. St. Louis, Mosby, 1993.
6. Nakano K: Characteristics of human papillomavirus (HPV) infection in papilloma of the head and neck—detection of HPV according to clinical features and type specificity. Nippon Jibiinkoka Gakkai Kaiho 97:1381-1392, 1994.
7. Thawley SE, O'Leary MO: Malignant neoplasms of the oropharynx. In Cummings CW, et al (eds): Otolaryngology–Head and Neck Surgery, 2nd ed. St. Louis, Mosby, 1993.

41. ODONTOGENIC CYSTS, TUMORS, AND RELATED JAW LESIONS

Ethan Lazarus, M.D., and R. Casey Strahan, M.D.

1. What is the differential diagnosis for a mass in the jaw (mandible or maxilla)?

Like any other swelling in the body, masses of the jaw can be classified into three categories: neoplastic, infectious/inflammatory, and congenital. In addition, the jaws are unique in that they contain teeth, and therefore, each category can be broken down further into masses related to the teeth (odontogenic) and masses not related to the teeth (nonodontogenic).

Differential Diagnosis of Jaw Mass

Neoplastic diseases
Odontogenic
  Malignant
    Primary intraosseous carcinoma
    Ameloblastic fibrosarcoma
    Ameloblastic dentinosarcoma
    Ameloblastic odontosarcoma
  Benign
    Ameloblastoma
    Calcifying epithelial odontogenic tumor
      (Pindborg tumor)
    Odontogenic adenomatoid tumor
    Calcifying odontogenic cyst
    Ameloblastic fibroma, fibro-odontoma,
      or odontoma
    Odontoma
    Odontogenic fibroma or myxoma
    Cementoma
    Dentinoma
Nonodontogenic
  Malignant
    Osteosarcoma
    Chondrosarcoma
    Metastatic malignancies
  Benign
    Ossifying fibroma
    Fibrous dysplasia
    Cherubism
    Osteoma
    Osteoblastoma

Inflammatory/infectious diseases
Odontogenic
  Radicular cyst (periapical or lateral perio-
    dontal cysts
  Residual cyst
Nonodontogenic
  Retention cyst
  Traumatic bone cyst
  Idiopathic bone cavity
  Aneurysmal bone cyst
  Stafne's mandibular lingual cortical defect

Developmental diseases
Odontogenic
  Follicular (or dentigerous) cyst
  Odontogenic keratocyst
  Eruption cyst
  Alveolar cyst of infants
  Gingival cyst of adults
  Developmental lateral periodontal cyst
Nonodontogenic
  Nasopalatine duct cyst
  Midpalatal cyst of infants
  Nasolabial cyst
  Globulomaxillary cyst
  Medial mandibular and palatal cysts

2. **Name the two most common cystic lesions of the jaw.**

Periapical cysts are the most common, representing approximately 55% of jaw cysts. These are inflammatory and odontogenic in origin and are secondary to inflammation at the apex of a nonvital tooth. They are thus related to overall poor dental hygiene, and additional dental disease is usually noted in other teeth. Although often asymptomatic, patients may report pain either with biting or percussion. Radiographically, these cysts present as an area of radiolucency attached to a root apex.

Follicular (or dentigerous) cysts are developmental and odontogenic in origin, accounting for about 10% of jaw cysts. These cysts form around the crown of an unerupted but fully formed tooth. Radiographically, they present as a radiolucency at the crown of an unerupted tooth, usually a third molar or canine. Follicular cysts may be quite large (up to 5 cm in diameter).

3. **Why is an odontogenic keratocyst (OKC) often difficult to diagnose? Why is its differentiation from other types of cysts important?**

OKCs can be difficult to diagnose because they often have a radiologic and/or histologic appearance consistent with other less aggressive cysts. It may occur in association with the crown of an unerupted tooth, thus resembling a follicular cyst, or it may occur in association with a tooth root, thus resembling a periapical cyst. Histologically, OKCs can easily be mistaken for follicular cysts, as both have a thin connective tissue wall lined by a thin layer of stratified squamous epithelium. There are, however, specific criteria for the diagnosis of OKC, and these must be evaluated by an experienced pathologist.

The importance of differentiating an OKC from other cysts is that OKCs have a very high recurrence rate. Treatment consists of enucleation and curettage, but recurrence rates of 10–60% can be expected. Therefore, the postoperative followup for these cases must be much more vigilant and long-term.

4. **A patient presents with multiple odontogenic keratocysts and basal cell carcinomas. What genetic syndrome do you suspect?**

Basal cell nevus syndrome is associated with the development of multiple odontogenic keratocysts and basal cell carcinomas. This autosomal dominant syndrome affects patients at a young age. The syndrome may be associated with bifid ribs, a wide nasal bridge, and mandibular prognathism, and 85% of patients have calcification of the falx cerebri and 65% have palmar pitting.

5. **A patient presents with a swelling in the upper buccal-gingival sulcus. The patient's history is significant for a Caldwell-Luc procedure 1 year ago. What lesion should you consider?**

This patient has probably developed a **retention cyst**. This is an inflammatory nonodontogenic cyst with an iatrogenic cause. A Caldwell-Luc procedure may result in the entrapment of sinus epithelium within the incision tract, forming a retention cyst. Typically, retention cysts are lined with ciliated, columnar (i.e., respiratory) epithelium. Simple excision is usually curative.

6. **The oral cavity counterpart to basal cell carcinoma of the skin is what?**

Ameloblastoma. The ameloblastic cell resembles the basal cell of basal cell carcinoma. The clinical behavior of an ameloblastoma also resembles that of basal cell carcinoma, as both show local growth and invasion but limited metastatic potential.

7. **Describe the characteristics of an ameloblastoma.**

Ameloblastomas are benign neoplasms of odontogenic origin. They are rare tumors, accounting for only 1% of all tumors and cysts of the jaws. They arise from odontogenic epithelium or the enamel organ and thus are classified as benign epithelial odontogenic tumors. About 20% of ameloblastomas are associated with impacted teeth or dentigerous cysts. There are several types of ameloblastomas. These lesions may occur at any age, though those associated with a dentigerous cyst or impacted tooth typically occur before the age of 40. The average age at presentation is 34–38 years. The usual symptom is a painless swelling. Radiologically, a multiloculated, radiolucent area resembling "soap bubbles" or "honeycomb" is pathognomonic. These tumors are benign but locally invasive, and the treatment of choice is wide local excision. Histologically, they show a characteristic pattern of follicles lined by tall columnar cells with reversed nuclear polarity. The epithelium is supported by a mature collagenous stroma.

8. How does a malignant ameloblastoma differ from an ameloblastic carcinoma?

In a **malignant ameloblastoma**, the cells retain their benign histologic pattern, but these cells are found to metastasize to lung and lymph nodes. In an **ameloblastic carcinoma**, the cells appear cytologically malignant and metastasize to lung and lymph nodes. Both have a very poor prognosis.

9. What is an ossifying fibroma?

An ossifying fibroma is a slow-growing, nonodontogenic, benign tumor of the mandible and, less frequently, maxilla. This lesion is most common in women in their third to fourth decades. It presents as a well-circumscribed, marble-like mass in the bone. The tumor follows an expansile course and can attain a substantial size. It usually grows slowly, destroying the normal bone and producing facial asymmetry. Radiologically, it can be radiopaque or radiolucent. Normal radiologic landmarks are distorted. With large masses, there can be evidence of both bone destruction and bone formation. The histologic picture demonstrates collagenous stroma and cementoid deposits. Treatment involves excision and curettage.

10. How does fibrous dysplasia affect the jaw?

This benign, hamartomatous lesion affects the maxilla more frequently than the mandible. It most commonly presents in the first or second decade of life. Patients are generally asymptomatic, but this painless swelling may lead to a unilateral facial deformity. Normal bone is replaced by fibrous tissue that calcifies in an abnormal pattern. Radiographically, this lesion has diffuse margins and a "ground-glass" appearance. Fibrous dysplasia is generally associated with a good prognosis. However, a **juvenile aggressive** type of fibrous dysplasia is associated with a rapidly destructive lesion that obliterates tooth buds and is refractory to treatment. Polyostotic fibrous dysplasia may be associated with **Alport's syndrome**.

11. What is cherubism?

Cherubism is a benign, self-limited disease of the jaw bones. This rare congenital disorder displays an autosomal dominant inheritance pattern. It is more common in males and usually presents prior to age 5 with premature tooth displacement and loss. Symmetric mandibular enlargement may lead to a mild cosmetic deformity, giving these children a round, cherub-like face. Radiographically, the lesions are bilateral, multiple, multilocular, well-defined radiolucencies with a thin or absent cortex. The prognosis is generally favorable. Although some patients may require facial contouring, these features generally regress spontaneously by puberty.

12. What history and physical findings are useful in evaluating a patient with jaw swelling?

A complete history and physical is the first step in the workup of a patient with swelling in the jaw. A slow-growing, painless, nonspecific swelling is the usual scenario. Pain or paresthesia may be an indication of neural invasion or compression and must raise the suspicion of a malignant process. Alternatively, pain may be an indication of recent infection of a benign process. Other indicators that raise the suspicion for malignancy include pathologic fractures, malocclusion, and trismus. A bruit over the mass or in the common carotid raises the suspicion of a vascular malformation or tumor.

13. Which tests are basic in the workup for a swelling in the jaw?

The **panoramic** (Panorex) **radiograph** is indispensable in the workup of a swelling in the jaw. The location of the lesion, density of the lesion, presence or absence of septa or loculations, and reaction of surrounding bone and teeth all give specific clues as to the etiology. Well-demarcated lesions surrounded by sclerotic bone are most likely slow-growing and benign. Proximity to teeth, especially diseased teeth, suggests an odontogenic origin. Ill-defined lytic lesions with resorption of bone and neighboring teeth are more likely malignant or at least locally aggressive. A **CT scan** will more accurately identify cortical thinning and local invasion.

A **fine-needle aspiration** (FNA) may be helpful prior to open biopsy. Although the FNA likely will not identify the tumor, it may aid in the identification of a vascular malformation or tumor, preventing the disastrous result of an open biopsy of such a lesion. The final diagnosis usually requires an **open biopsy,** which can be combined with curative procedures, such as curettage or enucleation.

14. Name the three basic treatment modalities for these cysts and tumors of the jaw.

Odontogenic cysts and tumors can be treated by one of three different modalities:

1. **Simple enucleation**, with or without curettage, can be used to treat the more benign lesions.

2. A **marginal or segmental resection** of the lesion and surrounding bone is usually used for benign but more locally invasive tumors and cysts.

3. **Composite resection** of bone and surrounding soft tissues is used for malignant tumors.

15. Which lesions can be treated with enucleation and curettage?

Enucleation and curettage is adequate treatment for virtually all odontogenic cysts and many odontogenic tumors. Odontogenic tumors in this category include odontoma, ameloblastic fibroma and fibro-odontoma, adenomatoid odontogenic tumor, calcifying odontogenic cyst, cementoblastoma, and central cementifying fibroma. The odontogenic keratocyst is a notable exception in this category (see below).

16. What lesions can be treated with marginal or segmental resection of the mandible?

Marginal resection of the mandible involves the resection of only a margin of the mandible, usually the alveolar margin. Segmental resection, on the other hand, involves the resection of a complete segment, i.e., the full height of the mandible is resected along a certain portion. Either of these modalities may require reconstruction using some type of bone graft. This modality is appropriate for persistent or locally invasive lesions, including odontogenic keratocyst (especially if recurrent), ameloblastoma, Pindborg tumor, odontogenic myxoma, ameloblastic odontoma, and squamous odontogenic tumor.

17. Which lesions require a composite resection?

Composite resection of bone and surrounding soft tissues may be required for malignant tumors of the jaws, especially if there is obvious involvement of the adjacent tissues. A CT scan is helpful in delineating the extent of involvement and in the preoperative planning. These tumors include malignant ameloblastoma, ameloblastic carcinoma, ameloblastic fibrosarcoma or odontosarcoma, or primary intraosseous carcinoma.

18. A patient with an adenomatoid odontogenic tumor undergoes surgery, but portions of the tumor are difficult to access and are left in the maxilla. Should a "second-look" operation be performed to assess recurrence?

Surprisingly, the answer is no. Adenomatoid odontogenic tumors occur in females under the age of 20. Two-thirds occur in the mandible, and most are anterior to the permanent molars. These tumors have a rapid life cycle which culminates in amyloid and calcific material replacing the cells. Therefore, recurrence is rare, even if the entire tumor is not removed at the time of surgery.

19. What complications may be associated with these masses?

1. Recurrence
2. Infection
3. Rapid increase in size
4. Pathologic fracture of the mandible

CONTROVERSIES

20. How is fibrous dysplasia of the jaw managed?

Treatment of fibrous dysplasia generally consists of conservative surgery, involving shaving and recontouring of the bone. The treatment is cosmetic in nature. No attempt should be made to remove all of the diseased bone, as there is no distinct border. Controversy arises as to the timing of this surgery, and even its necessity. Fibrous dysplasia nearly always "burns itself out" around the age of puberty. Malignant transformation, although rare, can occur.

21. Can a patient wear false teeth if the mandible is reconstructed?

In general, yes. However, the patient may or may not be able to chew food, depending on the size and location of the defect in the mandible and on the type of reconstruction. Controversy exists as to how and when mandibular reconstruction is performed. If the resected segment of the mandible is relatively short and is located at the angle, then some surgeons argue that no reconstruction is necessary. The patient may wear a denture but will not be able to chew with any significant force. Other surgeons favor reconstructing this defect with one sort of bone graft or another, with the goal of giving the patient a strong enough mandible to chew. Similar controversy exists for defects in other segments of the mandible.

22. Which cysts are known to be "fissural"?

In the past, several types of nonodontogenic, developmental cysts were thought to arise from epithelium trapped between fusing embryonic processes. Today, it is known that the **median palatal cyst** is the only true fissural jaw cyst. It is formed by the growth of epithelium that is trapped between the fusing embryonic palatal shelves. Median palatal cysts are rare and present as a prominent midline palatal mass. In the past, it was argued that nasopalatine duct cysts, globulomaxillary cysts, and nasoalveolar cysts were also fissural. However, these arguments have been disproved.

BIBLIOGRAPHY

1. Dierks EJ, Bernstein ML: Odontogenic cysts, tumors, and related jaw lesions. In Bailey BJ (ed): Head and Neck Surgery–Otolaryngology. Philadelphia, J.B. Lippincott, 1993, pp 1176–1191.
2. Han MH, et al: Cystic expansile masses of the maxilla: Differential diagnosis with CT and MR. Am J Neuroradiol 16:333–338, 1995.
3. Larsen PE, Hegtvedt AK: Odontogenesis and odontogenic cysts and tumors. In Cummings CW, et al (eds): Otolaryngology–Head and Neck Surgery. St. Louis, Mosby, 1993, pp 1414–1442.
4. Lee KJ (ed): Essential Otolaryngology–Head and Neck Surgery, 6th ed. Norwalk CT, Appleton & Lange, 1995, pp 624–631.
5. Slootweg PJ: Bone and cementum as stromal features in Pindborg tumor. J Oral Pathol Med 20(2):93–95, 1991.

42. TUMORS OF THE NOSE AND PARANASAL SINUSES

Mark R. Mount, M.D.

1. What are the most common benign tumors of the nose and sinuses?

Osteomas are the most common benign tumors, followed by hemangiomas and papillomas.

2. An inverting papilloma is a benign tumor often misdiagnosed as a nasal polyp. Why is it important to make the correct diagnosis?

10–15% of inverting papillomas will transform into squamous cell carcinoma. If the polyp is simply excised, it may recur aggressively with bony destruction and intracranial extension. Overall, recurrence rates vary from 27–73%.

3. When should one suspect an inverting papilloma?

These tumors are less translucent than polyps. They are usually unilateral and more commonly present with epistaxis. As a rule, one should biopsy all unilateral nasal polyps in the clinic before surgery unless they are obviously vascular.

4. Which strains of human papilloma virus (HPV) are associated with sinonasal papillomas?

As with genital condylomas, skin warts, and laryngeal papillomas, sinonasal papillomas often contain HPV. HPV types 6 and 11 are associated with benign papillary tumors, while types 16 and 18 are weakly associated with malignant degeneration.

5. Unilateral epistaxis in a teenage boy should alert the physician to rule out what tumor?

A **juvenile angiofibroma** is a benign vascular tumor that occurs almost exclusively in adolescent males. The presenting symptoms are usually unilateral epistaxis and obstruction. The tumor appears as a smooth lobulated mass. Because it is highly vascular, biopsies should be avoided. Diagnosis is made by inspection and CT scan. Treatment is primarily surgical, as the tumor may be quite aggressive.

6. Why is juvenile angiofibroma rarely seen in men over 30?

It's unknown. However, this type of tumor is thought to regress spontaneously in many or all patients. There are several reports of residual tumor completely regressing after surgery. Despite the good prognosis, resection of the mass is prudent. This expansive tumor may invade the cranial vault or orbit with devastating consequences before it regresses.

7. What is a pyogenic granuloma?

A pyogenic granuloma is a common benign polypoid lesion of the mucosa, usually seen on the septum. It is vascular and may bleed spontaneously. Although it may involute spontaneously, treatment revolves around excision.

8. Histiocytosis X may present as a nasal mass and/or epistaxis. What are the three types of histiocytosis X?

1. Eosinophilic granuloma
2. Hand-Schüller-Christian disease
3. Letterer-Siwe disease

These diseases, of unknown etiology, consist of an infiltration of differentiated histiocytes. They often present with ulcerations or granulation tissue. These three diseases are known collectively as histiocytosis X.

9. Which of these histiocytoses is most likely to be fatal? Least likely?

Letterer-Siwe disease, which occurs in children under 2 years old, is uniformly fatal. It is a disseminated disease, presenting with hepatosplenomegaly, fever, rash, and anemia. In contrast, an **eosinophilic granuloma** is a chronic disease that is treated with surgical excision and, occasionally, radiation therapy.

10. What is epiphora?

Epiphora is the symptom of **excessive tearing** caused by blockage of the nasolacrimal duct. It is most often a surgical complication. If this symptom presents in a patient who has had no facial surgery, nasal or maxillary sinus tumors obstructing the duct should be considered.

11. Which is the most common malignancy of the nose and paranasal sinuses?

Squamous cell carcinoma accounts for 70% of these cancers, followed by adenocarcinoma (5–10%) and adenoid cystic carcinoma (5–10%). Less common tumors include undifferentiated transitional cell carcinoma, olfactory esthesioneuroblastoma, and malignant melanoma.

12. Where do nose and sinus cancers typically originate?

The maxillary sinus is the most common site (55%), followed by the nasal cavity (35%), ethmoid sinus (9%), and, rarely, sphenoid sinus. Septal cancers are exceedingly rare.

13. Are there any risk factors associated with developing nasal or sinus malignancies?

Certain industrial workers have a predisposition for sinonasal malignancies. **Nickel workers** have an increase of 100–870 times the normal rate of sinus squamous cell carcinoma. These cancers may develop after 10 or more years of exposure and after 20 years of latency. **Wood dust** and, to a lesser extent, **leatherworking and furniture-making** are exclusively associated with adenocarcinoma. Other inhalants associated with these malignancies include chrome pigment, radium dial paint, mustard gas, and hydrocarbons. Tobacco has shown no association with nasal and sinus cancers. The incidence of nasal and sinus malignancies in males is twice that of females.

14. How do maxillary tumors present?

Usually, patients experience prolonged sinusitis, especially unilateral. Patients may develop epistaxis, numbness, swelling, or nasal congestion. They may have loose upper teeth or suddenly poor-fitting dentures. Rarely, a patient may experience trismus, palatal numbness, or diplopia. Pain is often a late and therefore ominous symptom.

15. How do ethmoid sinus tumors present?

Ethmoid sinus tumors usually spread into vital structures before causing symptoms. They may invade the anterior cranial fossa, orbits, maxillary sinuses, or sphenoid sinuses. Usual symptoms include unilateral nasal obstruction, severe headache, and/or diplopia.

16. How do sphenoid sinus tumors present?

The sphenoid sinus lies just inferior and anterior to the optic chiasm and pituitary gland. It lies between the carotid arteries. Tumors in this area present as headache, diplopia, or vision loss. Invasion of the skull base exists in 50% of cases.

17. Does CT or MRI better evaluate nasal and maxillary tumors?

CT is much better at evaluating bony invasion and destruction. Therefore, it is essential for proper evaluation and preoperative planning. MRI is also useful if there is possible CNS or orbital involvement, as MRI is better at distinguishing dura from tumor.

18. What is Ohngren's line?

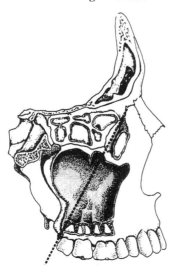

Ohngren's line is an imaginary line extending from the medial canthus of the eye to the angle of the jaw. Tumors above the line have a poorer prognosis because of their tendency to metastasize superiorly and posteriorly. Tumors below the line are more easily resected and carry a better prognosis.

Ohngren's line. (From Spiessl B, et al (eds): UICC TNM Atlas, 3rd ed. Berlin, Springer-Verlag, 1989, with permission.)

19. Where do nose and sinus tumors metastasize?

To cervical or retropharyngeal nodes. The incidence of cervical metastases on presentation is about 10%, although up to 44% of cases will eventually metastasize to the cervical area. Only 10% of patients ever develop distant metastases.

20. What are the most accepted therapies for cancer of the nose and paranasal sinuses?

Surgery is the mainstay therapy and can be curative if resection is complete. Obviously, surgery is more easily performed on small tumors. Most centers use postoperative **radiation** therapy for large tumors, positive margins, perineural or perivascular invasion, or lymph node metastases. However, considering the morbidity of radiation in this area, its use is controversial—100% of eyes receiving 5,800 rad will develop severe panophthalmopathy with severe corneal ulceration, and 86% of eyes receiving 2800–5400 rad will develop cataracts and visual disturbances. Due to the low overall incidence of nose and paranasal cancer, few studies have adequately compared various therapies. The eventual mortality for all nose and sinus tumors is > 50%.

21. Is there any role for chemotherapy?

As in many head and neck cancers, chemotherapy's use is expanding. Because it alone does not improve survival, it has been traditionally reserved for end-stage palliation. New protocols show promise for combination chemotherapy with surgery or radiation.

CONTROVERSIES

22. How should an inverting papilloma be removed at its initial presentation?

Aggressive: The traditional and proven approach for treating an inverting papilloma or early carcinoma has been a lateral rhinotomy incision with a **medial maxillectomy**. Because the incidence of malignant change is > 10%, complete removal of the tumor is imperative. Even benign tumors have recurrence rates of up to 70% after conservative resection. Intranasal endoscopic techniques are simply inadequate for total excision and have no data to support their use.

Conservative: Many surgeons advocate **endoscopic removal** of an inverting papilloma whenever possible. If the tumor does not extend into the maxillary sinus, it may be easily and completely removed with this procedure. A medial maxillectomy is a major procedure with definite morbidity and leaves the patient with a visible deformity. If the tumor can be removed without this operation, it is to the patient's advantage. If HPV types 6 or 11 are found in the tumor, there is little likelihood of malignant degeneration. Therefore, it may not always be necessary to perform large aggressive surgeries. Most studies that criticize conservative techniques are flawed in that the newer endoscopic techniques were not available at the time of the study.

23. Should orbital exenteration be performed routinely for advanced sinus cancers?

Yes: Despite the obviously unpleasant effect of removing the entire orbit, there is evidence, presented by Ketcham and VanBuren, that this procedure may double the survival of patients with ethmoid tumors (50% vs. 30%). Even if exenteration is avoided, the patient will surely go blind in the same eye after radiation therapy.

No: Although a tumor that invades the orbit is difficult to remove curatively while still sparing sight, the decision to remove the eye should be heavily weighed. The Ketcham study is contradicted by at least two other studies, including Perry and Weymuller. One must seriously consider the cosmetic and psychological devastation to the patient before proceeding with exenteration.

BIBLIOGRAPHY

1. Bielamowicz S, Calcaterra TC, Watson D: Inverting papilloma of the head and neck: The UCLA update. Otolaryngol Head Neck Surg 109:71–76, 1993.
2. Buchwald C, Franzmann MB, Jacobsen GK, Lindeberg H: Human papillomavirus in sinonasal papillomas: A study of 78 cases using in situ hybridization and polymerase chain reaction. Laryngoscope 105:66-71, 1995.

3. DeSanto L: Neoplasms [of the nose]. In Cummings CW, et al (eds): Otolaryngology–Head and Neck Surgery, 2nd ed. St. Louis, Mosby, 1993.
4. Hill JH, Soboroff BJ, Applebaum EL: Nonsquamous tumors of the nose and paranasal sinuses. Otolaryngol Clin North Am 19:723–739, 1986.
5. Ketcham AS, VanBuren JM: Tumors of the paranasal sinuses: A therapeutic challenge. Am J Surg 150:406–413, 1985.
6. Kenady D: Cancer of the paranasal sinuses. Surg Clin North Am 66:119–131, 1986.
7. Lee KJ (ed): Essential Otolaryngology–Head and Neck Surgery, 6th ed. Norwalk, CT, Appleton & Lange, 1995.
8. Meyers EN, Carrau RL: Neoplasms of the nose and paranasal sinuses. In Bailey BJ (ed): Head and Neck Surgery–Otolaryngology, Philadelphia, J.B. Lippincott, 1993.
9. Perry C, et al: Preservation of the eye in paranasal sinus cancer surgery. Arch Otolaryngol Head Neck Surg 114:632–634, 1988.
10. Spiessl B, et al (ed): UICC TNM Atlas, 3rd ed. Berlin, Springer-Verlag, 1989.
11. Weymuller EA: Neoplasms [of paranasal sinuses]. In Cummings CW, et al (eds): Otolaryngology–Head and Neck Surgery, 2nd ed. St. Louis, Mosby, 1993.
12. Weymuller EA, Reardon EJ, Nash D: A comparison of treatment modalities in carcinoma of the maxillary antrum. Arch Otolaryngol Head Neck Surg 106:625, 1980.

43. LARYNGEAL CANCER

Vincent D. Eusterman, M.D., D.D.S., and Mark R. Mount, M.D.

1. How frequently does laryngeal cancer occur?

Laryngeal cancer comprises **1–5% of all malignancies** diagnosed annually, or about 3–8/100,000 population. In the United States, this represents about 11,000 new cases annually, with 3,700 deaths annually for a mortality rate of 1.6/10,000. Laryngeal cancer is more common in men (8:1), having a peak incidence in the sixth to seventh decades with an average age of onset at 60–62 years.

2. Where do these cancers form?

Generally, 67% are glottic, 31% supraglottic, and 2% subglottic. 95% of glottic cancers arise from the true vocal cords. When diagnosed, laryngeal cancer is confined to the larynx in 60% of the cases, 25% have regional metastasis, and 15% have distant metastasis. The incidence of multiple synchronous primary tumors (occurring at the same time) is 0.5–1%, and the incidence of metachronous tumors (occurring at different times) is 5–10%, with lung the most common site.

3. What types of cancers are found in the larynx?

Squamous-cell carcinoma (carcinoma in situ; well, moderately, and poorly differentiated; spindle-cell variant)	94%
Verrucous carcinoma	2–4%
Adenocarcinoma (nonspecific adenocarcinomas, adenoid cystic carcinomas, mucoepidermoid carcinomas)	1%
Sarcomas (fibrosarcoma, chondrosarcoma, malignant fibrous histiocytoma, rhabdomyosarcomas)	1%
Metastatic tumors (melanoma, renal-cell, prostate, breast, lung, stomach)	Rare

4. What risk factors predispose to laryngeal carcinoma?

The most important risk factors are **smoking** and **alcohol abuse**. When these two factors are both present, the risk is 50% greater than the additive risk of each. Smokers are 6–39 times more likely to get laryngeal carcinoma than nonsmokers. Less than 5% of laryngeal cancer patients have *no* smoking history. Less important risk factors include esophageal reflux, radiation, presence of laryngocele, and history of juvenile papillomatosis.

5. Describe the anatomic divisions of the larynx. What is their significance?

The larynx is subdivided into three divisions: **supraglottis, glottis, and subglottis**. The supraglottis extends from the tip of the epiglottis to the ventricular fold, the glottis begins at the ventricular fold and extends 1 cm inferior to the vocal cord, while the subglottis begins there and proceeds to the inferior border of the cricoid cartilage.

Each division is affected by cancer differently, with each requiring different treatment and each having its own prognosis. Accurate diagnosis of cancer in each of these regions is important.

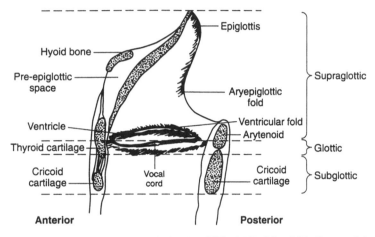

Anatomic subdivisions of the larynx. (From Eisele DW, Clifford AR, Johns ME: Cancer of the larynx, paranasal sinuses, and temporal bone. In Lee KJ (ed): Essential Otolaryngology, 6th ed. Norwalk, CT, Appleton & Lange, 1995, p 556, with permission.)

6. How does cancer differ among these three subdivisions?

The **supraglottis** has extensive lymphatics that feed the pre-epiglottic space and the neck bilaterally. The incidence of nodal metastasis varies from 25–50% depending on the tumor stage of the primary; 20–35% are bilateral. Tumors on the epiglottis that invade the pre-epiglottic space through cartilage perforations access the "paraglottic space," which communicates with the entire larynx.

Glottic cancers occur more frequently, but fortunately this region has limited lymphatic drainage. Tumors are detected early because of hoarseness, and spread to the neck nodes occurs in < 10% of cases. Glottic cancers are usually slow-growing, well-differentiated tumors that extend in predictable ways.

Subglottic carcinoma is often silent and poorly differentiated and extends into or through the cricoid cartilage to involve the paratracheal and cervical lymphatics in a large number of the cases. Prognosis is poor because of the advanced stage at the time of diagnosis.

7. What barriers exist in the larynx to check the spread of cancer?

The **quadrangular membrane** above the false cords and the **conus elasticus** between the true cords and cricoid cartilage act as barriers to the spread of cancer. The thyroid and cricoid cartilage is lateral to these structures, and when they become invaded, it suggests a poor prognosis (T4).

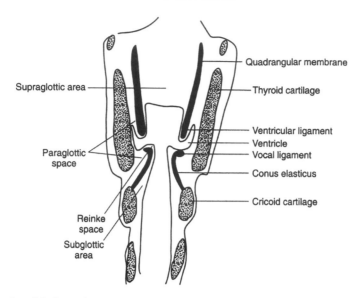

Coronal section of the larynx illustrating the barriers to the spread of cancer. (From Eisele DW, Clifford AR, Johns ME: Cancer of the larynx, paranasal sinuses, and temporal bone. In Lee KJ (ed): Essential Otolaryngology, 6th ed. Norwalk, Connecticut, Appleton & Lange, 1995, p 557, with permission.)

8. How is laryngeal carcinoma staged?

The American Joint Committee on Cancer (AJCC) uses the TNM classification for laryngeal cancer by anatomic region. Nodal and metastatic staging is identical to that for other forms of head and neck cancers. A hoarse patient with a left fixed cord and a single left 2-cm neck mass would have at least a T3N1Mx classification.

Staging System for Laryngeal Carcinoma

Glottis

T1	Tumor limited to vocal cords (involving anterior or posterior commissure) with normal mobility
T1a	Tumor limited to one vocal cord
T1b	Tumor involving both cords
T2	Tumor extending to supra- or subglottis with impaired vocal cord mobility
T3	Tumor confined to larynx with vocal cord fixation
T4	Tumor invading through thyroid cartilage and/or with direct extralaryngeal spread

Supraglottis

T1	Tumor limited to 1 subsite of supraglottis with normal vocal cord mobility
T2	Tumor involving > 1 subsite of supraglottis or glottis, with impaired vocal cord mobility
T3	Tumor limited to larynx with vocal cord fixation; tumor may invade postcricoid area, medial pyriform sinus, or pre-epiglottic space
T4	Tumor invades beyond thyroid cartilage and/or with extralaryngeal spread

Subglottis

T1	Tumor limited to subglottis
T2	Tumor extending to glottis with or without impaired vocal cord mobility
T3	Tumor limited to larynx with vocal cord fixation
T4	Tumor invading beyond cricoid or thyroid cartilages, with extralaryngeal tissue spread

9. What diagnostic techniques are used to evaluate laryngeal cancer?

The single most valuable technique for imaging the larynx is the **CT scan**. It can identify tumor in the intermedullary space, loss of the internal laryngeal fat plane, breaks or fenestrations in cartilage, and demineralization of calcified cartilage. **MRI scans** have longer scan times, producing greater artifact due to laryngeal and carotid movement. Gadolinium-enhanced MRI is superior to CT in detecting tumor recurrences. **Direct laryngoscopy** (microlaryngoscopy) is preferable to imaging for ventricular tumors or small lesions at the free margin of the vocal fold and is necessary for obtaining a tissue diagnosis. Nasopharyngoscopy, direct esophagoscopy, bronchoscopy, and chest radiographs are important to rule out synchronous lesions.

10. How does laryngeal cancer present?

Glottic carcinoma presents with **hoarseness** as the cardinal symptom. Sore throat, dysphagia, otalgia, and odynophagia may exist alone or with other symptoms. Airway obstruction and hemoptysis are late findings, less common in glottic cancer, and often require emergency treatment.

Supraglottic carcinoma presents with **hoarseness** (laryngeal fixation, mass effect), odynophagia, dysphagia, otalgia (tongue base, pharyngeal extension), and neck mass.

11. What is a "fixed cord"?

Vocal cords that have motor neural injury or tumor invasion into the thyroarytenoid muscle or arytenoid cartilage can be "fixed in place," or immobile. A nonworking cord is considered "fixed," and the alert clinician should evaluate the patient for cancer, either in or around the larynx or over the pathway of the vagus and recurrent laryngeal nerve. There are many other causes of vocal cord paralysis (traumatic, infective, congenital, idiopathic, iatrogenic), but neoplastic sources should be ruled out first. Laryngeal cancers with mobile cords are usually staged T1 or T2; however, when cord fixation is present, the stage increases to T3, which drops 5-year survival from 80–95% to 30–57%.

12. Where is Reinke's space?

Reinke's space is a potential space beneath the epithelium of the vocal fold. It contains loose connective tissue and can transport cancer throughout the cord. Once through the space, cancer can invade the thyroarytenoid muscle (vocalis muscle), causing cord paralysis.

13. What is the significance of the paraglottic space?

This space surrounds the glottis and acts as a conduit for cancer to spread between all divisions of the larynx. Cancers that extend between regions are considered **transglottic tumors** and have a high incidence of cartilage invasion and a poorer prognosis.

14. What happens when the recurrent nerve or superior laryngeal nerve to the larynx is injured?

A recurrent nerve paralysis causes loss of motor function to all intrinsic muscles of the ipsilateral larynx. The vocal cord will assume a midline position due to adduction of the cricothyroid muscle (the only extrinsic muscle of the larynx), which is supplied by the superior laryngeal nerve.

Bilateral recurrent nerve paralysis results in bilateral midline cords and airway obstruction which may require tracheostomy. The superior nerve supplies motor (cricothyroid) and sensation to the supraglottis.

When both superior and recurrent nerves are paralyzed, the cord assumes a "cadaveric," or intermediate, position as is seen under general anesthesia. Loss of sensory function associated with the superior nerve may result in chronic aspiration and, when severe enough, could ultimately lead to laryngectomy.

15. How do the survival rates for laryngeal cancer vary by T stage?

Survival is measured as the percent 5-year cure rate. Increased nodal disease reduces these figures significantly, depending on nodal stage.

Supraglottic

T1–T2	75% with either surgery or radiation alone
T3–T4	23% with radiation alone, 52–83% with surgical salvage or surgery alone

Glottic

T1–T2	70–95% with either modality alone
T3	30–40% with radiation with surgical salvage, 50–80% with surgery alone
T4	20% with radiation, 40% with surgery and neck dissection, 50% for combined surgery and radiation

Subglottic

T1–T2	70% with combined therapy
T1–T4	36% with radiation and surgical salvage, 42% with surgery alone

16. How is laryngeal cancer treated?

Current thought for laryngeal cancer is "organ-sparing" therapy for voice preservation. **Radiation therapy** is ideal for organ-sparing and works well for lower stages of the disease. **Surgical therapy** has evolved organ-sparing techniques to include partial laryngectomy (horizontal supraglottic, vertical hemilaryngectomy), laryngofissure and cordectomy, and laser cordectomy. Controversy arises with higher stages of disease; patients who do not want to lose their voices can undergo an organ-sparing protocol with **combination therapy** (chemotherapy and radiation). However, these and lower-staged radiation failures generally result in total laryngectomy. Near-total laryngectomy is a surgical procedure to treat advanced-stage disease by constructing a physiologic mucosal shunt with the remaining arytenoid to produce speech and requires a tracheostomy.

17. Are laryngeal cancer and lung cancer related?

Yes. In all probability, the inciting factor for laryngeal cancer has a similar effect on lung mucosa. A laryngeal cancer patient has about a 5–10% chance of developing a second primary cancer in the lung after laryngeal therapy and should be followed closely with laryngeal exams and chest radiographs.

18. Discuss the patient criteria for performing a horizontal supraglottic laryngectomy.

Important to any conservative surgery for laryngeal cancer is that control of the tumor takes precedence over voice preservation. Physiologic parameters are an important consideration with supraglottic laryngectomy. The patient should have near-normal pulmonary function testing and be under age 65 years. Som and Sisson have described criteria that include a 5-mm anterior commissure clearance, normal vocal cord mobility, no cartilage invasion, no tongue extension within 5 mm of the circumvallate papillae, and no extension to postcricoid, arytenoid, interarytenoid, prevertebral fascia, or pyriform sinus apex. Lesions > 3 cm or with fixed cervical nodes are also a contraindication to surgery.

19. What is pyriform sinus cancer? What is its significance to the larynx?

The pyriform sinus is the inferior extent of the hypopharynx just before it turns into the cervical esophagus. It is a funnel-shaped mucosa-lined sinus that invaginates between and around the thyroid and cricoid cartilages. It opens during swallowing to direct food into the esophagus. It is also the site of hypopharyngeal cancer which is often silent. Medial-wall pyriform sinus cancers invade the larynx through the paraglottic space. Laterally, they invade the thyroid cartilage or pharyngeal wall. They often present late as a neck mass, often with a history of referred ear pain, and require aggressive combined therapy. Three-year survival is about 40% with treatment.

20. What are the patterns of endolaryngeal lymphatic drainage?

There is a rich superficial lymphatic system throughout the mucosa that is not compartmentalized. The deep system, however, arises from midline structures in the supraglottis and subglottis that form lateral cell masses in the glottis. The deep system drains ipsilaterally, except at the subglottis and pre-epiglottic space, where bilateral drainage occurs.

CONTROVERSIES

21. How is T1 carcinoma of the larynx treated?

There are two methods of treatment, surgery and radiation, and each works effectively. However, surgical proponents feel that radiation should be held in reserve, as failure of radiation often results in laryngectomy. Radiation therapy requires 6 weeks of therapy and is expensive. Surgery may only require one treatment as an outpatient. Voice quality is an issue that may have better results with radiation, although some surgeons feel that postoperative voice is comparable. Also, the surgical patient has less post-treatment swelling and no chance of radiation-induced chondronecrosis.

22. Is total laryngectomy the surgery of choice for advanced laryngeal cancer?

A Veterans Cooperative study recently showed similar results at 1 year between an induction chemo-radiation protocol and total laryngectomy with radiation. Long-term 5-year survival figures are not available. However, this new model may represent a chance to preserve the larynx with advanced cancers. The older proven technique of total laryngectomy is still a primary modality for patients who are not candidates for the experimental protocol.

23. Should the N0 neck in glottic cancer be treated when using primary radiation therapy?

Controversy persists as to the indication for treatment of the N0 neck. Recommendations vary depending on the site, location, and extent of tumor. In glottic cancer, occult metastasis occurs in 14–16% of patients, while a higher incidence of 20–38% occurs in those with supraglottic tumors. The highest rate of occult metastasis is seen in patients with pyriform sinus neoplasms. When the risk of occult cervical metastasis is high (> 15%), consideration should be given to include regional nodes in the planned radiation fields for the primary tumor. Patients with positive clinical adenopathy should have a neck dissection.

24. What is the treatment for anterior commissure glottic cancer?

No natural barrier exists to the spread of cancer from the anterior vocal commissure into the thyroid cartilage where it attaches. Often, these tumors are understaged, and deep invasion diminishes the effectiveness of radiation therapy. Zohar et al. found local control rates of 90% with conservation surgery versus 72% with radiation. There are no well-controlled prospective studies that compare radiation therapy for this site. Woodhouse and others feel that anterior commissure involvement does not affect the outcome for radiation therapy and believe it remains the preferred method of initial treatment.

BIBLIOGRAPHY

1. American Joint Committee on Cancer: Manual for Staging Cancer, 4th ed. Philadelphia, J.B. Lippincott, 1992.
2. Bailey BJ: Early glottic carcinoma. In Bailey BJ (ed): Head and Neck Surgery–Otolaryngology. Philadelphia, J.B. Lippincott, 1993.
3. Boyd JH, Johnson JT, Curtin H: Carcinoma of the Supraglottic Larynx [Self-instructional package]. Rochester, MN, American Academy of Otolaryngology-Head and Neck Surgery Foundation, 1993.
4. Eisele DW, Clifford AR, Johns ME: Cancer of the larynx, paranasal sinuses, and temporal bone. In Lee KJ (ed): Essential Otolaryngology, 6th ed. Norwalk, CT, Appleton & Lange, 1995.
5. Leach JL, Schaefer SD: Diagnosis and Treatment of Cancer of the Glottis and Subglottis [Self-instructional package]. Rochester, MN, American Academy of Otolaryngology–Head and Neck Surgery Foundation, 1993.
6. Veterans Affairs Laryngeal Cancer Study Group: Induction chemotherapy plus radiation compared with surgery plus radiation in patients with advanced laryngeal cancer. N Engl J Med 324:1685–1690, 1991.
7. Woodhouse RJ, Quively JM, Fu KK, et al: Treatment of carcinoma of the vocal cord: A review of 20 years of experience. Laryngoscope 91:1155–1162, 1981.
8. Zohar Y, Rahima M, Shvili Y, et al: The controversial treatment of anterior commissure carcinoma of the larynx. Laryngoscope 102:69–72, 1992.

44. TUMORS OF THE TRACHEA AND TRACHEOBRONCHIAL TREE

Douglas M. Sorensen, M.D.

1. Describe the anatomy of the trachea.

The adult trachea averages 11 cm in length and is composed of 18–22 incomplete cartilaginous rings. Each incomplete ring has a posterior membranous segment. Posteriorly, the trachea lies against the esophagus, while anteriorly, the thyroid isthmus crosses at the level of the second or third tracheal ring. The innominate artery crosses the trachea inferiorly. The trachea begins 2 cm below the vocal cords and extends inferiorly to the carina.

2. Which arteries supply the trachea?

The inferior thyroid, subclavian, internal thoracic, supreme intercostal, innominate, and superior and middle bronchial arteries.

3. Describe the histologic features of the tracheobronchial tree epithelium.

The tracheobronchial tree is lined by a pseudostratified, columnar, ciliated epithelium that rests on an elastic lamina propria. The ciliated cells are dominant and are interfoliated by goblet cells. The epithelial layer also consists of two or three layers of undifferentiated basal cells that may become either goblet or ciliated cells.

4. What is the differential diagnosis of a tracheal neoplasm in the adult?

Tracheal tumors are rare, representing 2% of all upper airway tumors. 90% of tracheal neoplasms in the adult population are malignant, while 10% are benign.

Squamous cell carcinoma
Adenoid cystic carcinoma
Heterogeneous group
    Malignant: adenocarcinoma, adenosquamous carcinoma, small-cell carcinoma, mucoepidermoid carcinoma, sarcoma, melanoma
    Benign: squamous papillomata, pleomorphic adenoma, granular cell tumor, fibrous histiocytoma, leiomyoma, chondroma, chondroblastoma

5. Name the two most common malignant primary tracheal tumors. How do they differ?

Squamous Cell Carcinoma	Adenoid Cystic Carcinoma
Strongly associated with smoking	Not associated with smoking
Lymph node metastasis common	Lymph nodes rarely involved
Grows rapidly and aggressively	Grows slowly, indolent
Invades mediastinal structures	Displaces mediastinal structures

6. What are the most common secondary tracheal tumors?

A secondary tracheal tumor is a malignant tumor that involves or invades the trachea from an adjacent site. These tumors are often incurable. They are (in order of frequency):

1. Laryngeal carcinoma
2. Bronchogenic carcinoma, from a main bronchus
3. Esophageal carcinoma, commonly associated with a fistula
4. Metastatic breast carcinoma, lymphoma, or other head and neck cancer
5. Thyroid carcinoma of any variety, usually anaplastic

7. How does the differential diagnosis of a primary tracheal neoplasm differ in a child?

While 90% of tracheal tumors in the adult are malignant, the opposite is true in children—90% of tracheal tumors in children are benign. Of the benign pediatric neoplasms, squamous papilloma and hemangioma are the most common. Chondroma, osteochondroma, osteoma, and fibroma are much less common. Although rare, reported malignant pediatric tracheal neoplasms include squamous cell carcinoma, adenoid cystic carcinoma, sarcoma, and adenocarcinoma.

8. What is a bronchogenic cyst?

A congenital cyst of the bronchi, usually located near the bifurcation of the trachea. This cyst often causes compression of the bronchus, most commonly on the left side. Diagnosis is achieved with chest radiography and ultrasonography. The treatment of choice is cyst excision.

9. How does the patient with a tracheal tumor present clinically?

Tracheal tumors are rare, and therefore, a tracheal tumor is usually not the first diagnosis considered when a clinician sees a patient with dyspnea, cough, or wheezing. However, a high index of suspicion is required. Because these tumors often are initially diagnosed as chronic bronchitis or asthma, most tracheal neoplasms are not detected until they are in an advanced stage. Common signs and symptoms include cough, dyspnea, hemoptysis, stridor, and wheezing. A patient with recurrent bilateral pneumonia and no evidence of chronic aspiration should be considered to have a tracheal tumor until proven otherwise. Any patient who has been diagnosed with adult-onset asthma should also be evaluated for a tracheal tumor.

10. A patient has stridor and is in moderate respiratory distress. A chest x-ray is suspicious for a tracheal mass. How do you manage this patient?

The patient may have a foreign body in the airway or, worse, an obstructing tracheal tumor. If you try to intubate this patient, it is likely that tumor will be found obstructing the tracheal lumen; attempts at intubation will only aggravate the patient's airway, causing swelling. A tracheotomy will be fraught with problems for the same reasons.

To avoid these problems, take the patient immediately to the operating room. After the anesthesiologist has mask-ventilated the patient with general anesthesia, rigid bronchoscopy should be performed. No muscle relaxants should be administered, as this may cause complete collapse of the airway. After the bronchoscope has been placed through the vocal cords, the patient may be ventilated through this device. An obstructing endotracheal tumor can be partially removed via the bronchoscope.

11. Describe the work-up of a tracheal tumor.

When a tracheal tumor is suspected, *plain films* should be obtained initially, including a chest x-ray (anteroposterior and lateral views) and plain films of the neck. A neck *CT scan* may further delineate the tumor's extension. To evaluate esophageal extension, a *barium swallow* may also be helpful. *Rigid bronchoscopy with biopsies* should be performed in the operating room.

12. How are benign tracheal tumors treated?

Respiratory papillomas are the most common benign tumors of the trachea. About 1500 patients are treated annually for this disorder, with most cases being children. The disease is probably of viral origin. In the pediatric patient, multiple sites are involved throughout the laryngotracheobronchial tree. In contrast, the adult patient usually has a single lesion or discrete site of involvement. Treatment of symptomatic, benign tracheal lesions primarily involves endoscopic ablation. Currently, the CO_2 laser may be used to vaporize benign neoplasms from the tracheal wall. It is generally not indicated to resect the entire tracheal segment that is associated with a benign tumor.

13. What is the role of surgery in treating malignant tracheal tumors?

Most malignant tracheal tumors carry a poor prognosis, and treatment is directed toward palliation. Tracheal resection is the mainstay of therapy, with a primary anastomosis performed on the free ends of the trachea. Most tumors can be approached through a low collar incision in the neck. Tumors located at or near the carina require a combination approach, which involves a neck incision and a right posterolateral thoracotomy incision.

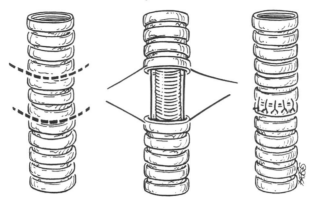

End-to-end reanastomosis of the trachea. (From Cardoso et al. In Cummings CW, et al (eds): Otolaryngology–Head and Neck Surgery. St. Louis, Mosby, 1993, p 2369; with permission.)

14. How much of the trachea can be resected?

Up to one-half of the trachea can be resected and still be reconstructed with a primary anastomosis. The trachea is 10–11 cm in the adult. Therefore, roughly 5–6 cm can be resected.

15. What are the complications of a tracheal resection and reconstruction?

1. Wound infection is a potential complication, as with any surgery. Drainage should be implemented and appropriate antibiotics should be administered.
2. Anastomotic dehiscence may be caused by ischemia or undue tension on the anastomosis.
3. Aspiration may be due to transection of one or both recurrent laryngeal nerves.
4. A tracheal–innominate artery fistula is a rare but serious complication.
5. A suture-line granuloma can usually be treated successfully by endoscopy.
6. Restenosis is caused by ischemia or undue tension on the anastomosis.

16. Name two maneuvers to prevent dehiscence of the tracheal anastomosis.

Most commonly, dehiscence at the tracheal anastomosis is caused by local ischemia or excessive tension.

• To prevent ischemia, the surgeon should avoid circumferentially dissecting around two or more consecutive tracheal rings.

• To avoid excessive tension, the surgeon should perform a suprahyoid laryngeal release. In this procedure, the suprahyoid muscle is severed to allow the neck to easily flex. The patient's neck should remain in such a flexed position to avoid excessive tension.

17. How are radiation and chemotherapy used in treating malignant tracheal tumors?

Both squamous cell carcinoma and adenoid cystic carcinoma are radiosensitive. Therefore, most patients are treated with postoperative irradiation. Radiation therapy alone will not provide a cure, but when radiation is combined with surgery, a 3-fold increase in survival time results as compared to surgery alone. Chemotherapy has not been shown to be effective in treating tracheal tumors.

18. What is the long-term survival for patients with tracheal tumors?

Patients with adenoid cystic carcinoma who are treated with tracheal resection and postoperative radiation have a 5-year survival of 75%. Patients with squamous cell carcinoma who receive the same treatment have a 5-year survival of 49%.

BIBLIOGRAPHY

1. Glazer HS, Siegel MJ: Imaging of tracheal tumors. In Cummings CW, et al (eds): Otolaryngology–Head and Neck Surgery. St. Louis, Mosby, 1993, pp 2243–2257.
2. Grillo HC: Management of tracheal tumors. Am J Surg 143:697, 1982.
3. Frist WH, Ossoff RH, Duncavage JA: In Gates GA (ed): Current Therapy in Otolaryngology–Head and Neck Surgery. St. Louis, Mosby, 1994, pp 305–308.
4. Cardoso PFG, Pearson FG: Diagnosis and management of tracheal neoplasms. In Cummings CW, et al (eds): Otolaryngology–Head and Neck Surgery. St. Louis, Mosby, 1993, pp 2339–2348.
5. Grillo HC: The trachea. In Shields TW (ed): General Thoracic Surgery. Philadelphia, Lea & Febiger, 1989.

45. TUMORS OF THE ESOPHAGUS

John P. Campana, M.D.

1. What are the major categories of esophageal tumors?

Esophageal tumors are either benign (0.5–0.8%) or malignant. The most common benign tumor is leiomyoma, and the most common malignant tumor is squamous cell (epidermoid) carcinoma. Esophageal malignancies represent 1% of all malignancy and 4% of GI malignancies. Esophageal cancer accounts for 4% of cancer deaths. In the United States, 92–95% of esophageal malignant tumors are squamous cell cancers, and 3–5% are adenocarcinomas.

Benign	*Malignant*
Nonepithelial	**Carcinoma**
Myomas	Squamous cell carcinoma
Leiomyoma	Adenocarcinoma
Fibromyoma	Adenoid cystic carcinoma
Lipomyoma	Mucoepidermoid carcinoma
Fibroma	Small-cell carcinoma
Vascular tumors	Undifferentiated
Hemangioma	**Sarcoma**
Lymphangioma	Leiomyosarcoma
Mesenchymal tumors	Fibrosarcoma
Reticuloendothelial	Osteosarcoma
Lipoma	Synovial sarcoma
Myxofibroma	Hemangiopericytoma
Giant cell tumor	Kaposi's sarcoma
Neurofibroma	Rhabdomyosarcoma
Osteochondroma	Liposarcoma
Epithelial	Malignant mesenchymoma
Papilloma	**Lymphoproliferative**
Polyp	Malignant lymphoma
Adenoma	Hodgkin's disease
Mucous cyst	Plasmacytoma
Heterotopic tumors	**Mucosal melanoma**
Gastric mucosal tumor	**Metastatic or direct invasion from:**
Melanoblastic tumor	Lungs/bronchi
Sebaceous gland tumor	Larynx
Granular cell myoblastoma	Thyroid
Pancreatic gland tumor	
Thyroid nodule	

Adapted from Wurster CF, Sisson GA: Neoplasms of the trachea/esophagus. In Cummings CW, et al (eds): Otolaryngology–Head and Neck Surgery. St. Louis, Mosby, 1986; and Begin LR: The pathobiology of esophageal cancer. In Roth JA (ed): Thoracic Oncology. Philadelphia, W.B. Saunders, 1989.

2. What are some of the presenting complaints of esophageal tumors?

Small benign lesions may be asymptomatic or present with mild dysphagia. Patients sometimes feel the sensation of pressure in the chest or neck. These neoplasms can occasionally bleed, resulting in hemoptysis. Rare pedunculated lesions can be regurgitated into the mouth and occasionally into the region of the vocal cords, causing airway obstruction. Cancers of the esophagus tend to grow rapidly. They usually present with progressive dysphagia, pain, weight loss, and malaise. Hemoptysis may be a recurrent problem. Fatal hemorrhage can occur from invasion into major mediastinal vessels. Tumor invasion can also cause hoarseness from the involvement of the recurrent laryngeal nerve or aspiration from a tracheoesophageal fistula. Unrelenting cough and regurgitation plague some patients.

3. Which patients are at high risk for esophageal cancer?

In the United States, esophageal cancer is mostly a disease of **men** between the **ages 50–70** who use **alcohol** and **tobacco**. Men are affected 3–4 times more often than women and have mortality rates 4–6 times higher than women. **African-Americans** are 4–5 times more likely than whites to get esophageal cancer. The overall annual incidence of esophageal squamous cell cancer in the United States is 2.6/100,000, with approximately 10,000 new cases diagnosed each year. In certain parts of China, Iran, and the former Soviet Union, the incidence is over 100/100,000 males.

Nutritional, vitamin, and mineral deficiencies, radiation exposure, chemical exposures (nitrates, nitrites, petroleum oils), and repeated ingestion of extremely hot liquids have all been associated with an increased incidence of esophageal malignancy. A history of achalasia, chronic esophagitis, and caustic ingestion increase the risk of these cancers. Human papillomavirus and genetic predisposition may also play a role in their development.

4. What is Plummer-Vinson syndrome? How does it relate to esophageal cancer?

Plummer-Vinson syndrome is characterized by dysphagia due to degeneration of the esophageal musculature, microcytic hypochromic anemia, and splenomegaly. It is also associated with achlorhydria with atrophy and inflammation of the mouth, pharynx, and upper end of the esophagus. Fissures at the corners of the lips (cheilitis) may be present. Pharyngoesophageal webs can occur which sometimes require dilation. This disorder is more prevalent in women than men. Patients have an increased risk of developing a pharyngeal or upper esophageal squamous cell carcinoma.

5. Which diagnostic methods are most often used to evaluate esophageal tumors?

Chest x-rays, barium swallows, esophagoscopy with and without endoscopic ultrasonography, and CT scan.

6. What information can a chest x-ray reveal to the clinician regarding esophageal tumors?

A chest x-ray for a benign lesion is usually unremarkable, but it can show a mediastinal density if the mass is large. In malignancies, chest x-rays can reveal tumor and lymph node densities in the mediastinum, displacement of normal mediastinal structures, aspiration pneumonitis and pneumonia, air/fluid levels in the esophagus, pulmonary metastasis, and pleural effusions.

7. Describe the characteristic findings for esophageal tumors on barium swallow.

A barium swallow can usually delineate extraluminal from intraluminal tumors. Leiomyomas are intramural neoplasms that narrow the lumen extrinsically. Although the mucosa can ulcerate with leiomyomas, it is usually intact with a smooth outline, and the tumor does not affect peristalsis. Dilation proximal to a benign lesion is rare. Malignancies of the esophagus usually have an irregular, ulcerated mucosa with luminal narrowing in a "shelf-like" or concentric, annular fashion and dilation proximal to the mass. Metastatic lymph nodes often displace or leave an impression on the esophagus. A barium swallow may also reveal tracheoesophageal fistulas.

8. What nontumor findings can be confused with tumors on esophageal barium studies?

Normal extrinsic impressions from the aortic arch, left mainstem bronchus, and left atrium can occasionally mimic tumors, especially if these structures are dilated or tortuous. Reflux stenosis (Schatzki's ring), scleroderma strictures, Barrett's esophagus with ulceration and stricture, cricopharyngeal spasm with and without associated diverticula (Zenker's), foreign bodies, diffuse esophageal spasm, lower esophageal spasm due to achalasia and reflux, congenital bands, webs, cysts, duplications, and vascular rings can all occasionally be confused with esophageal tumors.

9. What can endoscopy add to the workup?

Esophagoscopy can provide tissue for histopathologic evaluation, help dilate stenoses, and aid in the placement of endoprosthetic stents for palliation in advanced cases. Ulcerated, fungating, polypoid, pedunculated, and verrucous lesions should be biopsied. Small cancers confined to the mucosa without lymph node metastasis can be resected endoscopically. However, conventional wisdom dictates that intramural lesions with intact mucosa should not be biopsied. These are usually benign leiomyomas, and biopsies make subsequent thoracotomy excision more difficult. This issue has recently been questioned, and some centers are finding endoscopic aspiration lumpectomy to be safe and effective for small esophageal leiomyomas.

10. Can other diagnostic modalities supplement the endoscopic evaluation?

Endoscopic ultrasonography (EUS) is a valuable diagnostic tool for local tumor and nodal staging. Usually, EUS can correctly determine the T and N stage of an esophageal malignancy. Occasionally, laryngoscopy and bronchoscopy are added to the endoscopic workup to check for second primary malignancies and to evaluate the trachea and bronchi for invasion or fistulization. Some centers add thoracoscopy and a minilaparotomy or laparoscopy to the staging workup. This allows evaluation of the esophagus, other mediastinal structures, regional lymph nodes, lungs, and pleura for invasion or metastasis. At this time, biopsies of suspicious tissue can also be performed.

11. When evaluating an esophageal malignancy, is any additional information obtained from a CT scan that can justify the cost?

Absolutely yes. Esophageal cancer spreads directly to surrounding structures, through the bloodstream, and via lymphatic channels. Most of these malignancies directly involve a major mediastinal structure (trachea, left mainstem bronchus, or aorta) and have already spread to regional lymphatics (cervical, mediastinal, or celiac nodes) at the time of diagnosis. CT scans of the chest and abdomen reveal invasion of mediastinal structures, nodal metastasis, and distant metastasis to the liver, lungs, pleura, adrenals, and other sites. MRI does not usually add anything significant to the workup of these malignancies.

12. Where do cancers usually occur in the esophagus?

Most cancers of the esophagus are squamous cell carcinomas. A recent paper from China with a total of 3,603 patients revealed that 0.9% of malignancies were in the cervical esophagus, 15.9% were in the upper mediastinum, 60.9% were in the middle third, and 22.2% were in the lower thoracic esophagus. In the West, lower-third malignancies seem to be more common than those in the middle third of the esophagus. Adenocarcinomas are frequently found in the lower esophagus and are often thought to be extensions from gastric malignancies.

13. What are the survival rates for patients with esophageal cancer?

The overall 5-year survival rate for squamous cell cancer of the esophagus is usually < 15%, regardless of treatment modality. For small stage I lesions (T1N0M0 = tumor that invades the lamina propria or submucosa, without evidence of nodal or distant metastasis), 5-year survival rates are usually 50–70%, regardless of the therapeutic intervention. Patients with evidence of lymph node involvement have one-half to one-fifth the chance of surviving 5 years. The 5-year survival rates for stage IV malignancies (any T, any N, M1 = any tumor size and any lymph node status with known distant metastasis) are 0–7%. Most patients with distant metastasis die within several months. Survival rates for cancers between stages I and IV decrease with increasing stage, although there are some provocative exceptions to these grim statistics.

14. Does chemotherapy play a role in therapy for esophageal malignancies?

Used alone, chemotherapy cannot cure and is considered palliation only. Although there are sporadic reports of reasonable palliation using chemotherapy, no randomized studies are available that reveal statistically significant improvements in survival. The response is usually poor. Most regimens are cisplatin-based combinations. Chemotherapy-related morbidity and mortality are problems in themselves. As part of multimodality therapy, there is a definitive role for chemotherapy.

15. Is radiation therapy helpful in treating esophageal malignancies?

Yes. Squamous cell cancers of the esophagus are moderately radioresponsive. When radiotherapy is used alone for the definitive treatment of cancers at all esophageal levels, the best reported results yielded a 5-year survival of 20% (20/99 patients). Most reports are not as good and have rates below 10%. This disparity may be due to the fact that radiation therapy has been historically considered palliation, and more advanced tumors may have been selected for this treatment. Radiation therapy can be used as palliation in selected patients, with many getting relief of their dysphagia for the remainder of their lives. There is evidence indicating that the use of concurrent chemotherapy and radiation is superior to radiation therapy alone for palliation of locally advanced esophageal carcinoma. Pre- and postoperative radiotherapy has been shown to increase locoregional control, but there is no demonstrable increase in overall survival after this combination therapy is used.

16. What are the complications of radiation therapy used for esophageal carcinoma?

Radiation therapy is not without its own complications. It can cause bleeding, tracheoesophageal fistulization, perforation into the mediastinum, radiation pneumonitis and fibrosis, myelitis of the spinal cord, and strictures. If radiation is followed by surgery, increased operative complications, such as anastomotic leakage, and increased perioperative mortality from high doses to the lungs are observed. These negative effects are counterbalanced by the observation that often there is no residual tumor left in the esophagus in surgical resection specimens after preoperative radiation therapy.

17. Does surgery alone, as a single modality therapy, have much to offer these patients?

If the malignancies are detected early and confined to the mucosa or submucosa, aggressive surgery involving esophagectomy and cervical, mediastinal, and abdominal lymph node dissection can lead to 5-year survival rates of up to 73.2% with a 2.3% operative mortality rate. Unfortunately, most lesions are more advanced at presentation, and surgery alone is similar to radiation alone with overall 5-year survivals mostly < 15%. Perioperative mortality can be significant, with most series reporting rates of up to 20%. These results may be skewed because they often include procedures done for palliation as well as for cure—only 30–50% of patients are considered "resectable" at presentation, but many more are considered "operable" for palliation. Most patients have been losing weight and have coexistent chronic lung disease. It is important to try and optimize both their nutritional and pulmonary status for a week or two prior to surgery.

18. What types of surgery are employed in esophageal carcinoma?

Cervical esophageal carcinomas often require bilateral neck dissections and complete laryngopharyngectomy with gastric pullup, colon interposition, jejunal free flap, or lateral cutaneous thigh free flap for reconstruction. Resections for "cure" of all other esophageal cancers usually require a "three-hole" technique, combining a cervical approach, laparotomy, and right thoracotomy. Left thoracotomies are anatomically more difficult due to the physical interference offered by the heart and aortic arch. A transhiatal esophagectomy via cervical and abdominal incisions is usually considered a palliative procedure because midesophageal segments are dissected without direct vision and complete mediastinal lymph node dissection is difficult, if not impossible. Reconstruction after esophagectomy is usually accomplished using a gastric pullup or colon interposition. If the patient has had previous gastric surgery or if there is tumor involvement of the stomach, colon interposition is the procedure of choice.

19. Does combining all three treatment modalities do anything to improve survival in this grim disease?

Trimodality therapy involving preoperative radiation and chemotherapy followed by curative surgery holds promise. The best results published demonstrate a 34% five-year survival rate.

20. What is anatomically unique about the esophagus that leads to increased postoperative complications?

The esophagus is the only part of the alimentary canal that does not have a fibrous serosal layer. Anastomosis with esophageal remnants tends to heal poorly, resulting in more anastomotic leaks and postoperative morbidity and mortality.

21. What can be offered as palliation to patients with esophageal malignancies?

Chemotherapy, radiation therapy, and transhiatal esophagectomy were mentioned above. Unresectable tumors can occasionally be palliated by dilation and placement of an esophageal endoprosthesis or stent, including the newer expansile metal stents. A stent can also be employed in the presence of a tracheoesophageal fistula to help prevent continued pulmonary contamination. Iatrogenic perforation is not uncommon with the placement of a stent. An occasional tumor can be debulked using endoscopic laser techniques, intraluminal brachytherapy, or photodynamic therapy. Selected patients may benefit from surgical bypass of an obstructed esophagus without actual tumor removal, usually using a substernal gastric pullup. Tracheotomy, gastrostomy, and jejunostomy do not give good palliation in most patients but must be considered in selected cases.

22. Is there anything beyond procedural palliation that you can offer terminally ill patients?

Yes. Most patients have advanced disease at diagnosis. Palliation, pain control, and emotional support are what you can do for them. Most pain can be well-relieved with appropriate doses of narcotics. Addiction is obviously not an issue in these very sick, terminal patients. Adequate patient and family counseling regarding terminal issues, such as resuscitation status, should be provided. Hospice programs may be of great benefit to both the patient and family. To ensure that analgesia is adequate and to provide emotional support, frequent follow-up is indicated.

BIBLIOGRAPHY

1. Begin LR: The pathobiology of esophageal cancer. In Roth JA (ed): Thoracic Oncology. Philadelphia, W.B. Saunders, 1989.
2. Forastiere AA, Orringer MD, et al: Preoperative chemoradiation followed by transhiatal esophagectomy for carcinoma of the esophagus: Final report. J Clin Oncol 11:1118–1123, 1993.
3. Haddad NG, Fleischer DE: Neoplasms of the esophagus. In Castell DO (ed): The Esophagus, 2nd ed. Boston, Little, Brown, 1995.
4. Kato H, Tachimori Y, et al: Cervical, mediastinal, and abdominal lymph node dissection (three-field dissection) for superficial carcinoma of the thoracic esophagus. Cancer 72:2879–2882, 1993.
5. Pearson JG: The value of radiotherapy in the management of esophageal cancer. Am J Roentgenol 105: 500–513, 1969.
6. Wurster CF, Sisson GA: Neoplasms of the trachea/esophagus. In Cummings CW, et al (eds): Otolaryngology–Head and Neck Surgery. St. Louis, Mosby, 1993.
7. Zhang DW, Cheng GY, et al: Operable squamous esophageal cancer: Current results for the east. World J Surg 18:347–354, 1994.

46. THYROID AND PARATHYROID TUMORS

Catherine Winslow, M.D., and Margaret K.T. Squier, M.D.

1. What is a thyroid nodule?

A thyroid nodule is a discrete mass in the thyroid gland. The prevalence of thyroid nodules on physical exam has been estimated at approximately 6% in women and 1–2% in men. These statistics increase up to 10-fold when ultrasonographic or necropsy data are considered. The conditions that produce nodules may be benign, such as a solitary cyst, or life-threatening, such as an undifferentiated carcinoma. Because thyroid nodules are common and also potentially serious, the clinician must be prepared to evaluate and treat them methodically.

2. What are some common benign causes of focal thyroid enlargement?

About half of clinical thyroid nodules are due to a nodular goiter with one dominant nodule. A benign goiter is a common response of the thyroid gland to inadequate thyroid hormone levels. It can occur for physiologic reasons (during puberty, menses, and pregnancy), because of low iodine intake, from congenital defects in thyroid hormone production, or secondary to "goitrogenic" foods and drugs. Other benign causes of focal enlargement include cysts, teratomas, granulation bodies, and lymphadenopathy. Unilateral lobe agenesis can also produce an asymmetric thyroid gland. Focal enlargement can be produced by abscesses, as in acute suppurative (pyogenic) thyroiditis, an uncommon complication of upper respiratory infection or of pyogenic infection elsewhere in the body, which is treated by surgical drainage and antibiotics. The autoimmune diseases Hashimoto's thyroiditis and Graves' disease, in contrast, are relatively common causes of diffuse thyroid enlargement. Other forms of thyroiditis include subacute, painless, and Riedel's thyroiditis.

3. Which is the most common benign tumor of the thyroid?

Most benign tumors of the thyroid are follicular adenomas. Histologically and functionally, they are similar to normal thyroid tissue, but they take up radioactive iodine and can be distinguished as "warm" or "hot" spots on a radioiodine scan. Eventually, they can overwhelm the normal function of the thyroid and produce chemical thyrotoxicosis. They can also undergo hemorrhagic necrosis and produce localized pain. A necrosed adenoma may appear as a cold nodule on a radioiodine scan and therefore be mistaken for a carcinoma.

4. What percentage of thyroid nodules are malignant?

Malignant tumors are the main concern when evaluating a thyroid nodule. It has been reported that 5–20% of thyroid nodules are malignant. The major malignancies include papillary adenocarcinoma, follicular adenocarcinoma, medullary carcinoma, and undifferentiated (anaplastic) adenocarcinoma as well as lymphomas and metastases from kidney, lung, esophagus, and breast.

5. Describe the major characteristics of papillary adenocarcinoma.

Eighty-five percent of thyroid cancers are papillary adenocarcinoma. Metastasis is generally through the lymphatics, first to the subcapsular and pericapsular lymph nodes. Eighty percent of children and 20% of adults will have palpable lymph nodes at diagnosis. Distant metastatic sites include lung and bone. Papillary adenocarcinoma carries a good prognosis for survival, even if disease is metastatic.

6. Are there prognostic indicators in papillary thyroid cancer?

Age, sex, and extent of tumor are the main prognostic indicators. Females under age 40 with minimal invasion and nuclear euploidy tend to have a more favorable prognosis.

7. What are the major characteristics of follicular adenocarcinoma?

Follicular adenocarcinoma accounts for 10% of thyroid cancers. Like its benign counterpart, this carcinoma can be detected by radioactive iodine, which may be used to image metastases. Microscopically, one feature that distinguishes follicular adenocarcinoma from a benign follicular tumor is invasion to the thyroid capsule and vessels. Only 7% of follicular carcinomas spread to the lymph nodes, but this cancer often spreads through the blood to the lungs, bone, and liver. Follicular adenocarcinoma carries a poorer prognosis than papillary adenocarcinoma.

8. What is a Hürthle cell tumor?

This subtype of follicular adenocarcinoma tends to occur in older patients and is associated with a more aggressive course. It tends to be more invasive and carries a worse prognosis. The Hürthle cell has eosinophilic cytoplasm, the function of which is unknown. It may or may not take up radioactive iodine on a scan.

9. What are the major characteristics of medullary carcinoma?

Medullary carcinoma accounts for 2–5% of thyroid cancers. This cancer may arise from the calcitonin-secreting parafollicular cells of the thyroid, or C-cells. These cells are neuroectodermal in origin and join the thyroid gland as it descends from the base of the tongue. Because they secrete calcitonin, calcitonin immunoreactivity can be used as an identifier of this type of cancer. Serum calcitonin and CEA levels can also prove useful. Twenty percent of medullary carcinomas are familial.

10. How do the various multiple endocrine neoplasia (MEN) syndromes differ?

• MEN I (Wermer's syndrome)—hyperparathyroidism, pancreatic islet cell tumors, pituitary tumors, gastric carcinoid
• MEN IIA (Sipple's syndrome)—thyroid medullary carcinoma, pheochromocytoma, hyperparathyroidism
• MEN IIB—thyroid medullary carcinoma, pheochromocytoma, mucosal neuromas, ganglioneuromas, marfanoid habitus

11. What are the major characteristics of undifferentiated (anaplastic) adenocarcinoma?

Undifferentiated (anaplastic) adenocarcinoma usually affects older adults, often women. This uncommon tumor is nonencapsulated, rapid-growing, often invasive and metastatic, and may arise from a preexisting papillary or follicular tumor. It usually recurs after resection. External radiation and chemotherapy may be palliative, but most patients die within months due to local recurrence or metastasis to the lung or both.

12. A diagnosis of papillary-follicular carcinoma was returned on a thyroid specimen. Does this just indicate an indecisive pathologist?

A papillary-follicular carcinoma is a tumor with microscopic evidence of both types. It behaves clinically as a papillary carcinoma, with lymphatic metastasis and a favorable prognosis.

13. Which type of thyroid cancer cannot be found in a lingual thyroid? Why?

Lingual thyroid carcinomas are exceedingly rare but do occur. Medullary carcinoma is not found in a lingual thyroid, as the parafollicular cells only join the gland on its descent.

14. In the evaluation of a patient with a thyroid nodule, what should the history address?

The history should assess the awareness of a neck mass, pain, dyspnea, voice changes, or dysphagia. Patients may identify symptoms of infection, hyper- or hypothyroidism, or impingement on neck structures. The clinician should ask about the duration of symptoms, recent growth of the mass, and the patient's age, place of birth, history of radiation exposure, and the personal and family history of thyroid ailments and cancer. High risk factors for malignant disease include a family history of medullary carcinoma and rapid growth of the nodule; moderate risk factors include age < 20 or > 60, history of irradiation to the neck, and male gender.

15. When evaluating a patient with a thyroid nodule, what should you check on physical exam?

The physical exam is a key aspect of the thyroid nodule evaluation. It should emphasize whether the thyroid is enlarged symmetrically or asymmetrically; the number, size, smoothness, fixation, and hardness of any nodules palpated; and whether local structures, such as the trachea, have been displaced. Regional lymphadenopathy should be noted. High risk factors include firm consistency of the nodule, dysphonia (suggesting vocal cord paralysis), fixation of the nodule to adjacent structures, and regional lymphadenopathy. A nodule > 4 cm in diameter is a moderate risk factor.

16. What is a Delphian node?

Also known as the **cricothyroid node**, the Delphian node is a common site of thyroid carcinoma metastases.

17. How is fine-needle aspiration cytology used in evaluating a thyroid nodule?

The most used test for thyroid nodules is **fine-needle aspiration cytology** (FNAC). Given a qualified cytologist and an adequate specimen, this is often the test of choice. Early fears that this technique would lead to seeding of the needle track with malignant cells and contribute to spread of the disease have not been borne out clinically. FNAC is also relatively simple to perform and less expensive than either ultrasonography or radioiodine scanning.

18. Are thyroid function tests useful in evaluating a thyroid nodule?

Thyroid function tests include triiodothyronine (T_3) resin uptake, serum thyroid hormone, and TSH levels. These tests are generally not considered to be effective discriminators between benign and malignant nodules. In both cases, thyroid function may be normal. One test that may be useful, however, is a serum calcitonin level for patients with a family history of medullary carcinoma.

19. What is the role of ultrasound when evaluating a thyroid nodule?

This technique can distinguish solid from cystic lesions. Though it cannot discriminate benign from malignant status with reliability, solid nodules are generally more likely to be cancerous. This noninvasive, nonradioactive technique carries a low risk and makes it attractive for use in populations such as children and pregnant women.

20. When is radioiodine scanning used in evaluating a thyroid nodule?

Again, this is not a sensitive discriminator between benign and malignant processes, but this test helps to determine whether a lesion is single or multiple and whether it is functioning (warm to hot) or not (cold). A solitary, "hot" nodule may cause symptoms of hyperthyroidism but is usually nonmalignant. In contrast, 20% of solitary "cold" nodules are malignant. In children, a solitary cold nodule has a 40% chance of indicating thyroid cancer.

21. If a thyroid cyst can be easily aspirated, is there a need for further intervention?

Aspirates should always be sent for pathologic examination, as papillary carcinoma can be cystic. If the aspirate is negative for malignancy, careful observation with or without thyroid suppression will suffice. A positive or suspicious result warrants further treatment.

22. How do you manage a thyroid nodule?

Most physicians agree that management is based on FNAC results:

Result	Management
Benign	Follow-up with exam, FNAC in 1 year
Malignant	Surgical resection
Intermediate	Other diagnostic tests (e.g., radioiodine scan), consider resection based on test results and high clinical suspicion
Inadequate sample	Repeat FNAC

23. What treatment modalities are available for thyroid cancer?

Partial thyroidectomy, total thyroidectomy, neck dissection, radioactive iodine, thyroid suppression, or irradiation.

24. What are some potential risks of thyroidectomy for carcinoma?

Because surgery poses a risk to the recurrent laryngeal nerve, a baseline preoperative evaluation of vocal cord function should be obtained. The potential need for life-long thyroid replacement should be discussed with patients. Also, inadvertent parathyroidectomy may occur and require life-long calcium and vitamin D replacement therapy. Voice changes may occur either from damage to the recurrent laryngeal nerve or to the superior laryngeal nerve. The superior laryngeal nerve supplies the cricothyroid muscle, a tensor of the vocal cord.

25. What can be done if the patient is hoarse postoperatively?

To avoid injury to the recurrent laryngeal nerve, the surgeon should always expose and identify the nerve before removing tissue. Damage to the nerve, either by traction or transection, needs to be evaluated postoperatively by laryngoscopy. If unilateral vocal cord paralysis is present, it should be documented and followed. Such complication should be followed for at least 6 months before medialization is considered. Recovery from traction injury is common during this period of time.

26. What is a nonrecurrent laryngeal nerve?

The recurrent laryngeal nerve, a branch of the vagus nerve, embryologically loops around the fifth arch. On the left side, the fifth arch is represented by the aortic arch and ductus arteriosus. On the right, the fifth and sixth arches disappear, and the nerve loops around the subclavian artery. In patients with anomalous subclavian arteries, the nerve arises directly from the vagus, hence, a nonrecurrent nerve. A nonrecurrent laryngeal nerve is more likely to be injured during surgery due to its location.

27. How can potential traction injury to the nerve be decreased?

Steroids given preoperatively or postoperatively decrease the incidence of recurrent laryngeal nerve injury from 10% to 3%.

28. What should be done if a patient has respiratory distress postoperatively?

An immediate evaluation of the wound should be made. If evidence of a hematoma exists, the wound should be opened. Immediate intubation or urgent tracheotomy may be necessary.

29. Should thyroid replacement be started if radioactive iodine scan is planned for a patient postoperatively?

Although thyroid replacement will lower the TSH and therefore cause less iodine uptake, thyroid replacement with a short-acting preparation can be started postoperatively and withheld 1 week prior to the planned thyroid scan.

30. Do patients undergoing thyroid lobectomy for cancer need postoperative thyroid replacement?

Postop replacement is advocated by most surgeons, regardless of thyroid levels, to decrease TSH stimulation of any remaining thyroid tissue.

31. How is the parathyroid gland identified?

The glands are tan and oval-shaped, and they weigh approximately 35 mg. The adenomatous gland has been noted to sink in normal saline, as opposed to fat and normal parathyroids, which float. Ultimate identification should be pathologic.

32. Can anything be done if a parathyroid is accidentally removed?

If the surgeon suspects that parathyroid has been removed with the thyroid tissue, a small sample can be sent for pathologic verification. If parathyroid tissue is identified, the gland can be reimplanted in the sternocleidomastoid muscle or forearm. Calcium levels should be followed closely postoperatively.

33. How can a parathyroid carcinoma be detected?

Parathyroid carcinoma is often associated with hypercalcemia (usually >15 mg/dl), pathologic fractures, nephrocalcinosis, or a palpable neck mass.

34. How aggressive is a parathyroid carcinoma?

Metastasis at the time of presentation is unusual, although local visceral invasion is common. Parathyroid carcinoma commonly recurs, and death is often secondary to hypercalcemia with these recurrences. The 5 year survival is about 50%.

BIBLIOGRAPHY

1. Ackerstrom G, Malmaeus J, Bergstrom R: Surgical anatomy of human parathyroid glands. Surgery 95:14, 1984.
2. Belfiore A, Rosa GL, Giuffrida D, et al: The management of thyroid nodules. J Endocrinol Invest 18:155–158, 1995.
3. Boigon M, Moyer D: Solitary thyroid nodules: Separating benign from malignant conditions. Postgrad Med 98:73–80. 1995.
4. Clark OH: Thyroid and parathyroid. In Way LW (ed): Current Surgical Diagnosis and Treatment, 10th ed. Norwalk, CT, Appleton & Lange, 1994, pp 274–292.
5. Gharib H: Fine-needle aspiration biopsy of thyroid nodules: Advantages, limitations, and effect. Mayo Clin Proc 69:44–49, 1994.
6. Hung W: Nodular thyroid disease and thyroid carcinoma. Pediatr Ann 21:50–57, 1992.
7. Friedman M, Lore JM, Paloyan E, Skolnik EM: Difficult decisions in the management of thyroid carcinoma. Otolaryngol Clin North Am 19:463, 1986.
8. Friedman M, Toriumi DM: Malignant diseases of the thyroid gland. In Paparella MM, et al (eds): Otolaryngology, 3rd ed. Philadelphia, W.B. Saunders, 1991.
9. Hamburger JI: Diagnosis of thyroid nodules by fine-needle biopsy: use and abuse. J Clin Endocrinol Metab 79:335–339, 1994.
10. Kahn NF, Perzin KH: Follicular carcinoma of the thyroid. Pathol Ann 18(pt 1):221, 1983.
11. Lore JM: An Atlas of Head and Neck Surgery. Philadelphia, W.B. Saunders, 1988, pp 726–810.
12. Lore JM, Kim DJ, Elias S: Preservation of the laryngeal nerves during thyroidectomy lobectomy. Ann Otol Rhinol Laryngol 86:777, 1977.
13. Mazzaferri EL: Management of a solitary thyroid nodule. N Engl J Med 328:553–559, 1993.
14. Noyek A, Friedberg J: Thyroglossal duct and ectopic thyroid disorders. Otolaryngol Clin North Am 14:187, 1981.
15. Rifat SF, Ruffin MT: Management of thyroid nodules. Am Fam Physician 50:785–790, 1994.
16. Ross DS: Evaluation of the thyroid nodule. J Nucl Med 32:2181–2192, 1991.
17. Segal K, Fridental R, Lubin E, et al: Papillary carcinoma of the thyroid. Otolaryngol Head Neck Surg 113:356, 1996.
18. Sheppard MC, Franklyn JA: Management of the single thyroid nodule. Clin Endocrinol 37:398–401, 1992.
19. Sreenivas VI, Radakrishna SM: Thyroid and parathyroid glands. In Lee KJ (ed): Essential Otolaryngology: Head and Neck Surgery, 5th ed. New York: Elsevier Science Publ., 1991, pp 537–563.
20. Tennvall J, et al: Prognostic factors of papillary, follicular, and medullary carcinomas of the thyroid gland. Acta Radiol Oncol 23:(fasc 1), 1985.
21. Wanebo HJ, Andrews W, Kaiser DL: Thyroid cancer: Some basic considerations. Am J Surg 142:474, 1981.
22. Ward PH: The surgical treatment of thyroid cancer. The primary disease. Arch Otolaryngol Head Neck Surg 112:1204, 1986.
23. Wartofsky L: Diseases of the thyroid. In Isselbacher KJ, et al (eds): Harrison's Principles of Internal Medicine, 13th ed. New York, McGraw Hill, 1994, pp 1930–1953.
24. Wiersinga WM: Is repeated fine-needle aspiration cytology indicated in (benign) thyroid nodules? Eur J Endocrinol 132:661–662, 1995.
25. Woeber KA: Cost-effective evaluation of the patient with a thyroid nodule. Surg Clin North Am 75:357–336, 1995.

47. VASCULAR TUMORS OF THE HEAD AND NECK

Catherine Winslow, M.D.

1. What is the most common head and neck tumor in children?

Hemangiomas are the most common congenital disorder in humans and the most common head and neck tumor in children. Overall, these lesions occur more often in females than males (3:1).

2. What is a strawberry hemangioma?

Strawberry hemangiomas are lesions that are raised above the skin and blanch to touch. They comprise 90% of hemangiomas, and about 80% involute by age 5.

3. What is a port-wine stain?

A port-wine stain, also known as **nevus flammeus**, is a dark-purple, irregularly shaped patch that usually occurs on the face or neck. It grows with the skin and is not elevated. They also frequently involute, although laser surgery has had promising results.

4. Describe the Sturge-Weber syndrome.

This congenital syndrome, of unknown etiology, is characterized by venous angioma of the cerebral leptomeninges and port-wine nevi in a distribution of the first and second trigeminal branches. The mouth and nasal mucosa are frequently involved with angiomas. The occipital and posterior lobes may have calcifications, and patients may exhibit ophthalmologic problems. Seizure disorders are also associated.

5. A child develops a rapidly enlarging cavernous hemangioma on her face. Her parents beg you to remove the lesion surgically. What is the appropriate treatment?

Certain lesions may be associated with severe cosmetic or functional deformities. For example, the surgeon may consider removing lesions on the eyelid, lip, or nasal tip. Very large lesions may ulcerate, become infected, or hemorrhage. In general, however, most uncomplicated hemangiomas involute over several years with no treatment.

6. How do you evaluate a child with a facial hemangioma who presents with stridor?

Hemangiomas may occur in the larynx as well as on the skin. In adults, most laryngeal hemangiomas are supraglottic, while in children most are subglottic. About 50% of children with subglottic hemangiomas also have cutaneous lesions. Therefore, a child with a cutaneous hemangioma and stridor should be evaluated for a laryngeal tumor. These children frequently need tracheostomies to protect their airways.

7. What is a cystic hygroma?

A cystic hygroma, also known as a cystic lymphangioma, is a benign neck mass due to lymphatic dilation. Most often presenting by the second year of life, cystic hygromas are commonly painless, soft, and compressible. Although these lesions may be small and unrecognized for long periods of time, patients often present after the lesions have undergone rapid enlargement.

8. How is a cystic hygroma treated?

The child may suffer airway compromise if a cystic hygroma is associated with pharyngeal compression or laryngeal involvement. Therefore, a tracheotomy may be necessary. Complete surgical excision is the only successful treatment. Surgery may require a multi-staged procedure, and recurrence is uncommon if all visible disease is excised; a 50% recurrence is cited with partial excision alone.

9. A 13-year-old male presents with a history of unilateral nasal congestion, epistaxis, and anosmia. Physical exam reveals a large purplish mass in the symptomatic nasopharynx. What diagnosis should you consider?

Juvenile nasopharyngeal angiofibromas occur exclusively in males, often presenting with nasal congestion, epistaxis, or anosmia. These tumors are hormonally responsive and usually occur during adolescence. Although they are histologically benign, they may be locally invasive and have the potential to spread intracranially. A suspected nasopharyngeal angiofibroma can be evaluated with carotid arteriography, CT, and biopsy. Treatment involves surgery, often with preoperative embolization. Radiation therapy is reserved for unresectable cases. These vascular tumors are associated with a high recurrence rate.

10. An adolescent female is diagnosed with juvenile nasopharyngeal angiofibroma. How should you proceed?

This diagnosis is unlikely. Although nasopharyngeal angiofibroma is the most common vascular lesion in the nasal cavity, it occurs only in males. If there is doubt, chromosomal analysis may be pursued.

11. How are carotid body tumors diagnosed?

A firm, nontender, slow-growing pulsatile mass that moves horizontally but not vertically may be identified on physical exam. A bruit may be auscultated over it. Angiography will reveal a widening of the bifurcation of the internal and external carotids, a finding known as the **lyre sign**.

12. Is the carotid body tumor a true vascular tumor?

No. A carotid body tumor is actually a tumor of the neural crest cells that comprise the carotid body, the neurovascular structure located at the bifurcation of the carotid. This body is sensitive to pH, PO_2, and PCO_2 changes.

13. Are carotid body tumors malignant?

About 10% are malignant. Remembering the **rule of 10's** will help in recalling that 10% of these lesions are familial, 10% are malignant, 10% are multicentric, and up to 10% secrete catecholamines.

14. Where else do carotid body tumors occur?

Carotid body tumors, also known as *chemodectomas*, usually occur in the head and neck. They may also be found in the mediastinum, femoral areas, and retroperitoneal areas. These tumors arise from parasympathetic nerves in the adventitia of vessels.

15. A patient presents with hearing loss, bloody discharge, and pain in one ear. Otoscopic exam reveals a bluish discoloration of the tympanic membrane. What diagnosis should you consider?

The glomus jugular complex is a type of paraganglioma found in the jugular bulb and temporal bone. They are named by location—**glomus jugulare** for tumors of the jugular ganglion of CN IX and **glomus tympanicum** for those of the tympanic plexus of CN IX. These can present with otic complaints of pain, discharge, tinnitus, hearing loss, and infection. Of course, a high-riding jugular bulb, a normal variant, may also appear as a discoloration of the eardrum.

16. What is the next diagnostic step in glomus tympanicum?

Due to the risk of bleeding, a biopsy should never be performed on these lesions. If a CT scan of the region with fine cuts or digital subtraction angiography is consistent with the lesion, angiography or magnetic resonance angiography should be performed. Due to the association with catecholamine secretion, blood pressure should be documented and consideration should be given to checking urinary catecholamines, vanillylmandelic acid, and metanephrines.

BIBLIOGRAPHY

1. Adams GL, Latchaw RE: Carotid body tumor. In Gates GA (ed): Current Therapy in Otolaryngology–Head and Neck Surgery, 5th ed. St. Louis, Mosby, 1994.
2. Garfinkle TJ, Handler SD: Hemangiomas of the head and neck in children—A guide to management. J Otolaryngol. 9:439–450, 1980.
3. Kaplan MJ, Deschler DG: Angiofibroma. In Gates GA (ed): Current Therapy in Otolaryngology–Head and Neck Surgery, 5th ed. St. Louis, Mosby, 1994.\
4. Karmody CS, Fortson JK, Calcaterra VE: Lymphangiomas of the head and neck in adults. Otolaryngol Head Neck Surg 90:283, 1982.
5. Lee KJ, Anand V: Carotid body tumor, hemangioma, lymphangioma, melanoma, cysts, and tumors of the jaw. In Lee KJ (ed): Essential Otolaryngology, 5th ed. East Norwalk, CT, Appleton & Lange, 1991.
6. Lore JM: An Atlas of Head and Neck Surgery. Philadelphia, W. B. Saunders, 1988, pp 874–875.
7. Myer CM: Congenital neck masses. In Paparella MM, Shumrick DA, Gluckman JL, Meyerhoff WL (eds): Otolaryngology, 3rd ed. Philadelphia, W. B. Saunders, 1991.
8. Nissen AJ: Laser applications in otologic surgery. Ear Nose Throat J 74:477–482, 1995.
9. Ward PH, et al: Diagnosis and treatment of carotid body tumors. Ann Otol Rhinol Laryngol 87:614, 1978.
10. Yanagisawa E , Hausfeld J: The larynx. In Lee KJ (ed): Essential Otolaryngology, 5th ed. East Norwalk, CT, Appleton & Lange, 1991.

48. CUTANEOUS NEOPLASMS OF THE HEAD AND NECK

Tyler M. Lewark, M.D.

1. Describe the appearance of seborrheic keratoses. Are these lesions concerning?

Seborrheic keratoses are very common skin lesions. They usually present as well-defined, elevated plaques that have a "stuck-on" appearance. Waxy, soft scale may be present. Seborrheic keratoses have no malignant potential and are unrelated to sun exposure. Treatment is not necessary but may be requested for cosmetic reasons. Bothersome lesions may be effectively removed with cryosurgery.

2. What are actinic keratoses? How are they diagnosed?

Actinic keratoses are scaly or warty growths that appear on sun-exposed regions of skin. They are well-circumscribed patches or papules that are usually skin-colored or brown. When inflamed, they are often pink or red. Diagnosis requires careful observation with adequate illumination and palpation. The most distinctive feature on clinical exam is their sandpaper-like scale. The amount of scale varies considerably and may be detectable only with palpation. Lesions may also appear markedly hyperkeratotic with very thick scale. Definitive diagnosis requires biopsy with histopathologic examination.

3. Who is most at risk for actinic keratoses?

Actinic keratoses occur most commonly on fair or light-skinned individuals who tan poorly and sunburn easily. Persons of Northern European descent who have blonde or red hair, blue eyes, and scant pigmentation are especially at risk. Deeply tanning persons and those with black or brown skin usually develop these lesions only with extreme, long-standing sun exposure. Actinic keratoses are caused by exposure to ultraviolet (UV) light, and it is clear that the intensity and duration of sun exposure are important to their development. However, the mechanism that leads to this disordered regulation of growth is unknown.

4. How are actinic keratoses treated?

Actinic keratoses are thought to be premalignant because of their histologic cellular feature of epidermal dysplasia. When these lesions undergo malignant degeneration, they usually become squamous cell carcinoma. Because it is difficult to predict which lesions will develop into malignancies, many clinicians will perform a biopsy or treat prophylactically. Effective treatments include superficial shave excision, cryotherapy, trichloroacetic acid peel, and topical 5-fluorouracil.

5. What is the most common skin malignancy?

Basal cell carcinomas (BCCs) are the most common, accounting for > 75% of nonmelanoma skin cancers. In addition, they are by far the most common malignant tumor of any organ. More than 25% of diagnosed cancers in the United States each year are BCCs.

6. What are the risk factors for BCC?

Light skin and the duration of UV radiation exposure are the major risk factors for BCC. However, because the distribution of BCCs does not correlate directly with degree of sun exposure, the relationship between BCC and UV radiation is unclear. Additional risk factors include ionizing radiation, scars, and arsenic exposure. Immunosuppressed patients have a modestly increased risk for developing BCCs, which may be more aggressive in this population.

7. What is the basal cell nevus syndrome?

Also called Gorlin's syndrome, basal cell nevus syndrome is an autosomally dominant genetic condition that predisposes the affected individual to multiple BCCs, cysts of the jaw, and rib abnormalities. Affected patients usually present with multiple BCCs between puberty and their mid-30s. The number of lesions varies from patient to patient and ranges from a few to thousands. They can become locally invasive and cause significant destruction. Complete cutaneous examinations every 3–6 months are required for early diagnosis and treatment.

8. Describe the clinical types of BCC.

Clinical Types of Basal Cell Carcinomas

Nodulo-ulcerative	Most common type. Begins as small, pearly telangiectatic papule and slowly enlarges. Forms central ulcer surrounded by rolled, pearly border.
Pigmented	Similar to noculo-ulcerative, but with brown pigmentation.
Superficial	Occurs predominantly on trunk. Appears as slightly indurated, erythematous patches with scaling. May resemble patches of eczema, psoriasis, tinea, or excoriation.
Morpheaform	Occurs almost exclusively on face; often mistaken as scar. Flat or slightly depressed, indurated, yellowish plaques without defined borders.
Fibroepitheliomas	Raised, moderately firm, slightly pedunculated or sessile lesions. Mildly erythematous with smooth skin surface.

9. Are BCCs aggressive? What factors suggest that a BCC will be aggressive?

In general, BCCs are locally invasive, slowly spreading, and have very low metastatic potential. **Morpheaform tumors** are undoubtedly the most aggressive type and also have the highest recurrence rate. **Local nerve involvement** by neurophilic spread has been associated with increased aggressiveness. This occurs in approximately 1% of BCCs, most of which are of the infiltrating type. **Tumor location** also seems to influence BCC behavior, with central face tumors tending to be more aggressive and having an increased recurrence rate. Greater recurrence risk has also been seen with **large tumors**.

10. Why is Mohs' micrographic surgery performed for BCC?

Originally devised by Frederick Mohs in the 1930s, this technique significantly decreases the recurrence rate of certain skin cancers. Completeness of excision is assessed with intraoperative histopathologic tumor examination. The usual approach today involves freezing a surgical speci-men, cutting horizontal sections from its base, and examining these sections for residual tumor. Mohs' surgery is most effective for tumors that invade by direct extension from the primary site. Accordingly, BCCs are excellent candidates. The overall 5-year recurrence rate for primary BCCs is estimated at 1%. This technique should be considered when a BCC is recurrent or possesses a diameter > 2 cm, aggressive histology, or ill-defined border. It also should be considered when a BCC of the head and neck region occurs in a high-risk location, such as the nose, periorbital area, ears, or lips.

11. Are additional treatments available for BCC?

Effective management of primary BCC usually involves early diagnosis and surgery. Surgical excision, curettage with electrodesiccation, and cryosurgery have 5-year recurrence rates of 10.1%, 7.7%, and 7.5%, respectively. Radiation therapy also is effective in treating BCC, with a 5-year recurrence rate of approximately 9%. Less aggressive treatment with topical 5-flu-orouracil has received recent support. In addition to primary tumor treatment, adequate follow-up is important for early diagnosis of recurrence. Because they are at risk for developing a second lesion, patients should be taught to recognize the early features of skin cancer.

12. How prevalent are cutaneous squamous cell carcinomas of the head and neck?

Cutaneous squamous cell carcinoma (CSCC) is the second most common skin cancer. It ac-counts for 20% of all cutaneous malignancies, over 95% of which arise on the head and neck. The diagnosis is typically made during the seventh decade of life, and males are more likely to develop these lesions.

13. What factors predispose to CSCC development?

The etiology of CSCC seems to involve an interplay between intrinsic and extrinsic factors. The most commonly implicated extrinsic factor is long-term unprotected exposure to **ultraviolet light**. The wavelengths of light responsible for skin erythema and sunburn are associated with car-cinogenesis. **Chemical exposure** is another extrinsic factor implicated in CSCC development. Inciting chemicals include arsenic, soot, coal tar, paraffin oil, petroleum oil, and asphalt. **Immunosuppression** appears to be an important intrinsic factor for CSCC development, with the patient's ability to respond immunologically to UV radiation perhaps being one of the most im-portant carcinogenic mechanisms. **Age** is clearly a risk factor for CSCC development. However, some argue that aging may be a manifestation of altered immunologic function and therefore not an independent etiologic factor. A high incidence of **human papillomavirus** presence has been detected in certain cases and may be another extrinsic factor in CSCC carcinogenesis. This finding also may be related to immune system dysfunction and not an independent etiologic factor.

14. How often is CSCC cured?

The 5-year cure rate for CSCC ranges from 75–90%. Of the approximately 5,000 deaths that occur yearly from nonmelanoma skin cancer, 75% are due to head and neck CSCCs. The incidence of metastasis varies between 0.3–3.7%, and the 5-year survival rate for these patients is only 25%.

15. What factors affect recurrence and prognosis?

Factors affecting recurrence and prognosis of CSCCs include anatomic site, etiology, histo-logic features, tumor size, depth of invasion, and the patient's immune status. Lesions arising from the external ear, lip, and temple are more likely to recur. Increased recurrence is also seen when lesions arise from areas previously exposed to gamma radiation or from chronic lesions in-cluding wounds, burn scars, and ulcers. Survival and cure rate decrease as lesion size increases, especially when lesions are > 2–3 cm in diameter. Invasion below the coiled region of the sweat glands or penetration into muscle, cartilage, bone, parotid gland, or perineurium increases the re-currence risk. Patients with lesions containing a larger percentage of well-differentiated cells have increased survival. Immune factors also affect prognosis. The amount of immune dysfunction varies directly with metastasis incidence. In addition, this population has a higher incidence of multiple primaries and a poorer prognosis.

16. What is Bowen's disease?

Bowen's disease is an intraepidermal squamous cell carcinoma that usually spreads along the epidermal plane. It may invade the dermis and metastasize in 20–25% of cases. On exam, it is a slowly growing, reddened, scaly patch that may become nodular with invasion. These lesions usually occur on sun-exposed areas, although they may occur on nonexposed areas in blacks. When involving the oral mucosa, it appears as a velvety, reddened macule that becomes elevated and may ulcerate. Approximately 30% of these patients develop invasive squamous cell carcinoma.

17. A patient in the clinic has a 3-cm lesion over his right temple, which he states has tripled in size over the last month. You suspect CSCC. Are you likely to be correct?

Although this lesion may be CSCC, it is most likely a **keratoacanthoma**. This lesion is often difficult to distinguish from CSCC, both clinically and histopathologically. Unlike CSCCs, keratoacanthomas rapidly enlarge, reaching their full size in about 2 months. They are usually smooth, firm, dome-shaped, verrucous nodules filled centrally with keratin craters. Involution usually occurs within 2–6 months and may leave a depressed scar. Large central face or lip lesions may be aggressive. Deep tissue invasion has been reported, and metastases may be seen in cases with multiple lesions refractory to treatment.

18. How are BCC and CSCC staged? Graded?

The American Joint Committee on Cancer has developed a classification system for skin carcinoma that applies to both clinical and pathologic staging. Bowen's disease is included and should be classified as Tis.

Clinical and Pathologic TNM Classification and Histopathologic Grading for Squamous Cell Carcinoma and Basal Cell Carcinoma*

STAGE	DEFINITION
Primary tumor (T)	
TX	Primary tumor cannot be assessed
T0	No evidence of primary tumor
Tis	Carcinoma in situ
T1	Tumor ≤ 2 cm in greatest dimension
T2	Tumor 2–5 cm in greatest dimension
T3	Tumor > 5 cm in greatest dimension
T4	Tumor invades deep extradermal structures (cartilage, skeletal muscle, bone)
Regional lymph nodes (N)	
NX	Regional lymph nodes cannot be assessed
N0	No regional node metastasis
N1	Regional lymph node metastasis
Distant metastasis (M)	
MX	Presence of distant metastasis cannot be assessed
M0	No distant metastasis
M1	Distant metastasis
Histopathologic grade (G)	
GX	Grade cannot be assessed
G1	Well differentiated
G2	Moderately well differentiated
G3	Poorly differentiated
G4	Undifferentiated

* Excluding eyelid, vulva, and penis.
From Haydon RC: Cutaneous squamous carcinoma and related lesions. Otolaryngol Clin North Am 26:67, 1993, with permission.

TNM Stage Grouping

Stage 0	Tis	N0	M0
Stage I	T1	N0	M0
Stage II	T2	N0	M0
	T3	N0	M0
Stage III	T4	N0	M0
	Any T	N1	M0
Stage IV	Any T	Any N	M1

19. Describe the clinical features of xeroderma pigmentosum.

Xeroderma pigmentosum is an autosomal recessive disorder in which patients have a defect in the DNA-repair system responsible for detecting and excising damaged DNA segments. The most common cause of DNA damage is UV radiation. The initial clinical manifestation is an abnormal response to sunlight, with patients having a delayed-onset erythema and prolonged response after sun exposure. Early freckling and pigment abnormalities also occur. The incidence of skin malignancies in this population is very high. The median age that patients present with a skin cancer is 8 years. Malignancies include BCC and CSCC, and the overwhelming majority occur on the face, head, or neck. Melanomas have been estimated to occur 2,000 times more often than expected in the general population.

20. What are the risk factors for malignant melanoma of the head and neck?
- Prolonged sunlight exposure, particularly when it occurs during early childhood and leads to sunburning
- Preexisting pigmented lesions—About 70% of melanomas arising on the head and neck develop from a preexisting mole.
- Race and skin complexion—Fair-skinned, poorly tanning individuals with red or blonde hair are more likely to develop melanoma.
- Age—Most melanomas are diagnosed in the 5th and 6th decades of life.
- Family history
- Immunosuppression

21. What physical findings of a pigmented lesion suggest malignant melanoma?

The distinction between melanoma and nonmelanoma pigmented lesions can be difficult.

Characteristics of Pigmented Lesions Suggestive of Melanoma

1. Mild itch or slightly altered skin sensation
2. Maximum diameter > 1 cm
3. Increasing size
4. Irregular lateral margin
5. Multiple shades of brown-black, red, and blue (color variation)
6. Inflammation
7. Bleeding or crusting within the lesion

Adapted from MacKie RM: Skin Cancer. Chicago, Year Book, 1989, p 130, with permission.

22. What preventive measures should be taken for individuals who are at risk?

Patients with multiple pigmented nevi should be taught to recognize suspicious lesions and encouraged to see a physician when one is discovered. At risk individuals should be followed by a dermatologist.

23. Describe the clinical appearance of the subdivisions of malignant melanoma.

Clinical Types of Malignant Melanoma

Lentigo maligna	Occur predominantly on sun-exposed skin in older persons, with 90% on head and neck.
	Appear initially as macular areas with increased pigmentation (neoplastic melanocytes confined to epidermis).
	Lesions expand laterally across skin and may regress centrally.
	Invasive phase shows densely pigmented, raised nodules within preexisting macular area (melanoma cell present in dermis).
Superficial spreading melanoma	40–50% of melanomas in United States.
	Usually occur on calf or back, less common on head and neck.
	Present as irregulary shaped pigmented areas, usually > 1 cm in diameter.
	Border and pigmentation tend to be irregular.
	Central nodules may develop over time.
Nodular malignant melanoma	Occur predominantly on trunk, but may occur on head and neck.
	Blue-black nodule with normal surrounding skin.
Acral lentiginous melanoma	Occur on hand and soles of feet, usually not found on head and neck.
	Raised, densely black nodular lesions within a pigmented macular area.

24. In addition to appearance, what physical features are important in assessing a possible malignant melanoma?

Thorough examination of the neck with careful palpation for **enlarged lymph nodes** is essential when assessing melanotic lymphatic metastasis. In addition, the preauricular, retroauricular, suboccipital, and buccinator regions should be evaluated when the location of a pigmented lesion suggests lymph node involvement.

25. How is the diagnosis made?

Diagnosis of melanoma is made primarily on histopathologic examination of **biopsy tissue**. Whenever possible, excisional biopsy should be performed so that the entire lesion may be examined microscopically. Shave biopsy with curettage should not be performed on any lesion suspicious for melanoma. In cases when the lesion is large or excisional biopsy is impractical, a full-thickness elliptical incision or punch biopsy provides adequate sample for diagnosis.

26. What is Breslow thickness? What are Clark levels?

Tumor thickness in malignant melanoma is often reported according to **Breslow thickness**. This measurement is obtained by selecting the thickest portion of a given tumor and cutting a section. After hematoxylin-eosin staining, the distance between the granular layer of the epidermis and the deepest identified tumor cell is measured. Reported in millimeters, this value is inversely proportional to survival.

Tumor invasion is indicated by **Clark levels**, which relate the most deeply invading tumor cells to surrounding structures. Like Breslow thickness, these levels also have prognostic significance.

Level 1	Intraepidermal or in situ melanoma
2	Invasion of papillary dermis
3	Invasion of papillary dermis to reticular dermis
4	Invasion of reticular dermis
5	Invasion of fat

27. How are malignant melanomas staged?

Staging of malignant melanoma uses lesion thickness to determine the tumor stage.

Staging of Melanomas

STAGE	DEFINITION
Primary tumor (T)	
TX	Primary tumor cannot be assessed
T0	No evidence of primary tumor
Tis	Carcinoma in situ
T1	Tumor ≤ 2 cm in greatest dimension
T2	Tumor 2–5 cm in greatest dimension
T3	Tumor > 5 cm in greatest dimension
T4	Tumor invades deep extradermal structures (cartilage, skeletal muscle, bone)
Regional lymph nodes (N)	
NX	Regional lymph nodes cannot be assessed
N0	No regional node metastasis
N1	Regional lymph node metastasis
Distant metastasis (M)	
MX	Presence of distant metastasis cannot be assessed
M0	No distant metastasis
M1	Distant metastasis
Histopathologic grade (G)	
GX	Grade cannot be assessed
G1	Well differentiated
G2	Moderately well differentiated
G3	Poorly differentiated
G4	Undifferentiated

From Medina JE: Malignant melanoma of the head and neck. Otolaryngol Clin North Am 26:76, 1993, with permission.

28. How is malignant melanoma treated?

The primary tumor is treated by **surgical removal**. The amount of normal skin margin resected around a malignant melanoma is determined by tumor thickness. A 1-cm margin of normal skin around the resected lesion is appropriate for tumors < 2 mm thick. Thicker melanomas require wider margins, but no more than 3 cm is necessary. Adequate margins are often difficult to obtain in the head and neck region because of the proximity of important structures, such as the eye.

Primary treatment is followed by evaluation and treatment of possible **regional and distant metastasis**. Patients with localized melanoma are at risk for regional lymphatic metastases, and elective neck dissection is advocated by many clinicians. Patients with palpable lymph nodes should undergo regional lymph node dissection. Involved nodes and those at risk for containing metastases should be removed. When multiple nodes are involved, a radical neck dissection is frequently necessary. It is not clear at present whether adjuvant radiation or systemic therapy is helpful, but initial data indicate that radiation may increase survival for patients with proven neck metastases.

29. What is the familial dysplastic nevus syndrome?

The familial dysplastic nevus syndrome is an autosomal dominant heritable disorder with variable penetrance and a wide range of expressivity. Affected individuals have a large number of pigmented nevi, many of which are dysplastic. Persons who have dysplastic nevi, either familial or nonfamilial, are predisposed to developing malignant melanoma. A patient with familial dysplastic nevi is approximately 400 times more likely to develop melanoma. Individuals with dysplastic nevi with no family history are 6–7 times more likely to develop melanoma.

Dysplastic nevi tend to appear on sun-exposed areas and are commonly found on the head and neck. When compared to benign nevi, these lesions are larger and more numerous with more variegated color, irregular borders, and papular surface. Affected individuals require careful monitoring every 3–6 months. Lesion removal with histopathologic examination should be performed when clinical features are consistent with malignant transformation.

30. How prevalent are neoplasms of the adnexa?

The adnexa are the skin appendages and include eccrine and apocrine sweat glands, hair follicles, and sebaceous glands. Malignancies of these structures are very different from those of the epidermis, and most are highly malignant. They account for approximately 0.005% of all skin lesions.

31. Which are more common—sarcomas of the skin or deeper tissue sarcomas?

Sarcomas of the dermis and subcutaneous tissue are much less common than deeper tissue sarcomas. They comprise approximately 0.003% of soft tissue sarcomas. Sarcomas of the skin are usually histologically identical to deeper tumors and thus are a diagnostic challenge. Sarcomas confined to superficial structures, particularly the dermis, have a better prognosis than deeper tissue sarcomas.

32. Does Kaposi's sarcoma often occur on the head and neck?

Kaposi's sarcoma (KS), a superficial skin sarcoma, has had a dramatic increase in the number of cases in young AIDS patients, especially homosexual men. It is the initial manifestation of AIDS in 18–30% of patients. The classic KS type usually involves the lower extremities and affects elderly men of Mediterranean or Jewish descent. AIDS-associated KS differs in appearance and distribution. Lesions occur commonly on the head and neck, as well as on the arms and trunk and in all areas of the upper aerodigestive tract. Early lesions can be small and subtle, often resembling a simple bruise. These pink macules have a surrounding white halo and progress within days to indurated papules with a yellow-green halo. They usually cease growing when they attain a size of 8–15 mm and turn gray with maturation. KS lesions are highly radiosensitive, and single-agent chemotherapy regimens have been effective in treating the disease.

CONTROVERSIES

33. Should elective lymph node dissection (ELND) be performed with localized malignant melanoma?

The role of ELND is probably the most controversial aspect of malignant melanoma treatment. Proponents cite studies that demonstrate effective control of regional metastases and more accurate staging with ELND. It removes a possible source of tumor burden and allows early treatment of metastatic disease. Opponents argue that the patient undergoes unnecessary morbidity from ELND.

Tumor thickness is the measure most often used to determine if ELND is indicated. Most investigators argue that it should not be performed when the lesion is < 1.0 mm thick, but it has little benefit when the lesion is > 4.0 mm thick. Several studies indicate that ELND confers survival advantage for intermediate-thickness melanomas. However, other trials support the concept that positive lymph nodes are a systemic disease manifestation and show that survival is the same for patients who wait until a therapeutic lymph node dissection is necessary.

Selective lymphadenectomy following **sentinel node identification** has received recent support. The sentinel node is the first node into which the primary lesion drains. Theoretically, if this node is negative, the remaining nodes should also be negative. The procedure can be performed as an outpatient, using local anesthesia and small incisions. Proponents of the procedure argue that it can be used as a prognostic indicator, identifying the subgroup of melanoma patients who would be candidates for complete ELND and therefore reducing unnecessary morbidity.

34. How is distant metastatic melanoma treated?

Complete resection of a single distant metastatic melanoma can usually be achieved in two-thirds of cases. Complete resection of melanoma metastatic to multiple sites can be achieved in about one-third of cases, but 5-year survival in this group is < 10%. Soft tissue and extraregional nodal lesions are resectable in 70% of cases. Pulmonary, extrahepatic abdominal, and osseous lesions can be resected in only 40% of cases.

35. Are mucosal melanomas different from cutaneous melanomas?
Mucosal melanomas behave differently than cutaneous melanomas. They are more aggressive and usually are associated with a grave prognosis. Lymph node metastases from a mucosal primary are infrequent. They occur more commonly on Orientals, primarily the Japanese, than on whites. The overall incidence of head and neck mucosal melanomas is 2%.

BIBLIOGRAPHY

1. Godellas CV, Berman CG, Lyman G, et al: The identification and mapping of melanoma regional nodal metastases: Minimally invasive surgery for the diagnosis of nodal metastases. Am Surg 61(2):97–101, 1995.
2. Harris MN, Shapiro RL, Roses DF: Malignant melanoma: Primary surgical management (excision and node dissection) based on pathology and staging. Cancer 75(2 suppl):715–725, 1995.
3. Haydon RC: Cutaneous squamous carcinoma and related lesions. Otolaryngol Clin North Am 26:57–71, 1993.
4. MacKie RM: Skin Cancer. Chicago, Year Book, 1989.
5. Marenda SA, Otto RA: Adnexal carcinomas of the skin. Otolaryngol Clin North Am 26:87–115, 1993.
6. Marks VJ: Actinic keratosis. Otolaryngol Clin North Am 26:23–35, 1993.
7. Medina JE: Malignant melanoma of the head and neck. Otolaryngol Clin North Am 26:73–85, 1993.
8. Nguyen AV, Whitaker DC, Frodel J: Differentiation of basal cell carcinoma. Otolaryngol Clin North Am 26:37–55, 1993.
9. Shumrick KA, Coldiron B: Genetic syndromes associated with skin cancer. Otolaryngol Clin North Am 26:117–137, 1993.

49. RADIATION THERAPY FOR HEAD AND NECK CANCER

Rachel Rabinovitch, M.D.

1. What is radiation therapy (RT)?
RT involves the use of various forms of ionizing radiation to treat benign and malignant tumors. This radiation commonly includes photons (deeply penetrating radiation) and/or electrons (superficial radiation). These forms of radiation can be delivered in one of two ways. **External-beam radiation therapy** (EBRT) is the delivery of radiation from a source external to the patient (i.e., a linear accelerator or cobalt machine) and directed at a target tissue within the patient. **Brachytherapy** involves implantation of permanent or temporary radioactive sources into the tumor or tissues at risk.

2. How does RT work?
Ionizing radiation causes damage to the DNA of the target cells through a complicated series of atomic interactions. Most of the nuclear damage is due to the interaction of DNA with free radicals, which are formed by the interaction of the radiation with water molecules. Normal cells in the body are better able to repair DNA damage, whereas tumor cells are less efficient at DNA repair. Following RT, damaged cells undergo mitotic cell death.

3. What are the advantages of RT in comparison with surgery?
RT, like surgery, is a local therapy. It is delivered as an outpatient treatment, usually allowing the patient to continue daily activities without interruption. The overall medical condition of the

patient does not inhibit the ability to receive RT, as there is no concern with the risks of anesthesia, bleeding, etc. RT, when delivered as the primary treatment modality, is less physically deforming than surgery since it does not result in large scars or organ resection. Furthermore, it allows continued organ preservation and therefore function, resulting in improved quality of life. This advantage is most significant in the treatment of tumors of the tongue and larynx, where RT can preserve normal speech, swallowing, and eating.

4. Are there disadvantages of RT in comparison with surgery?

On the downside, RT is generally delivered on a daily basis over 6–8 weeks, requiring a longer time commitment than surgery. This duration can be problematic for noncompliant patients or those who live long distances from a radiation oncology facility. Tumor control depends on the site of the tumor and the maximum tolerable doses. Thus, large tumors or those situated near sensitive structures (i.e., mandible, spinal cord, visual apparatus) may be difficult to control with RT.

5. Will RT make the patient radioactive?

Patients undergoing EBRT are not radioactive. However, with certain brachytherapy procedures, they are if radioactive sources of sufficient energy are implanted into them. This therapy generally implies use of a temporary implant, and patients are then admitted to single-bed rooms for the duration of the brachytherapy treatment. Once the implant is removed, the patient is no longer radioactive. \

6. What tumors can be definitively treated with radiation as the sole treatment modality?

Nearly all head and neck cancers that are T1–T2 (< 4 cm) and N0–N1 (single ipsilateral lymph nodes < 3 cm) are candidates for definitive RT. These include primary tumors of the tongue, tonsil, larynx, and hypopharynx. Exceptions include cancers of the nasopharynx, where EBRT is the standard treatment regardless of T or N stage. Tumors of the salivary glands and floor of the mouth are generally managed primarily with surgery, even if diagnosed at an early stage.

7. What are the standard indications for adjuvant RT following surgical resection of a head and neck tumor?

- Primary tumor > 4 cm, invading bone or beyond the primary site (T3–T4)
- Multiple positive neck nodes
- Extracapsular nodal extension
- Positive resection margins of either the primary tumor or neck disease
- Recurrent disease

8. Who cannot be treated with RT?

Patients with collagen-vascular diseases, pregnant women, and those who have previously received RT to the head and neck region.

9. What are the common acute side effects of RT?

During treatment, erythema, dryness, pruritus, and mild desquamation of the skin within the treatment field are typically encountered. Hoarseness, serous otitis, mucositis, odynophagia, and xerostomia are also common. The acute side effects of RT usually become manifest by the second to third week of treatment and resolve within 4–6 weeks after completing RT. The main exception is xerostomia, which is permanent if the major salivary glands are included within the treatment field.

10. How are these side effects managed during the course of treatment?

Lanolin-based skin care products or other moisturizers minimize and soothe the dermal symptoms. Mild odynophagia is lessened with anesthetic mouth rinses. Oral analgesics (including narcotics) are indicated for more severe mucositis. On occasion, gastric tube feeding is required to maintain adequate nutrition.

11. Are there potential long-term complications of RT?

Complications related to RT are unusual (with an incidence of < 10%) but are more difficult to manage when they occur. The likelihood of a given patient developing long-term complications depends on the total dose of radiation delivered, the time frame over which it was given, and the anatomic sites included within the radiation portal. In general, the risk increases with increasing doses delivered over shorter time periods to greater volumes of tissue. Complications include xerostomia, skin changes, osteonecrosis, bone exposure, laryngeal edema, and induction of secondary cancers. The incidence of osteonecrosis can be greatly diminished by meticulous dental care both before, during, and after RT.

12. What is the most common long-term side effect of RT?

Xerostomia is the most common and bothersome long-term side effect and results whenever both major salivary glands are treated to doses > 2000 cGy. Intake of large amounts of liquids between and during meals and use of artificial saliva preparations are the most common means of managing the problem. Use of pilocarpine can improve salivary function in irradiated patients.

13. What long-term skin changes are associated with RT?

Male patients may experience permanent facial alopecia in regions treated to > 6,000 cGy. Other skin changes may include mild atrophy, pigmentation changes, and submental edema.

14. What is the standard treatment for a T1N0M0 squamous cell carcinoma of the glottic larynx?

EBRT delivered to the larynx, to a total dose of 6,600 cGy in 6.5 weeks, results in a cure rate of >90%. Since the radiation is delivered to the larynx only, and not to regional lymph nodes, xerostomia does not result.

15. Is a total laryngectomy necessary in the curative management of advanced larynx cancer?

No. The Veterans Affairs Laryngeal Cancer Study Group performed a randomized trial involving 332 patients with stage III or IV larynx cancer in which patients received either total laryngectomy followed by RT or 3 cycles of chemotherapy (cisplatin and 5-fluorouracil) followed by RT. The results from this study demonstrated no difference in the survival rate between the two groups. Sixty-four percent of the patients in the chemo-radiation arm were able to preserve laryngeal function. This trial established the curative role of chemo-radiation as an organ-preserving treatment for advanced cancers of the larynx. All patients being evaluated for advanced laryngeal cancer should be offered both treatment options.

16. When planning treatment for a patient, what factors should be taken into consideration?

It is critical to manage both the primary tumor and regional lymph nodes with one treatment modality whenever possible. This approach minimizes the toxicity and complications of combined modality therapy. Therefore, if the primary tumor is to be managed with surgical resection, then the neck(s), if at risk, should be treated with a neck dissection. Postoperative RT is added only if indicated. Likewise, when the primary is to be treated with RT alone, the neck(s) should be managed with EBRT, followed by a neck dissection if necessary. If both surgery and RT are clearly necessary from the outset (i.e., large and/or multiple neck nodes), the treatment modality addressing both the primary and neck(s) should be delivered first. It is unsound oncologic practice first to manage the neck with surgery, leaving the primary tumor untreated. Any wound complication would further delay initiation of definitive RT and/or potentially result in aberrant contralateral nodal drainage.

17. Explain the general dosing guidelines for treatment of the neck with RT.

A clinically negative **undissected** neck will be controlled with a probability of > 90% when a total dose of 5,400 cGy is delivered in daily fractions of 180 cGy. **Postoperative** doses are higher, due to the presence of fibrous scarring within the operative bed, resulting in decreased blood flow to the tissues at risk which renders them less sensitive to EBRT. A minimum of 5,760 cGy is therefore indicated, increasing to a total dose of 6,300 cGy whenever the neck dissection demonstrates extracapsular extension or other high-risk features. These dose recommendations are the result of a randomized trial from the M.D. Anderson Cancer Center that demonstrated increased failures with postoperative doses of 5,400 cGy.

18. What are the dental effects of RT?
Saliva normally bathes and cleanses the teeth, providing a partial barrier to the formation of dental caries. Caries, in the nonirradiated mouth, develops at the tips of teeth where saliva is least abundant. Radiation caries, however, occurs at the bases of teeth, where xerostomia has caused a changed pH environment and less inherent salivary cleansing.

19. What is the role of pre-RT dental evaluation?
Radiation-induced caries can be completely avoided by the combination of routine oral hygiene with daily fluoride treatments. As part of the pre-RT evaluation, all patients are fitted by their dentist for custom fluoride trays. Dental evaluation before treatment initiation also determines if any oral extractions are indicated and ensures that they are managed with adequate time for healing before RT begins. Healing of the gingiva and mandible is impaired following standard doses of RT, and dental extractions or invasive surgical procedures following RT predispose patients to chronic and painful bone exposure and tissue necrosis.

BIBLIOGRAPHY
1. Cancer Facts and Figures—1995. Atlanta, American Cancer Society, 1995.
2. Department of Veterans Affairs Laryngeal Cancer Study Group: Induction chemotherapy plus radiation compared with surgery plus radiation in patients with advanced laryngeal cancer. N Engl J Med 324:1685–1690, 1985.
3. Johnson JT, Ferretti GA, Nethery WJ, et al: Oral pilocarpine for post-irradiation xerostomia in patients with head and neck cancer. N Engl J Med 329:390–395, 1993.
4. LeVeque FG, Montgomery M, Potter D, et al: A multicenter, randomized, double-blind, placebo-controlled, dose-titration study of oral pilocarpine for treatment of radiation-induced xerostomia in head and neck cancer patients. J Clin Oncol 11:1124–1131, 1993.
5. Peters LJ, Goepfert H, Ang KK, et al: Evaluation of the dose for postoperative radiation therapy of head and neck cancer: First report of a prospective randomized trial. Int J Radiat Oncol Biol Phys 26:3–11, 1993.

50. CHEMOTHERAPY FOR HEAD AND NECK CANCER
Allen L. Cohn, M.D.

1. In what situations is chemotherapy given for head and neck cancer?
Neoadjuvant chemotherapy
Adjuvant chemotherapy
Chemotherapy for recurrent or metastatic disease
In combination with radiation therapy
Chemo-prevention

2. What is neoadjuvant chemotherapy?
Neoadjuvant chemotherapy, also referred to as induction chemotherapy, is chemotherapy used prior to a definitive treatment modality such as surgery or radiation therapy. Most commonly, it is used prior to surgical intervention.

3. What are the potential benefits of neoadjuvant chemotherapy?

Neoadjuvant chemotherapy may decrease the size of the tumor, which may lead to less extensive surgery. Hopefully, this effect may increase survival rates, decrease local relapse rates, or decrease the morbidity associated with surgery. Other potential benefits include determining the response to a chemotherapy regimen when measurable disease is present to predict its efficacy in an adjuvant setting.

4. Are there negative theoretical considerations to neoadjuvant chemotherapy?

If neoadjuvant chemotherapy is given and the primary tumor has a dramatic response, it may be difficult to determine the margins that are necessary at surgery. If there is tumor progression when neoadjuvant chemotherapy is given, the tumor may become noncurable with surgery, or more extensive resection, creating increased morbidity, may be required.

5. Define adjuvant chemotherapy.

Adjuvant chemotherapy is chemotherapy that is given after a primary treatment modality such as surgery or radiation therapy. All known disease should be removed or eradicated by the primary treatment, and the intent of adjuvant chemotherapy is hopefully to eradicate any microscopic tumor that is left behind and thus decrease the relapse rates, both locally and systemically.

6. Has adjuvant chemotherapy been proved to be beneficial to patients with resected head and neck cancer?

Although there is a theoretical rationale as to why this approach should benefit patients, no randomized clinical trials have shown a survival or disease-free survival benefit. Ongoing clinical trials with new agents hopefully will prove some benefit in the future.

7. When should chemotherapy be considered in patients with metastatic or locally recurrent head and neck cancer?

Patients with metastatic head and neck cancer who have a good performance status and are symptomatic are excellent candidates for chemotherapy. Patients should be staged to determine the extent of disease and their general physical condition. Laboratory assessment of renal and hepatic function must be carried out so that the least toxic chemotherapy regimen can be employed. Response rates of 30–70% are often seen.

8. Has chemotherapy for metastatic disease been shown to extend survival?

No. No randomized clinical trials to date have shown an increase in survival in patients with metastatic head and neck cancer treated with chemotherapy. Often, patients will have a dramatic response in terms of tumor shrinkage. Although this shrinkage may not lead to increases in survival, it can be fairly effective at palliating symptoms caused by metastatic or locally recurrent disease.

9. Which drugs have single-agent activity in head and neck cancer?

Methotrexate   Bleomycin
5-fluorouracil (5-FU)   Mitomycin-C
Cisplatin   Paclitaxel (Taxol)
Carboplatin

10. What are the most commonly used combination chemotherapy regimens for patients with head and neck cancer?

Cisplatin + 5-FU
Cisplatin + 5-FU with leucovorin modulation
Carboplatin + 5-FU

11. Name the common side effects of the most commonly used chemotherapeutic agents in head and neck cancer.

Cisplatin	Nausea and vomiting, renal failure, potassium and magnesium wasting, peripheral neuropathies, hearing loss, anorexia, anemia
5-FU	Mucositis, slight alopecia, potential for neutropenia and thrombocytopenia, and skin reactions
Methotrexate	Mucositis, neutropenia, anemia, thrombocytopenia
Carboplatin	Neutropenia, thrombocytopenia, anemia, nausea and vomiting
Bleomycin	Allergic reactions, pulmonary toxicity, and fevers
Mitomycin C	Nausea, bone marrow suppression, potential for hemolytic uremic syndrome
Paclitaxel (Taxol)	Allergic reactions, bone marrow suppression, alopecia, and neuropathies

12. What factors can increase the toxicity of methotrexate?

Methotrexate is cleared via the kidneys, and thus patients with decreased creatinine clearance must receive appropriate dose reductions to avoid excessive toxicity. Because methotrexate is concentrated in fluids in body cavities and is slowly released later, it can cause severe side effects. Thus, it should be avoided in patients with ascites or pleural effusions.

13. Why does radiation therapy used in conjunction with chemotherapy have increased side effects?

Radiation therapy and most chemotherapy for head and neck cancers have similar and overlapping side effects. Combined-modality treatment most likely increases the incidence and severity of mucositis as well as bone marrow suppression. Mucositis is the dose-limiting toxicity when combined-modality treatment is employed.

14. Why is the mucositis so severe?

Most of the active agents used in the treatment of head and neck cancers cause mucositis. This side effect can be potentiated with previous radiation therapy that may decrease salivary gland function.

15. What is meant by chemo-prevention?

Chemo-prevention is treatment with an agent to decrease the chances that the patient will develop a cancer. Isotretinoin (13-*cis*-retinoic acid) has been shown in some studies to decrease the likelihood of developing new primary cancers in patients previously treated for head and neck cancers.

16. Why is nutrition so important in patients undergoing chemotherapy for head and neck cancer?

For the most part, these patients are nutritionally deficient secondary to morbidity from previous surgery and radiotherapy. Mucositis, nausea, vomiting, and anorexia from chemotherapy compound this nutritional depletion, resulting in severe weight loss. Often, tube feedings or total parenteral nutrition are required to supplement patients' dietary needs.

17. What new investigational agents show promise in their early phases of research?

Taxotere, Topotecan, and Thymitaq have all shown promise in preliminary studies in the treatment of patients with head and neck cancer. Further Phase II and Phase III studies will determine their ultimate place in the armamentarium of chemotherapeutic agents in otolaryngology.

18. What is meant by organ-preservation chemotherapy?

Many clinical trials have been conducted to determine if the combination of chemotherapy and radiation therapy can be used to avoid the need for extensive operations in patients with head and neck cancer. A recently completed VA cooperative study looked at chemotherapy and radiation compared to surgery in T3 and T4 laryngeal tumors. Patients were randomized to either surgery alone or chemotherapy and radiation followed by surgical salvage if necessary. Survival rates were the same in both groups. Two-thirds of the patients in the chemotherapy and radiation group had excellent local control; however, one-third of the patients still required a laryngectomy. Systemic relapse rates were slightly higher in the surgery-alone arm. Other clinical trials are ongoing with other organ-preservation protocols.

BIBLIOGRAPHY

1. DeConti RC: Perspectives on chemotherapy of head and neck cancer. Cancer Control (Jan):24–34, 1994.
2. Department of Veterans Affairs Laryngeal Cancer Study Group: Induction chemotherapy plus radiation compared with surgery plus radiation in patients with advanced laryngeal cancer. N Engl J Med 324: 1685–1690, 1991.
3. Head and Neck Contracts Program: Adjuvant chemotherapy for advanced head and neck squamous carcinoma: Final report of the head and neck contracts program. Cancer 60:301–311, 1987.
4. Hong WK, Lippmann SM, Itri LM, et al: Prevention of second primary tumor with isotretinoin in squamous cell carcinoma. N Engl J Med. 323:795–801, 1990.
5. Lee KJ: Chemotherapy of Head and Neck Cancer. In Lee KJ (ed): Essential Otolaryngology. Norwalk, CT, Appleton & Lange, 1995, pp 393-407.
6. Vokes EE: Interactions of chemotherapy and radiation. Semin Oncol 20:70, 1993.
7. Vokes EE, Weichselbaum RR, Lippmann SM, Hong WK: Head and neck cancer. N Engl J Med 328:184–193, 1990.

VII. Facial Plastic Surgery

51. PRINCIPLES OF GRAFTS AND FLAPS

Gregory E. Krause, M.D., and Michael L. Lepore, M.D.

1. How do grafts and flaps differ?

A **graft** is a segment of tissue, often skin, that is transplanted en bloc to a recipient site where it is required to obtain nutrients and, eventually, a blood supply from the recipient tissue. A **flap** is a segment of tissue (skin, subcutaneous tissue, muscle, bone, etc.) that is transplanted to the area of defect while maintaining attachment to its own vascular supply. A **microvascular free flap** is a segment of tissue dissected deep with its arterial and venous blood supply that is transplanted to the area of defect. The vessels (arterial and venous) are grafted to vessels in the area of the proposed defect.

2. What are the commonly used grafts in head and neck surgery?

1. A **full-thickness skin graft** (FTSG) contains the epidermis and entire dermis.
2. A **split-thickness skin graft** (STSG) contains the epidermis and a variable amount, but not all, of the dermal layer. STSGs can be further classified as thin, intermediate, or thick.
3. A **dermal graft** contains dermis without any overlying epidermis. It is obtained by harvesting a STSG and then removing the overlying epidermis.
4. **Mucosal grafts** are obtained from mucosal-lined surfaces, such as the conjunctiva, oral cavity, or nasal cavity.
5. **Bone grafts** are used for mandibular and calvarium reconstruction.
6. **Composite grafts** contain more than one type of tissue, such as dermis-fat grafts and skin-cartilage-skin grafts.

3. Discuss the advantages and disadvantages of FTSGs and STSGs.

STSGs have less nutrient demand and therefore survive more readily. However, they result in more graft contracture and poorer color match and are less resistant to trauma. FTSGs, conversely, have greater nutrient demand due to the increased thickness of the graft and, therefore, do not "take" as easily. They do, however, suffer less contracture, are more resistant to trauma, and result in a better texture and color match than do STSGs. An additional disadvantage of FTSGs is that because the entire dermis is removed, the donor bed requires an STSG unless the defect is very small and can be closed primarily.

4. What are the steps involved in the survival of a skin graft?

It takes 3–4 days before blood flow to the graft is achieved. In the interim, survival of the graft depends on the arrival of nutrients and the removal of metabolic waste by diffusion. A **fibrin exudate** between graft and recipient bed is initially formed, which establishes adherence, allows for diffusion of metabolites, and establishes a framework through which vascular anastomoses will occur. After 3–4 days, **capillary beds** from both graft and recipient bed will anastomose to create a neovasculature capable of supporting the graft. After 4–5 days, the infiltration of **fibroblasts** within the fibrin exudate will have created a more permanent fibrin attachment.

5. What aspects of the recipient bed enhance survival of a skin graft?

The recipient bed should be level. There should not be active bleeding in the bed as this will result in hematoma formation and limit attachment of graft to bed. However, excessive cautery of the bed will result in diminished vascular supply to the graft. Healthy granulation tissue in the bed is necessary for the creation of the fibrin exudate. In addition, the graft should be sutured in place to reduce shearing. To help reduce tenting, movement, and fluid accumulation under the graft, a bolster dressing may be used. A skin graft will not "take" if placed on bare bone, cartilage, or tendon and will often fail if placed on radiated tissue or infected granulation tissue. If bone, cartilage, or tendons need coverage or if radiated tissue is involved, a flap or microvascular free flap would be a better option.

6. Name some donor sites for skin grafts used in the head and neck.

The color and thickness of skin vary for different areas of the body. The color and texture of facial skin are most closely approximated with skin from the face. The skin of the nasolabial fold and postauricular area have excellent color and texture matches to most areas of the face. The eyelids have particularly thin skin, and grafting in this area is usually best achieved by use of an upper eyelid graft from the same or contralateral eye. The donor sites for these facial grafts are almost always closed primarily, except for large postauricular grafts which require STSGs. The supraclavicular area can provide large amounts of donor skin with texture and color matches that are reasonable but not quite as good as from nasolabial and postauricular donor sites. FTSGs from areas of the body below the clavicle are usually too thick and the color match is poor. STSGs are usually taken from the abdomen, thigh, and back.

7. How are skin grafts harvested?

FTSGs are usually harvested with a scalpel and are cut in a plane between the dermis and subcutaneous tissue. Any subcutaneous tissue remaining should be trimmed to reduce the thickness of the graft and decrease its metabolic needs. STSGs are harvested with free-hand knives and, more commonly, dermatomes. With a dermatome, the exact thickness of the graft can be regulated. Thin (0.008–0.01 inch), intermediate (0.012–0.014 inch), or thick (0.016–0.018 inch) grafts can be harvested based on the surgeon's need. A STSG can be meshed so that it will then be able to cover a larger area.

8. When are FTSGs and STSGs used in head and neck reconstruction?

FTSGs are most commonly used for reconstruction following cutaneous malignancies that cannot be closed primarily. STSGs are often used in head and neck surgery to reconstruct oral cavity and pharyngeal defects following ablative oncologic surgery. Defects that cannot be closed primarily and that do not require a large flap are often best treated with a STSG. In these situations, STSGs close the defect while still allowing adequate tongue mobility.

9. Describe the various types of bone grafts.

1. **Autologous grafts** (from the same person) are most popular and can be divided into three groups. **Cancellous** bone grafts consist of bone marrow and medullary bone. These grafts have the quickest revascularization and highest percentage of surviving transplanted cells. **Cortical** bone grafts consist of cortex (lamellar) bone. Revascularization is slower and cell survival is low. **Cortico-cancellous** bone grafts contain both types. This graft has the advantage of using the quickly revascularized cancellous bone while possessing the strength of cortical bone.

2. **Allogeneic bone grafts** do not actually provide viable cells. Instead, these grafts induce proliferation of native osteogenic cells. The most common use of allogeneic bone grafts is for mandibular reconstruction. A hollowed-out crib of mandible or iliac crest which is filled with autologous cortico-cancellous bone chips may be used.

3. **Xenografts** are no longer used.

10. When is a flap needed?

There are many instances in which a flap provides a better result than a graft. A flap can often provide an optimum result when the defect is too large for a FTSG, when the defect possesses poor vascularity (e.g., following irradiation), or when it is used to approximate color and texture match with the surrounding tissue. In addition, when bulk or composite tissue is needed, flaps are usually the best choice.

11. What are some of the basic categories of flaps?
   1. **Local skin flaps** are harvested from skin in close proximity to the defect.
   2. **Regional pedicled flaps** are larger flaps and can contain skin, subcutaneous tissue, muscle, and/or bone. Regional pedicled flaps are rotated into the area of the defect along their pedicle from a greater distance than local flaps.
   3. **Microvascular free flaps** can originate from sites distant from the head and neck. Like regional pedicled flaps, free flaps can be composed of multiple tissue types. However, the vascular and sometimes nervous supply of the flap is isolated and then anastomosed with vessels and nerves in proximity to the defect.

12. What are random and axial pattern flaps?
   The blood supply to the epidermis and dermis is derived from the dermal-subdermal plexus. The vascular supply to the flap plexus may involve an artery that directly communicates with the plexus at the proximal end of the flap (**random pattern**). In contrast, it may also involve a segmental artery that runs the length of the flap, sending multiple branches to the plexus throughout the length of the flap (**axial pattern**). The blood supply to muscle can be characterized similarly. A random pattern has a random distribution of blood vessels throughout the muscle. An axial pattern, on the other hand, has a segmental artery that courses along the fascia deep to the muscle and sends perforating branches along its distribution into the muscle. Almost all local skin flaps have a random pattern. Regional skin flaps can have either random or axial patterns. Microvascular free flaps, by their very nature, are dependent on a particular arterial and venous supply.

13. Describe the various types of local flaps.
   Advancement flap—Skin adjacent to the defect is directly advanced into the defect. Incisions are made in the lateral aspects of the flap to allow advancement of the flap. Burow's triangles are made along the proximal aspect of the flap to prevent dog-earing.
   Rotation flap—As the name suggests, a flap is rotated along an arc into the defect. As with advancement flaps, Burow's triangles are often needed.
   Transposition flap—The flap is passed over an incomplete bridge of skin.
   Interpolated flap—The flap is passed either over or under a complete bridge of skin, which separates the flap from the defect.

14. Which anatomic structures must be considered with local flaps?
   The distribution of the **facial nerve** should be clearly understood by the reconstructive surgeon. Of particular note is the temporal branch as it traverses the zygoma midway between the lateral canthus and the external auditory canal. The marginal mandibular branch, which can be located near the mandibular notch, is also an important consideration. The **parotid duct** also resides in a superficial location. The course of the duct is located midway between a line drawn from the tragus to the oral commissure.

15. When using local flaps, it is important to avoid excess tension on what structures?
   Avoid placing excessive tension on the hairline, medial, or lateral canthus or the oral commissure when raising a local flap. Excessive tension will result in cosmetic deformity and loss of symmetry.

16. Which tissues are commonly used in a regional flap?
   There are three major types of regional pedicled flaps that are used for head and neck reconstruction: cutaneous, myocutaneous, and osteomyocutaneous flaps. **Cutaneous flaps** are composed of skin elements only and are used in the reconstruction of skin loss secondary to malignancy, radiation, or infection. **Myocutaneous flaps** are composed of skin and underlying muscle, provide more bulk than cutaneous flaps, and are used when a defect requires the additional bulk for enhanced return of form and function. **Osteomyocutaneous flaps** are used for reconstruction of the mandible and overlying soft tissue defects. In many instances, microvascular free flaps provide superior reconstructive results to regional pedicled flaps.

17. Name some commonly used regional cutaneous flaps and their vascular supply.

Regional cutaneous flaps are used for large facial defects and were commonly used for oral cavity and oropharyngeal reconstruction before the advent of more sophisticated reconstructive methods.

1. The **deltopectoral flap** is based on the first four perforating branches of the internal mammary artery and is an axial pattern flap. The skin and underlying superficial fascia of the pectoralis major and deltoid muscles are contained in this medially based flap.

2. The **midline forehead flap** is a pedicled axial-pattern flap based on the supratrochlear artery. It could also be classified as a local flap and is used for reconstruction of dorsal nasal defects.

3. The **temporal flap** is an axial flap based on the superficial temporal artery.

Other regional cutaneous flaps include the thoracoacromial, nape of neck, and cervicofacial flaps, which are all random-pattern flaps based on several arteries.

18. Name some commonly used regional myocutaneous flaps and their vascular supply.

1. The most commonly used myocutaneous flap for head and neck reconstruction is probably the **pectoralis major flap**. This flap is an axial-pattern flap based on the thoracoacromial artery. The lateral thoracic artery also provides blood to this flap, and the flap is laterally based. A skin paddle between the nipple and sternum is harvested, and the paddle and underlying pectoralis muscle are then tunneled above the clavicle and used as needed.

2. The **latissimus dorsi myocutaneous flap** is an axial-pattern flap based on the thoracodorsal artery. The muscle and skin paddle are tunneled either above or below the pectoralis major muscle and into the neck.

3. The **trapezius myocutaneous flap** is also an axial flap based on the transverse cervical artery which originates from the thyrocervical trunk.

4. The **sternocleidomastoid muscle flap** is a random-pattern flap. Its vascular supply is derived from the occipital artery superiorly, the superior thyroid artery, and the transverse cervical artery inferiorly.

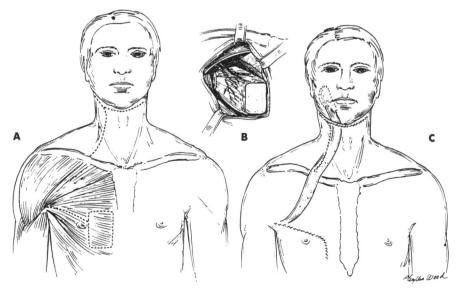

Pectoralis major flap. *A,* The cutaneous island is incised down to the pectoralis major muscle. An incision is carried laterally from this island along the anterior axillary line. *B,* The medial and lateral muscle cuts are made, freeing up the pedicle and allowing the necessary arc for reconstruction in the head/neck. *C,* The flap in place and the donor area is closed primarily. (From Panje WR, Morris MR: Oral cavity and oropharyngeal reconstruction. In Cummings CW, et al (eds): Otolaryngology–Head and Neck Surgery, 2nd ed. St. Louis, Mosby, 1993, p 1485, with permission.)

19. Describe the blood supply to bone.

The blood supply to bone comes from three main sources:

1. The **nutrient artery** is the major vascular supply for long bones. This artery penetrates the cortex, enters the marrow, distributes blood to most of the internal portion of the bone, and then forms anastomoses with the other vascular sources.

2. The **periosteal vessels** travel along the periosteum and send perforating branches within the cortex. The periosteal vessels are felt to supply one-third to one-fourth of the nutrient needs of the cortex.

3. **Epiphyseal metaphyseal vessels** are separated in children and unite after fusion. Most long bones are dependent on the nutrient artery, while flat bones rely more on the periosteal vessels.

20. Name some of the regional osteomyocutaneous flaps.

Osteomyocutaneous flaps are similar to previously described myocutaneous flaps except that bone is included in these flaps. The pectoralis major flap includes an adjacent portion of rib, the sternocleidomastoid muscle flap includes an adjacent portion of clavicle, and the trapezius muscle includes an adjacent scapular spine. These have all been used for reconstructive purposes.

Because both the rib and clavicle are long bones, their blood supply is more dependent on the nutrient artery. Therefore, removal of a portion of these bones results in a more tenuous bone flap. The scapula is a flat bone; therefore, harvesting part of the scapula results in a more reliable flap because its blood supply is more dependent on periosteal vessels. Microvascular bone flaps, however, have been shown to be more reliable and are most often utilized if a flap is necessary for mandibular reconstruction.

21. What are the major advantages of microvascular free flaps over regional pedicled flaps?

Microvascular free flaps hold a number of advantages over regional pedicled flaps:

1. Many different postoncologic surgery defects confront the reconstructive surgeon, and the wide variety of free flaps enables the surgeon to tailor the flap to the defect much more closely than could be accomplished with regional flaps.

2. Microvascular free flaps provide reliable well-vascularized donor tissue.

3. Regional flaps are limited in where they can be used by the length of the pedicle.

4. The donor site defect, on the whole, is greater with regional flaps than with free flaps.

5. Microvascularized free flaps can also withstand subsequent radiation therapy if needed.

22. List some of the fasciocutaneous microvascular free flaps and their vascular pedicles.

1. The arterial supply of the **radial forearm fasciocutaneous flap** is the radial artery. Venous drainage is though the venae comitantes. The medial or lateral cutaneous nerves of the forearm may be used to create a sensate flap.

2. The **lateral thigh fasciocutaneous flap** is based on the third perforating branch of the profunda femoris artery. Venous drainage is through accompanying venae comitantes which drain into the profunda femoris vein. The lateral femoral cutaneous nerve of the thigh may be harvested to provide sensation.

3. The **scapular and parascapular fasciocutaneous flaps** are based on the cutaneous scapular and cutaneous parascapular arteries, respectively, which are branches of the circumflex scapular artery. These flaps can be raised as one large flap if necessary. Venous drainage is through accompanying veins.

4. The **lateral arm fasciocutaneous flap** relies on the radial collateral artery, cephalic vein, and venae comitantes and the lateral cutaneous nerve of the arm.

23. Name two myocutaneous microvascular free flaps.

1. The **rectus abdominis myocutaneous free flap** is based on the deep inferior epigastric vessels. Multiple superficial perforating arteries radiate out from the periumbilical area, enabling generous amounts of skin to be taken with the graft. Sensation is not possible with this graft.

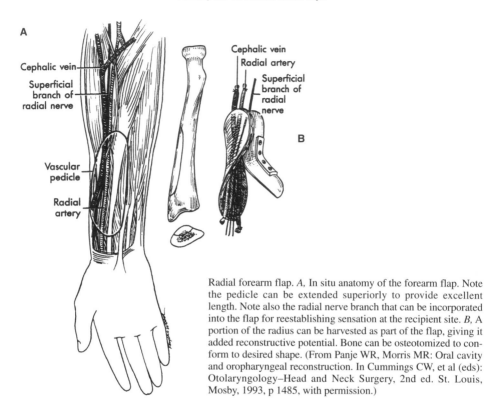

Radial forearm flap. *A,* In situ anatomy of the forearm flap. Note the pedicle can be extended superiorly to provide excellent length. Note also the radial nerve branch that can be incorporated into the flap for reestablishing sensation at the recipient site. *B,* A portion of the radius can be harvested as part of the flap, giving it added reconstructive potential. Bone can be osteotomized to conform to desired shape. (From Panje WR, Morris MR: Oral cavity and oropharyngeal reconstruction. In Cummings CW, et al (eds): Otolaryngology–Head and Neck Surgery, 2nd ed. St. Louis, Mosby, 1993, p 1485, with permission.)

2. The **latissimus dorsi myocutaneous free flap** is based on the thoracodorsal artery and accompanying venae comitantes. Sensation is possible through the thoracodorsal nerve. This flap can provide a large amount of both muscle and skin.

24. What is the purpose of the gracilis myogenous microvascular free flap?

The gracilis myogenous flap is used for facial reanimation. The motor nerve to the muscle can be anastomosed with the nerve to the masseter muscle. This results in facial movement when the teeth are clenched. The motor nerve may also be anastomosed with the contralateral facial nerve to improve symmetry of movement in the midportion of the face.

25. How are flaps and grafts used in the reconstruction of the mandible?

The reconstructive method depends on the location and size of the defect, the need for additional soft-tissue reconstruction in the oral cavity, and the desire for dental implants. Bone grafts and plates are often sufficient for small lateral mandibular defects. Larger defects and anterior "Andy Gump" deformities often require microvascular free flap reconstruction. Options include iliac crest, fibula, radial forearm, and scapular-based microvascular free flaps.

BIBLIOGRAPHY

1. Bailey BJ, Calhoun KH: Basic principles of plastic surgery in the head and neck. In Paparella MM, Shumrick DA, Gluckman JL, Meyerhoff WL (eds): Otolaryngology, 3rd ed. Philadelphia, W.B. Saunders, 1991.
2. Hayden RE, Fredrickson JM: Microvascular surgery for head and neck reconstruction. In Paparella MM, Shumrick DA, Gluckman JL, Meyerhoff WL (eds): Otolaryngology, 3rd ed. Philadelphia, W.B. Saunders, 1991.

3. Hoffmann JF, Cook TA: Reconstruction of facial defects. In Cummings CW, et al (eds): Otolaryn-gology–Head and Neck Surgery, 2nd ed. St. Louis, Mosby, 1993.
4. Levine HL: Skin, dermal, and mucosal grafting. In Paparella MM, Shumrick DA, Gluckman JL, Meyerhoff WL (eds): Otolaryngology, 3rd ed. Philadelphia, W.B. Saunders, 1991.
5. Panje WR, Morris MR: Oral cavity and oropharyngeal reconstruction. In Cummings CW, et al (eds): Otolaryngology–Head and Neck Surgery, 2nd ed. St. Louis, Mosby, 1993.
6. Petruzzelli GJ, Johnson JT: Skin grafts. Otolaryngol Clin North Am 27:25, 1994.
7. Shindo ML, Sullivan MJ: Muscular and myocutaneous pedicled flaps. Otolaryngol Clin North Am 27:161, 1994.
8. Shindo ML, Sullivan MJ: Soft-tissue microvascular free flaps. Otolaryngol Clin North Am 27:173, 1994.
9. Shumrick DA, Savoury LW: Local flaps. In Paparella MM, Shumrick DA, Gluckman JL, Meyerhoff WL (eds): Otolaryngology, 3rd ed. Philadelphia, W.B. Saunders, 1991.
10. Shumrick DA, Savoury LW: Distal flaps. In Paparella MM, Shumrick DA, Gluckman JL, Meyerhoff WL (eds): Otolaryngology, 3rd ed. Philadelphia, W.B. Saunders, 1991.
11. Urken ML, Buchbinder D: Oromandibular reconstruction. In Cummings CW, et al (eds): Otolaryn-gology–Head and Neck Surgery, 2nd ed. St. Louis, Mosby, 1993.

52. PRINCIPLES OF SKIN RESURFACING

Arlen D. Meyers, M.D., M.B.A.

1. What are the indications for skin resurfacing?

Skin resurfacing may be considered for patients with actinic keratoses, rhytids, pigmentary dyschromias, superficial scarring, radiation dermatitis, acne vulgaris, and rosacea.

2. What are the different techniques of facial skin resurfacing?

Treatment is either medical or surgical. The application of retinoic acid (Retin-A) is the most common medical treatment. Surgical treatments include chemical face peels, dermabrasion, laser selective photothermolysis, and injectable fillers.

3. What are the different skin types?

Fitzpatrick Skin Classification System

Type I	Eastern European descent	Extremely fair skin, little melanin, red hair, green eyes
Type II	Eastern European or Scandinavian descent	Fair skin, blond hair, blue eyes
Type III	Mediterranean descent	Light brown skin, brown hair, brown eyes
Type IV	Asian descent	More pigmentation, with greater sun tolerance
Type V	Nonwhites	Light black skin
Type VI	Blacks	Very dark skin

4. How does the sun change the skin?

Sun exposure, or actinic radiation, primarily results in changes of the dermis. Collagen in the papillary dermis becomes disorganized as elastic fibers increase (elastosis).

5. How does aging change the skin?

The epidermis tends to remain the same thickness throughout the aging process. However, the rete ridges, which are pronounced in young healthy skin, become flattened and give the appearance of skin thinning. The papillary and reticular dermis thins with age. Likewise, elastin, ground substance, dermal cells, the microcirculation, and cutaneous nerves decrease with aging. Thicker skin will require more treatments than thinner skin to achieve the same degree of tissue removal.

6. How do you classify aged skin?
The Glogau classification groups patients as having mild, moderate, advanced, and severe damage.

7. What is Retin-A?
Topical tretinoin (all-*trans*-retinoic acid) is not a true chemical wounding agent. It is often mixed with a moisturizer and applied at home. The cream can be used alone or in preparation for a dermabrasion or face peel. When it is used for > 6 months, it has been demonstrated to reduce rhytids, actinic keratoses, and pigmentary actinic changes.

8. What is a skin peel?
Skin peels are administered in an attempt to reverse the histologic damage created by actinic radiation, preneoplastic conditions, and the aging process. Acids or other substances are applied to the skin to destroy progressively deeper layers of epidermis and papillary dermis.

9. Are there different kinds of face peels?
Yes. Face-peeling solutions are usually classified according to the depth of burn that they create. Superficial peeling solutions (e.g., glycolic acids) create damage that is limited to the epidermis and papillary dermis. Medium-depth peels (e.g., trichloroacetic acid) create a burn through the upper reticular dermis. Deeper peeling solutions (e.g., phenol or "Baker's solution") create tissue damage through the mid-reticular dermis. There are different indications for the use of each of these solutions.

10. What are the indications for a deep peel?
Actinic keratoses	Rhytids
Photoaging	Epidermal growth
Lentignes	Acne management
Pigment changes	Acne scarring

11. How is a peel performed?
Peels are usually performed in an outpatient setting with the patient under mild sedation. The skin is degreased and prepped, and the wounding agent is applied. The application is sometimes covered with tape or ointment. The acid often creates a facial burn that takes several weeks to heal.

12. What are the complications of face peeling?
Pigmentary changes	Milia
Scarring	Cold sensitivity
Infection	Cardiac arrhythmias
Prolonged erythema or pruritus	Laryngeal edema
Textural changes	Poor patient/physician relationship
Atrophy	

13. What kind of pigmentary changes can occur?
Pigmentary changes include hyperpigmentation, hypopigmentation, depigmentation, lines of demarcation, and nevi accentuation.

14. Should a patient with a history of herpes be given a face peel?
These patients should be pretreated with acyclovir before the peel. After the peel, they should strictly avoid sun exposure.

15. What is dermabrasion?

Dermabrasion is performed with an abrasive wheel that is attached to an electrically driven handpiece. Layers of skin are literally "sanded off" to the proper depth for the clinical problem. An eschar forms over the dermabraded area. It takes several weeks for the eschar to detach and the underlying skin to heel.

16. What is a laser?

LASER is an acronym for light amplification by stimulated emission of radiation. A laser is a light that is collimated (has parallel rays), coherent (has all waves of the same frequency and periodicity), and monochromatic (is a single wavelength). A laser may be used in a defocused mode to treat superficial lesions, or it may be used in a focused excisional mode much like a scalpel is used.

17. Define selective photothermal epidermolysis.

Selective photothermal epidermolysis refers to the ability of a laser to selectively destroy small layers of cells with little peripheral tissue damage. The most frequently used lasers for this purpose are the CO_2 laser and the flash pump dye laser.

18. What happens to the skin when it is treated with a CO_2 laser?

When the CO_2 laser contacts skin, it immediately boils intracellular water and leads to tissue vaporization. The effect of the laser depends on the anatomy, thickness of the skin, and dose of the laser. When eyelid skin is treated with 100 mJ/cm², there is complete loss of the epidermis, minimal coagulation of the papillary dermal collagen, and minimal degeneration of the necks of adnexal structures. The deep dermal layers are unaffected. When the tissue is treated with 200 mJ/cm², there is complete loss of the epidermis, moderate coagulation of the papillary dermal collagen, and moderate degeneration of the necks of adnexal structures. The deep dermal structures remain unaffected. When eyelid tissue is treated with 300 mJ/cm², there is complete loss of the epidermis and moderate to severe coagulation of the papillary and reticular dermis. At this dose, there is extensive degeneration of the adnexal structures and coarse cystic changes throughout the deeper dermis.

19. What is rhinophyma, and how is it treated?

Rhinophyma is a form of rosacea that is caused by sebaceous hyperplasia. Common in elderly men, this hyperplasia leads to an erythematous, swollen, nodular nose. Currently, the CO_2 laser is the treatment of choice. It can be used much like a scalpel to sculpt the soft tissue, and it can be used more superficially to vaporize excess hypertrophic tissue. Re-epithelialization begins about 1 week after laser treatment.

20. How are injectable fillers used?

Fillers can be injected under the skin to elevate depressed scars or wrinkles. The most commonly used substance is collagen. Unfortunately, the material can cause allergic reactions. Injectable fillers need to be reinjected at 6–9-month intervals to maintain the result.

21. Is one method of skin resurfacing surgery better than another?

Each technique has its advantages and disadvantages. It is often difficult to achieve controlled results with dermabrasion. Chemical peeling around areas such as the eyelids can cause sensitivity problems. Some procedures are safer to do in combination with other aging-face procedures, such as blepharoplasty or facelift surgery.

BIBLIOGRAPHY

1. Brody H: Chemical Peeling. St. Louis, Mosby Year Book, 1992.
2. Fitzpatrick TB: The validity and practicality of sun reactive skin types I through VI. Arch Dermatol 124:869–871, 1988
3. Schoenrock LD, Chernoff WG, Rubach BW: Cutaneous ultrapulse laser resurfacing of the eyelids. Int J Aesthetic Restor Surg 3:31–36, 1995.

53. RHINOPLASTY

David A. Hendrick, M.D.

1. What is rhinoplasty?

Rhinoplasty is plastic surgery that involves the repositioning and/or refinement of the nasal skeleton and soft tissue. This surgery serves to improve function, facial aesthetics, or both. Obstruction is the most commonly addressed functional problem. Often, a septoplasty is incorporated into the surgery. Aesthetic concerns often focus on a dorsal nasal hump, a poorly defined nasal tip, or an acquired deformity from trauma.

2. What should be considered in the preoperative planning of rhinoplasty?

The importance of thorough preoperative planning cannot be overemphasized. The most important part is listening to the patient's concerns about appearance and expectations about the surgery. With a mirror, it is important that the surgeon and patient mutually understand exactly what the patient likes and dislikes about his or her nose. Preoperative photography is extremely helpful in assessing the patient's desires and in planning the operative steps. In addition, the physical examination should include a complete functional assessment of the nose.

3. Which types of anesthesia are used for rhinoplasty?

Rhinoplasty may be performed with general or local anesthesia. Most surgeons prefer local anesthesia in combination with IV sedation. This combination tends to provide better hemostasis, hastens recovery, and decreases cost. Lidocaine with epinephrine is the most commonly used injectable anesthetic. Topicals include ephedrine, oxymetazoline, and cocaine. If a general anesthetic is used, the surgeon often uses additional injected anesthetic to enhance vasoconstriction.

4. What is the Frankfort horizontal plane? Why is it important?

On x-ray, the Frankfort horizontal plane is a line drawn from the top of the bony external auditory canal to the bony infraorbital rim. On facial photographs, it is approximated as a line from the top of the tragus to the infraorbital rim. This line is important because it provides a good, reproducible, reference plane for facial photography and analysis.

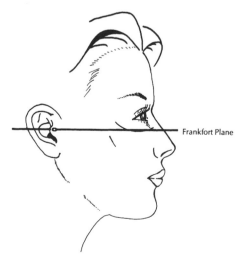

Frankfort Plane

The Frankfort plane. (From Powell N, Humphries B: Proportions of the Aesthetic Face. New York, Thieme-Stratton, 1984, p 8, with permission).

5. When analyzing the nose in proportion to the face, what are some of the most important aesthetic relationships?

Nasal length—generally the middle ⅓ of facial length

Nasal width—approximately the intercanthal distance of the eyes, or about ⅕ facial width.

Nasofacial angle—the slope of the angle of the nose compared to the plane of the face; about 30–40°

Nasofrontal angle—the angle between the frontal bone and nose taken at the nasal root, or "radix"; about 120°

Nasolabial angle—the angle between the upper lip and nasal columella; a generic "unisex" value is 95–100°

6. When analyzing the nose, what are some of the important components to assess?

Dorsal profile—In addition to assessing the various nasal-facial relationships, assess the amount of dorsal hump, presence of a desirable "supratip break" and infratip "double break," and the amount of "columellar show"(2–4 mm normal). On AP view, the brow line should blend smoothly with the dorsal sides, forming a smooth arc.

Basal view—generally an equilateral triangle that can be broken into thirds

Tip projection—the distance the tip projects away from the face

Tip rotation—the relative position of the tip along a caudal-cephalic arc

Tip volume—the amount of tip lobule bulbosity

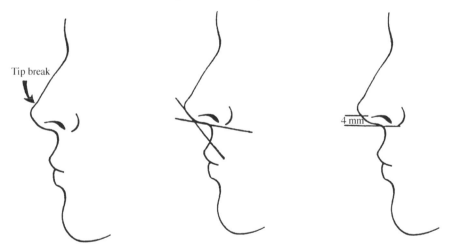

| The supratip break. | The "double-break" of the nasal tip. | There is 3 to 5 mm of columella exposed seen on lateral view. |

The supratip break, infratip double break, and columellar show of the nasal dorsal profile. (From Powell N, Humphries B: Proportions of the Aesthetic Face. New York, Thieme-Stratton, 1984, p 32, with permission.)

7. What is the "sellion"? How is this different from the "nasion"?

The **sellion** is a soft-tissue landmark representing the deepest point of the nasofrontal angle. The **nasion** is a bony landmark at the nasofrontal suture. It is usually slightly higher than the sellion. Other useful landmarks of the nasal profile include the rhinion, radix, and glabella. The **rhinion** is a point representing the bony-cartilaginous junction of the nasal dorsum. The **radix** is the region that is considered to be the "root" of the nose. This area contributes to the nasofrontal angle. The sellion and nasion exist within the radix. The **glabella** is a frontal prominence between the brows above the root of the nose.

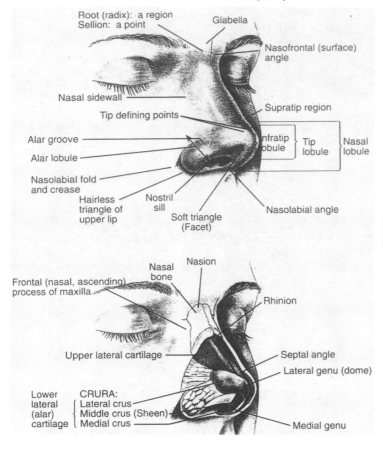

Landmarks and anatomy of the nose. (From Burget GC, Menick FJ: Aesthetic Reconstruction of the Nose. St. Louis, Mosby, 1994, p 7, with permission.)

8. What are nasal "aesthetic units"? What is their role in reconstructive rhinoplasty?

The complex contours of the nose can be divided into units based on natural boundaries of shadowed valleys and lighted ridges. Each unit is generally convex or concave. A defect in a given aesthetic unit is best reconstructed with skin from the same unit. Incisions that follow unit boundaries heal with the least perceptible scar, while incisions that cross unit boundaries heal with the most noticeable scars. When defects involve most of an aesthetic unit, it is best to resect and reconstruct the entire unit as a single entity. Aesthetic units include the sidewall, tip, columella, dorsum, alar-nostril sill, and soft triangle.

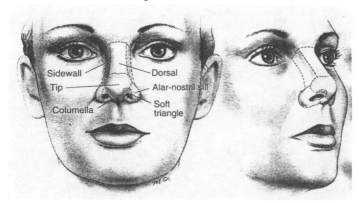

Nasal aesthetic units. (From Burget GC, Menick FJ: Aesthetic Reconstruction of the Nose. St. Louis, Mosby, 1994, p 7, with permission.)

9. Name the three major anatomic areas that are addressed in rhinoplasty.

The septum, tip, and dorsum. Each of these areas may be addressed separately during the operation.

10. Describe the important incisions employed in rhinoplasty.

Several incisions are possible to gain access to the tip and dorsum. Most incisions in rhinoplasty are situated around the lower lateral cartilage.

1. **Transcartilaginous incision**—This incision is made directly beneath the alar cartilage to "split" the cartilage. It is used only for conservative volume reduction of the lower lateral cartilage.

2. **Intercartilaginous incision**—This incision is made between the lower lateral and upper lateral cartilage to gain access to the nasal dorsum in closed rhinoplasty. It may be extended down onto the septum as a hemitransfixion or even full transfixion incision for access to the septum.

3. **Marginal rim incision**—This incision is made along the caudal edge of the lower lateral cartilage to gain access to the nasal tip. In closed rhinoplasty, where the lower lateral cartilage is "delivered" into direct view, this incision is combined with an intercartilaginous incision. In open rhinoplasty, in which the nose is to be degloved, this incision is combined with a transcolumellar incision.

4. **Transcolumellar incision**—This incision is made through the skin of the columella and extends up along both anterior edges of the medial crura of the lower lateral cartilage. Incisions then extend into marginal rim incisions to permit degloving the nose for open rhinoplasty. This technique is usually performed at the narrowest portion of the columella in a broken-line fashion (typically an upward directed dart of skin in the midline) for best cosmetic results.

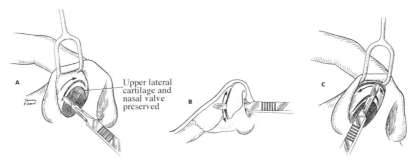

The intercartilaginous incision (*A*) and marginal rim incision (*C*) are made on either side of the lateral crura of the alar cartilage. The intercartilaginous incision permits good access to the nasal dorsum (*B*). (From Tardy ME JR: Rhinoplasty. In Cummings CS (ed): Otolaryngology–Head and Neck Surgery. St. Louis, Mosby, 1993, p 830, with permission.)

11. Where is the "soft triangle" of the nose? What complication is associated with it?

The soft triangles are the apices of the nostrils beneath the lobules. Iatrogenic injury to these areas can result in notching of the nostril rim. These areas should not be violated, especially during marginal incisions, delivery of the lower lateral cartilages during closed rhinoplasty, or open rhinoplasty skin elevation.

12. Name the three major tip support mechanisms.

1. Cartilage of the medial and lateral crura
2. Attachments of the medial crura to the caudal septum (an overlapping connection)
3. Attachments of the lateral crura to the upper lateral cartilage (a "scrolled" intercartilage connection)

Most tip rhinoplasty techniques deliberately alter one or more of these major tip supports. "Minor" tip support mechanisms that can be altered in rhinoplasty include: (a) interdomal ligaments, (b) dorsal cartilaginous septum, (c) attachments of the lower lateral crura to the piriform aperture (the "sesamoid complex," or "hinge" area), (d) attachments of the alar cartilage to the overlying skin and subcutaneous tissues, (e) membranous septum, and (f) nasal spine.

13. How is the nasal "tripod" used in planning tip rhinoplasty?

The nasal tripod is a model for the alar cartilage and tip support mechanisms. The middle leg represents the medial crura, and the two lateral legs the lateral crura. The tripod apex (which acts as a floating hinge) is the nasal tip. The tripod legs are held in place by the various forces of tip support described earlier. In this manner, one can analyze how altering some aspect of the tripod or its support will affect the nasal tip.

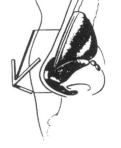

In this figure, a fourth leg is depicted for the influence of the nasal dorsum on tip support. (From Toriumi DM, Johnson CM Jr: Open structure rhinoplasty. Fac Plast Surg Clin North Am 1:2, 1993, with permission.)

14. What is the most important technique for upward tip rotation?

Tip rotation involves movement of the tip either up or down along an arc such that the nasolabial angle is altered without a significant change in tip projection. The most dramatic amount of upward tip rotation is achieved by using tip suspension sutures to pull the alar cartilage lobules in the cephalic direction. More subtle rotation is achieved by simply resecting cartilage from the cephalic portion of the alar cartilage or from the caudal edge of the upper lateral cartilage. The key to this method of tip rotation is in understanding the dynamics of healing and scar contracture. Postoperative fibrosis will form in the resected void and contract to cause tip rotation in the cephalic direction. Finally, one can simply redefine the nasolabial angle and achieve tip rotation by resecting a wedge out of the caudal septum.

Besides actually rotating the tip, one can also create an illusion of tip rotation. Angulating the infratip lobule in a cephalic direction (i.e., enhancing the "double break") using tip grafts or blunting the nasolabial angle using "plumping" grafts can both achieve the illusion of upward tip rotation.

15. How is tip projection measured? What is the most important technique for increased tip projection?

Tip projection refers to the distance the tip projects from the face and can be measured in a number of ways. The **Simon method** is the simplest to remember: the projected length of the nasal base should be approximately equal to the length of the upper lip (a 1:1 ratio). Most rhinoplasty techniques risk loss of projection through interruption of tip support mechanisms.

Tip projection is most effectively augmented using a **medial crural strut graft**. The use of various tip grafts can also enhance projection and may be necessary when using strut grafts to avoid a "tent pole" appearance to the projected tip.

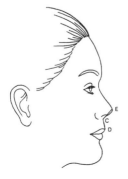

Measuring nasal tip projection. Simon's method simply notes that the length of the lower nasal contour (CE) and the length of the upper lip (CD) should exist in about a 1:1 ratio. (From Kridel RWH, Konior RJ: The underprojected tip. In Krause CJ, Pastorek N, Mangat DS (eds): Aesthetic Facial Surgery. Philadelphia, J.B. Lippincott, 1991, p 193, with permission.)

16. Describe the three basic methods for reducing alar cartilage volume (lobule modification).

Volume reduction of the lobules involves excising some portion of the cephalic border of the alar cartilage. This residual strip can be left intact as (1) a **complete strip**; it can be cut strategically to create (2) an **interrupted strip**; or it can be weakened in various ways to create (3) a **weakened complete strip**. In general, the greater the resection, the more dramatic the tip narrowing and rotation up. Conversely, the greater the strip weakening (or interruption), the more severe the loss of tip support and the greater the potential for undesirable tip retrodisplacement or postoperative tip asymmetries. Most surgeons believe that a minimum of 4–8 mm of residual strip must be preserved to avoid significant loss of tip support.

17. How can the nasal base be reduced?

The nasal base may be narrowed through some form of wedge excisions of the alar base, such as the Weir incision. These excisions can be fashioned in various ways such that in addition to narrowing the alar base, the nostrils can be narrowed and/or the tip can be retrodisplaced.

18. What techniques can be used to shorten nasal length?

Nasal length is modified by causing the nasal tip to be rotated up or down. This maneuver can be performed with or without altering the nasolabial angle, depending on what is done with the caudal edge of the septum. The septum plays a major role in tip and columellar position. Tip rotation up will shorten the dorsum and increase the nasolabial angle. Resecting caudal septum will change columellar position to alter or preserve the original nasolabial angle while permitting this dorsal shortening.

19. What other techniques can be used to alter the nasolabial angle?

Aside from the caudal septum resection techniques, the nasolabial angle can be changed through the use of caudal septal grafts, medial crura stay sutures, columellar strut grafts, or, for overly acute angles, "softened" through the use of "plumping" grafts anterior to the nasal spine. To make the angle more acute, resection of procerus muscle and/or the nasal spine can be performed.

20. What are some important factors in determining how much dorsal hump to remove?

A straight nasal dorsum is the generic "unisex" norm. However, a slightly concave dorsum is considered a desirable feminine trait, while a slightly convex dorsum is considered a distinctive masculine characteristic. Long-term postoperative results may be slightly more concave than the intraoperative result. This phenomenon is due to the thinner skin overlying the middle one-third of the nose which is more easily distorted with local anesthetic and edema. This distortion may take some time to resolve and must be considered when performing a dorsal reduction. In general, some amount of convexity to the cartilage and bone must be preserved to achieve a straight or concave dorsal profile.

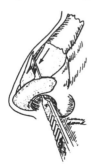 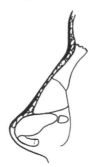 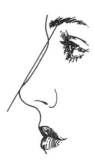

A, Reducing a cartilaginous dorsal hump. *B,* Nasal dorsal skin is thinnest over the rhinion. The bony-cartilaginous dorsum must still be convex to achieve a straight dorsum. *C,* In females, a slightly concave dorsum is aesthetically desirable. (Panel *A* from Tardy ME Jr: Rhinoplasty. In Cummings CW, et al (eds): Otolaryngology–Head and Neck Surgery. St. Louis, Mosby, 1993, p 847; Panels *B* and *C* from Gunter JP: Deformities of the nasal dorsum. In Krause CJ, Pastorek N, Mangat DS (eds): Aesthetic Facial Surgery. Philadelphia, J.B. Lippincott, 1991, p 342, with permission.)

21. What is a "pollybeak" deformity?

Pollybeak is a postsurgical convexity of the supratip relative to the rest of the nose such that the lower two-thirds of the nose takes on the convex profile of a parrot's beak. It is classically a complication of over-resection of the nose. Over-resecting the nasal dorsum or the nasal tip supports can lead to relative protrusion of the supratip region. Paradoxically, over-resection of the supratip itself may lead to excessive "dead space," especially if the overlying skin is thick and inelastic. Subsequently, excessive scar tissue can lead to a supratip prominence. Corrective measures are directed at either resecting the prominent tissues, grafting the nasal dorsum, augmenting tip support and projection, or a combination of these methods.

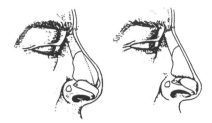

Correcting a pollybeak deformity by supratip excision of dorsal septal cartilage. (From Walter C: Surgical approaches to problems of the nasal valve area and the extramucosal rhinoplasty. In Rees TD, Baker DC, Tabbal N (eds): Rhinoplasty: Problems and Controversies. St. Louis, Mosby, 1988, p 207, with permission.)

22. Why are osteotomies used in rhinoplasty?

It is important to free the nasal bones so that they may be manipulated into their desired positions. **Medial** osteotomies free the nasal bones from the nasal septum. **Lateral** osteotomies free the nasal bones from the maxilla. For example, once the dorsal hump has been removed, the nose has no anterior roof. Although it may look very straight on the patient's profile, the nose looks very broad and misshaped on the frontal view. With osteotomies, the nasal bones are surgically broken and bent medially so that they are once again in continuity with the midline.

23. How are splints used in the postoperative care of the rhinoplasty patient?

Both internal and external nasal splints may be used. External splints are placed over the nasal dorsum and may be constructed of a number of different materials. In general, splints for the nasal dorsum are first prepared using a skin prep solution such as benzoin. Tape is then applied to the nasal dorsum to protect the skin. The splint is shaped and placed over the tape. This splint is used to maintain the nasal bones in their desired position during early healing. The splint is usually removed about 7 days postoperatively. If a septoplasty has been performed, internal nasal splints are often placed along either side of the nasal septum. These are usually made of a flexible material such as Silastic and are usually held in place with sutures through the septum. The purpose of these splints is to maintain the septum in the midline and to assist in the prevention of a septal hematoma. They are also removed about 7 days postoperatively.

24. When is the rhinoplasty result in its final form?

The results should not be considered final until at least 6 months postoperatively. Although the bones may heal in about 6 weeks, the soft tissue swelling that is associated with rhinoplasty will take months to resolve completely. Swelling in the nasal tip is especially slow to dissipate. Patients should be made aware of this fact preoperatively so that they are not disappointed by their immediate postoperative results. Also, if revisions are necessary, the surgeon should wait at least 6 months between operations.

CONTROVERSIES

25. Which surgical technique is superior, open, or closed rhinoplasty?

Open rhinoplasty involves a transcolumellar incision to deglove the nose for optimal exposure of the nasal structures. Although exposure is superb, it requires more dissection trauma with more postoperative edema, and it results in an external scar that may or may not be easily visible on close inspection. **Closed rhinoplasty** involves intranasal incisions (intercartilaginous, marginal, transcartilaginous) to gain access to the nasal structures through the nostrils. Exposure is limited and tip work requires "delivery" of the lower lateral cartilages into view. Although this method leaves no external scar, it does disrupt more of the nasal tip support mechanisms than does the open approach. Most experienced rhinoplastic surgeons prefer (and preach) one approach over the other for general rhinoplasty. Nevertheless, few surgeons will argue against using the closed approach for addressing minimal defects and using the open approach for correcting significant, severe deformities of the nose.

26. What implant materials should be utilized in rhinoplasty?

Rhinoplasty frequently requires the implantation of materials to strengthen or augment the nasal structures. Using the patient's own cartilage and bone (**autogenous grafts**) is certainly the most biocompatible and perhaps most enduring material that can be used. However, harvesting autogenous graft material can be time-consuming and costly, and it risks morbidity to a separate operative site. Furthermore, available autogenous material may be limited, especially in the case of revision rhinoplasty since septal or conchal cartilage may have already been harvested. Finally, autogenous material may be unsuitable for some applications since conchal cartilage and even septal cartilage or bone may have too much curvature or "memory" to provide a good long-term graft result.

Some surgeons have sought to circumvent these problems by using irradiated rib cartilage (**homograft**) or synthetic materials (**allografts**) such as silicone, Gore-Tex, and Medpore. These materials all represent compromises in terms of biocompatability and endurance but are faster and easier to use and capable of producing excellent postoperative results. However, the rate of graft infection (requiring removal), graft extrusion (a devastating complication), and graft resorption (requiring later revisions) for these materials continues to be a source of ongoing debate and investigations. The recent events surrounding silicone breast implants have caused many rhinoplastic surgeons to avoid the use of alloplastic implants completely.

BIBLIOGRAPHY

1. Adamson PA: Open rhinoplasty. In Papel ID, Nachlas NE (eds): Facial Plastic and Reconstructive Surgery. St. Louis, Mosby, 1992, pp 295–300.
2. Davidson TM, Murakami WT: Rhinoplasty Planning: Aesthetic Concepts, Dynamics, and Facial Construction. Alexandria, VA, American Academy of Otolaryngology–Head and Neck Surgery Foundation, 1986.
3. Farrior RT, Farrior EH: Special rhinoplasty techniques. In Cummings CW, et al (eds): Otolaryngology–Head and Neck Surgery. St. Louis, Mosby, 1993, pp 857–886.
4. Larrabee WF Jr, Sherris DA: Principles of Facial Reconstruction. Philadelphia, Lippincott-Raven, 1995, pp 8, 68–69.
5. Tardy ME Jr: Surgical Anatomy of the Nose. New York, Raven Press, 1990.
6. Tardy ME Jr: Rhinoplasty. In Cummings CW, et al (eds): Otolaryngology–Head and Neck Surgery. St. Louis, Mosby, 1993, pp 807–856.
7. Toriumi DM, Johnson CM Jr: Open structure rhinoplasty. Fac Plast Surg Clin North Am 1:1–22, 1993.
8. Walter C: Supratip and related deformities. In Rees TD, Baker DC, Tabbal N (eds): Rhinoplasty: Problems and Controversies. St. Louis, Mosby, 1988, pp 359–361.
9. Willett JM, Hirokawa RH: Facial plastic surgery. In Lee KJ (ed): Essential Otolaryngology–Head and Neck Surgery, 6th ed. Norwalk, CT, Appleton &Lange, 1995, pp 909–915.
10. Willett JM, Lee KJ: Otolaryngology: 630 Questions & Answers. Norwalk, CT, Appleton & Lange, 1995.

54. BLEPHAROPLASTY

R. *Casey Strahan*, M.D.

1. Define blepharoplasty.

Blepharoplasty is a facial plastic procedure intended to improve eyelid appearance and/or function. When performed for cosmetic reasons, a blepharoplasty attempts to give to the eyes a more youthful and attractive appearance. Occasionally, the upper lids become so redundant that they actually drape over the upper lashes and obstruct the patient's view. In these cases, the procedure is done to improve the upper lid function.

2. Which eyelid abnormalities can be corrected with a blepharoplasty?

In general, four abnormalities can be corrected with a blepharoplasty. These may be isolated abnormalities, or they may be present in combination. These are
Blepharochalasis
Dermatochalasis
Pseudoherniation of fat
Orbicularis muscle hypertrophy

3. What is blepharochalasis?

Redundancy and draping of eyelid skin that occurs in the aged face. This is first noticed laterally where redundant skin becomes apparent only during animation (e.g., smiling). With time, this redundancy becomes a permanent feature, noticed even during repose. Blepharochalasis may progress such that skin actually drapes over the upper eyelashes and causes visual field defects in superior and superior-lateral gaze.

4. What is dermatochalasis?

Dermatochalasis refers to hereditary hypertrophy of skin and orbularis muscle that occurs in a young individual. It is thus unrelated to aging and occurs early in life. This hypertrophy results in a hooded appearance of the upper lid, and the upper lid fold is totally obscured.

5. What is the cosmetic effect of pseudoherniation of fat?

Pseudoherniation of orbital fat is a common cause of baggy lids and results from laxity in the orbital septum combined with continued gravitational force on the orbital fat. Orbital fat migrates anteriorly, causing a bulge that gives the appearance of a puffy or baggy lid. This may result in the objectionable look of sleepiness or weariness.

6. Is there any importance to orbicularis muscle hypertrophy?

The orbicularis muscle may become hypertrophied in the lower lid, adding to the bagginess associated with fat pseudoherniation. Unless recognized, this hypertrophy may result in residual bagginess after a blepharoplasty in which only the fat was addressed.

7. How do an upper and a lower blepharoplasty differ?

Just as you would think, an upper blepharoplasty addresses the upper eyelid, and a lower blepharoplasty addresses the lower eyelid. These procedures may be performed together or singularly, depending on the needs of the individual patient.

8. What tissues are excised during a blepharoplasty?

In both upper and lower lid blepharoplasty, three tissues need to be addressed: the skin, orbicularis muscle, and orbital fat. Depending on the pathology present, any combination of these three tissues may be excised.

9. Which features of the eyelid can be altered with a blepharoplasty?

Because a blepharoplasty addresses the skin, orbicularis muscle, and fat pockets of the upper and lower eyelids, only the features associated with these structures can be altered. Redundant skin (blepharochalasis or dermatochalasis) is usually the most obvious feature to be addressed. Redundant or hypertrophied orbicularis muscle (made obvious by having the patient squint) can also be resected. Lastly, pseudoherniation of fat in the upper and/or lower lid can also be corrected.

10. Which features of the eyelid cannot be altered with a blepharoplasty?

A patient may have complaints about some features around the eyelid that cannot be altered by a blepharoplasty alone, and these must be pointed out and addressed during the preoperative visit. Problems that cannot be altered by a blepharoplasty alone include brow ptosis, lateral crow's feet, fine wrinkles of the lower lid, and cheek or malar bags.

11. What must the surgeon consider in the preoperative evaluation of a blepharoplasty candidate?

In addition to receiving a complete history and physical, each patient must be carefully evaluated for the particular aesthetic problem(s) present. Here, the surgeon and patient must work together to ensure that both agree on what features are undesirable and how these can be corrected. The surgeon must examine the skin of the eyelids, noting the presence of wrinkles, lesions, or abnormal pigmentations. Any asymmetries in the eyelids or palpebral fissures are noted and pointed out to the patient. These asymmetries may or may not be correctable. The eyes are examined for proptosis, and, if there is any doubt, the eyes are viewed from above and behind the patient in order to view both corneas as they relate to the upper lid margins. Next, the amount of excess skin in the upper and lower lids is estimated by pinching the skin together with blunt forceps until the lids are taught, but not so much so that complete eye closing is hindered. The snap test (see below) gives an indication of excessive lid laxity and the need for lid-shortening procedures. The fat pockets are then examined individually, and the location and relative volume of each pocket are noted. The orbicularis muscle is then examined while the patient squints, and any hypertrophy or "festooning" of the muscle is noted.

12. What is the snap test? How is it useful in the preoperative evaluation for blepharoplasty?

The snap test is a test for laxity in the lower lid. In this test, the patient looks directly forward, and the lower lid is grasped gently in the examiner's fingers. The lid is then pulled forward, off the globe, and then quickly released. The normal lid "snaps" immediately against the globe. A normal snap test is a reliable sign that the usual skin resection in a lower blepharoplasty will not result in scleral show or ectropion. If the lower lid remains off the globe for a few seconds or returns only after blinking, then a lid-shortening procedure may be indicated to avoid ectropion.

13. What should be included in the preoperative ophthalmologic evaluation?

A basic ophthalmologic examination is essential, including tests of visual acuity (both near and far vision), visual field testing, and tests of corneal protective mechanisms. These later tests include Bell's phenomenon, lagophthalmos, facial nerve weakness, corneal sensitivity, and decreased tear production (Schirmer's test).

14. Describe the relationship of the brow to the upper eyelid.

The medial half of the brow normally lies at or just above the palpable superior orbital rim, and the lateral half lies slightly higher above the rim. The infrabrow skin differs from the delicate eyelid skin in that the infrabrow skin is thicker and more sebaceous.

15. How might the position of the brow affect your decision to perform a blepharoplasty?

The position of the eyebrows in relation to the superior orbital rim and upper eyelids is a critical factor in blepharoplasty planning. If brow ptosis goes unrecognized, the amount of skin excised in an upper blepharoplasty may be overestimated. This can lead to the reapproximation of delicate eyelid skin to the thicker and less pliable infrabrow skin, resulting in an unnatural appearance of the upper lid, and possibly even persistent lagophthalmos. In addition, uncorrected brow ptosis may also result in a facial appearance dominated by the low-set brow, giving the face an angry or depressed look. Therefore, the preoperative evaluation of the blepharoplasty patient must include palpation of the superior orbital rims and assessment of brow position. If brow ptosis is present, then it must be taken into account when planning the amount of skin excised and in possibly combining the blepharoplasty with some type of brow lift.

16. What other factors must be considered in the decision to proceed with a blepharoplasty?
    In addition to the technical details regarding the aesthetic problems to be addressed during the surgery, the preoperative evaluation must also address the psychosocial issues present in each patient. These include the motivations of the patient as well as his or her psychological and medical background. Questionable motivations that should raise a red flag include early revision surgery to correct an unsatisfactory result, surgery at the insistence of a close family member or mate, sudden decisions, and a history of psychiatric illness. Medical factors that may influence the decision to proceed with surgery include a history of bleeding problems, history of ophthalmologic problems, any general or systemic disease, and alcohol and/or tobacco use.

17. Describe the anatomy of the upper eyelid.

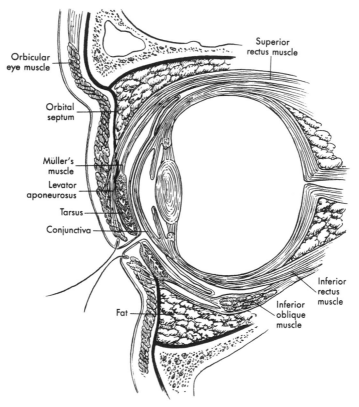

Cross section of orbit and eyelids. (From Colton JJ, Beekhuis GJ: Blepharoplasty. In Cummings CW, et al (eds): Otolaryngology–Head and Neck Surgery, 2nd ed. St. Louis, Mosby, 1993, with permission.)

    To understand the steps in a blepharoplasty and to avoid injury to the lid levator mechanism, you must have a comprehensive understanding of the upper lid anatomy. In the lid, just deep to the skin lies the orbicularis muscle, and just deep to this muscle lies the orbital septum. Orbital fat lies deep to the septum. This essentially describes the anatomy of the lower lid in its entirety, but in the upper lid, the levator mechanism is also present, making the anatomy more complicated. In the upper lid, the levator muscle originates from the orbital periosteum and passes forward above the superior rectus muscle. As the levator approaches the lid, its fibers fan out to form the levator aponeurosis, which extends the full width of the lid. This aponeurosis then fuses with the orbital septum several millimeters above the superior margin of the tarsal plate. These fibers then continue forward to insert into the orbicularis muscle, subcutaneous tissue, and skin, forming the lid crease.

18. What is Müller's muscle?

Müller's muscle is a smooth muscle that arises from the belly of the levator and inserts onto the superior border of the tarsal plate. This muscle receives sympathetic innervation off the oculomotor nerve and is responsible for the opening tone of the upper eyelid. Injury to either the levator or Müller's muscles may result in ptosis.

19. Describe the incision for an upper blepharoplasty.

An upper blepharoplasty usually involves the excision of an ellipse of skin from the upper eyelid. The lower limb of this ellipse is placed horizontally in the upper lid crease. This crease represents the upper anatomic boundary of the tarsal plate. This line should be at least 8 mm above the upper lid margin. Medially, this incision ends 1–2 mm medial to the upper lid puncta. Carrying the incision more medially, onto the concavity of the orbital rim or onto the nasal skin, risks a webbed scar. Laterally, the incision is carried to the sulcus between the lateral orbital rim and lid. If there is redundant skin lateral to this point, the incision is extended lateral to this point and is angled upward. The upper limb of the incision is then made such that it encompasses all of the redundant skin. This amount of skin is estimated by having the patient close his or her eyes; you then gently grasp the skin between the blades of a forceps, including enough skin such that the skin across the lid is tensed but the eyelid remains closed. This process is repeated medially and laterally so that the upper incision mimics the curvature of the lower incision. Because the marks for these incisions are made with the patient in the supine position, care must be taken to push down gently on the brow during marking in order to mimic the effects of gravity in the upright position. If this is not done, the amount of skin excised may be underestimated.

20. Outline the steps in an upper blepharoplasty.

Most surgeons prefer to perform a blepharoplasty under local anesthesia with intravenous sedation. The incisions are first marked with ink (see above). The skin is then infiltrated with 1% lidocaine with 1:100,000 epinephrine. The outlined ellipse of skin is then sharply excised from the underlying muscle using a no. 15 blade. Some surgeons prefer to excise the skin and muscle as a single unit. Muscle is excised only if indicated, i.e., if it is redundant or if enhancement of the lid crease is desired.

If excision of pseudoherniated fat is indicated, this is performed next. Additional lidocaine (some surgeons prefer plain lidocaine here) is infiltrated into the orbital septum and anterior fat compartments. The orbital septum is then opened sharply, and the central and medial fat pads are dissected. Gentle pressure on the closed eyelid and upward traction on the medial brow will assist in exposing the medial fat pad. The superior oblique muscle must be identified prior to clamping the fat. Once the amount of fat to be removed has been teased into the field, the fat is clamped and excised. Prior to releasing the proximal stub of tissue, meticulous hemostasis is achieved. The central fat compartment is addressed in a similar fashion.

The skin is then draped over the wound, and any additional skin excision is performed so as to prevent any redundancy that may be apparent after the fat excision. The wound is then closed with a running subcuticular monofilament suture.

21. What techniques can be used for a lower blepharoplasty?

Skin-muscle flap technique   Transconjunctival technique
Skin flap technique

22. Describe the skin-muscle flap technique for a lower lid blepharoplasty.

A subciliary incision is made 2–3 mm below the lashes and is extended laterally in a horizontal natural skin crease over the orbital rim. The initial incision is carried through the skin only, and a 3-mm-wide flap of skin is elevated inferiorly over the pretarsal portion of the orbicularis muscle. The incision is then carried through the orbicularis muscle, and a skin-muscle flap is elevated to the inferior orbital rim. This technique has the advantages that the plane of dissection behind the muscle is easy to identify and is avascular, there is minimal risk of button-holing the flap, and additional tightening of skin and muscle can be achieved by placing lateral suspension sutures. This is the preferred method when there is fat pseudoherniation with minimal skin excess.

23. Describe the skin flap technique for a lower lid blepharoblasty.

The same incision is used, but the plane of dissection is between the skin and muscle all the way to the inferior orbital rim. This technique is advantageous when there is extremely wrinkled or redundant skin and when plication or resection of orbicularis muscle is desired.

24. When is the transconjunctival approach used for a lower lid blepharoplasty?

In the transconjunctival approach, an incision is made in the conjunctiva on the inner aspect of the lower lid. This technique is useful when only fat removal is desired and there is no need for modification of the skin or muscle. However, this is rarely the case.

25. How do the fat compartments of the upper and lower orbital compartments differ?

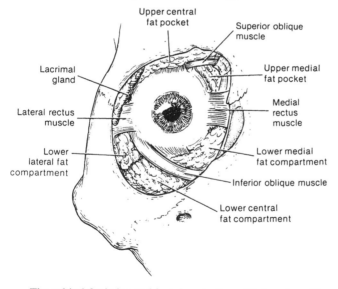

Fat compartments of right orbit and lacrimal gland. (From Colton JJ, Beekhuis GJ: Blepharoplasty. In Cummings CW, et al (eds): Otolaryngology–Head and Neck Surgery, 2nd ed. St. Louis, Mosby, 1993, with permisson.)

The orbital fat is located just deep to the orbital septum. There are three distinct compartments in the lower lid and two in the upper lid. In the **lower lid**, the *medial* and *central* compartments are separated by the inferior oblique muscle. Thus, this muscle must be identified prior to the cauterization or removal of fat from these compartments. The fat of the medial compartment is also lighter in color than that of the other compartments, which aids in its identification. The *lateral* pocket of the lower lid is separated from the central by a band of fascia.

In the **upper lid**, the *medial* and *central* compartments are separated by the superior oblique muscle, which also must be identified prior to fat removal. The lateral compartment in the upper lid is occupied by the lacrimal gland. During the removal of pseudoherniated fat from these compartments, hemostasis must be achieved prior to letting go of the remaining fat, as a bleeding vessel will be difficult to isolate after the fat has retracted back into the orbit. An alternative to fat removal is simply to apply cautery to the orbital septum.

26. What is the most frequent complication of blepharoplasty? How is it treated?

Milia are the most frequent complication in blepharoplasty. These are white globular nodules that form along the suture tracks. They are easily and effectively treated with either pinpoint cautery or marsupialization with a knife.

27. What are some other possible complications of blepharoplasty?

Serious complications following blepharoplasty are rare. Lesser and usually self-limited complications are not so rare and can usually be managed simply with local care measures and good communication with the patient. The more common complications include milia, scleral show or frank ectropion, hematoma, subconjunctival ecchymosis, chemosis, lagophthalmos, and ptosis.

28. How are scleral show and ectropion managed?

Scleral show is not uncommon following blepharoplasty and may be considered almost a normal variant in the postoperative period. It usually resolves as the edema and induration resolve in the first week or two. However, significant **ectropion** (the eversion or turning out of the lower lid) may be an indication of either too much skin excision or unrecognized lid laxity. Ectropion is first managed conservatively, with taping and eyelid massage. If it persists, either a lid-shortening procedure or a lower lid skin graft, depending on the etiology, may be required.

29. How are hematomas, subconjunctival ecchymoses, and chemosis managed?

Hematoma is rare following blepharoplasty and must be differentiated from normal ecchymosis. If a hematoma is detected, it must be drained and the bleeding vessel cauterized.

Subconjunctival ecchymosis is a rare problem, the cause of which remains unexplained. Although it may be quite disturbing to the patient, it usually resolves completely in about 3 weeks. No treatment is necessary.

Chemosis is a marked swelling of the bulbar conjunctiva that may occur after a lower lid blepharoplasty. It also resolves on its own but may take as long as 6 weeks to do so.

30. How are lagophthalmos and postoperative ptosis managed?

Lagophthalmos is the inability to close the eyelid completely, and it may follow upper lid blepharoplasty, especially secondary procedures. It is usually mild and is also temporary. Artificial tears and ointments may be necessary to protect the cornea until complete healing occurs. **Postoperative ptosis** is due either to unrecognized preoperative ptosis or to injury to the levator mechanism during upper lid blepharoplasty. It is more common after procedures to elevate and deepen the upper lid fold. If it persists for > 6 months, surgical correction may be required.

31. Can emergencies arise in the postoperative period?

Yes. The most common is **retrobulbar hematoma**. This rare complication is usually heralded by a sudden intense increase in pain associated with lid swelling and proptosis. This bleeding is usually arterial and represents a surgical emergency. If not treated promptly, it can lead to increased intraocular pressure and blindness. Treatment consists of opening the wound to express any clots, lateral canthotomy to decompress the orbit, and emergent ophthalmologic consultation to measure intraocular pressure. The wound must be explored, and the bleeding vessel identified and controlled.

Another rare but potentially devastating problem is severe **dry eye syndrome**. This condition may be due either to unrecognized preoperative dry eyes or to lagophthalmos. If it occurs, it must be recognized and treated aggressively with lubricating drops and ointment.

Vision loss in the postoperative period is a very rare (occurring in 1 in 25,000–50,000 cases) and very disturbing problem. Most commonly, it is related to a retrobulbar hematoma. In the absence of hematoma, cases are suspected to be related to unpreventable problems, such as idiopathic optic nerve atrophy or retrobulbar optic neuritis. To date, these problems have always been unilateral.

CONTROVERSY

32. What is "westernization" of the Oriental eyelid?
The Oriental eyelid differs from the Western or Occidental eyelid in that the Oriental upper lid lacks a lid crease and is more full, without a deep superior sulcus. In addition, the Oriental eye often has an epicanthal fold located medially. The absence of an upper lid crease is due to the levator aponeurosis fusing with the orbital septum below the superior tarsal border (whereas in occidentals, this fusion takes place a few millimeters above the superior tarsal border, creating the crease). The upper lid fullness is due to the presence of a thicker subcutaneous areolar layer as well as an additional layer of fat located between the orbicularis muscle and orbital septum.

Westernization of an Oriental eyelid involves the creation of an upper lid crease, thinning of the upper lid, and removal of the epicanthal fold. These three procedures may be performed together, singularly, or in any combination. These procedures are controversial because they may or may not be desired by a particular patient. The patient should be the one to decide what is done.

BIBLIOGRAPHY

1. Colton JJ, Beekhuis GJ: Blepharoplasty. In Cummings CW, et al (eds): Otolaryngology–Head and Neck Surgery, 2nd ed. St. Louis, Mosby, 1993.
2. Liu D: Oriental eyelids: Anatomic difference and surgical considerations. In Hornblass A (ed): Oculoplastic, Orbital and Reconstructive Surgery: Vol 1. Eyelids. Baltimore, Williams & Wilkins, 1988, p 513.
3. Pastorek N: Blepharoplasty. In Bailey BJ (ed): Head and Neck Surgery–Otolaryngology, vol 2. Philadelphia, J.B. Lippincott, 1993, p 2205.

55. OTOPLASTY

David A. Hendrick, M.D.

1. What anatomic landmarks of the external ear are important in otoplasty?
The circumference of the external ear consists of the tragus, helix, and lobule. The inner folds of the ear consist of the antihelix and its two crura. Between the two crura lies the fossa triangularis. Between the helix and antihelix is the scaphoid fossa. The "bowl" of the ear is the concha. Most otoplasty techniques are designed to augment the antihelical folds and/or reduce the conchal bowl. (See also chapter 8.)

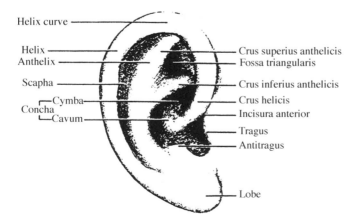

Helix curve
Helix
Anthelix
Scapha
Cymba
Concha
Cavum

Crus superius anthelicis
Fossa triangularis
Crus inferius anthelicis
Crus helicis
Incisura anterior
Tragus
Antitragus
Lobe

Important anatomic landmarks of the external ear. (From Siegert R, Weerda H, Remmert S: Embryology and surgical anatomy of the auricle. Fac Plast Surg 10:236, 1994, with permission.)

2. How are external ear malformations classified?

Various grading systems have been proposed for congenital malformations of the auricle. The best known system is Tanzer's 5-stage system, ranging from stage I (complete anotia) to stage IV (prominent ear). The simplest system is Aguilar's 3-stage system, where stage I is normal, II is deformed, and III is microtia or anotia. The most comprehensive may be the 3-stage Weerda system. Each stage is determined by the degree of surgical reconstruction required:

1. **Weerda Stage I:** First-degree dysplasia where most structures of the normal auricle are recognized. No additional skin or cartilage is needed for reconstruction. This category includes prominent ears, macrotia, minor deformities, and mild to moderate cup-ear deformities.

2. **Weerda Stage II:** Second-degree dysplasia where some structures of the normal auricle are recognized. Partial reconstruction here requires additional skin and/or cartilage. Severe cup-ear and mini-ear are included in this category.

3. **Weerda Stage III:** Third-degree dysplasia where no structures of the normal auricle are recognized. Reconstruction here is total, requiring additional skin and large amounts of cartilage. Microtia and anotia fall under this heading.

3. What head and neck syndromes commonly have auricular malformations?

Treacher Collins syndrome
Hemifacial microsomia
Goldenhar syndrome ("eye-ear-spine" dysplasia)

4. What is a "prominent" ear?

The normal ear has an angle between the auricle and head of 25–30°. The helical rim extends < 20 mm from the mastoid, and a well-defined antihelical crus is present. The prominent or protruding ear is abnormal in one or more of these areas. Typically, the protruding ear has an auriculocephalic angle approaching 90°, a helical rim > 20 mm from the mastoid, and a scaphoid fossa deficient in antihelical folds or crura.

5. When should prominent ears be corrected?

The best time to correct prominent ears is between the ages of 4–6. At this age, ear growth is essentially complete, and correction is completed prior to school age, when children become subject to peer ridicule. For the same reasons, 6 years is also the most appropriate age for microtia reconstruction.

6. When assessing an ear for otoplasty, what are the important considerations on anteroposterior or posteroanterior views?

When assessing an ear for otoplasty, the following deficiencies should be anticipated:
1. Poor antihelical fold
2. Deficient superior and inferior crus around the fossa triangularis
3. Abnormal scapha
4. Overdeveloped concha
5. Abnormal helix definition and curvature

The first four deficiencies involve assessment for a prominent ear. The last assessment involves ensuring that the helix is visible lateral to most of the antihelical fold and that the helix is an appropriate distance from the head. A horizontal line drawn through the inferior orbital rims should intersect the top of the two tragi (the "Frankfort horizontal plane"). A horizontal line drawn through the two pupils should pass through the maximum width of the auricles. A horizontal line drawn through the lateral brows should transect the upper helical rims.

7. When assessing an ear for otoplasty, how should the ear appear on the lateral view?

In general, the slope of the ear should approximate the slope of the nasal dorsum. More precisely, the "line of balance" of the auricle should be about 20° from the vertical. The ear should sit slightly posterior to the midcoronal plane on the head, a distance said to be about one ear width from the lateral orbital rim. Ear width is normally about 60% of its height. Ear height in an adult is about 60 mm. Ear position with respect to the orbit, eye, and brow should be as described for the AP view.

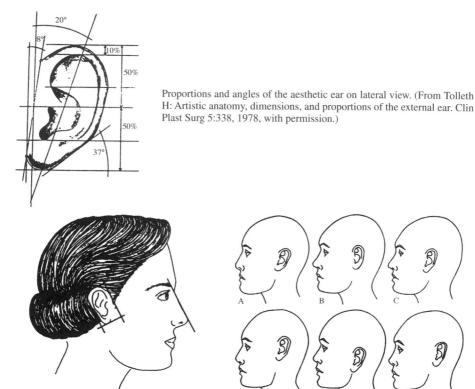

Proportions and angles of the aesthetic ear on lateral view. (From Tolleth H: Artistic anatomy, dimensions, and proportions of the external ear. Clin Plast Surg 5:338, 1978, with permission.)

The angle of the external ear on the head should approximate the angle of the nasal dorsum. Schematic *A* demonstrates the proper location of the auricle on the side of the head. (Left panel from Ridley MB: Aesthetic facial proportions. In Papel ID, Nachlas NE (eds): Facial Plastic and Reconstructive Surgery. St. Louis, Mosby, 1992, p 107; right panel from Tolleth H: Artistic anatomy, dimensions, and proportions of the external ear. Clin Plast Surg 5:339, 1978, with permission.)

8. Describe the major goals of otoplasty.
The six major goals of otoplasty are described by McDowell:
1. Correct protrusion of the upper $^1/_3$ of the ear (the most critical $^1/_3$).
2. Allow helix to be visible beyond the antihelix on AP view.
3. Give the helix a smooth contour.
4. Avoid a decreased or distorted postauricular sulcus.
5. Achieve appropriate distances from mastoid to helical rim.
6. Achieve symmetry between the two ears within 3 mm at any given point.

9. The varied techniques of otoplasty can be divided into what general groups?
1. Removal of postauricular skin
2. Weakening of antihelical cartilage
3. Shaping the antihelical cartilage into folds
4. Reduction of the conchal bowl if indicated

Most otoplasty techniques can be grouped according to how steps 2 and 3 are performed. Weakening of the antihelical cartilage can be achieved through scoring, thinning (e.g., drilling), or cutting. Shaping of the folds can be accomplished passively after weakening or actively through the use of mattress sutures.

10. What is the Mustardé technique of otoplasty?

The Mustardé technique was described in 1960 and again in 1963 with modifications. This method is the best known and perhaps easiest for correcting prominent ears. The technique essentially involves a postauricular skin excision and placement of permanent horizontal mattress sutures in the cartilage to shape the deficient antihelical fold. Suture placement is planned by using needles through the front of the auricle. When the ink-tipped needles are withdrawn from the cartilage, ink spots are left on the posterior side for suture placement. The primary disadvantages of the Mustardé technique are the possibility that the mattress sutures can become visible under the skin if they are poorly placed. The method also fails to address any excess of conchal bowl cartilage. Most surgeons also will do cartilage weakening techniques and conchal setback sutures (Furnas sutures) to correct the prominent ear more fully.

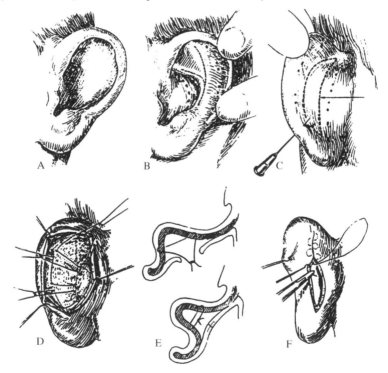

The Mustardé technique of otoplasty. (From Wood-Smith D: Otoplasty. In Rees TD (ed): Aesthetic Plastic Surgery. Philadelphia, W.B. Saunders, 1980, p 851, with permission.)

11. What are other popular methods of otoplasty?

Converse: This method creates an "island" of antihelical cartilage which sits anterior to the rest of the auricular cartilage. This method is technically more complicated than the Mustardé technique but is better suited for thicker cartilage.

Farrior: This method refines the "island" of cartilage. The cartilage island itself is scored to allow additional rolling of the cartilage. This method is technically complicated.

Furnas: This simple technique sets the conchal bowl back to the mastoid periosteum using sutures. It is often used in conjunction with other methods of otoplasty to fully correct the prominent ear. Its main disadvantage is the tendency for the conchal cartilage to protrude into the os of the external auditory canal. Resection of cartilage may be necessary.

12. How can auricular reduction be accomplished?

Auricular reduction is usually only employed when trying to match a smaller reconstructed ear on the opposite side. Such a reduction may be easier than trying to reconstruct the deficient ear to a larger size. Historically, many methods have been described for reducing the auricle. All of these methods involve a geometric excision and closure.

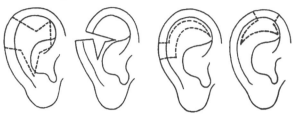

Resection methods for auricular reduction. (From Adamson PA, Tropper GJ, McGraw BL: Otoplasty. In Krause CJ, Pastorek N, Mangat DS (eds): Aesthetic Facial Surgery. Philadelphia, J.B. Lippincott, 1991, p 719, with permission.)

13. How can a protruding lobule be corrected?

The protruding lobule is usually a product of a flared caudal helical cartilage. Resecting this tail of cartilage will make the lobule less protruding. Excessive lobule skin can also be elipsed out on the postauricular side to further reduce the ear lobe. As with auricular reductions, very large lobules can be reduced with a geometric excision and closure of skin. Simple wedge excisions here can be associated with scar contracture and lobule notching.

14. How can a deeply cupped, protruding concha be managed?

An excessively large conchal cartilage must be reduced by removing a crescent of cartilage from the bowl. This can be done through the postauricular incision, or it may be done through a separate, anterior incision hidden in the crease of the antihelix. The protruding concha is laid back on the head using conchamastoid sutures.

15. How can a "cup ear" be corrected?

The cup ear has a constriction of the helix and scapha which requires helical rim unfurling, expansion, and redraping of skin over the expanded cartilage. Most describe techniques which involve dividing the helical-scaphoid cartilage into interdigitating fingers that can then be expanded open in a fanlike manner. Conchal cartilage can be used to stabilize the tips of the framework. Severe cases may require skin grafts or flaps to cover the expanded cartilage. Other techniques of correcting the cup ear deformity involve wedging open the cupped helical rim and rotating a composite flap of skin and cartilage into the opening from the postauricular area.

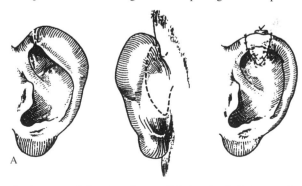

A, Correction of a moderate cup-ear deformity using a pedicled postauricular composite flap. (From Walter C, Trenité JN: Revision otoplasty and special problems. Fac Plast Surg 10:303, 1994, with permission.)

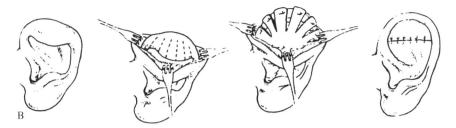

B, Correction of severe cup ear deformity. (From Converse JM: Congenital deformities of the auricle. In Converse JM (ed): Reconstructive Plastic Surgery, 2nd ed. Philadelphia, W.B. Saunders, 1977, p 1708, with permission.)

16. What is a "telephone ear"?

Telephone ear is a deformity caused by overcorrecting the middle third of a prominent ear such that the ear takes on the appearance of a telephone on AP view. Such overcorrection can be due to excessive removal of postauricular skin or mastoid soft tissue or by overtightening conchamastoid sutures.

17. Should a completed otoplasty be covered in dressings?

The completed otoplasty requires a soft cast to support and help define the remodeled cartilaginous folds. Cotton soaked in glycerol or antibiotic ointment will mold well for this purpose. A mastoid dressing should be applied over this cast and maintained for a week. After removal of this dressing, an elastic headband should be used to splint the ears back for an additional 4–6 weeks.

18. Describe the major early complications of otoplasty.

Hematoma is the most worrisome postoperative complication. Failure to investigate the persistent postop pain associated with otoplasty hematoma can lead to perichondritis and a disastrous loss of cartilage. Treatment is immediate evacuation of clot and debridement of necrotic tissue. Other early complications of otoplasty include skin hypersensitivity to pressure or temperature, dressing pressure necroses, and suture spitting.

19. What are the significant late complications?

The most common late complication is inadequate correction. Asymmetries and deformities may require revision otoplasty. Other late complications include scar hypertrophy and keloid formation.

20. What are the five stages of microtia reconstruction otoplasty?

Stage I: **Auricular reconstruction**—Autogenous rib is harvested, fashioned into an auricular cartilage framework, and implanted beneath the skin of the scalp. Usually done at age 6.

Stage II: **Lobule transposition**—A pedicle of preauricular skin is rotated into position at the caudal end of the neoauricle. Done as an outpatient procedure about 2 months after stage I.

Stage III: **Atresia repair**—An otologist corrects the atretic external auditory canal for functional improvement. This stage follows the previous two stages to avoid compromising skin elasticity and vascularity for graft placement.

Stage IV: **Tragal reconstruction**—A composite graft of skin and cartilage is taken from the contralateral ear to create the tragus.

Stage V: **Auricular elevation**—A postauricular incision and skin graft are done to elevate the auricle away from the mastoid.

BIBLIOGRAPHY

1. Adamson PA, Tropper GJ, McGraw BL: Otoplasty. In Krause CJ, Pastorek N, Mangat DS (eds): Aesthetic Facial Surgery. Philadelphia, J.B. Lippincott, 1991, pp 707–720.
2. Aguilar EA III: Major congenital malformations of the auricle. In Bailey BJ (ed): Head and Neck Surgery–Otolaryngology. Philadelphia, J.B. Lippincott, 1993, pp 1535–1541.
3. Aguilar EA III: Otoplasty. In Bailey BJ (ed): Head and Neck Surgery–Otolaryngology. Philadelphia, J.B. Lippincott, 1993, pp 2276–2283.
4. Brent B: The correction of microtia with autogenous cartilage grafts: I. The classic deformity. Plast Reconstr Surg 66:1–12, 1980.
5. Converse JM: Congenital deformities of the auricle. In Converse JM (ed): Reconstructive Plastic Surgery, 2nd ed. Philadelphia, W.B. Saunders, 1977, pp 1707–1719.
6. Lee KJ: Facial plastic and reconstructive surgery: Otoplasty. In Lee KJ (ed): Essential Otolaryngology—Head and Neck Surgery, 6th ed. Norwalk, CT, Appleton & Lange, 1995, pp 824–826.
7. Nachlas NE, Smith HW, Keen MS: Otoplasty. In Papel ID, Nachlas NE (eds): Facial Plastic and Reconstructive Surgery. St. Louis, Mosby, 1992.
8. Ridley MB. Aesthetic facial proportions. In Papel ID, Nachlas NE (eds): Facial Plastic and Reconstructive Surgery. St. Louis, Mosby, 1992, pp 99–109.
9. Siegert R, Weerda H, Remmert S: Embryology and surgical anatomy of the auricle. Fac Plast Surg 10:232–243, 1994.
10. Stark RB: Otoplasty for prominent ears. In Stark RB (ed): Plastic Surgery of the Head and Neck. New York, Churchill Livingstone, 1987, pp 472–483.
11. Tolleth H: Artistic anatomy, dimensions, and proportions of the external ear. Clin Plast Surg 5:337–345, 1978.
12. Walter C, Trenité JN: Revision otoplasty and special problems. Fac Plast Surg 10:298–308, 1994.
13. Weerda H, Siegert R: Complications in otoplastic surgery and their treatment. Fac Plast Surg 10:287–297, 1994.
14. Willett JM, Lee KJ: Otolaryngology: 630 Questions & Answers. Norwalk, CT, Appleton & Lange, 1995.
15. Wood-Smith D: Otoplasty. In Rees TD (ed): Aesthetic Plastic Surgery. Philadelphia, W.B. Saunders, 1980, pp 833–861.

56. RHYTIDECTOMY

Richard A. Mouchantat, M.D.

1. What is rhytidectomy?

Rhytidectomy is the excision, *-ectomy*, of skin to prevent wrinkles, *rhytid*. Or, as commonly known, a facelift.

2. How does the skin age?

Most aging changes occur in the dermal layer of the skin, although there is also atrophy of the facial skeleton and subcutaneous fat. The dermis contains collagen, elastin, and ground substance, all of which diminish with age. The normal collagen in the skin contains types I and III in a ratio of 6:1. This ratio decreases with age. The total amount of elastin, normally 2–4% of the entire volume, also decreases. Wrinkles occur in areas of muscle insertion and facial animation, probably due to a multitude of factors including decreased elasticity and cutaneous thinning.

3. How does ultraviolet radiation affect the skin?

UVA is associated with actinic damage, and UVB is associated with DNA damage and skin cancer. Actinic damage is not simply an acceleration of the aging process. The dermis becomes thickened, and overall, the amount of elastin increases. While there is a decreased amount of type I collagen, there is an increased amount of immature type III collagen. The histologic changes, referred to as **elastosis**, are the result of degraded elastic fibers, which accumulate and thicken the dermis. Common sources of UVA include sunlight, tanning lights, and fluorescent bulbs.

4. What is the SMAS?

The **superficial musculo-aponeurotic system** includes the platysma and risorius, triangularis, and auricularis posterior muscles and is connected to the dermis by fibrous septa. It is a fibrous dissectable layer that can be used to provide traction on facial tissues during rhytidectomy. Although there is some controversy, the SMAS is likely contiguous with the frontalis muscle and may insert into the nasolabial crease. The significance of this structure is its relationship to the nerves in the face, deeper facial motor nerves, and more superficial sensory nerves.

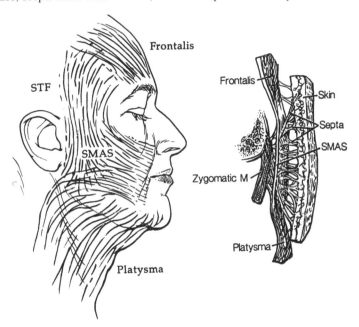

Anatomy of the SMAS. The SMAS is continuous with the platsyma below and the superficial temporal fascia (STF) above. On the right, fibrous septa that connect the skin to the underlying SMAS are demonstrated. (From Rees TD, Aston SJ, Thorne CHM: Blepharoplasty and facialplasty. In McCarthy JG (ed): Plastic Surgery. Philadelphia, W.B. Saunders, 1990, with permission.)

5. Describe the anatomy of the nasolabial fold.

The nasolabial fold is formed by the insertion of muscles originating on the zygoma and the insertion of the thinned SMAS. This fold arises above the nasal ala and descends toward the mandible lateral to the parasymphysis. Of clinical significance, dissection anterior to the fold during facialplasty produces little change in the contour of the nasolabial fold. Patients must be aware of this preoperatively.

6. What are the osseocutaneous retaining ligaments in the face?

These are areas where the skin is attached to the underlying bone or fascia directly. The areas of the bony ligaments are the zygoma and the mandible at the parasymphysis. The ligaments to fascia are to the platysma, the platysma-auricular ligament, and the parotid and masseter area. The significance of these ligaments is that they must be released in order to adequately redrape the skin in a facialplasty.

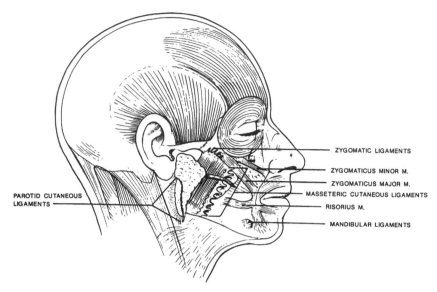

Retaining ligaments of the cheek. (From Stuzin JM, Baker TJ, Gorden HL: The relationship of the superficial and deep facial fascias: Relevance to rhytidectomy and aging. Plast Reconstr Surg 89:441, 1992, with permission.)

7. What are the variations and significance of the platysma muscle anatomy in the midline?

The anatomy of the platysma muscle in the anterior midline has three variations with respect to the decussation of its fibers. In general, fibers either cross at the level of the thyroid cartilage, submentally, or at the mentum. The "turkey gobbler" appearance is caused by a laxity in the platysma that does not decussate across the midline.

8. How do the frontal and mandibular branches of the facial nerve differ anatomically?

The frontal and mandibular branches are terminal branches of the seventh cranial nerve. In only 15% of cases, is there crossover communication between these branches and adjacent branches. The crossover in the rest of the face is approximately 70%. Injury to either the frontal or mandibular branch leaves little chance for alternative pathways to innervate the end motor unit.

9. Describe the course of the frontal and mandibular branches of the facial nerve.

The facial nerve exits the stylomastoid foramen and enters the substance of the parotid gland where it typically divides into five main branches: temporal, zygomatic, buccal, mandibular, and cervical. The **frontal branch** traverses the zygoma deep to the SMAS and through the temporal region on the temporoparietal fascia deep to the superficial temporal fascia. The nerve usually lies within 2 cm of the lateral brow and enters the frontalis muscle on the deep surface.

The **mandibular branch** courses within 1 cm of the inferior border of the mandible, posterior to the facial artery. This relationship changes when the head is turned away, as in surgery, and the nerve may be as far as 3–4 cm below the mandible. The mandibular branch is at risk during an anterior dissection deep under the skin flap because it becomes more superficial. This nerve lies deep to the platysma and superficial to the facial artery.

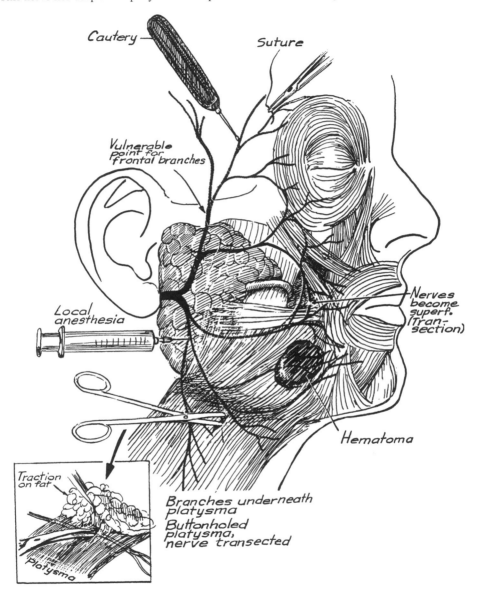

Causes of facial nerve palsy in rhytidectomy. (From Baker DC, Conley J: Avoiding facial nerve injuries in rhytidectomy: Anatomical variations and pitfalls. Plast Reconstr Surg 64:781, 1979, with permission.)

10. Which nerve is injured most commonly in a rhytidectomy?

The greater auricular nerve, which supplies sensation to the skin of the ear and nearby skin, is most commonly injured. The nerve lies deep to the SMAS about 6.5 cm inferior to the external auditory canal in close proximity to the external jugular vein. After emerging from the posterior border of the sternocleidomastoid, it lies on the surface of this muscle.

11. How should nerve injury be treated?
If the injury is noted intraoperatively, the nerve, whether the greater auricular or a facial nerve branch, should be repaired under appropriate magnification. The patient who is recognized postoperatively to have a facial nerve injury can be observed for spontaneous recovery. Recovery may occur in weeks to months, depending on whether the injury is partial and whether it occurs from traction or cautery.

12. What are reasonable goals of rhytidectomy?
Rhytidectomy addresses only the lower two-thirds of the face and neckline. Skin redundancy in the lower face, jowls, laxity of the neck, turkey gobbler deformity, and an obtuse cervicomental angle are all improved. Adjunctive procedures, such as foreheadplasty, blepharoplasty, and skin resurfacing, can often be done in conjunction with rhytidectomy for more complete facial rejuvenation.

13. What four basic types of rhytidectomy are done?
Superficial plane
Sub-SMAS plane
Subperiosteal plane
Composite

14. Discuss some of the advantages and disadvantages of the first three rhytidectomy techniques.
The subcutaneous, or **superficial plane rhytidectomy**, lifts the skin only, which is then safely dissected beyond the nasolabial fold. This technique is one of the oldest and most reliable. This technique provides versatility of access to the SMAS for adjunctive procedures with little risk to the facial nerve. However, it does not provide the improved blood supply to the skin via the SMAS. In addition, the vectors of pull are limited.
The **sub-SMAS technique** offers improved blood supply to the skin, which may be an advantage to smokers. However, the facial nerve is at greater risk, the nasolabial fold is not addressed, and the vectors of pull are limited.
The **subperiosteal dissection** provides vertical lift, redraping of the periorbital area, and good blood supply, and it preserves the relationships between tissues. However, this lifting is less effective in the lower face and does not address the jowls. The subperiosteal procedure can be combined with a cervicoplasty to address these issues.

15. What is a composite rhytidectomy?
The composite rhytidectomy is a combination of sub-SMAS dissection to the masseter and subcutaneous dissection anterior to the lateral border of the masseter to protect the facial nerve. The dissection of both subcutaneous and sub-SMAS planes allows for the skin and SMAS to be re-draped separately, providing multiple directions of pull. However, this technique does not provide the improved blood supply through the SMAS.

16. How is the "turkey gobbler" corrected?
Through a submental incision, the area extending along the inferior border of each mandible is defatted, and the anterior platysma muscle is dissected to define the anatomy. The muscle is then approximated in the midline to eliminate the "cords." There are several methods to achieve this, but most only close the muscle to the level of the hyoid bone. Releasing incisions or transections of the platysma on each side has been described to sling the upper neck and to achieve an acute cervicomental angle.

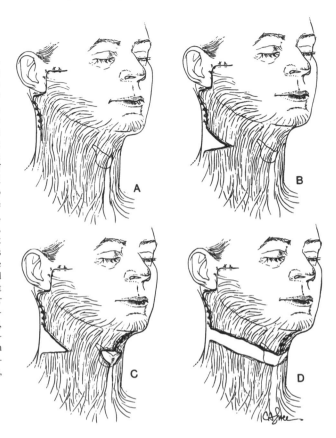

Variations of platysma surgery. *A,* Cephaloposterior advancement of the SMAS-platysma flap without cutting the platysma laterally and without midline alteration. *B,* Rotation of the SMAS-platysma flap with a partial cut across the lateral platysma. *C,* Rotation of the SMAS-platysma flap with a partial lateral cut, plication of the medial platysma borders, and excision of a midline wedge to interrupt the continuity of the bands. *D,* SMAS-platysma flap, full-width platysma transection, and midline plication. Note that full-width transection extends from a level 6 cm below the mandibular angle to the thyroid cartilage. In addition, the cut muscle edges are contoured under direct vision to avoid irregularities in the neck. (From Rees TD, Aston SJ, Thorne CHM: Blepharoplasty and facialplasty. In McCarthy JG (ed): Plastic Surgery. Philadelphia, W.B. Saunders, 1990, with permission.)

17. What is the role of suction lipectomy in facial rejuvenation? What dangers are involved?

Suction lipectomy has been used for contouring the cheeks and submandibular area. Many experts caution against fat excision in the cheeks because of further atrophy during the aging process. It has been useful in the supraplatysmal plane below the mandible to de-fat the anterior neck and improve the cervicomental angle. This can be done through a small submental incision as well as from a lateral approach under the skin flaps. Deep to the platysma, fat excision is dangerous, owing to the location of the mandibular branch of the facial nerve and vascular structures.

18. What are the complications of facelifts?

Major	Minor
Hematoma (4%)	Deformity of the earlobe
Facial nerve palsy (0.8%)	Hypertrophic scarring
Greater auricular nerve injury (5%)	Small hematomas
Skin slough (3.6%)	Infection
Alopecia (1.6%)	Pain

19. How are these complications treated?

Hematoma is heralded by complaints of unusual pain and swelling. Hematomas must be drained surgically in the operating room under sterile conditions. Small hematomas can be aspirated by syringe, and small infections can be drained locally. Skin slough is generally treated expectantly by minimal debridement, as the eschar separates to allow maximal wound contraction and re-epithelialization.

20. What is the effect of smoking on patients undergoing facial rejuvenation?

The rate of skin slough in patients who smoke has been reported to be 12 times that in non-smokers. The effects of nicotine have been studied experimentally and clinically. Nicotine triggers the release of epinephrine and increases platelet adhesiveness, leading to vasospasm and microclots. Cigarette smoke contains carbon monoxide, which impairs oxygen delivery, and hydrogen cyanide, which inhibits oxidative metabolism and oxygen transport. Many surgeons require that a patient abstain from smoking for 2 or more weeks before performing facialplasty.

21. What is the ideal position of the eyebrows in women? In men?

The ideal brow level in women lies just above the superior orbital rim. The shape of the brow individually varies but tends to be a gentle arc with the apex corresponding to the lateral aspect of the limbus. The horizontal level, both medially and laterally, is even. In men, the brow is similar in shape but lies over, not above, the orbital rim.

22. Describe the indications for brow lift.

Brow-lifting is used in patients with eyebrows that are ptotic and to improve lateral upper lid ptosis. The glabellar and transverse frown lines that cause a stern appearance are also improved. Blepharoplasty is frequently performed in conjunction with a brow lift. However, the blepharoplasty must be done after the brow lift to avoid overresection of upper lid skin, leading to lagophthalmos and corneal exposure.

23. Describe the incision and dissection for brow-lifting.

A coronal incision is placed just anterior to the ear and is carried across the top of the head to the opposite side. In variations, the incision follows along the hairline or just posterior to it. The dissection is carried in the subgaleal plane down to 2 cm above the orbital rim. Here, the plane is deepened to the subperiosteal plane to protect the frontal branch of the facial nerve. The dissection is carried over the orbital rim and, on occasion, onto the dorsum of the nose. The frontalis, corrugator supercilii, and procerus are thus exposed and resected as needed. Muscle resection will weaken the forces that contribute to the wrinkling. It also creates a raw surface that can adhere to the periosteum, fixing the flap in position.

24. Are there alternatives to the coronal approach to brow rejuvenation?

Direct full-thickness skin and galea excision can be done on the forehead within the wrinkle lines, but these procedures may leave prominent scars. The glabellar area muscles are accessible through upper blepharoplasty incisions when the indications are hyperactivity of the corrugator supercilii and procerus. A new alternative, endoscopic brow-lifting, appears promising. This may be the procedure of choice for balding men and, as experience grows, may be as versatile as current conventional brow lifts.

25. What additional complications are reported in endoscopic facial plastic surgery?

Recurrence of the ptotic deformity has been reported in endoforehead lifts due to excessive skin and galea redundancy or inadequate fixation. Full-thickness skin burns from the use of cautery during endoscopic surgery and injury from the light source have also been reported.

26. What are the emotional and social considerations when evaluating a patient for rhytidectomy?

Several books have been written on the psychologic aspects of esthetic plastic surgery, as many psychologic considerations accompany this field. The surgeon must assess the patient's motivation for and expectations of surgery. Patients with recent dramatic life changes, such as marital separation, loss of a loved one, or children leaving home, can have unreasonable expectations about what the surgery will do for them. Beware of patients with a long history of plastic surgery. One should also be cautious of patients who denigrate the previous surgeon while praising the current surgeon.

BIBLIOGRAPHY

1. Baker DC, Conley J: Avoiding facial nerve injuries in rhytidectomy: Anatomical variations and pitfalls. Plast Reconstr Surg 64:781, 1979.
2. Barton FE Jr: Esthetic surgery of the face. In Selected Readings in Plastic Surgery. 7(19): 1994.
3. Cardoso de Castro C: The anatomy of the platysma muscle. Plast Reconstr Surg 66:680, 1980.
4. Duffy MJ, Friedland JA: The superficial plane rytidectomy revisited. Plast Reconstr Surg 93:1392, 1994.
5. Goin JM, Goin MK: Changing the Body: Psychological Effects of Plastic Surgery. Baltimore, Williams & Wilkins, 1981.
6. Hamra ST: Composite rhytidectomy. Plast Reconstr Surg 90:1, 1992.
7. Isse NG: Endoscopic forehead lift evolution and update. Clin Plast Surg 22:4, 1995.
8. Mitz V, Peyronie M: The superficial musculo-aponeurotic system (SMAS) in the parotid and cheek area. Plast Reconstr Surg 58:80, 1976.
9. Ramirez OM: The subperiosteal rhytidectomy: The third generation face lift. Ann Plast Surg 28:218, 1992.
10. Rees TD, Aston SJ, Thorne CHM: Blepharoplasty and facialplasty. In McCarthy JG (ed): Plastic Surgery. Philadelphia, W.B. Saunders, 1990.
11. Rees TD, Liverett DM, Guy CL: The effect of cigarette smoking on skin flap survival in the face lift patient. Plast Reconstr Surg 73:911, 1984.

VIII. Trauma and Emergencies

---

57. PRINCIPLES OF TRAUMA

James F. Benson, Jr., M.D.

---

1. What is meant by the trimodal distribution of death?

Death from trauma generally occurs in one of three time frames:

1. Within seconds to minutes after the injury: These patients die as a result of overwhelming trauma and/or head and brain injury. They can rarely be saved.

2. From minutes to hours after the injury: This period is known as the "golden hour," and modern trauma care focuses on these victims.

3. From days to weeks after injury: These patients often succumb to progressive organ failure or sepsis.

2. When approaching a trauma victim, what steps should immediately run through your mind?

The ABCs (or ABCDEs) should immediately be considered and acted upon. This is the initial survey. Next is the resuscitation phase, which is done both after and simultaneously with the initial survey. During this time, the patient receives IV fluids, nasogastric tube, cardiac monitors, necessary x-ray studies, urinary catheter, and laboratory studies. Next is the secondary survey, a head-to-toe exam of the patient. Finally, the patient is definitively treated.

3. What does "ABCDE" stand for?

A—Airway	D—Disability
B—Breathing	E—Exposure
C—Circulation	

4. What do you mean by "airway" in the ABCDEs?

The initial treatment step of the trauma victim involves assessing and stabilizing the airway. This step must be done while maintaining control of the cervical spine. During support of the airway, the airway must be constantly monitored. If the patient's condition deteriorates, the airway management can be adapted.

5. Describe the most common, nonsurgical ways to manage the airway.

- **Chin lift**—The mandible is lifted to bring the chin anteriorly.
- **Jaw thrust**—The entire mandible is displaced forward. This maneuver is an excellent way to ventilate a patient when combined with a facemask and an Ambu bag.
- **Oropharyngeal airway**—This tube is inserted by using either a tongue blade or by inserting it upside down and rotating 180°. It should never be inserted and rotated in children because of the risk of extensive soft tissue injury.
- **Nasopharyngeal airway**—This method is very well tolerated in the awake patient.
- **Orotracheal intubation**—This is the most common of definitive ways to manage the airway. Spinal immobilization must be maintained during intubation.
- **Nasotracheal intubation**—This method is useful in patients with known cervical spine injuries, but should not be used in patients with extensive midface fractures.

6. **Describe two common surgical ways to manage the airway.**

• **Needle cricothyroidotomy**—A large-bore IV catheter (12–16 gauge) is inserted into the cricothyroid membrane. After insertion, high-pressure oxygen is used to ventilate and oxygenate the patient.

• **Surgical cricothyroidotomy**—A skin incision is made over and down to the cricothyroid membrane. By use of either the knife handle or a hemostat, the incision is widened, and a tracheostomy tube is inserted. This procedure is not recommended in children under 12 because of potential damage to the cricoid cartilage.

7. **What is meant by "breathing" in ABCDE?**

Breathing refers to maintaining and aiding ventilation and oxygenation. 100% oxygen should be provided, with the minimum being a tight-fitting reservoir mask. A nasal cannula alone is not sufficient. Proper ventilation can be prevented by correctable injuries to the chest. Pneumothorax (both open and tension), flail chest segments, hemothorax, pulmonary contusion, and diaphragm rupture need to be recognized immediately.

8. **What is meant by "circulation"?**

Circulation refers to the recognition of shock, identification of its probable cause, and the subsequent treatment. Shock is defined as inadequate perfusion of end organs. In the trauma patient, shock is almost always caused by hemorrhage. If an obvious source of bleeding is not found in a patient suffering with shock, an undiagnosed abdominal source should be sought.

9. **How is organ perfusion assessed in the acutely injured patient?**

In the acutely injured patient, pulse, blood pressure, urinary output, skin color, and mental status reflect organ perfusion.

10. **Should CVP monitoring be used in the acutely injured patient?**

While central venous pressure (CVP) monitoring is extremely useful when evaluating patients hemodynamically, it should not be used routinely in the initial management of a trauma patient. It can be time-consuming to set up and cumbersome. In the acutely injured patient, enough information often can be gleaned clinically.

11. **What are the different classes of blood loss? What do they mean?**

Blood loss can be classified as Class I through IV.

Class I	15% of total blood volume
Class II	15–30% of total blood volume
Class III	30–40% of total blood volume
Class IV	> 40% of total blood volume

12. **How do you treat shock?**

The cornerstone to management is vascular access and rapid infusion of warm, isotonic, crystalloid fluids. Two large-bore (18 gauge or larger) lines should be established. In adults, 1–2 liters of IV fluid is the usual initial dose, with 20 ml/kg being the initial dose for pediatric patients. Acutely, it takes approximately 3 ml of crystalloid to replace each 1 ml of blood loss. If more fluid is required, a careful search should be made for an otherwise occult injury. Patients with Class III and IV blood loss often require blood transfusions.

13. **What kind of blood should be given?**

There are three general "flavors" of blood available. Type O blood, the so-called "universal donor," should be used as a last resort in the face of exsanguinating hemorrhage. Specific blood (i.e., B, O, AB, rH+, or rH−) is available in < 15 minutes in most hospitals and is usually the best choice. Fully typed and cross-matched blood most closely resembles the patient's own blood. However, typing and crossing can be a time-consuming task (> 1 hour in many institutions).

14. How is the EKG used in the trauma patient? What should you look for?
All trauma victims should have an EKG acutely. Cardiac contusions can result in a myriad of dysrhythmias, including premature ventricular contractions (PVCs), atrial fibrillation, and ST-segment changes. Electromechanical dissociation can result from a tension pneumothorax, cardiac tamponade, or severe hypovolemia.

15. What is meant by "disability" in ABCDE?
Disability refers to the patient's neurologic status. During the initial survey of the patient, pupil size and reactivity are noted, and the victim's level of consciousness assessed. This is easily done by the AVPU method:
   A—alert
   V—responds to verbal stimuli
   P—responds to painful stimuli
   U—unresponsive
Later, the patient should be assigned a Glasgow Coma Score. Any lateralized extremity weakness should be noted. The patient should constantly be reassessed for any deterioration in the neurologic status.

16. How is the Glasgow Coma Scale measured?
The Glasgow Coma Scale is a standardized assessment of the neurologic impairment of a patient. It assigns a number to a patient's level of consciousness. This number allows comparison to later changes in mental status, at the same or different medical centers. It is the sum of the best verbal, eye opening, and motor scores. Scores of < 8 suggest severe head injury, 9–12 suggest moderate head injury, and > 13 suggest mild head injury.
   Eye Opening
   4   Normal
   3   Responds to speech
   2   Responds to pain
   1   No eye opening
   Verbal
   5   Oriented
   4   Confused
   3   Inappropriate words
   2   Incomprehensible sounds, grunts, groans, etc.
   1   None
   Motor (measured in best extremity)
   6   Moves best extremity to command
   5   Localizes best extremity to pain
   4   Withdraws best extremity from pain
   3   Decorticate posturing
   2   Decerebrate posturing
   1   No movement

17. What is meant by "exposure" in ABCDE?
The patient should be completely undressed to allow for examination of any previously unrecognized injuries.

18. When should monitors be applied and nasogastric tubes and urinary catheters be placed? When should they not?
The placement of catheters and monitors (EKG leads, pulse oximeter) should be done as a routine part of the resuscitation. The initial assessment (ABCDEs) and resuscitation (IV fluids, airway control, and monitors) should proceed simultaneously. Urinary catheters should also be placed unless there is evidence of urethral injury. Evidence of blood at the meatus, blood in the

scrotum, and a high-riding or nonpalpable prostate are contraindications to catheter placement. If a cribriform plate fracture or severe midfacial fractures are present, a nasogastric tube should not be placed.

19. At a minimum, which x-rays should be obtained in a blunt trauma victim?
   An AP chest film, a lateral cervical spine, and an AP pelvis should be obtained as early as possible. Other films should be ordered as the mechanism of trauma suggests. However, any x-ray study should not interfere with the resuscitation of the patient.

20. What should you do when a previously stabilized patient begins to deteriorate?
   Go back to your ABCDEs. Often, an injury is unrecognized, or a previously treated injury remanifests itself. For example, just because a patient did not have a clinically significant pneumothorax on admission, such an injury could declare itself hours later and compromise the patient's life.

BIBLIOGRAPHY

1. Advanced Trauma Life Support: Program for Physicians. Chicago, Committee on Trauma, American College of Surgeons, 1993.
2. Bowen TE: Emergency War Surgery, 2nd ed. Washington, DC, U.S. Department of Defense.
3. Sabiston DC: Textbook of Surgery, 13th ed. Philadelphia, W.B. Saunders, 1986.

58. EPISTAXIS

Anne K. Stark, M.D.

1. A patient presents with epistaxis. What are the key questions in your initial history?
   1. On which side did the bleeding begin?
   2. Has the patient experienced isolated nasal bleeding, or is the patient spitting excessive blood? (The latter may suggest a posterior bleed.)
   3. What has been the duration of bleeding? What is the estimated blood loss?
   4. Is the patient experiencing symptoms of orthostasis or hypovolemia?
   5. Has the patient had a history of previous epistaxis? How has it been treated in the past?
   6. Does the patient have any significant medical problems, such as hypertension, liver disease, alcoholism, or cardiopulmonary disease?
   7. Does the patient take aspirin, warfarin, or nonsteroidal anti-inflammatory drugs (NSAIDs)?

2. What percentage of the U.S. population has had at least one episode of epistaxis in their lifetime?
   About 10%. Therefore, proper and effective treatment skills are obviously of great value.

3. What are the etiologies of epistaxis?
   1. **Local disorders:** Trauma, infection, foreign body, surgical procedures, inflammatory reaction to respiratory tract infections, sinusitis, or chemical irritants
   2. **Neoplastic disorders:** Malignant or benign neoplasms, juvenile nasopharyngeal audiofibromas
   3. **Systemic disorders:** Arteriosclerotic disease associated with hypertension, hepatic disease, chronic nephritis

4. **Hematologic disorders:** Myelomas, leukemias, hemophilias, lymphomas, anemias, hypovitaminoses, chemotherapy, aspirin use, warfarin use, NSAID use

5. **Other:** Sudden pressure changes, hemodialysis

4. Which genetic disorder predisposes patients to severe recurrent nosebleeds?

Osler-Weber-Rendu disease is an autosomal dominant disorder in which vessel walls lack contractile elements and mucosal telangiectasias are present throughout the respiratory and gastrointestinal systems. This condition requires repeated laser coagulation treatment of vessels or skin grafting of the nasal cavity.

5. When does epistaxis become a critical care issue?

Epistaxis, although common, should never be approached casually. Initial clinical assessment should always include ABCs (airway, breathing, circulation) with correction of hypovolemia, as patients may lose over 40% of their blood supply with serious epistaxis.

6. Where is Kiesselbach's plexus located?

Kiesselbach's plexus, also known as Little's area, is a rich anastomosis on the anterior septum. The ophthalmic branch of the internal carotid artery branches into the anterior and posterior ethmoidal arteries, supplying the superior posterior septum. The internal maxillary branch of the external carotid artery branches into the sphenopalatine and descending palatine arteries, supplying the posterior septum. The superior labial branch of the facial artery supplies the vestibule and lower anterior septum. These arteries all join to form Kiesselbach's plexus, where 90% of all nosebleeds occur.

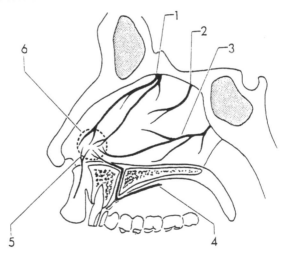

Kiesselbach's plexus: 1 and 2, anterior and posterior ethmoid arteries; 3, septal branch of the sphenopalatine, 4, greater palatine; 5, branch from superior labial; 6, Kiesselbach's plexus. (From Coleman BH: Diseases of the Nose, Throat, and Ear, and Head and Neck. London, Churchill Livingstone, 1992, p 7, with permission.)

7. Does arteriosclerosis predispose to anterior or posterior epistaxis?

Posterior epistaxis is most commonly associated with arteriosclerotic disease. Although this association remains unexplained, it is known that arterial disease is present in these posterior vessels.

8. The patient is bleeding profusely. What initial measures are used to determine the origin of the hemorrhage?

First, position the patient so that you have adequate light and both you and the patient are comfortable. Protect yourself with adequate gowns and eye wear. Remove all clots with suction and bayonet forceps. The application of vasoconstrictive agents such as phenylephrine hydrochloride 0.25% or cocaine 4% will decrease edema and slow active bleeding.

9. You localize the source of bleeding to the anterior septum. Describe your initial treatment.

The patient should be seated, leaning slightly forward, in a position that maximizes visualization of the site. Advise the patient to spit out, not swallow, the blood. Apply local anesthetic, such as 2% lidocaine, prior to cauterization. While visualizing the source with a nasal speculum and a headlight, lightly cauterize the area with a silver nitrate stick. The stick should be held or lightly rolled over the mucosa until a gray residue appears. Because this technique is difficult in the face of heavy active bleeding, electrical suction cauterization may be more effective. One should avoid deep or bilateral cauterization, as it may lead to cartilage damage and subsequent septal perforation.

10. Bleeding persists. What next?

Consider placing an anterior pack.

11. How do you place an anterior pack?

The entire length (72 inches) of a ½-inch Vaseline gauze is coated with antibiotic ointment. With bayonet forceps, the gauze should be grasped 4 or 5 inches from the end. Firmly slide the tip of the forceps along the cavity floor and into the nasopharynx, releasing the forceps only when the tip has reached the extreme posterior nose. Grab the next layer 4 inches from the nostril, positioning it upon the first. Continue to layer these 4-inch strips until the nose is tightly packed. Sufficient tamponading pressure will undoubtedly be uncomfortable for the patient. Taping a 2 × 2-inch sponge at the nostril will secure the packing and collect residual secretions and blood.

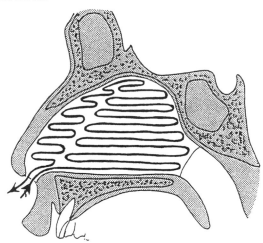

Anterior pack placement. (From Coleman BH: Diseases of the Nose, Throat, and Ear, and Head and Neck. London, Churchill Livingstone, 1992, p 37, with permission.)

12. Is antibiotic treatment indicated with a pack?

Yes. An anterior pack may occlude the sinus ostia, resulting in a sinus effusion. A posterior pack may predispose patients to sinus and middle ear effusions, and there have been several reported cases of staphylococcal toxic shock syndrome associated with packs. Therefore, prophylactic antibiotics with activity against nasal flora and *Staphylococcus aureus* should be used. A cephalosporin or amoxicillin with clavulanic acid is an appropriate choice.

13. A 26-year-old woman presents with severe unilateral epistaxis that requires an anterior pack. She has no prior history of trauma and no family history of bleeding. What studies or lab tests should be done to evaluate her condition prior to unpacking her nose?
- Prothrombin time (PT), partial thromboplastin time (PTT), and bleeding time, as indicated with any diffuse bleeding disorder
- Complete blood count with platelet count to assess for a hematopoietic malignancy
- Sinus x-rays to rule out bone destruction from an occult neoplasm

14. When is a posterior pack indicated?
A posterior pack is indicated in three situations:
1. When the chief complaint is bleeding into the throat,
2. When a posterior nosebleed is visualized, or
3. When an anterior pack cannot be correctly placed to tamponade flow.

15. How do you construct and place a posterior pack?
A posterior pack can be constructed from finely rolled gauze or a 1-in length of vaginal tampon with a $^1/_2$–$^3/_4$-in diameter. In the center, three lengths of 2–0 silk are securely placed. A 14 French catheter is passed through the affected nostril into the nasopharynx and subsequently into the mouth. Two of the three silk ends are secured to the catheter in the mouth. By withdrawing the catheter, the pack may be placed in the affected choana. The combination of traction on the extruded nasal silk with forward finger pressure in the nasopharynx should firmly lodge the pack in place. When properly placed, the pack should not depress the soft palate. One should maintain traction on the two nasal silk ties as an anterior pack is placed. Finally these sutures are secured with a dental roll at the nostril.

Because disfiguring pressure necrosis may develop, the sutures should never be tied across the columella. The third silk suture, protruding from the mouth, may be taped to the cheek for easy pack removal. Alternatively, a no. 14 French Foley catheter with a 30-ml balloon may be used as a posterior pack. The Foley catheter should be inflated with 10–15 ml of saline as air leaks and is ineffective. A balloon catheter is easier to place and is better tolerated than the standard pack, but unfortunately, it is usually less effective.

16. What are the complications of a posterior pack?
Posterior packs may lead to eustachian tube dysfunction, pain, aspiration, and difficulty swallowing. More critical, these patients often have hypoventilation, hypoxia, and hypercapnia, possibly leading to respiratory failure and cardiac arrhythmias. Posterior epistaxis usually occurs in the elderly and is frequently associated with hypertension, atherosclerosis, and conditions that decrease platelets and clotting function. Hospitalization is therefore necessary, and such situations usually mandate intensive care.

17. How long should a posterior pack be left in place?
For 3–5 days.

18. A patient with facial trauma presents with epistaxis. What should be considered before a pack is placed?
Facial bone fractures should be ruled out prior to pack placement. The pressure from a nasal pack or balloon might displace any unstable fractures.

19. Unfortunately, the nose of an otherwise healthy patient continues to bleed despite all packing measures. What is your next step?
Sometimes patients continue to bleed through the packing or rebleed when the packing is removed. At this point, arterial ligation should be considered. If you have localized the bleeding to the superior nose, it is appropriate to ligate the anterior and posterior ethmoidal arteries. If the bleeding originates from the inferior or posterior nose, consider internal maxillary ligation to terminate hemorrhage from the sphenopalatine artery.

20. How is anterior and posterior ethmoidal ligation performed?

An incision is initiated halfway between the inner canthus of the eye and midline of the nose. Carefully cutting through skin, subcutaneous tissue, and periosteum, the surgeon extends the incision superiorly toward the eyebrow. To prevent bleeding, the angular vein should be ligated. The periosteum of the ascending process of the maxillary bone and the anterior lacrimal crest is then elevated. The frontoethmoidal suture should be identified at the superior edge of the lacrimal bone. With the lacrimal sac and orbital periosteum retracted laterally, the frontoethmoidal suture may be traced posteriorly until the anterior ethmoidal artery is identified. The surgeon doubly ligates this vessel with neurosurgical clips, then divides the vessel as it enters the anterior ethmoidal foramen. The posterior ethmoidal artery is then identified. Because it is located about 1 cm from the optic nerve, extreme caution should be used when ligating this artery. The skin is closed, and a pressure dressing is applied to the incision to prevent excessive postoperative edema and ecchymosis.

21. How is internal maxillary artery ligation performed?

The maxillary sinus is entered with a sublabial antrostomy, or Caldwell-Luc approach. First, an incision is made in the gingivobuccal sulcus. The surgeon proceeds to elevate soft tissue and periosteum from the maxilla, thus exposing the canine fossa. Carefully avoiding the infraorbital nerve and vessels, the surgeon opens the maxillary antrum. An opening is made into the pterygopalatine visualization of the vessels. A blunt, right-angle hook may be used to elevate the vessels, which are subsequently clipped. This procedure is more comfortable than packing for the patient, lessening the need for extensive critical care hospitalization. In addition, the complication rate of this procedure is lower than that of posterior packing. For these reasons, several surgeons advocate this procedure when epistaxis can be visually isolated to a sphenopalatine origin and cannot be easily controlled in the emergency room.

BIBLIOGRAPHY

1. Josephson GD, Godley FA, Stierna P: Practical management of epistaxis. Med Clin North Am 75:1311–1320,1991.
2. Lepore ML: Epistaxis. In Bailey BJ (ed): Head and Neck Surgery–Otolaryngology. Philadelphia, J. B. Lippincott, 1993, pp 428–446.
3. Randall DA, Freeman SB: Management of anterior and posterior epistaxis. Am Fam Physician 43:2007–2014, 1991.
4. Rude SW, Parnes SM, Myers EN, Schramm VL: The Management of Epistaxis: A Self-Instructional Package. Rochester, NY, American Academy of Otolaryngology–Head and Neck Surgery Foundation, 1977.
5. Wurman LH: Epistaxis. In Gates GA (ed): Current Therapy in Otolaryngology–Head and Neck Surgery. St. Louis, Mosby, 1990, pp 354–357.
6. Wurman LH, Sack JG, Flannery JV, Lipsman RA: The management of epistaxis. Am J Otolaryngol 13:193–209, 1992.

59. NASAL TRAUMA

James F. Benson, Jr., M.D.

1. Which bone in the body sustains the most fractures?

The clavicle is the most commonly fractured bone in the body, followed by the wrist. The nasal bones are the most commonly fractured facial bones and the third most commonly fractured bones in the body.

2. What are key questions to be asked during the history?

1. When did the trauma occur?
2. What was the mechanism?

3. Did the patient experience epistaxis?
4. Has the appearance of the nose changed?
5. Is the patient experiencing any new onset of nasal airway obstruction?

3. What should you evaluate on the physical exam?

The examiner should evaluate the nose, both internally and externally. Proper lighting (i.e., fiberoptic headlight) and suction are usually necessary. It is best to anesthetize and decongest the mucosa prior to the examination. The septum should be examined for fractures, deviation, perforation, hematoma, and mucosal tears. The lateral nasal wall should be examined in the same manner. The external nose should also be examined in a systemic approach. New nasal deviation should be noted. The nasal bones should be palpated for any instability, motion, or crepitus.

4. How do you confirm the presence of a septal hematoma?

A septal hematoma has a bluish or reddish hue. If someone is not familiar with intranasal exams, it can be easily confused with a deviated septum. A cotton-tipped swab is used to blot the suspected hematoma. A hematoma will blot; a deviated septum will not. If there is still doubt, the swelling can be aspirated to confirm the presence of blood.

5. How do you treat a septal hematoma?

The nasal mucosa is first anesthetized. A scalpel then is used to widely open the hematoma, and the hematoma is drained. A rubber band drain is inserted, and the mucosa is reapproximated with a 4-0 plain gut quilting stitch. The suture can be omitted if the nose is packed bilaterally with Vaseline gauze. If a drain is used, it is removed 24–72 hours after insertion.

6. What else should the physician be alert for in a patient with a nasal fracture?

If trauma to the face is sufficient to fracture the nasal bones, it can also injure surrounding structures. The eye, lacrimal system, paranasal sinuses, teeth, and oral cavity should also be examined. The possibility of a CSF leak should not be overlooked.

7. When should a nasal fracture be reduced?

Most agree that nasal fractures can be reduced in the first few hours after injury. After this, edema makes accurate judgment of the degree of deformity difficult. The next window of opportunity occurs after the edema has resolved but before bony healing has started, generally 3–14 days.

8. What is a closed nasal reduction? How is it performed?

A closed reduction is generally reserved for simple fractures with only minimal displacement. This procedure may be performed in the clinic. After the nose is anesthetized, the surgeon uses a blunt instrument to lift the displaced nasal bones. The bones are then reset into their normal anatomic position. A splint is applied to the dorsum of the nose, and Vaseline-impregnated gauze packing stabilizes the nasal cavity internally.

9. When is a closed reduction not advisable?

If there is severe deformity of the nose. In these cases, an open reduction may be necessary. Likewise, a fractured, displaced septum may best be treated with open reduction and septoplasty.

10. How is an open reduction performed?

An open reduction is performed in the operating room. First, the septum is addressed, and then the nasal pyramids. With the patient under local or general anesthesia, the surgeon makes a **hemitransfixion incision** (an incision along the caudal edge of one side of the septum), and a mucoperichondrial flap is elevated. The bony and cartilaginous septum are exposed and reduced. If the fragments are not reducible and protrude into the airway, the fragments may need to be removed. However, the surgeon should be very conservative when removing any cartilage or bone. At this point, the surgeon should attempt a closed reduction of the nasal pyramid.

If the nasal pyramid is not amenable to a closed reduction, then an open reduction is required. This procedure is similar to a normal rhinoplasty. **Intercartilaginous incisions** (between the upper and lower lateral cartilages) are made, and the periosteum over the dorsal nasal bones is elevated. **Stab incisions** are made laterally at the tips of the inferior turbinates, and the lateral periosteum is similarly elevated. The surgeon again attempts to reduce the nasal pyramid. If adequate reduction is not obtained, then formal medial and lateral **osteotomies** are performed. Osteotomies should free up the fragments adequately to allow proper reduction. When adequate reduction is obtained, the nose is splinted and packed with Vaseline-impregnated gauze.

11. A patient sustained an injury over 2 weeks ago. He now comes to your clinic desiring reduction. What is your next step?

First, examine the patient as you would a new fracture. However, careful attention should be directed to the septum to rule out a septal abscess. These patients usually cannot be adequately reduced at this time. Definitive management, usually a formal septorhinoplasty, should be considered but should not be performed for at least 6 months.

12. How do pediatric fractures differ from adult ones?

It is often necessary to reduce pediatric nasal fractures with the child under a general anesthetic. Pediatric fractures begin to heal more quickly than adult fractures, and reduction becomes difficult in 5–7 days. Injury to growth centers in the nose may become compromised by either the fracture itself or poor surgical management. Conservative management is the key to pediatric injuries. The mechanism of injury should be thoroughly investigated, and child abuse should not be overlooked.

13. What are some late complications of nasal fractures?
• Airway obstruction
• Nasal deformity (secondary to scar contracture/formation, altered growth centers)
• Septal perforation
• Recurrent epistaxis
• Recurrent sinusitis secondary to intranasal anatomic abnormalities

14. What are the most important outcomes in the management of nasal fractures?
Good cosmetic result
Good nasal airway
Normal nasal growth and development in pediatric patients

15. What is a septal abscess?

If a patient develops a hematoma that goes untreated, it may become infected and result in abscess formation. This can occur in as little as 24 hours. The cartilage can rapidly die and be resorbed, resulting in loss of dorsal support and a saddle-nose deformity. The best way to prevent this complication is to evaluate and treat septal hematomas aggressively before they progress.

16. How do you treat a septal abscess?

Like any other abscess. It is opened and drained just as a septal hematoma would be. A drain may or may not be used.

17. Which organisms most commonly cause a septal abscess?

The most common pathogen reported is *Staphylococcus aureus*. Group A streptococci, *Staphylococcus epidermidis*, *Streptococcus pneumoniae*, *Haemophilus influenzae*, and anaerobes have also been reported.

18. What is a good choice for antibiotic coverage in a septal abscess?

When selecting an antibiotic, it is important to consider the initial Gram stain. Because staphylococci are the most commonly encountered organism, a first-generation cephalosporin provides good coverage, even for penicillin-resistant strains. Obviously, the antibiotic should be altered according to the final microbiology report.

19. A little pus in the septum doesn't sound too bad. Can it really lead to serious complications?

Yes. Meningitis, brain abscesses, subarachnoid empyema, cavernous sinus thrombosis, and orbital abscesses have all been reported as complications of septal abscesses. Intercranial extension is believed to result from communication of the anterior septal veins with the veins of the upper lip and palate. In turn, these veins communicate with the facial angular and ophthalmic veins, which communicate with the cavernous sinus. The ethmoidal veins may also contribute with communication to the sagittal sinus.

CONTROVERSIES

20. Should plain films of the nasal bones be ordered?

Studies have shown that plain films of the nasal bones often do not add to or change the management of nasal fractures. In fact, they may be misleading. On the other hand, they may be of medicolegal importance when documenting an injury. Photographs of the nose are very helpful in documenting the nasal appearance before the nose is reduced or surgically modified.

21. Should antibiotics be prescribed for nasal fractures?

There is no evidence to support the routine use of prophylactic antibiotics, although some use antibiotics if the nose is packed. The antibiotic theoretically prevents toxic shock syndrome, although no studies have proved that the use of prophylactic antibiotics prevents toxic shock syndrome. The excellent vascular supply to the nose, in combination with a competent immune system, is usually sufficient to prevent infection.

BIBLIOGRAPHY

1. Ambrus PS, Eavey RD, Baker AS, et al: Management of nasal septal abscesses. Laryngoscope 91:575-582, 1981.
2. Bailey BJ (ed): Head and Neck Surgery–Otolaryngology. Philadelphia, J.B. Lippincott, 1993.
3. Close D, Guinness MDG: Abscess of the nasal septum after trauma. Med J Aust 142:472-474, 1985.
4. da Silva M, Helman J, Eliachar I, et al: Nasal septal abscess of dental origin. Arch Otolaryngol 108:380–381, 1982.
5. Ehrlich A: Nasal septal abscess: An usual complication of nasal trauma. Am J Emerg Med 11: 149–150. 1993.
6. Mathog RH: Atlas of Craniofacial Trauma. Philadelphia, W. B. Saunders, 1992.
7. Paparella MM, Shumrick DA (eds): Otolaryngology. Philadelphia, W.B. Saunders, 1991.
8. Waldron J, Mitchell DB, Ford G: Reduction of fractured nasal bones; Local vs. general anesthesia. Clin Otolaryngol 14:357, 1989.
9. Watson DJ, Parker AJ, Slack RWT: Local vs general anaesthetic in the management of the fractured nose. Clin Otolaryngol 13:491, 1988.

60. PENETRATING NECK AND FACIAL TRAUMA

James F. Benson, Jr., M.D.

1. What are the first management steps in caring for a victim with face and neck trauma?

As with any other trauma victim, the ABCDEs delineate the initial steps. However, patients who sustain injury to the neck and face have a high propensity for airway compromise.

2. Describe the anatomic divisions of the face.

Area 1—superior to the supraorbital rim; contains the forehead.
Area 2—from the commissary of the lips to the supraorbital rim
Area 3—from the hyoid to the commissure of the lips

3. What are the anatomic divisions of the neck?

Zone 1—extends from the sternal notch to the cricoid cartilage
Zone 2—extends from the cricoid cartilage to the angle of the mandible
Zone 3—extends from the angle of the mandible to the base of the skull

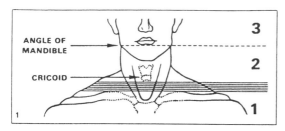

The three zones of the neck are seen on this frontal view. The shaded area represents the portion that some authors consider zone 1 but that others label zone 2. (From Carducci B, et al: Penetrating neck trauma: Consensus and controversies. Ann Emerg Med 15:208–215, 1986, with permission.)

4. What is the mandibular angle plane?

The mandibular angle plane (MAP) is an imaginary vertical plane that runs through the angle and neck of the mandible and through the base of the skull. Any injuries that cross this plane must be assumed to involve the carotid sheath.

5. In facial trauma, how are area 1 injuries evaluated and treated?

After a neurologic exam, a CT scan best evaluates damage to the brain and frontal sinus. Depending on the injury, craniotomy and/or a frontal sinus procedure (obliteration, cranialization, or repair) may be necessary.

6. In facial trauma, how are area 2 injuries evaluated and treated?

After a neurologic exam, ophthalmologic exam, and oropharyngeal exam, a CT of the brain, orbit, and sinuses should be obtained. Orbital involvement requires an ophthalmology consult. Involvement of the maxilla may require surgical exposure and debridement. Severe maxillary involvement may require rigid fixation with plates and/or intermaxillary fixation. Injuries that cross the MAP need to be evaluated with an arteriogram. Facial nerve function should also be carefully documented.

7. How should injury to the parotid duct be managed?

The two ends of the severed duct should be repaired over a small catheter. The catheter should be left in place as a stent for 10–14 days.

8. What treatment is required for transection of the facial nerve?

In general, only nerve injuries proximal to the lateral canthus need to be explored and repaired. If a tension-free reapproximation of the nerve edges is possible, then a primary repair is performed. If not, a cable interposition graft (great auricular or sural nerve) is used to repair the facial nerve. For any deep laceration to the parotid gland, injury to the facial nerve should be assumed until proved otherwise.

9. In facial trauma, how are area 3 injuries evaluated and treated?

After a complete oropharyngeal and neck exam, triple endoscopy should be performed. Again, injuries crossing the MAP need to be evaluated with an angiogram. Mandibular injuries are treated with either intermaxillary fixation or open reduction/internal fixation. A panoramic view (Panorex) is the single best plain film to diagnose mandibular injuries.

10. Which diagnostic test is used to evaluate zone 1 injuries of the neck?

Angiography is the mainstay of zone 1 evaluation. Surgical treatment is via a combined cervical/thoracic approach.

11. Can zone 2 neck injuries be treated without surgery?

These patients can be managed either operatively or nonoperatively. Nonoperative management consists of panendoscopy, angiography, and possibly esophagraphy. Otherwise, surgical exploration of the penetrating wound tract is performed. If the facilities to image the neck are not available, the wound should be explored, the patient's condition stabilized, and then the patient is transferred to another facility. Soft tissue films of the neck are also helpful. Air in the tissues may suggest injury to the aerodigestive tract. Radiopaque foreign bodies, such as bullets, can also be identified. Their location, in conjunction with the site of the entry wound, can be used to hypothesize the missile tract.

12. In neck trauma, how are zone 3 injuries evaluated and treated?

Angiography is the cornerstone of zone 3 evaluation. Zone 3 is a difficult area to evaluate. Cranial nerve injuries are common. Frequent intraoral exams may reveal an expanding retro- or parapharyngeal hematoma. This area is also a difficult one to explore surgically, and a craniotomy may be necessary. Displacing the mandible may also be necessary.

13. What are some signs and symptoms of laryngeal or tracheal injury?

Hoarseness	Voice change	Subcutaneous emphysema
Stridor	Airway obstruction	Hemoptysis

14. What are some signs and symptoms of esophageal or hypopharyngeal injury?

Dysphagia, odynophagia, hematemesis, and subcutaneous emphysema.

15. Vascular injury?

Expanding hematoma, active bleeding, neurologic deficit, and pulse abnormalities may all indicate injury to a major vascular structure in the neck.

16. Name some common mechanisms for blunt trauma to the neck.

Automobile, bicycle, motorcycle, and snowmobile accidents; assaults; and hanging or strangulation attempts.

17. What are some signs and symptoms of blunt laryngeal trauma?

Hoarseness, stridor, voice change, airway obstruction, cough, subcutaneous emphysema, and hemoptysis are often associated with blunt laryngeal trauma. Such trauma may also be associated with loss of the thyroid prominence and loss of the normal crepitus of the laryngeal framework.

18. How is blunt laryngeal trauma diagnosed?

Flexible fiberoptic laryngoscopy and CT scanning of the laryngeal framework are the mainstays of evaluation in these situations. Careful attention should be given to a posteroanterior and lateral chest film and to the anteroposterior and lateral soft tissue neck films. Rigid laryngoscopy and an esophagogram may also be indicated.

19. How is mild blunt laryngeal trauma managed?

Patients with mild cases of blunt laryngeal trauma, which involve only edema or simple mucosal lacerations, can be observed if they are in a monitored hospital bed. Treatment includes humidified air or oxygen, steroids, a soft diet, and frequent evaluations.

20. How is severe blunt laryngeal trauma managed?

Severe cases may require that the airway be secured with a tracheostomy. Intubation and cricothyrotomy may further compromise the airway. Open exploration is then undertaken. Thyroid cartilage fractures can be reduced and wired or sutured in place. If there is gross displacement of the vocal cords, the lumen should be explored either via the fracture itself or a midline laryngofissure. The mucosa should be repaired, the cartilage reapproximated, and the external perichondrium closed. Fracture of the cricoid cartilage is managed by reducing and securing the cartilage and then closing the external perichondrium. If the cricoid ring is too unstable, a stent may be necessary. Rarely, a formal laryngotracheoplasty using rib or auricular cartilage is required.

CONTROVERSIES

21. Should zone 2 injuries of the neck be explored routinely or selectively?

Routine exploration: Proponents base their stance on the low morbidity and mortality of neck exploration. They state that many patients who have sustained a neck injury do better if the injury is found and treated early. They also cite that hospital stays are equal in any case.

Selective exploration: Proponents look at the high rate of negative findings that is associated with mandatory exploration. They also cite the high cost of neck exploration. Studies have shown that the morbidity and mortality from penetrating neck wounds are closely associated with the mechanism of injury, not the style of management.

22. Should stents be used when managing laryngeal trauma?

After major trauma to the larynx and open reduction and fixation of the cartilage, a stent may be necessary to prevent anterior commissure webbing. Conversely, a stent may contribute to the formation of granulation tissue and scarring, especially anteriorly. Therefore, a stent can either help or harm the patient, and no blanket recommendations can be made regarding its use. A decision must be made on clinical grounds.

BIBLIOGRAPHY

1. Ayuyao AM, Kaledzi YL, Parsa MH: Penetrating neck wounds: Mandatory vs. selective exploration. Ann Surg 202:563–567, 1985.
2. Bailey BJ: Head and Neck Surgery–Otolaryngology. Philadelphia, J.B. Lippincott, 1993.
3. Cummings CW, et al (eds): Otolaryngology–Head and Neck Surgery. St. Louis, Mosby, 1993.
4. Gussack GS, Jurkovich GJ: Penetrating facial trauma: A management plan. South Med J 81:297, 1988.
5. Sankaran S, Walt AJ: Penetrating wounds of the neck: Principles and some controversies. Surg Clin North Am 57:139, 1977.

61. UPPER AIRWAY OBSTRUCTION

Tyler M. Lewark, M.D.

1. What is the differential diagnosis of upper airway obstruction?

The causes of upper airway obstruction may be classified in many ways, including by anatomic site. The site of obstruction may occur anywhere along the upper airway from the nose to the carina.

Origins of Upper Airway Obstruction by Anatomic Site

Nasal airway obstruction	**Pharyngeal obstruction**
Upper respiratory infections (bacterial, viral)	Infectious (tonsillitis, pharyngitis, parapharyngeal space
Allergy	abscess, peritonsillar abscess)
Rhinitis medicamentosum	Ludwig's angina
Sinusitis	Foreign bodies
Granulomatous diseases	Pharyngeal tumors (benign, malignant)
Deviated nasal septum	Allergic reactions, angioedema
Nasal trauma (septal hematoma)	**Laryngeal and tracheal airway obstruction**
Foreign bodies	Infectious (epiglottitis, laryngitis, croup, tracheitis, bronchitis)
Nasal tumors (malignant, benign)	Trauma
Choanal atresia	Foreign bodies
Nasopharyngeal obstruction	Laryngeal tumors (benign, malignant)
Adenoid hypertrophy/adenoiditis	Subglottic stenosis
Infectious (tuberculosis, mononucleosis,	Congenital lesions (laryngotracheal malacia)
syphilis)	Gastroesophageal reflux
Nasopharyngeal tumors (benign, malignant)	Tracheal compression
Cysts (Thornwaldt's, encephalocele)	Vocal cord paralysis

From Josephson GD, Josephson JS, Krespi YP, et al: Airway obstruction: New modalities in treatment. Med Clin North Am 77:540, 1993, with permission.

2. What is Ludwig's angina? How is it treated?

Ludwig's angina is cellulitis of the submandibular space and floor of the mouth. It presents as bilateral submandibular swelling with posterior and superior displacement of the tongue. It can result in complete upper airway obstruction, with symptoms of airway compromise occurring in 25% of patients. Additional symptoms include neck swelling with restricted neck movement, neck pain, and, sometimes, trismus. Poor dental hygiene is the most common predisposing condition. Treatment includes management of the airway, antibiotics, and surgical exploration with drainage when indicated.

3. What causes angioedema? How is it treated?

Angioedema can result in life-threatening upper airway obstruction. It is characterized by transient episode of painless, well-demarcated, nonpitting, asymmetric edema of the face, lips, tongue, mucous membranes, and eyelids. About 20% of patients with angioedema suffer severe upper airway obstruction. It has many causes, including allergic IgE-mediated reactions, hereditary angioneurotic edema, acquired deficiency of C1 esterase inhibitor, and many prescription medications. It may also be idiopathic. Treatment includes management of the airway with subsequent therapy directed toward the underlying cause, if known.

4. Describe the symptoms of upper airway obstruction.

The common symptoms of acute upper airway obstruction include dyspnea, dysphagia, local pain, coughing, choking, and voice change. These nonspecific symptoms can may be associated with any degree of airway obstruction. Progressive dyspnea suggests an increasing degree of obstruction. There may be deceptively few symptoms except progressive dyspnea with nearly complete airway obstruction.

5. List the signs of upper airway obstruction.

Physical examination is vital for the diagnosis of upper airway obstruction.

1. **Stridor**, or noisy respiration due to obstruction of airflow, is the hallmark finding. Stridor due to obstruction from the larynx or above is usually inspiratory, while distal obstruction is often expiratory, and midtracheal involvement may be biphasic.

2. **Suprasternal retractions** may be evident. All forms of airway obstruction may be accompanied by accessory respiratory muscle prominence. However, obstruction below the thoracic inlet does not result in suprasternal retractions. Retractions of the sternal notch and midline neck and muscle activity of the sternocleidomastoid indicate obstruction of the upper airway.

3. **Abnormal** voice may be present. Hoarseness suggests laryngeal involvement. A muffled voice may be due to supraglottic obstruction. Lack of the glottic stop or a weak cry implicates vocal cord paralysis.

4. **Fever** suggests an infectious cause.

5. **Restlessness** is a sign of airway obstruction and should be considered a sign of hypoxia.

6. **Drooling** may be caused by a decrease in the function of the pharyngeal neuromuscular apparatus when it is traumatized or infiltrated with blood.

7. **Bleeding** is a sign of mucosal disruption.

8. **Subcutaneous emphysema**, or air in the soft tissues, is diagnostic of a rupture in the continuity of the aerodigestive tract.

9. **Palpable fracture** involving any portion of the laryngeal or tracheal cartilage or facial skeleton may be present with trauma.

6. What is the definitive diagnostic tool for evaluating upper airway obstruction?

Abnormalities of the entire upper airway can be accurately assessed with endoscopy. **Nasopharyngoscopy** with a flexible nasopharyngoscope can assess the airway from the nasal alae to the level of the vocal cords or subglottic larynx. **Bronchoscopy** allows evaluation of the trachea and bronchi. A flexible bronchoscope can be used to assess the dynamic aspects of the upper airway without the distorting forces that occur during rigid bronchoscopy. The rigid bronchoscope permits active intervention in cases such as foreign body removal.

7. Are laboratory tests helpful when evaluating a patient with suspected upper airway obstruction?

In general, no. Blood gases may help define the degree of hypoxia or identify an acid-base disorder. However, decisions regarding the need for endotracheal intubation or tracheotomy should not be based solely on blood gas results in an acute situation, as a patient with near-obstruction may have normal-appearing blood gases.

8. Are plain film radiographs helpful when evaluating upper airway obstruction?

Plain chest films can be a useful screening study. They may identify tracheal deviation, compression, foreign bodies, or vascular abnormalities. A cervical spine film should be assessed early in management of the patient with upper airway trauma. The condition of the cervical spine should be known when making decisions regarding head positioning for intubation or tracheotomy. Croup and epiglottitis may be identified with neck films that are taken during inspiration. A lateral soft tissue film of the neck emphasizes the laryngeal and tracheal air column. Findings such as supraglottic edema and obliteration of the laryngeal ventricle may be identified. Radiographs of the face may be useful when evaluating the patient with trauma associated airway obstruction.

9. Which causes of upper airway obstruction may be identified with computed tomography (CT)?

CT scan may be helpful when evaluating the mediastinum in cases of tumors and compressive airway lesions. In addition, contrast enhancement can help define vascularity. A disadvantage of CT is its inability to image the trachea along its long axis.

10. When does spirometry play a role in the evaluation of upper airway obstruction?

Spirometry is often one of the first tests ordered when evaluating upper airway obstruction electively. Because it is relatively insensitive, it does not have a role when managing the patient in acute respiratory distress.

It has been estimated that luminal obstruction of > 80% is required before an abnormality is seen on a flow-volume loop. Although symptoms usually present when the obstruction is advanced, flow-volume loop analysis may indicate the functional severity of the obstruction. A sawtooth appearance is a nonspecific sign of upper airway obstruction seen in neuromuscular diseases, Parkinson's disease, laryngeal dyskinesia, and after upper airway burns. Sawtooth patterns are also seen in 10% of normals. A double-hump pattern in the expiratory portion of the loop may indicate an obstructing lesion that has an intrathoracic and then extrathoracic location, varying with the expiratory maneuver or with neck flexion and extension.

11. What therapeutic options are available for treating acute upper airway obstruction?

One possible option is **observation** without intervention. A mild to moderate airway problem may be judged to be clinically stable in cases of traumatic, infectious, or neoplastic disease. Various forms of **medical therapy** may be instituted with observation of the patient. This decision must be made with care, and the physician must be prepared to intervene rapidly if the patient's condition deteriorates. Observation must occur in an intensive care unit with personnel present who can capably assess the airway and intervene if necessary. Various types of **artificial airways** may be employed and can be quite useful. **Endotracheal intubation** may be necessary when medical therapy or simple measures fail. If intubation is unsuccessful, placement of a **surgical airway** is necessary to ensure adequate ventilation.

12. What pharmacologic agents may be useful when treating upper airway obstruction?

Increasing the amount of **oxygen** can be accomplished with a face mask. The addition of humidification may help to liquefy secretions and improve clearance of partially obstructing secretions.

Racemic epinephrine is useful when vasoconstriction and decreased mucosal edema are desired. In the treatment of croup, racemic epinephrine decreases morbidity, mortality, and length of hospital stay. Racemic epinephrine is usually not effective in treating epiglottitis and may, in fact, be deleterious. Some clinicians also use this drug as empiric treatment in laryngeal edema.

Corticosteroids are thought to reduce airway edema and are used in croup and to prevent post-extubation laryngeal edema. However, there appears to be no benefit of routine steroid use to prevent post-extubation laryngeal edema. There are no significant data suggesting that short-term corticosteroid use has a detrimental effect when delivered in bolus form.

Antibiotics should be administered with any suggestion of infection or transmucosal injury.

13. Are helium-oxygen treatments a definitive treatment for upper airway obstruction?

Helium-oxygen treatments involve administering an 80% helium/20% oxygen mixture to the patient with upper airway obstruction. The lowered density of this mixture reduces airway resistance to turbulent flow and thus decreases flow-resistive work. In addition, the decreased pressure gradient required to produce a specific flow may decrease the tendency of the airway to collapse distal to the obstruction. These treatments have been used in several upper airway obstruction conditions, including post-extubation stridor in children, tracheal stenosis or compression, status asthmaticus, and angioedema. Helium-oxygen treatments are not a definitive treatment for upper airway obstruction. They may, however, serve as a temporizing measure while awaiting resolution of the disorder or definitive therapy.

14. List the types of artificial airways that are available and their indications.

1. The **oral airway** is a curved, semirigid device that is usually plastic and is inserted through the oral cavity. It can be used to bypass an obstruction in the nose or mouth. The disadvantage is that it is not well tolerated and is easily dislodged by a struggling or semiconscious patient.

2. The **nasopharyngeal airway** is useful for maintaining an airway in the patient who is recovering from general anesthesia or obtunded after a mild to moderate head injury. The device is usually soft and trumpet-shaped. It is much more readily tolerated by patients than the oral airway.

3. The **esophageal airway** is inserted blindly into the esophagus, and a balloon is distended. Air insufflated through the device into the hypopharynx provides ventilation. Significant problems can occur with its use, including inappropriate placement in the larynx leading to complete airway obstruction following balloon distention. It can also lacerate the esophageal mucosa or worsen an evolving supraglottic edematous process.

15. What are the indications for endotracheal intubation?

Endotracheal intubation is indicated to improve respiratory toilet, assist ventilation, relieve obstruction, and prevent aspiration. Endotracheal intubation may be used for long periods of time in neonates and the extensively burned patient. In general, however, it should be considered a short-term solution over periods of 10 days to 2 weeks. To prevent damage to the larynx and trachea from prolonged intubation, tracheotomy should be performed if ventilatory support will be needed for longer than 2 weeks.

16. What are its contraindications?

The presence of a **cervical spine fracture** is a relative contraindication to transoral intubation. This is due to the concern that neck hyperextension with intubation may complete an unstable or incomplete neurologic injury. **Laryngeal trauma** is also a relative contraindication to endotracheal intubation, as passage of the tube through an injured larynx may be difficult and may further aggravate the injury. **Severe oral trauma** may preclude the surgeon's obtaining an adequate view of the vocal cords due to blood or trismus.

17. What are the advantages and disadvantages of orotracheal intubation?

Advantages: This procedure allows full control of ventilation and prevents aspiration.

Disadvantages: It requires expertise and proper equipment. It may cause injury to the larynx and/or pharynx.

18. How is orotracheal intubation performed?

To perform adequate orotracheal intubation, the clinician must have endotracheal tubes of varying sizes, a stylet to give rigidity to the tip of the tube, adequate suction, and a laryngoscope. Ideally, the patient is placed in the "sniffing position" with the neck flexed slightly on the chest and the head extended slightly on the neck. For the right-handed clinician, the laryngoscope is directed with the left hand into the right aspect of the mouth while pushing the tongue to the left. The curved-blade laryngoscope (MacIntosh) is directed into the vallecula, and the larynx is lifted anteriorly or ventrally to expose the glottis. The straight-blade laryngoscope (Miller) is introduced under the epiglottis, fixing the larynx at the petiole of the epiglottis and lifting the larynx anteriorly to expose the glottis. The endotracheal tube is inserted with the right hand. An assistant can provide slight cricoid pressure. This maneuver helps the clinician to visualize the larynx and helps to prevent the patient from aspirating gastric contents.

19. What are the advantages and disadvantages of nasotracheal intubation?

Advantages: Nasotracheal intubation maintains the airway, facilitates suctioning, is simple to perform, and is well tolerated by alert patients.

Disadvantages: It can cause epistaxis, and it requires normal ventilatory support.

20. What are the indications for nasotracheal intubation?

Nasotracheal intubation is used when:
1. It is important to leave the oral cavity clear of obstruction for operative procedures;
2. Cervical spine injury is suspected;
3. Prolonged intubation is expected; and
4. Orotracheal intubation is impossible.

21. How is nasotracheal intubation performed?

When this procedure is performed electively, the nasal cavity is topically anesthetized and decongested. Dilatation of the nasal cavity is performed with progressively larger nasal airways, which are coated with viscous lidocaine. The tube is then introduced transnasally into the pharynx, and a laryngoscope is inserted through the mouth. Magill forceps are then used to grasp the tube and insert it through the glottis.

Intubation over a fiberoptic bronchoscope may be attempted if a difficult intubation is expected. In these cases, the nose is prepared as described, and topical anesthesia may be applied to the larynx and pharynx. The bronchoscope is introduced through the tube and into the nose, larynx, and cervical trachea. The endotracheal tube is advanced over the bronchoscope and into the trachea with subsequent withdrawal of the bronchoscope.

Blind nasotracheal intubation may be attempted in patients with suspected cervical spine trauma and in patients who are awake when there is no time to administer anesthesia.

22. What are the acute complications of endotracheal intubation?

Acute pulmonary edema may be seen when the obstruction is relieved in the patient who has labored under partial airway obstruction for some time. This is thought to be due to the sudden loss of highly negative intrathoracic pressures during inspiration and positive pressures during expiration. The subsequent rapid increase in systemic venous return and pulmonary hydrostatic pressure creates an imbalance in pressure gradients across the alveolar membrane. Frothy fluid from the endotracheal tube or hypoxia with inadequate ventilation may be seen in the recovery room. Diuretics with institution of mechanical ventilation and positive end-expiratory pressure are the treatment for this complication.

Improper tube placement is a possible complication of endotracheal intubation. An endotracheal tube may be inadvertently placed into the esophagus, with ventilation resulting in gastric distention and hypoxia. The tube may also be passed through the pyriform sinus into the soft tissues of the neck during an intubation when excessive force is used. Often the tube is placed too far inferiorly, resting in the right mainstem bronchus. This presents as inadequate breath sounds on auscultation of the left chest.

23. List the complications of long-term endotracheal intubation.

Laryngeal stenosis may result from long-term endotracheal intubation, and most clinicians opt for timely tracheotomy to avoid this complication. Tube motion, infection, and high cuff pressures will exacerbate this injury. To minimize the chance of this complication, the smallest size tube that allows adequate ventilation should be used. In addition, the cuff should be inflated to the minimal occlusion volume. Chronic intubation may also lead to the formation of a **tracheoesophageal fistula**. The concomitant presence of both an endotracheal and a nasogastric tube may increase the incidence of this complication. **Recurrent laryngeal nerve injury** may occur from long-term intubation. The nerve is at risk because it may be pinched by the tube at its location near the articulation of the cricoid and thyroid cartilages. **Sinusitis** is common in patients who are nasotracheally intubated for more than several days. Obstruction by the tube at the normal drainage site of the paranasal sinuses predisposes to the development of purulent sinusitis.

24. A patient in the emergency room has upper airway obstruction and serious hypoxia. You are unable to secure an endotracheal tube. What do you do?

This patient requires a surgical airway to ensure adequate ventilation and relieve the hypoxia. **Transtracheal needle ventilation** is useful in the emergency setting and provides rapid ventilatory control while a patient is being stabilized prior to more definitive measures. A large-bore needle is directed through the cricothyroid membrane and attached to an oxygen line under pressure. The patient may be ventilated for at least 30 minutes.

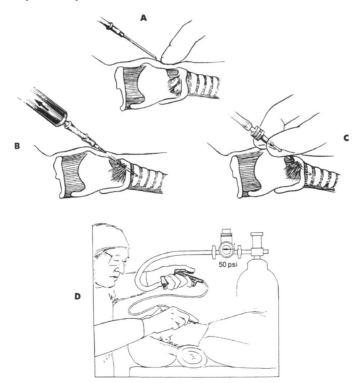

Transtracheal needle ventilation. *A,* Area of penetration identified. *B,* Sheathed needle inserted through cricothyroid membrane; trachea identified when air is aspirated. *C,* Needle removed; plastic cannula attached to jetting device; stabilized by hand. *D,* Transtracheal ventilation monitored by observing chest wall excursion. (From Weymuller EA: Airway management. In Cummings CW, et al (eds): Otolaryngology—Head and Neck Surgery. St. Louis, Mosby, 1986, p 2423, with permission.)

Cricothyroidotomy is the procedure of choice with total upper airway obstruction. A horizontal incision is made through the cricothyroid membrane and a tracheotomy tube is inserted into the trachea. The cricothyroidotomy may be converted to a formal **tracheotomy** at a later time if necessary. Urgent tracheotomies should be performed by the most experienced surgeon available.

CONTROVERSY

25. When is the placement of an airway stent necessary?
After laryngeal or tracheal stenosis reconstruction and after acute traumatic injury, airway stenting is done to counteract scar contracture and provide support for healing. While many advocate the use of stents in these circumstances, others argue that they cause additional trauma to the airway. The type of stent to use and duration of stenting are also controversial.

BIBLIOGRAPHY

1. Aboussouan LS, Stoller JK: Diagnosis and management of upper airway obstruction. Clin Chest Med 15:35–53, 1994.
2. Drake AF: Controversies in upper airway obstruction. In Bailey BJ (eds): Head and Neck Surgery–Otolaryngology. Philadelphia, J. B. Lippincott, 1993, pp 912–922.
3. Gallagher TJ: Endotracheal intubation. Crit Care Clin 8:665–677, 1992.
4. Josephson GD, Josephson JS, Krespi YP, et al: Airway obstruction: New modalities in treatment. Med Clin North Am 77:539–549, 1993.
5. Weissler MC: Tracheotomy and intubation. In Bailey BJ (ed): Head and Neck Surgery–Otolaryngology. Philadelphia, J. B. Lippincott, 1993, pp 711–724.
6. Weymuller EA: Airway management. In Cummings CW, et al (eds): Otolaryngology–Head and Neck Surgery. St. Louis, Mosby, 1986, pp 2417–2432.

62. THE MANDIBULAR FRACTURE

Kent E. Gardner, M.D., and Steven B. Aragon, M.D., D.D.S.

1. How are mandibular fractures classified?
1. Anatomic location of the fracture
2. Condition and position of the teeth relative to the fracture
3. The "favorability," or displacement, of the fracture
4. Type of fracture (e.g., greenstick, simple, compound, comminuted)
Each of these factors plays a role in choosing an approach to treatment.

2. Describe the anatomic classification of mandibular fractures.
The anatomic components of the mandible include the body, angle, ramus, coronoid process, condyle, alveolar process, and the symphysis/parasymphysis.
Symphyseal or parasymphyseal fractures occur anteriorly between the two lower canine teeth.
Body fractures occur between the distal aspect of the canines and a hypothetical line which corresponds to the anterior attachment of the masseter. This anterior border of the masseter is located at approximately the second or third molar.
Angle fractures occur in a triangular region located between the anterior border of the masseter and the posterosuperior insertion of the masseter, which is distal to the third molar.
Ramus fractures occur between the angle and the sigmoid notch.
Coronoid fractures simply involve the coronoid process.

Condylar fractures may involve the intracapsular portion of the condylar head, within the temporomandibular joint (TMJ), or the neck of the condyle, also known as the subcondylar region.

Alveolar process fractures are isolated to the teeth-bearing portion of the mandible.

3. What are the most commonly fractured sites of the mandible?

Weak areas of the mandible include the angle (especially when impacted third molars are present), the anterior body or parasymphyseal area (where the mental foramen exists), and the neck of the condyle (the subcondylar area) due to the small bone mass in this area. In order of decreasing frequency, the most common sites for fracture are the condyle (36%), body (21%), angle (20%), symphysis (1%), parasymphysis (14%), ramus (3%), alveolar process (3%), and coronoid process (2%).

4. How does the presence of teeth in the fracture segments affect treatment?

Teeth are important because they are the key to reduction, stabilization, and immobilization in fracture repair. In 1949, Kazanjian and Converse classified mandibular fractures according to the presence or absence of teeth in the fractured segments.

Class I fractures have teeth present in the fragments on both sides of the fracture and are therefore amenable to closed reduction with maxillo-mandibular fixation.

Class II fractures have teeth in only one of the two fracture segments. While the teeth can be used for fixation of that particular segment, the edentulous segment may require a splint or internal fixation if unstable.

Class III fractures occur in edentulous patients and are always treated with either open reduction with internal fixation or closed reduction with splints (e.g., dentures).

5. What muscles insert into the mandible? What is the action of each muscle?

Muscles that insert into the mandible can be divided into anterior and posterior groups. The **anterior group** consists of the mylohyoid, geniohyoid, genioglossus, platysma, and the anterior belly of the digastric. The anterior muscles depress and retract the mandible. The **posterior muscles** are the major muscles of mastication including the temporalis, masseter, and the medial and lateral pterygoids. The lateral pterygoid muscle inserts into the TMJ capsule and condylar neck. This muscle protrudes and depresses the mandible and causes the mandible to move toward the opposite side. The medial pterygoid inserts into the medial ramus. This muscle raises and protrudes the mandible and also causes the mandible to move toward the opposite side. The masseter inserts into the lateral ramus and coronoid process. This muscle raises and retracts the mandible. The temporalis inserts into the coronoid process and anterior border of the ramus. It also raises and retracts the mandible. Each of the anterior and posterior muscles can cause the distraction of fracture segments in unfavorable fractures.

6. Contrast favorable and unfavorable mandibular fractures.

Mandible fractures are described as favorable when muscles tend to draw the bony fragments together. They are unfavorable when the fragments are distracted or displaced by muscle forces. Fractures may be vertically or horizontally unfavorable. Vertically unfavorable fractures allow fracture segments to be distracted in a horizontal direction. Horizontally unfavorable fractures allow fracture segments to be distracted in a vertical direction. Favorable fractures can be treated with closed reduction, while unfavorable fractures tend to need open reduction with internal fixation.

Almost all fractures of the angle are unfavorable. This is due to the action of the masseter, temporalis, and medial pterygoid which distract the proximal segment superomedially. Subcondylar fractures tend to be unfavorable due to the action of the lateral pterygoid which distracts the condyle anteromedially. Most vertically unfavorable fractures tend to occur in the body and symphysis-parasymphysis region. The anterior segments of vertically unfavorable body and symphysis fractures are displaced posteromedially by the mylohyoid and other suprahyoid muscles.

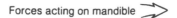

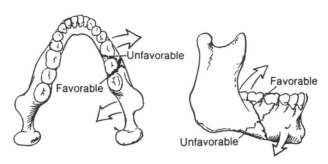

Forces acting on the mandible. Left, vertical plane; right, horizontal plane. (From Lowlich RA, Goodwin WJ: Facial and airway trauma. In Lee KJ (ed): Essential Otolaryngology, 6th ed. Norwalk, CT, Appleton & Lange, 1995, with permission.)

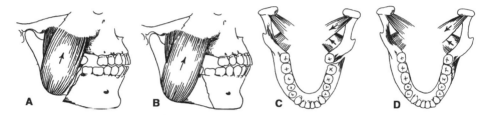

Mandibular fracture angulations and their relationship to muscle pulls. A, Horizontally unfavorable; B, horizontally favorable; C, vertically unfavorable; D, vertically favorable. (From Stanley RB: Pathogenesis and evaluation of mandibular fractures. In Mathog RH (ed): Maxillofacial trauma. Baltimore, Williams & Wilkins, 1984, with permission.)

7. When describing teeth, how does the universal numbering system work?

The **universal numbering system** assigns a number from 1 to 32 to each tooth in the adult permanent dentition. The number 1 is assigned to the right maxillary 3rd molar. Numbering then proceeds across the maxilla to the left maxillary 3rd molar, which is numbered 16. Similarly, numbering moves down to the left 3rd mandibular molar, number 17. Proceeding across the mandible to the right 3rd mandibular molar, number 32, the system completes a full circle.

In children, the **universal lettering system** assigns the letters A through T in a similar fashion to the 20 deciduous teeth.

8. Describe the course of the inferior alveolar nerve.

The mandibular nerve is the third division (V_3) of the trigeminal nerve, which exits the base of the skull through the foramen ovale. It then branches into the lingual and inferior alveolar nerves. The inferior alveolar nerve enters the mandible through the mandibular foramen near the lingula on the medial aspect of the ramus. It courses through the mandible and exits anteriorly through the mental foramen. The mental foramen is located just below the first or second bicuspids. After exiting the foramen, the nerve is referred to as the **mental nerve**. The mental nerve supplies sensation to the lower lip and chin.

9. What is the angle classification of occlusion?

The angle classification describes the dental relationship between the maxillary and mandibular first molars. In the **Class I** relationship, the mesiobuccal cusp of the maxillary first molar lies in the buccal groove of the mandibular first molar. This is accepted as the desired or normal occlusion. **Class II** occlusion is present when the maxillary cusp is anterior to the mandibular buccal groove. The maxilla protrudes more than the mandible (i.e., an overbite). This malocclusion may be due to a protrusive maxilla, a retrognathic mandible, or a combination of both. In **Class III** occlusion, the mesiobuccal cusp of the maxillary first molar is posterior to the buccal groove of the mandibular first molar. Thus, the maxilla is positioned more posteriorly than the mandible (i.e., an underbite). This condition may be due to a retrognathic maxilla, prognathic mandible, or a combination of both.

10. What are the most common signs and symptoms of mandibular fractures?
  1. Pain
  2. Malocclusion
  3. Paresthesia in the distribution of the mental nerve
  4. Mucosal lacerations
  5. Trismus
  6. Fracture step-off or crepitance
  7. Floor of the mouth hematoma (symphyseal fractures)
  8. Impaired translational mobility or protrusion of mandible (condylar fractures)
  9. Unilateral or bilateral open bite (unilateral or bilateral posterior mandibular fractures)
  10. Bloody otorrhea due to external auditory canal laceration

11. Do patients with mandibular fractures need antibiotics?
   Any fracture that communicates with the oral cavity via a laceration or is in contact with an erupted tooth is considered to be a compound fracture. Such fractures are contaminated and require antibiotic therapy. Penicillin or other antibiotics that cover the oral flora are the usual choice. Antibiotic prophylaxis should be continued until the gingiva, periodontia, and mucosa have completely healed, a process which can take from 24 hours to 2 weeks.

12. What x-rays should be taken if a mandibular fracture is suspected?
   Traditionally, the mandibular series has included several views of the mandible in order to view the entire mandible adequately. These have included anteroposterior and bilateral oblique views to assess the symphysis, parasymphysis, body, angle, and ramus. Special views (Towne projection) are often required to assess the medial or lateral displacement of the condyle. The panoramic view (Panorex) has become the single most useful radiograph for assessment of the entire mandible. While a good panoramic radiograph will show the anterior displacement of the condyle, it may not reveal medial displacement, which is seen more easily on the Towne view.

13. What techniques are used in the closed reduction and fixation of mandibular fractures?
   Many techniques of closed reduction have been utilized. Closed reduction techniques assume that a fracture is reduced when a patient is placed into normal occlusion. Fixing the teeth into their normal occlusion is known as **maxillomandibular fixation** (MMF), formerly known as intermaxillary fixation (IMF).
   One commonly used technique to achieve MMF involves Erich arch bars, which are stainless steel bars with small blunt hooks. The bars are applied to both the mandible and maxilla by a series of stainless steel wires which are wrapped around each of the patient's teeth. The upper and lower arch bars are then solidly fixed to each other by elastics or stainless steel wires.
   Other techniques used to achieve MMF include the use of wires without arch bars (e.g., Ivy loops, Risdon wires), dental splints, and dentures. Dentures are fixed to the mandible and maxilla with wires or screws and then are fixed to each other.

14. What techniques are available for open reduction and internal fixation (ORIF) of mandibular fractures?
   When performing ORIF, the surgeon uses metal plates with screws, interosseous wires, and lag screws. When using **metal plates with screws**, the surgeon first places the patient in MMF to reduce the fracture and obtain proper occlusion. Next, an intraoral or external approach is used to

expose the fracture, and metal plates are used to stabilize the fracture line. The mandible has complex stresses (compression and tension) due to its unique articulation to the skull at the TMJs and the effects of the muscles of mastication. In general, both compression and tension forces must be addressed to stabilize the fracture adequately. For example, in mandibular body fractures, **compression** stresses occur along the inferior border of the mandible and are managed by placing one plate across the inferior aspect of the fracture. These plates must conform perfectly to the contour of the mandible and ideally lie at right angles to the direction of the fracture. A variety of plates is available, including compression and noncompression plates. **Tension**, in body fractures, occurs along the superior border of the mandible and tends to cause distraction or separation of the fracture segments superiorly. This can be addressed with a smaller plate (placed along the superior mandible), wires, or an arch bar to resist tension and maintain proper reduction. Because metal plates can impart total stabilization of the fractured mandible, patients may actually function without MMF when rigid internal fixation is used.

When utilizing **intraosseous wiring**, the surgeon threads stainless steel wire through holes which are drilled in the bone segments on either side of the mandibular fracture. This wire is then twisted onto itself until the fracture segments are held in close approximation. Interosseous wires do not provide rigid internal fixation and total stability of the fractured segment. Therefore, patients require additional stabilization and immobilization, which can be provided with MMF or splints, for 4–6 weeks.

15. How are lag screws used?

Lag screws are long bicortical screws that are placed through the superficial cortex of one fracture segment, across the fracture line in an oblique direction, and into the deep cortex of the opposite fracture segment. The proximal segment and cortex are overdrilled so that the diameter of the hole is larger than the screw. The threads of the lag screw then engage the distal fragment only. As the screw is tightened the distal segment is drawn into tight approximation with the proximal segment. Often, more than one lag screw is used to avoid rotation of the fracture line. Because lag screws can provide rigid internal fixation and total stabilization and prevent interfragment mobility, patients do not require additional periods of MMF. Lag screws are best used in oblique fractures, which may occur in the symphysis, parasymphysis, and anterior body of the mandible.

16. How do you treat a patient with a symphyseal or parasymphyseal fracture?

Fractures in the symphysis-parasymphysis region are often unstable due to the forces of the suprahyoid musculature. Unfavorable fractures can be associated with collapse of the mandibular arch and therefore usually require ORIF or MMF in combination with an acrylic lingual splint. The lingual splint prevents collapse of the mandibular fragments. ORIF can be performed with a variety of techniques through either an intraoral or external approach. The most common technique is the placement of a dynamic compression plate along the inferior border in combination with a tension band arch bar or a miniplate for superior stabilization. An alternative is the placement of an intraosseous wire at the inferior border followed by MMF for 6 weeks. Stable, favorable fractures can be treated with MMF for 6 weeks with or without an acrylic lingual splint.

17. How would you treat a patient with a body fracture?

Nondisplaced favorable fractures of the body may be treated with either 6 weeks of MMF or by ORIF. For displaced unfavorable fractures, ORIF with plates, interosseous wires in combination with MMF, or lag screws are required. These internal fixation techniques can be performed through intraoral or external approaches. However, the intraoral approach is difficult due to the location of the mental foramen and nerve. Oblique fractures can be treated nicely with lag screws via a transoral or transcutaneous approach.

18. Which techniques are used to treat an angle fracture?

Patients with nondisplaced fractures can be treated with closed reduction and MMF. However, angle fractures tend to be horizontally unfavorable and displaced due to the forces of the muscles of mastication. Unfavorable fractures require internal fixation. The options for internal fixation include:

1. Dynamic compression plates with or without a second miniplate through an external skin incision

2. Intraosseous wiring, placed either transorally or through an external skin incision, in association with MMF for 6 weeks

3. Lag screw fixation with no MMF for unilateral fractures or 1 week of MMF for bilateral fractures

4. Two tension band miniplates, one placed at the superior border, the second placed on the buccal cortex.

External fixation devices are also an option.

19. How do you treat a patient with a ramus fracture?

Fractures of the ramus are uncommon. They are usually nondisplaced due to the protective and splinting effect of the pterygoid and masseter muscles. Generally, these fractures can be managed with closed reduction. However, open reduction may be employed if multiple fragments or marked displacement is present.

20. A coronoid process fracture?

Patients with isolated fractures of the coronoid process require only pain medication, a soft diet, and stretching exercises. Such exercises are used to prevent trismus from scar tissue. Occasionally, patients with severe trismus that does not respond to physical therapy require resection of the coronoid. Rarely, the fractured coronoid segment can cause a physical obstruction to mandibular movement and thus require removal.

21. A condylar fracture?

A patient with a nondisplaced or minimally displaced, unilateral condylar fracture with normal occlusion may be managed with a soft diet and close observation. A patient with bilateral condylar fractures or unilateral fractures with significant displacement is generally managed with IMF for 2–3 weeks followed by physiotherapy for jaw mobility. Early jaw mobility is essential to avoid ankylosis of the TMJ. When the patient is taken out of IMF, the arch bars are left in place for approximately 3 more weeks. During this time, the patient can be placed in fixation at night with elastics if necessary.

22. Why is the treatment of mandibular fractures in children more complicated?

A child's mandible has tooth buds and growth regions that can be damaged during the treatment of a mandible fracture. For this reason, mandibular fractures in children are treated conservatively. The last deciduous tooth appears between 20–30 months of age. This deciduous dentition continues until about 6 years of age. Children under 6 years of age are treated with closed reduction techniques. ORIF in this age group puts developing tooth buds at risk. From age 6 until 12, a child has a mixed dentition of deciduous and permanent teeth. After age 12, only permanent teeth are generally present. In children with mixed and permanent dentition, ORIF with miniplates can be considered due to the increase in distance from the inferior border of the mandible to the tooth buds. Mandible growth occurs due to elongation in the condylar region and remodeling and growth in the region of the ramus and body. Injuries in the condylar region are particularly concerning because they can affect mandible growth and lead to facial asymmetry.

23. How are condylar fractures managed in children (under age 12)?

Children with condylar fractures who are under age 12 and exhibit no malocclusion are treated with analgesics and a liquid or soft diet. They are closely observed for the development of malocclusion. Children with malocclusion require a short period of immobilization followed by soft diet, physiotherapy, and close observation. The condyles of children undergo rapid healing and remodeling; with closed management, very few long-term sequelae are reported. ORIF of condylar fractures in children is rarely indicated and should only be considered when closed reduction is not possible. Children over age 12 can be considered for ORIF if indicated.

24. How should the edentulous patients with a mandibular fracture be managed?
    The edentulous mandible undergoes significant atrophy and becomes susceptible to fractures. Classically, these fractures have been managed with closed reduction and MMF, which is accomplished by applying arch bars to the patient's dentures or by using Gunning splints. The dentures or Gunning splints are then secured to the maxilla by circumzygomatic and anterior nasal spine wiring, Kirschner pinning through the alveolus, or screws placed into the palate. Fixation to the mandible is accomplished by three circum-mandibular wires. However, IMF in combination with dentures or splints is more problematic than traditional IMF. ORIF is commonly used in edentulous fractures if advanced mandibular atrophy is not present. Complications of fractures of severely atrophic mandibles are not uncommon and include nonunion or malunion, often requiring bone grafting for optimum repair and return to function.

CONTROVERSIES

25. Contrast the advantages and disadvantages of open and closed reduction of mandibular fractures.
    Much controversy exists over open versus closed reduction techniques for mandible fractures. Traditionally, MMF has been the workhorse of mandibular fracture repair. However, plating techniques and materials have improved and the indications for open reduction are evolving. The advantages of **closed reduction** include proven efficacy, low complication rate, and short operating time. The disadvantages include fixation in MMF for 2–8 weeks, difficulty in maintaining adequate nutrition, risk to airway, and the possibility of TMJ ankylosis. Advantages of **ORIF** include more exact bone-fragment reapproximation and early mobilization. Disadvantages include cost, time in the operating room, and a higher reported complication rate.

26. Which condylar fractures should be managed with ORIF?
    The controversial indications for open surgical treatment of condylar fractures have been argued in the literature for over 50 years. The desired results after treatment of a condylar fracture include lack of pain, good interincisal opening, functional jaw movement in all directions, stable TMJs, and facial symmetry. Most of the time, good results are obtainable with closed treatment of condylar fractures. The difficulty lies in determining which patients will have a poor outcome without an open reduction. Zide and Kent have proposed that open reduction is absolutely indicated if:
    1. The condyle is displaced into the middle cranial fossa.
    2. Lateral extracapsular displacement of the condyle is present.
    3. Good occlusion cannot be obtained with closed techniques.
    4. A foreign body in the TMJ is present.
Other indications might include:
    1. Bilateral condylar fractures with an associated comminuted, unstable midfacial fractures
    2. Bilateral condylar fractures in an edentulous patient when a splint is unavailable or the alveolar ridge is atrophic
    3. Unilateral or bilateral fractures when closed reduction is not indicated for medical reasons

27. What should be done with a tooth that is located in the fracture line?
    In the preantibiotic era, most teeth located in a fracture line became infected. However, with proper antibiotic therapy, many of these teeth can be retained, and some retained teeth may even be useful in reduction and stabilization of the fractured segments. Teeth should be removed if they have significant periodontal disease, are grossly carious with periapical pathology, or interfere with proper reduction and stability of the fractured segments.

BIBLIOGRAPHY

1. Bruce B, Fonseca RJ: Mandibular fractures. In Fonseca RJ, Walker RV (eds): Oral and Maxillofacial Trauma. Philadelphia, W.B. Saunders, 1991.
2. Calloway DM, Anton MA, Jacobs JS: Changing concepts and controversies in the management of mandibular fractures. Clin Plast Surg 19:59-69, 1992.
3. Clark WD: Management of mandibular fractures. Am J Otolaryngol 13(3):125–132. 1992.
4. El-Degwi A, Mathog RH: Mandible fractures—Medical and economic considerations. Otolaryngol Head Neck Surg 108:213–219, 1993.
5. Dierks EJ: Management of associated dental injuries in maxillofacial trauma. Otolaryngol Clin North Am 24:165–179, 1991.
6. Dierks EJ: Mandibular Fractures. In Bailey BJ (ed): Head and Neck Surgery–Otolaryngology. Philadelphia, J.B. Lippincott, 1993.
7. Hall MB: Condylar fractures: Surgical management. J Oral Maxillofac Surg 52:1189–1192, 1994.
8. Hayward JR, Scott RF: Fractures of the mandibular condyle. J Oral Maxillofac Surg 51: 57–61, 1993.
9. Lowlicht RA, Goodwin WJ: Facial and airway trauma. In Lee KJ (ed): Essential Otolaryngology, 6th ed. Norwalk, CT, Appleton & Lange, 1995.
10. Mathog RH: Atlas of Craniofacial Trauma. Philadelphia, W.B. Saunders, 1992.
11. Stanley RB: Maxillofacial Trauma. In Cummings CW, et al (eds): Otolaryngology–Head and Neck Surgery, 2nd ed. St. Louis, Mosby, 1993.
12. Walker RV: Condylar fractures: Nonsurgical management. J Oral Maxillofac Surg 52: 1185–1188, 1994.

63. ZYGOMATIC, MAXILLARY, AND ORBITAL FRACTURES

Philip C. Fitzpatrick, M.D., and R. Casey Strahan, M.D.

1. What is the buttress system of the midface?

The middle one-third of the skull is composed of a lattice of vertical and horizontal buttresses. These structural adaptations provide strength to the midfacial skeleton, maintaining its dimensions under pressure.

The **vertical buttresses** maintain the vertical dimensions of the midface and are quite strong due to their role in bearing the forces of mastication. These include the nasomaxillary, zygomaticomaxillary, and pterygomaxillary buttresses.

The weaker **horizontal buttresses** maintain the horizontal dimensions or projection of the midface and must absorb horizontal impact forces directed to the middle third of the face. These buttresses are essentially reinforcing connections between the stronger vertical buttresses, and they include the frontal bar, inferior orbital rims, maxillary alveolus and palate, zygomatic process of the temporal bone, greater wing of the sphenoid, and medial and lateral pterygoid plates.

2. Why is this buttress system important?

The disruption of a single buttress may weaken the entire lattice and lead to its collapse. The importance of this system comes in the repair of midfacial fractures. These buttresses must be reconstituted to their original positions to reconstruct the original midfacial dimensions and to ensure structural integrity. Modern repair techniques use titanium plates to realign the bone fragments precisely and to provide support until bony healing has occurred.

3. What are LeFort fractures?

In 1901, the French surgeon Rene LeFort used low-velocity impact forces on fresh cadavers to describe the "great lines of weakness in the face." He described three typical patterns of fracture. These fractures are usually bilateral, and they may be mixed. That is, a patient may have a

LeFort I on the right and a LeFort II on the left side. All three types involve a fracture of the pterygoid plates.

LeFort I fracture—transverse maxillary fracture. The fracture line passes along the floor of the maxillary sinuses at the junction of the thin sinus cortex with the dense palatal bone and extends posteriorly along the maxillary tubercle and into the pterygoid plates.

LeFort II fracture—also called a pyramidal fracture because of its triangular appearance. The fracture line extends across the nasofrontal suture line, down the thin lamina papyracea of the ethmoid bone, across the floor of the orbit near the infraorbital canal, and around the zygoma to the pterygoid plates.

LeFort III fracture—also known as craniofacial disjunction because the fracture line involves all of the buttresses linking the maxilla to the skull. The fracture line begins across the root of the nose near the cribriform plate, goes across the frontoethmoidal suture line and superior orbit, involves the frontozygomatic suture, goes through the root of the zygoma, and crosses the temporal fossa to the pterygomaxillary space. The pterygoid plates are usually fractured free at the base of the skull.

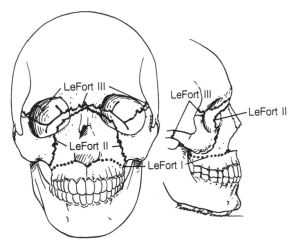

LeFort fractures. (From Lowlicht RA, Goodwin WJ: Facial and airway trauma. In Lee KJ (ed): Essential Otolaryngology–Head and Neck Surgery. Norwalk, CT, Appleton & Lange, 1995, p 850, with permission.)

4. Describe the signs of a LeFort fracture.

A **mobile palate** is pathognomonic of a LeFort fracture. The examiner stabilizes the forehead with one hand and attempts to move the palate and upper teeth with the other. If the palate is mobile, then there is certainly a LeFort fracture of one type or another. Facial edema, ecchymosis, and malocclusion are commonly associated with LeFort fractures. A patient may also exhibit epistaxis, step-offs or movement of the facial skeleton at the fracture site, and midface elongation or compression. Severe manifestations of a LeFort fracture include blindness, CSF rhinorrhea, and airway obstruction. Airway obstruction is more commonly associated with LeFort II and III fractures.

5. What is a tripod fracture?

A tripod fracture is the most common fracture of the malar bone. It is called a tripod fracture because of the three main fracture sites: the frontozygomatic suture line, the face of the maxilla, and the zygomatic arch. However, this term is a misnomer because it overlooks a fourth component, the zygomatic contribution to the floor of the orbit. The direction of displacement of the malar complex depends on the direction of the blow that caused the fracture. Usually the entire complex is displaced posteriorly and inferiorly, giving rise to a flattened appearance in the malar region. The region of the lateral orbital rim that contains the attachment of the lateral canthal tendon will thus be displaced inferiorly and will give rise to an oblique slant of the palpebral fissure.

6. Why is a tripod fracture typically left-sided?

The tripod fracture is typically left-sided because most of the population is right-handed. The etiology of this fracture is typically a fist fight, and the typical right-handed assailant strikes the opponent in the left cheek.

7. Name the seven bones that compose the orbit. Which one is the weakest?

The orbit is formed by the frontal, lacrimal, ethmoidal, zygomatic, maxillary, sphenoidal, and palatine bones. The weakest bone is the lamina papyracea of the ethmoid bone. Fractures of the ethmoid portion of the orbit are thus quite common, including traumatic and iatrogenic causes.

8. What is a blowout fracture?

A blowout fracture is a fracture of the orbital wall caused by a blunt, nonpenetrating force. The most common causes include a baseball, fist, hockey puck, or champagne cork. The direct blunt trauma to the globe increases intraorbital pressure, causing the thin bones of the orbit to "blow out." Typically, the inferior orbital wall is most commonly involved, probably because the floor of the orbit is inherently weak as a result of its thinness and the dehiscence caused by the infraorbital canal. The ocular globe is protected from this blunt trauma by the surrounding orbital fat.

9. How do pure and impure blowout fractures differ?

A **pure** blowout fracture involves a downward displacement of any part of the orbital floor without damage to the orbital rim. The patient may present with pain that is confined to the orbit, ecchymosis, enophthalmos, and/or diplopia. **Impure** blow-out fractures, also known as **rim fractures**, differ only in that they involve the inferior orbital rim as well as the floor of the orbit. Impure fractures are typically the result of an automobile injury in which the passenger's face strikes the dashboard. These fractures typically present with a palpable step-off deformity in addition to possible diplopia (if entrapment is present), and/or sensory changes (if the infraorbital nerve is involved).

10. When is forced duction testing indicated?

Forced duction testing has classically been used in the evaluation of possible muscle entrapment seen in blowout fractures. This technique measures the freedom of movement of the extraocular muscles. After the conjunctiva is topically anesthetized, fine-toothed forceps are used to grasp the episcleral tissues in the region where the inferior oblique muscle attaches to the globe. Attempts are then made to rotate the globe superiorly. This test can similarly be performed for the medial oblique muscle if necessary. When complete restriction of passive motion exists, it is said to be a 4+ positive forced duction test and the muscle is very likely entrapped in the fracture. Complete freedom of motion is a negative result, indicating no entrapment. Forced ductions can and should be performed in the operating room after repair of a blowout fracture to determine if adequate reduction of prolapsed orbital contents has been achieved.

11. Which imaging techniques are useful for maxillofacial trauma?

Plain films are usually ordered for the facial trauma patient in the emergency department due to their low cost and wide availability. The routine x-ray films include the Waters, Caldwell posteroanterior, and lateral facial views. The submental vertex and "jug-handle" views are frequently added as part of the routine films but should be obtained only after cervical spine injury has been ruled out.

CT scanning has long been the modality of choice in evaluating facial trauma patients. When the orbits are examined, the study should include soft tissue settings for the evaluation of the intraorbital structures. Coronal imaging is suggested for orbital studies but only when spine injury has been completely ruled out. Coronal imaging is ideal for evaluating horizontal structures, such as the hard palate, orbital floor and roof, and cribriform plate. Axial images are useful in evaluating the zygomatic arch and pterygoid plates and are the only images that can be obtained in a patient with a suspected or proven cervical spine injury. In general, both coronal and axial images are obtained (if possible) for the evaluation of any complex facial fracture.

12. What is the teardrop sign?

The teardrop sign is defined as a teardrop-shaped opacification seen hanging from the roof of the maxillary sinus on a Waters view. It is said to represent orbital contents (i.e., fat) that have herniated down into the maxillary sinus and is an indication of an orbital blowout.

Another reliable indication of a blowout fracture on a Waters view is loss of the double cortical lines representing the orbital rim and floor. If the patient has these abnormal plain radiographic findings coupled with clinical evidence, the presumptive diagnosis of a blowout fracture can be made. However, often the Waters view simply shows complete opacification of the maxillary sinus. In this case, one cannot tell if this opacification is herniated orbital fat or simply blood in the sinus from a mucosal tear. A CT scan would be necessary for a definitive diagnosis.

13. What is the significance of enophthalmos?

Enophthalmos associated with midfacial trauma is a good indicator that a blowout fracture has occurred. Enophthalmos may not be seen immediately, even after severe orbitozygomatic fractures. If the body of the zygoma is intact, it may be impacted medially to compensate for the decreased orbital volume caused by blowout fractures of other walls. When the zygomatic component of the injury is repaired, it may unmask a previously undiagnosed blowout fracture by revealing enophthalmos. Alternatively, swelling associated with an acute blowout fracture may also mask enophthalmos. As the swelling subsides with time, the enophthalmos may become apparent and may necessitate surgical correction. Enophthalmos is said to be the most difficult problem to correct in a blowout fracture.

14. Describe the surgical approaches used to repair tripod fractures.

Modern surgical approaches to tripod fractures involve directly visualizing the fractures so that accurate reduction can be achieved and rigid internal fixation applied. Since the tripod fracture involves several different fracture sites, several separate incisions are needed to view these sites. Studies have shown that at least two fracture sites must be visualized in order to obtain adequate reduction and stabilization:

1. Lateral brow incision (along the inferior border of the lateral eyebrow) or an upper blepharoplasty incision for visualization of the frontozygomatic suture
2. Subciliary or transconjunctival incision for visualization of the inferior orbital rim and orbital floor
3. Upper gingival-buccal sulcus incision (under the upper lip) for visualization of the face of the maxilla
4. Bicoronal approach for visualization of the lateral orbital rim and zygomatic arch.

Precisely which and how many incisions are necessary will be dictated by the location and severity of the fractures and by the surgeon's preferences. In general as many incisions are made as is necessary to ensure precise reduction of the fragments. Various sized and shaped plates are then applied across the fractures to stabilize the fragments during healing.

15. Describe the Gillies approach.

The Gillies approach is a limited-exposure reduction technique that is used to repair isolated zygomatic arch fractures. A 2.5-cm incision is made in an oblique direction, behind the hairline and above the helix of the auricle. This incision is carried through the superficial temporalis fascia and through the fibers of the superior auricularis muscle, avoiding the superficial temporal artery. Deep to the superior auricularis muscle lies the deep temporal fascia, which envelopes the temporalis muscle. This fascia is incised, and the fibers of the temporalis muscle identified. A blunt and sturdy elevator is inserted between the fascia and muscle such that a tunnel is made toward the zygomatic arch. By staying beneath this very tough fascia, the elevator will end up just deep to the arch, and injury to the zygomatic branch of the facial nerve will be avoided. The elevator is then used to lift up and slightly overcorrect the depressed arch. For an isolated arch fracture, internal fixation is rarely needed.

16. What materials are used to restore the orbital floor in the repair of a blowout fracture?

During the repair of an orbital blowout fracture, the herniated orbital contents are first placed back into the orbital cavity, and the floor is then reconstructed. This reconstruction is performed by sliding a thin piece of material along the bony floor (i.e., between the bone and periosteum of the orbit) such that this material acts as a sling to support the orbital contents. This material can be either an autogenous graft or an inorganic implant, again depending on the surgeon's preferences. Autogenous grafts include bone (harvested from the face of the maxilla or from the outer table of the calvarium) and cartilage (harvested from the nasal septum or conchal bowl). Inorganic implants include Gelfilm, Silastic, Teflon, Marlex mesh, and titanium mesh.

17. What is the most common error in orbital wall reconstruction?

Failure to repair the posterior orbital floor. The defect in the orbital floor can extend as much as 40 mm posterior to the inferior orbital rim. If the entire defect is not explored and the posterior edge of stable bone is not identified, the surgeon may not adequately repair the defect and the orbital contents may continue to herniate, resulting in persistent enophthalmos. It is important to recall that the optic nerve is approximately 50 mm posterior to the inferior orbital rim at the infraorbital grove. A graft material that is ideally suited for reconstruction of large orbital floor defects is outer table calvarial bone, as a very large graft may be harvested. The graft may be stabilized by attaching it to the orbital floor with lag screws or to the reconstructed orbital rim with miniplates and screws.

18. Name some other complications of maxillary and periorbital fracture repair.

Malocclusion (most common complication)
Facial asymmetry
Increased scleral show or gross ectropion
Lip distortion
Damage of the globe or optic nerve with resultant loss of vision
Forward positioning of globe by an oversized implant (causing acute increase in IOP)
Lid distortion (due to plate on inferior orbital rim)

19. What is the medial canthal tendon (MCT)?

This structure in the naso-orbito-ethmoid (NOE) region has importance both cosmetically, in shaping the medial aspect of the palpebral opening, and functionally, in protecting and supporting the globe and in pumping the lacrimal sac. The MCT has three attachments to the medial orbital wall: anterior horizontal, anterior vertical, and posterior horizontal. If any or all three of these attachments is disrupted, the severity of the deformity in the medial canthus increases, with the deformity increasing as the number of disrupted components increases. Also, the lacrimal sac is located within the three components of the MCT. The MCT thus functions as a pumping mechanism to pump tears out of the lacrimal sac. Disruption of these tendons thus may lead to epiphora by disrupting the pump mechanism. Signs of a MCT disruption include telecanthus, narrowing of the palpebral fissure (distance from the medial canthus to the lateral canthus), and epiphora. If the MCT is disrupted, this must be recognized and addressed during the initial repair of any facial fractures. Failure to do so will lead to cosmetic and functional problems that are very difficult to fix secondarily.

20. What degree of telecanthus is diagnostic of an NOE fracture?

The intercanthal distance should be approximately half of the interpupillary distance, and when this distance is increased, telecanthus exists. In general, intercanthal distances > 35 mm are suggestive of a displaced NOE fracture, and distances > 40 mm are diagnostic. Diagnosis of telecanthus is important because it is the most compelling reason for open treatment of an NOE injury. Edema may make the diagnosis of MCT disruption difficult, as it may obscure signs of rupture such as blunting of the medial palpebral fissure and/or epiphora. Measuring the intercanthal and interpupillary distances may raise the suspicion of MCT rupture and may thus give compelling evidence for the need for a CT scan to evaluate the NOE region.

CONTROVERSIES

21. What are the indications, contraindications, and time frame for surgical repair of orbital blowout fractures?

The only indication for immediate exploration of the orbit is the rapid onset of serious intraorbital hemorrhage with decreased visual acuity. Current **indications** for surgical repair include enophthalmos and extraocular muscle entrapment causing a mechanical restriction of gaze. **Contraindications** include soft tissue injuries of the eye, such as hyphema, retinal tears, and globe perforation, as these injuries can be aggravated by exploration. In addition, blowout fractures should not be repaired in an only seeing eye. The **time frame** for repair must also be considered. If surgery is performed too early, it can be compromised by swelling and bleeding that obscure landmarks and anatomic planes. If surgery is performed too late, bones may fuse in an abnormal position, and scar tissue may hamper the repair. In general, it is preferable to perform surgery 7–10 days from the date of the injury.

22. Should a lacrimal collection system injury be repaired primarily with MCT repair?

Lacrimal collection system injury with subsequent dysfunction is a surprisingly uncommon sequela of all but the most severe NOE fractures. If lacrimal duct injury is suspected or recognized at the time of the initial fracture reduction and fixation, repair of the duct is probably best delayed. An attempt at simultaneous lacrimal system repair will invariably lead to a compromised MCT repair and may cause injury to the canaliculi. Secondary MCT repairs are much more difficult and much less successful than primary MCT repairs, whereas secondary lacrimal collecting system repairs are usually quite successful. Therefore, lacrimal system repair is usually delayed to maximize the MCT result. The reported incidence of lacrimal obstruction requiring dacryocystorhinostomy after treatment of NOE injuries varies from 5–10%.

BIBLIOGRAPHY

1. Duckert LG: Management of middle third facial fractures. Otolaryngol Clin North Am 24:103–118, 1991.
2. Ellis E: Sequencing treatment for naso-orbito-ethmoid fractures. J Oral Maxillofac Surg 51:543–558, 1993.
3. Leipziger LS, Manson PN: Nasoethmoid orbital fractures—Current concepts and management principles. Clin Plast Surg 19:167–193, 1992.
4. Lowlicht RA, Goodwin WJ: Facial and airway trauma. In Lee KJ (ed): Essential Otolaryngology–Head and Neck Surgery. Norwalk, CT, Appleton & Lange, 1995.
5. Luce EA: Developing concepts and treatment of complex maxillary fractures. Clin Plast Surg 19:125–131, 1992.
6. Mathog RH: Management of orbital blow-out fractures. Otolaryngol Clin North Am 24:79–91, 1991.
7. O'Hare TH: Blow-out fractures—A review. J Emerg Med 9:253–263, 1991.
8. Stanley RB: Maxillary and periorbital fractures. In Bailey BJ, et al (eds): Head and Neck Surgery–Otolaryngology. Philadelphia, J.B. Lippincott, 1993.
9. Stanley RB: Maxillofacial trauma. In Cummings CW, et al (eds): Otolaryngology–Head and Neck Surgery. St Louis, Mosby, 1993.

64. TEMPORAL BONE TRAUMA

Kent E. Gardner, M.D., Mark Mount, M.D., and Ethan Lazarus, M.D.

1. What are the most common causes of temporal bone trauma?

Temporal bone trauma can be classified into **blunt** and **penetrating**. Penetrating trauma is almost exclusively due to gunshot wounds. Blunt trauma is most commonly the result of motor vehicle accidents but may include physical assault, falls, and bicycle accidents.

2. How are temporal bone fractures classified?

Temporal bone fractures are classified as longitudinal fractures or transverse fractures. **Longitudinal fractures** are the most common, occurring in 70–90% of temporal bone fractures. They result from lateral blunt trauma to the temporoparietal region of the skull. This type of fracture typically begins in the thin squamous portion of the temporal bone. The fracture line then runs across the superior external auditory canal, through the middle ear, and along the long axis of the petrous pyramid. Longitudinal fractures may involve the eustachian tube, foramen lacerum, or foramen ovale. They also may extend into the sphenoid bone or across the midline. Longitudinal fractures cross the midline or are bilateral 30% of the time. **Transverse fractures** result from a severe occipital or frontal blow. These fractures usually begin at the foramen magnum and run across the temporal bone perpendicular to the long axis of the petrous pyramid. Transverse fractures may involve the jugular foramen and almost always cause disruption of the otic capsule.

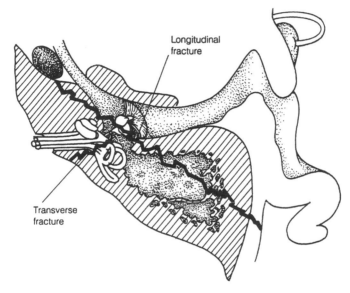

Temporal bone fractures. (From Pender DJ: Practical Otology. Philadelphia, J.B. Lippincott, 1992, p 160, with permission.)

3. What are the common complications associated with temporal bone fracture?

	Longitudinal	*Transverse*
Frequency	70–90%	10–20%
Mechanism of injury	Lateral skull trauma Minor injury	Frontal or occipital trauma Massive trauma
Complications	Ossicular damage common Conductive hearing loss Vertigo rare Bleeding in EAC Facial nerve paralysis rare CSF leak occasionally	Otic capsule and IAC rupture Sensorineural hearing loss Vertigo common Bleeding in middle ear cavity Facial nerve paralysis in 50% CSF leak common

EAC = external auditory canal; IAC = internal auditory canal.

Facial nerve injury, CSF leak, hearing loss, and vertigo are the most commonly recognized complications of temporal bone trauma. Cholesteatoma, vascular injuries, facial hypesthesia, diplopia, and other cranial nerve injuries may also occur. Cholesteatoma develops long after temporal bone trauma and occurs because of seeding of the mastoid cavity with squamous epithelium due to fracture of the external canal. Trauma patients are generally healthy and have well-pneumatized mastoid cavities which are conducive to rapid cholesteatoma growth. Facial hypesthesia occurs because of damage to the gasserian ganglion (CN V) at its location on the surface of the petrous bone. Diplopia can occur because of damage to abducens nerve (CN VI) as it courses through Dorello's canal.

4. How are blunt and penetrating temporal bone trauma different?

Over 6% of temporal bone trauma is due to penetrating trauma. Penetrating temporal bone trauma is generally more destructive than blunt trauma. The amount of destruction done by a gunshot wound is related to the kinetic energy of its missile, with high-velocity weapons causing more damage than low-velocity weapons. Vascular and other intracranial injuries are more common in penetrating trauma. Facial nerve trauma is present approximately half of the time and tends to be severe. Frequently, the nerve is transected, and large segments of the nerve may be missing or damaged.

5. What are the important questions to ask in the emergency department?

Important aspects of the history include the mechanism of injury, time of onset of symptoms, and presence or absence of hearing loss, vertigo, and facial weakness. In facial nerve trauma, the prognosis and approach to treatment depend partially on whether the onset of symptoms was immediate or delayed. Often, patients with severe head trauma resulting in temporal bone trauma are not conscious. In these cases, the history must be obtained from family, paramedics, and emergency department personnel.

6. What should one look for when examining a patient with suspected temporal bone trauma?

Facial nerve weakness—one of the most important physical findings to note. It is usually documented with the House-Brackman classification.

Hearing loss—may be conductive or sensorineural. Tuning forks can help distinguish between the two in the emergency room if the patient is conscious.

Hemotympanum—an indication of a transverse fracture

Tympanic membrane perforation—seen in longitudinal fractures

External auditory canal laceration with bloody otorrhea —seen in longitudinal fractures.

CSF otorrhea—occurs with longitudinal fractures

CSF rhinorrhea—occurs with transverse fractures. Rhinorrhea results from the intact tympanic membrane directing CSF down through the eustachian tube. CSF rhinorrhea worsens as the patient leans forward and the patient may complain of a salty taste in the mouth.

Nystagmus—implies damage to the vestibular system. Severe vertigo associated with nystagmus and sensorineural hearing loss implies otic capsule disruption.

Battle's sign

Raccoon sign

7. What is Battle's sign? A "raccoon" sign?

Battle's sign is postauricular ecchymosis that occurs due to fracture through the mastoid cortex. The **raccoon sign** is periorbital ecchymosis. Either of these signs seen in association with a history of head trauma is sufficient to make the diagnosis of temporal bone fracture.

8. Is CT or MRI more informative in temporal bone trauma?

Fine-cut temporal bone CT scan (1.0–1.5-mm cuts) with both coronal and axial views is the radiologic study of choice. These scans are extremely sensitive in evaluating the presence and extent of a temporal bone fracture. CT is also helpful in evaluating the presence of ossicular discontinuity and facial nerve lesions. MRI is less sensitive than CT in picking up fractures, ossicular discontinuity, and facial nerve trauma because bone does not show up well on MRI. Fractures are seen only because blood fills the fracture line. However, MRI is superior to CT in evaluating intracranial complications associated with temporal bone trauma. Therefore, MRI and CT can be complementary in some cases of temporal bone trauma.

9. When is an angiogram indicated in the management of penetrating temporal bone trauma?

Unless it can be determined by exam or radiologic study that the course of a bullet is lateral to the middle ear, an angiogram is always indicated in penetrating trauma of the temporal bone. Both the carotid and vertebral arteries should be studied. If an injury to the external carotid is noted, it is best treated with embolization at the time of angiography. Treatment of injuries to the internal carotid artery is controversial. Options include embolization, surgical revascularization, and ligation. For injuries in the petrous or intracranial portion of the internal carotid artery which are associated with life-threatening hemorrhage, immediate embolization should be attempted.

10. Most temporal bone fractures are not emergencies and do not require immediate otolaryngologic consultation. What sign may necessitate early surgical intervention?

Facial nerve paralysis. A patient with the immediate onset of facial nerve paralysis, especially in association with CT findings suggesting impingement or transection, may benefit from exploration. Surgical exploration is performed as soon as the patient's condition allows.

11. Are facial nerve injuries more commonly due to transverse or longitudinal fractures?

This is a trick question. A given transverse fracture is more commonly complicated by facial nerve injury than a given longitudinal fracture: 10–20% of longitudinal and 40–50% of transverse temporal bone fractures are associated with facial nerve injury. However, the overwhelming majority of temporal bone fractures are longitudinal. Therefore, because of the sheer number of longitudinal fractures, more often than not facial nerve injuries will be associated with longitudinal fractures.

12. What is the most commonly injured facial nerve site in blunt temporal bone trauma?

In longitudinal fractures, the perigeniculate ganglion region is involved in 80–93% of facial nerve injuries. The next most common site is just distal to the pyramidal eminence. In transverse fractures, the distal labyrinthine segment is most commonly injured. Transverse temporal bone fractures are generally associated with more severe injury to the facial nerve, including transection. Longitudinal fractures are more often associated with facial nerve injuries caused by edema and hematoma.

13. In penetrating temporal bone trauma, what is the most commonly injured facial nerve site?

Penetrating temporal bone trauma is synonymous with gunshot wounds. Bullets tend to enter the lateral or inferior temporal bone, and tissue injury is due to dissipation of kinetic energy from the bullet. The portions of the nerve closest to the entry site and tract receive most of the energy. Therefore, the most commonly injured sites include the extratemporal nerve, the stylomastoid foramen portion of the nerve, and the vertical segment of the nerve. Transection is common with penetrating trauma and commonly requires primary repair or grafting.

14. How common is a CSF leak after a temporal bone fracture?

11–27% of temporal bone fractures are complicated by a CSF leak. In longitudinal temporal bone fractures, this presents as CSF otorrhea. The diagnosis is sometimes difficult to establish due to the presence of bloody otorrhea. One way to identify a CSF leak is to check the glucose content of the otorrhea to see if it is consistent with CSF. Another way is to place some of the bloody otorrhea on a piece of gauze or paper. If CSF is present, it will diffuse more rapidly than the blood, and a "target" or "halo" sign will be present. In transverse fractures, a CSF leak presents as clear rhinorrhea.

15. What is the significance of a remote history of head trauma in a patient with recurrent meningitis?

Fractures of the otic capsule do not heal like long bone fractures, and incomplete healing is not uncommon. Incomplete healing of a fracture line can allow ingrowth of respiratory mucosa and lead to a microscopic fistula. The fistula then can act as a highway for infection and lead to meningitis. In patients with recurrent meningitis and a past history of head trauma, a fistula should be suspected. Localization of the fistula is accomplished by CT scans, radioisotope studies, or intrathecal dye injections. Treatment of the fistula is generally with a labyrinthectomy and obliteration of the pneumatized spaces and the eustachian tube.

16. How do you manage a patient with a CSF leak?

Most CSF leaks stop after a few days with only conservative therapy. Conservative treatment consists of bedrest, head elevation, and avoidance of activities that increase intracranial pressure (i.e., straining, lifting, or bending over). Some advocate fluid restriction and diuretics. The use of antibiotics is controversial. If the leak persists for several days (usually 3–5), then a lumbar drain may be added to conservative therapy. If leakage persists despite lumbar drainage, then consideration is given to surgery. Indications for surgery include persistent leak despite adequate conservative therapy, recurrent meningitis, and persistent pneumocephalus. In the rare case when surgery is necessary, localization of the leak can be aided by contrast-enhanced CT, radioisotope studies, and intrathecal dye instillation.

17. What is post-concussive syndrome? How is it treated?

Most patients experience some degree of balance disturbance after temporal bone trauma. Post-concussive syndrome is a constellation of symptoms including nonspecific dizziness, headache, inability to concentrate, and fatigue. These patients tend to have normal electronystagmographic (ENG) testing and a normal audiogram. After ruling out more serious injury, these patients are treated conservatively with gradual resumption of activity, nonsteroidal analgesics, and reassurance.

18. What are the causes of vertigo when it is associated with temporal bone trauma? How should vertigo be worked up?

Causes of post-traumatic vertigo include post-concussive syndrome, concussive injury to the membranous labyrinth, cupulolithiasis, massive and disruptive injury to the labyrinth, traumatic perilymph fistula, and trauma-induced endolymphatic hydrops. Patients with post-traumatic vertigo should undergo evaluation with an ENG and audiogram.

19. How are the different types of post-traumatic vertigo differentiated and treated?

Concussive injury to the membranous labyrinth is the most common form of post-traumatic vertigo. These patients have positional vertigo and usually have a normal ENG. Concussive injury to the labyrinth is almost always self-limited and requires only symptomatic treatment.

Cupulolithiasis is a more severe form of concussive injury. The onset of positional vertigo is usually delayed. ENG is usually normal except for a positive Dix-Hallpike provocative test. Treatment usually involves the Epley maneuver or Cawthorne exercises.

Massive injury to the vestibular labyrinth occurs as the result of an otic capsule-disrupting fracture. These patients have immediate severe vertigo with nausea and emesis. They also tend to have a horizontal nystagmus with the fast component away from the involved ear. Initial treatment consists of vestibular suppressants and antiemetics. Physical therapy is also helpful during vestibular rehabilitation. The symptoms of an otic capsule-disrupting fracture subside over days to weeks as the CNS begins to compensate.

A **perilymphatic fistula** is characterized by vertigo and a fluctuating or progressive sensorineural hearing loss. Initial treatment consists of bedrest with expectant management. If symptoms persist, consideration should be given to surgical exploration.

Trauma-induced endolymphatic hydrops usually develops months or years after head trauma. Symptoms include fluctuant hearing loss, tinnitus, and aural fullness. The possibility of perilymphatic fistula must be considered. Treatment is consistent with that used for other forms of endolymphatic hydrops.

20. What type of hearing loss is more common in patients after temporal bone trauma?

Patients with temporal bone trauma may suffer from either conductive hearing loss (CHL) or sensorineural hearing loss (SNHL), with CHL being the more common type. CHL is usually temporary and is caused by blood in the middle ear, edema, or tympanic membrane perforation. Sometimes CHL is more permanent. Persistent CHL is due to more severe injury to the middle ear structures. SNHL is less common and is usually the result of fracture of the otic capsule.

21. What is the most common reason for persistent CHL associated with temporal bone trauma?

The most common cause is **ossicular damage**. The most common form of ossicular injury is incudostapedial joint separation. The incudostapedial joint is prone to injury because the long process of the incus and the stapes suprastructure are at right angles to each other. When a severe blow strikes the temporal bone, the resultant torsional forces on the stapes suprastructure and long process of the incus are in opposite directions. The small surface area of the stapes cannot withstand these forces, and separation occurs. Other common ossicular injuries include massive dislocation of the incus, fracture of the stapedial arch, fracture of the malleus, and epitympanic fixation of the ossicular chain.

22. How does blunt trauma cause sensorineural hearing loss?

1. Disruption of the bony and membranous labyrinths from a fracture of the capsule
2. Concussion injury to the inner ear without evidence of labyrinthine fracture
3. Blast with noise-induced hearing loss
4. Perilymph fistula
5. Injury to the auditory CNS

23. When should patients with a CHL after temporal bone trauma be operated on?

Surgical intervention with exploration of the middle ear should be considered 3–6 months after temporal bone trauma. Some 75% of patients with CHL after trauma will return to normal within this 3–6-month waiting period. The rest have an unhealed tympanic membrane perforation or ossicular injuries. 78% of patients with ossicular discontinuity can have the air-bone gap closed to within 10 dB by using ossicular reconstruction techniques.

24. A patient sticks a Q-tip in his ear and notes severe pain and hearing loss. The emergency physician notes a small amount of blood in the external auditory canal as well as an anterior tympanic membrane perforation. How should this patient be managed?

Traumatic **tympanic membrane perforations** generally heal on their own in 3–6 weeks and require no treatment. However, there is an increased rate of persistent tympanic membrane perforation if infection develops in the ear. Therefore, any infection should be treated with antibiotic drops. If there is no evidence of infection, drops should not be used, and the ear should be kept dry. Hearing loss in this case is most likely a result of the tympanic membrane perforation causing a CHL. The presence of a CHL should be confirmed with tuning forks in the emergency department. An audiogram should also be obtained when available. If the patient has nystagmus, vertigo, and evidence of a SNHL, then a perilymphatic fistula may be present. Patients with posterosuperior tympanic membrane perforations are particularly susceptible to ossicular damage, facial nerve injury, and a perilymph fistula.

CONTROVERSIES

25. What are the indications for post-traumatic facial nerve exploration after intratemporal facial nerve injury?

There are no universally accepted indications for facial nerve exploration after temporal bone trauma. The spectrum of facial nerve injuries resulting from temporal bone trauma is broad. At one end of the spectrum is mild facial nerve paresis. These injuries are often delayed in onset and are usually secondary to nerve edema. At the opposite end of the spectrum is complete immediate paralysis due to transection of the nerve. Indicators of severe injury and possible benefits from surgical intervention include immediate onset of paralysis, poor prognosis by electrical testing, and evidence of nerve transection or impingement by CT scan. Patients with only a **paresis** of the facial nerve always have good return of function and do not require surgical intervention. Patients with **delayed paralysis** of the nerve also tend to have good return of function without surgical intervention. However, some authors advocate decompression of the facial nerve in patients with delayed onset of facial nerve paralysis if electrical testing indicates a poor prognosis. **Immediate-onset paralysis** with evidence of transection or impingement of the facial nerve by CT scan or **immediate-onset paralysis** in the setting of penetrating trauma are also indications for surgical exploration and repair of the nerve. The indications for exploration in cases of immediate paralysis without evidence of nerve transection or impingement by CT scan are controversial. Electrical testing can be helpful in predicting which of these patients have a poor prognosis and therefore may benefit from surgical exploration.

26. How is a perilymphatic fistula diagnosed and treated?

There are two approaches to handling a suspected perilymphatic fistula: early surgical exploration and noninvasive testing and observation.

Early surgical exploration: All noninvasive test batteries are ineffective in accurately diagnosing a perilymphatic fistula. By exploring an acutely dizzy patient early, the surgeon can both make the diagnosis and adequately treat the patient in a timely fashion. Delay may result in permanent labyrinthine dysfunction and deafness. Therefore, surgical exploration should not be delayed, especially in the patient with sudden hearing loss.

Noninvasive testing and observation: The diagnosis of perilymphatic fistula is difficult, even during surgery, and the incidence of fistulae due to indirect trauma is extremely low. Conservative therapy usually involves 1–2 weeks of bedrest with the head elevated. Many existing fistulae will heal spontaneously. Patients whose symptoms worsen should have surgery. A conservative approach saves many patients from an operation and the risks of complications.

27. Should patients with a CSF leak due to temporal bone fracture receive antibiotics?

Yes: Prophylactic antibiotics may prevent the development of meningitis in the patient with a CSF leak. Antibiotics are usually harmless. Moreover, the incidence of meningitis in head trauma patients with a CSF leak is as high as 20%.

No: Most patients with temporal bone fractures and an associated CSF leak will not develop meningitis. Most leaks heal spontaneously in 4–5 days without surgical intervention. Prophylactic antibiotics have not been clearly shown to prevent meningitis, and they are typically prescribed in doses that are too small to treat most infections. Furthermore, if clinically obvious meningitis develops in the presence of antibiotics, accurate diagnosis and identification of the organism may be difficult or impossible.

BIBLIOGRAPHY

1. Hansen MC, et al: Temporal bone fractures. Am J Emerg Med 13:211–214, 1995.
2. Kamerer DB: Middle ear and temporal bone trauma. In Bailey BJ (ed): Head and Neck Surgery–Otolaryngology. Philadelphia, J.B. Lippincott, 1993.
3. Kelly KE, Tami TA: Temporal bone and skull base trauma. In Jackler RK, Brackman DE (eds): Neurotology. St. Louis, Mosby, 1994.
4. Kinney SE: Trauma to the middle ear and temporal bone. In Cummings CW, et al (eds): Otolaryngology–Head and Neck Surgery, 3rd edition. St. Louis, Mosby, 1993.
5. Logan TC, Carrasco VN, Lee KJ: Facial Nerve Paralysis. In Lee KJ (ed): Essential Otolaryngology, 6th ed. Norwalk, CT, Appleton & Lange, 1995.
6. Shindo ML, et al: Gunshot wounds of the temporal bone: A rational approach to evaluation and management. Otolaryngol Head Neck Surg 112:533–539, 1995.
7. Vartiainen E, et al: Perilymph fistula—A diagnostic dilema. J Laryngol Otol 105:270–273, 1991.
8. Wall C III, Rauch SD: Perilymph fistula pathophysiology. Otolaryngol Head Neck Surg 112:145–153, 1995.

IX. Pediatric Otolaryngology

65. THE PEDIATRIC AIRWAY

Tyler M. Lewark, M.D., and Marshall E. Smith, M.D.

1. How does the airway of the infant differ anatomically from an adult's? Are these differences important for airway management?

Several important anatomic differences exist between the infant and adult airway. The infant has narrow nares, a relatively large tongue, elevated position of the larynx, a narrow cricoid ring, and a large occiput. Intubation of the child can be complicated by several factors, including the tongue obstructing the pharynx and difficulty with head positioning. Other considerations include the infantile larynx which, unlike the adult's, is funnel-shaped with the narrowest region at the cricoid ring, a difference that lasts up through 8 years of age. An endotracheal tube that easily passes through the glottis (space between the vocal cords) may not pass through the subglottic lumen of the cricoid.

2. What respiratory disadvantages make the infant more susceptible to difficulty in breathing than the adult?

1. **Narrow airways** become obstructed easily.
2. **Poor collateral ventilation** can complicate this obstruction.
3. **Less compliant lungs and thorax** result in a lower functional residual capacity.
4. **Horizontal rib position** (rather than angulated) yields less intercostal excursion.
5. **Easily fatigable respiratory muscles** are less able to compensate for stress placed on the respiratory system.

3. What percentage of infants are obligate nasal breathers?

Obligate nasal breathing is often seen in infants. The inability to tolerate nasal occlusion and to breathe by mouth is thought to be due to immature coordination of oral and respiratory function. Nasal breathing, combined with the high position of the larynx in the neck, allows infants to feed, swallow, and breathe simultaneously. About 92% of infants at 30–32 weeks' postconceptual age and 22% of term infants are obligate nasal breathers. Nearly all infants are able to coordinate oral and respiratory function by the age of 5 months.

4. What is stridor? What are its causes?

Stridor is a symptom term for noisy breathing. The noise is created by turbulent airflow or vibration of tissues in a structural or functional narrowing somewhere between the oral cavity and distal bronchi during respiration. The key to localizing the source of stridor is characterizing the occurrence of the sound with inspiratory and/or expiratory phases of respiration. **Inspiratory stridor** reflects airflow impairment above or at the level of the vocal cords. It is generally high-pitched when occurring at the vocal cords and may be low-pitched when obstruction is above the vocal cords (pharynx or supraglottic larynx). **Expiratory stridor** is usually produced from airflow limitation in the distal tracheobronchial (intrathoracic) tree and gives rise to a more prolonged, sonorous sound. This may be confused with wheezing, such as in asthma. Stridor that is both inspiratory and expiratory (**biphasic**) is usually due to obstruction immediately below the vocal cords or in the proximal (extrathoracic) trachea. About 60% of stridor in children is localized to the larynx, 15% to the trachea, and 5% to the bronchi; 5% have an infectious cause.

5. How do you evaluate a child with stridor?

Stridor may occur in a setting of acute respiratory distress or be a chronic condition. It may be due to one or more of a panoply of etiologies: congenital, inflammatory, traumatic, iatrogenic, and neoplastic.

The **history** is the major component of the evaluation, as it alone allows identification of the airway abnormality in up to 80% of cases. Onset and duration of symptoms as well as initiating and possible alleviating factors are ascertained. Associated factors such as fever, cough, apnea, swallowing or feeding difficulties, voice abnormality, and association of stridor with positioning, feeding, or crying are ascertained.

The **physical examination** documents the quality of stridor and its relation to phase of respiration. Respiratory effort is assessed by signs of tachypnea, tachycardia, suprasternal or intercostal retractions. Respiratory obstruction causes hypoventilation (decrease in PO_2 and increase in PCO_2), yielding signs of confusion or restlessness.

Radiographic studies are helpful to assess etiology of stridor in a noninvasive way. Plain films of the neck (anteroposterior and lateral) and chest during inspiration and expiration may document supraglotttic swelling, subglottic or tracheal narrowing, and shifts of the trachea and mediastinum. Barium swallow can delineate obstruction from a vascular ring causing extrinsic tracheal compression.

Definitive diagnosis of stridor generally requires **endoscopy** of the upper aerodigestive tract. Flexible fiberoptic laryngoscopy is well-tolerated in infants and young children and confirms the cause of stridor in most cases. Fiberoptic bronchoscopy identifies abnormalities of the distal airway. Rigid endoscopy is performed under general anesthesia and is used for diagnostic as well as therapeutic purposes (e.g., laser, foreign-body removal).

6. Which congenital disorders cause airway obstruction in the infant?

The most frequent causes of congenital airway obstruction are laryngeal anomalies, with laryngomalacia accounting for about 60%.

Laryngomalacia   Choanal atresia
Tracheomalacia   Congenital laryngeal webs
Vocal cord paralysis   Subglottic hemangioma
Congenital subglottic stenosis

7. What is the most common cause of childhood airway obstruction?

Acute laryngotracheobronchitis, or **croup**, is the most common cause of stridor in children. Patients are usually < 2 years old, ranging from 6 months to 5 years. It is often associated with upper respiratory tract infection and is characterized by a barking cough with inspiratory or biphasic stridor. The stridor is usually due to edema of the subglottic space, associated with the viral respiratory infection. Most cases are alleviated by simple home methods, such as humidification or walks in the cool night air. Only the most severe cases cause acute airway obstruction, and their therapy includes humidification, supplemental oxygen, fluids, and nebulized racemic epinephrine. The use of oral and/or parenteral steroids to treat croup has become widespread in recent years, avoiding many hospitalizations. Complications of croup include pulmonary edema, pneumonia, and cardiac failure.

8. What additional inflammatory conditions cause childhood airway obstruction?

Acute **epiglottitis** occurs much less commonly than croup in children. Prior to introduction of the HIB vaccine, *Haemophilus influenzae* type B used to be the most common inciting pathogen, but now, acute epiglottitis in children is frequently caused by other bacterial organisms. It is most frequent in patients aged 2–6 years. Signs and symptoms include rapidly developing sore throat, high fever, leukocytosis, restlessness, lethargy, and inability to control saliva. The patient's respiratory pattern is characterized by an excessively high rate with marked inspiratory stridor and retractions. Epiglottitis is a medical emergency, and intervention includes quick intubation by a skilled and experienced clinician who is prepared to perform tracheotomy if necessary. Direct laryngoscopy to obtain swab cultures from the epiglottis, followed by appropriate intravenous antibiotic therapy, is required. The epiglottis usually returns to normal size after 48 hours. Other inflammatory conditions leading to airway obstruction include bacterial tracheitis, spasmodic laryngitis, head and neck abscesses, inflammatory nasal obstruction, and oropharyngeal obstruction.

9. How are croup and epiglottitis differentiated pathologically and clinically?

Differentiation can be difficult. Generally, croup occurs in younger age groups, though there is considerable overlap. One of the more reliable signs is a spontaneous cough, which almost always indicates croup.

Distinguishing Features of Epiglottitis and Croup

	EPIGLOTTITIS	CROUP
Cause	Bacterial	Viral
Age	1 yr to adult	1–5 yrs
Obstruction	Supraglottic	Subglottic
Onset	Sudden (hours)	Gradual (days)
Fever	High	Low grade
Dysphagia	Marked	None
Drooling	Present	Minimal
Posture	Sitting	Recumbent
Toxemia	Mild to severe	Mild
Cough	Usually none	Barking, brassy, spontaneous
Voice	Clear to muffled	Hoarse
Respiratory rate	Normal to rapid	Rapid
Larynx palpation	Tender	Not tender
Clinical course	Shorter	Longer

From Berry FA, Yemen TA: Pediatric airway in health and disease. Pediatr Clin North Am 41:168, 1994, with permission.

10. Which iatrogenic disorders can lead to airway obstruction in the child?

The most common causes of iatrogenic stridor are from laryngeal obstruction and include intubation, instrumentation, and surgery. **Recurrent laryngeal nerve paralysis** may be secondary to surgical trauma or pressure-induced ischemia following routine intubation. Vocal cord paralysis due to the latter is usually self-limited. **Endotracheal intubation** may result in airway obstruction after removal due to the mechanical trauma and irritation of the tube. **Acquired subglottic stenosis** may be seen in neonates or older children subjected to long-term intubation. There are several causes of iatrogenic **nasal obstruction**, including scar tissue formation following tonsil or adenoid surgery, prolonged administration of topical nasal decongestants, and many systemically administered medications that cause nasal stuffiness as a side effect.

11. Which traumatic disorders cause childhood airway obstruction?

Foreign bodies can precipitate airway obstruction by lodging in virtually any region of the upper aerodigestive tract. Nasal foreign bodies often cause unilateral or, less commonly, bilateral purulent rhinorrhea. Foreign bodies in the larynx or hypopharynx often present with inspiratory stridor. In the trachea, they may mimic croup. Because many foreign bodies are radiolucent, radiographic techniques are often inadequate for identification, and endoscopy is often necessary for identification and removal of the inciting foreign body.

Many other types of trauma may cause airway obstruction, including mandibular fractures causing retrodisplacement of the tongue, blunt or penetrating cervical trauma, dislocation of the arytenoid cartilages, laryngeal fracture, and compression of the airway lumen secondary to hematoma. Traumatic injury to the nose may also precipitate airway obstruction. Exposure to hot air, smoke, or steam (thermal trauma) or inhalation/ingestion of caustic chemicals may lead to airway obstruction from massive mucosal edema.

12. Which neoplastic disorders most commonly cause airway obstruction in the child?

Hemangioma is the most common head and neck neoplasm in children and may appear anywhere in the upper aerodigestive tract. Hemangiomas of the larynx may cause inspiratory or biphasic stridor due to their subglottic location.

Juvenile nasopharyngeal angiofibroma is the most common vascular mass found in the nasal cavity. The condition is confined to males aged 7–21 years. Most present with nasal obstruction and recurrent epistaxis. The tumor is locally invasive and can lead to gross facial deformity or spread intracranially.

A **teratoma** is a neoplasm with tissue elements from all three germinal layers. The nasopharynx is a common location for such tumors, and the patient with a teratoma may present with varying degrees of nasal obstruction. Cervical teratomas may also cause airway obstruction due to extrinsic pressure, and surgical resection is necessary.

Lymphangiomas are soft, compressible masses that are areas of regional lymphatic dilation. Approximately 90% of these lesions present before age 3. Airway compromise may occur from intraoral or laryngeal extension.

Recurrent respiratory papillomatosis can be seen in any portion of the upper aerodigestive tract. The lesions, generally caused by the human papillomavirus (HPV), commonly present with respiratory obstruction, hoarseness, and even aphonia.

13. Are radiographic studies helpful in evaluating upper airway obstruction? Which ones?

An accurate diagnosis of the etiology of upper airway obstruction can usually be obtained from history, physical examination, and endoscopy. However, many lesions can be identified noninvasively with radiography. A lateral view **plain film** with the neck extended helps to identify adenotonsillar hypertrophy, epiglottitis, or retropharyngeal abscess. The anteroposterior view may show tracheal deviation, asymmetry or narrowing of the subglottis, and vocal cord paralysis when obtained during phonation and deep respiration. All views are helpful when evaluating radiopaque foreign bodies, although most of these foreign bodies are radiolucent. Chest x-rays help in diagnosing pneumonia, areas of hyperaeration, or atelectasis. **Upper gastrointestinal studies** identify tracheoesophageal fistulas, vascular rings, and gastroesophageal reflux. **Fluoroscopy** can identify dynamic obstructions, such as laryngomalacia, tracheomalacia, vocal cord paralysis, and foreign bodies, and it localizes the obstruction site in obstructive sleep apnea. **CT** and **MRI** help to identify and characterize pathology located within soft tissue structures. Anomalies of the great vessels are best visualized with noncontrast MRI.

14. What are the indications for endotracheal intubation and tracheostomy in children?

Indications for Endotracheal Intubation and Tracheostomy in Children

CLINICAL SETTING	ENDOTRACHEAL INTUBATION	TRACHEOSTOMY
Emergencies	Always, except →	Severe craniofacial or head and neck injuries
Neonates and infants < 6 mos	Oral intubation unless no hope of extubation →	When long-term intubation is required or when there is difficulty in maintaining intubation because of activity
Infants > 6 mos and children	Maintain for 7–14 days and then →	When long-term intubation or ventilatory support is required for conditions such as severe head injuries
Epiglottitis	Until infection has cleared	Usually not necessary
Croup or other severe glottic inflammatory diseases	If does not respond to inhalations of racemic epinephrine or with airway obstruction as a temporary measure before →	When glottic edema and inflammation are severe

From Otherson HB: Injuries of the airway: Extrinsic and intrinsic. In Gans SL (ed): The Pediatric Airway. Philadelphia, W.B. Saunders, 1991, p 69, with permission.

In general, prolonged endotracheal intubation is well-tolerated and managed more effectively than tracheostomy in infants from birth to 6 months of age. In the presence of severe inflammatory glottic or tracheal disease, edema in the area of the cricoid may cause pressure against the tube, and endotracheal intubation should be maintained only long enough for tracheostomy to be performed. To avoid subglottic injury, tracheostomy should be considered in a child over 6 months of age when intubation is required for > 10–14 days.

15. What surgical options are available when managing subglottic stenosis?
Mild to moderate laryngeal stenosis in infants and children may be managed with the **anterior cricoid split** procedure. It is performed only when the child has failed extubation and has discrete mild to moderate subglottic narrowing. The procedure is through an external neck incision and involves dividing the cricoid cartilage, upper tracheal ring, and lower portion of the thyroid cartilage anteriorly. The patient is intubated with a nasotracheal tube which serves as a stent. The stent is usually removed after 5–10 days. Endoscopic treatment of subglottic stenosis with laser and dilation has the advantage of avoiding a tracheotomy but is generally successful in treating stenosis of < 50%. When stenosis of the lumen is > 70%, **open reconstruction** is generally recommended. Several operative approaches are used. With anterior subglottic stenosis, an anterior **autogenous costal cartilage graft** is appropriate. With more circumferential stenosis, the cricoid may be divided anteriorly, posteriorly, and possibly laterally with placement of a stent and additional grafts.

BIBLIOGRAPHY

1. Berry FA, Yemen TA: Pediatric airway in health and disease. Pediatr Clin North Am 41:153–180, 1994.
2. Drake AF: Controversies in upper airway obstruction. In Bailey BJ (ed): Head and Neck Surgery–Otolaryngology. Philadelphia, J.B. Lippincott, 1993, pp 912–921.
3. Myer CM, Cotton RT, Shott SR: The Pediatric Airway: An Interdisciplinary Approach. J.B. Lippincott, Philadelphia, 1995.
4. Myer CM, Cotton RT: Pediatric airway and laryngeal problems. In Lee KJ (ed): Essential Otolaryngology–Head and Neck Surgery, 6th ed. Norwalk, CT, Appleton & Lange, 1995, pp 889–904.
5. Myer CM, Cotton RT: Cricoid split and cartilage tracheoplasty. In Gans SL (ed): The Pediatric Airway. Philadelphia, W.B. Saunders, 1991, pp 117–124.
6. Otherson HB: Medical diseases of the airway: A surgeon's role. In Gans SL (ed): The Pediatric Airway. Philadelphia, W.B. Saunders, 1991, pp 64–70.
7. Otherson HB: Injuries of the airway: Extrinsic and intrinsic. In Gans SL (ed): The Pediatric Airway. Philadelphia, W.B. Saunders, 1991, pp 107–114.
8. Shechtman FG: Office evaluation of pediatric upper airway obstruction. Otolaryngol Clin North Am 25: 857–865, 1992.

66. TONSILS AND ADENOIDS

Robert Pearson, M.D.

1. Where is Waldeyer's ring?
Waldeyer's ring is the lymphoid tissue located in the nasopharynx and oropharynx at the entrance to the aerodigestive tract. The structures composing this ring are the faucial (palatine) tonsils, pharyngeal tonsils (adenoids), lateral "bands" on the lateral wall of the oropharynx, and lingual tonsils at the base of the tongue.

2. What is Passavant's ridge? Why is it important?
Passavant's ridge is the bulge in the posterior pharyngeal wall formed by the interdigitating fibers of the superior constrictor muscle. The soft palate abuts against this portion of the posterior pharyngeal wall during swallowing and speech.

3. What is the function of the tonsils and adenoids?

The tonsils and adenoids are lymphoid structures and therefore play a role in immunology and host defenses, specifically of the aerodigestive tract. Their complete role is unknown. However, these structures have been shown to be involved in antibody production and, more notably, in secretory IgA production, which plays an important part in mucosal defense mechanisms.

4. Which blood vessels supply the tonsils?

The tonsils are supplied by several branches of the external carotid artery. These branches include the tonsillar and ascending palatine branches of the facial artery, the ascending pharyngeal artery, dorsal lingual branch of the lingual artery, and palatine branch of the maxillary artery.

5. The tonsillar pillars comprise which muscles?

The palatoglossus muscle forms the anterior pillar, while the palatopharyngeus muscle forms the posterior pillar.

6. What are the most common etiologic agents involved in tonsillitis?

Common bacterial pathogens include group A β-hemolytic streptococci (GABHS), non-GABHS bacteria, and β-lactamase-producing organisms such as *Bacteroides*, nontypable *Haemophilus, Staphylococcus aureus,* and *Moraxella catarrhalis*. Common viral pathogens include adenovirus, coxsackievirus, parainfluenza, enteroviruses, Epstein-Barr virus, herpes simplex virus, and respiratory syncytial virus.

7. Describe the nonsurgical treatment of tonsillitis.

It is often difficult to distinguish viral from bacterial tonsillitis/pharyngitis. Most viral infections are self-limiting. Throat cultures should always be performed but, in reality, often are not. Penicillin is the drug of choice for culture-positive streptococcal infections; the increased incidence of β-lactamase-producing organisms makes clindamycin a better choice for culture-negative infections.

8. At what age is adenotonsillar disease most prevalent?

Adenotonsillar disease is most often considered a disease of childhood. In fact, tonsillectomies are the most common major surgical procedure performed in children. The tonsils are most active between the ages of 4 and 10 years, at which time adenotonsillar disease most often occurs. Although involution begins after puberty, tonsillar disease frequently occurs in adults as well.

9. What is "quinsy?"

Quinsy is a peritonsillar abscess, or a loculation of pus in the potential space that surrounds the tonsil. This process develops as an infection in a peripheral tonsillar crypt, penetrates through the tonsillar capsule, and enters the peritonsillar space.

10. What are the etiologic factors that lead to a peritonsillar abscess?

Over half of patients who present with quinsy have a history of previous tonsillar infections. Allergy and dental caries have been postulated as contributing factors. The same organisms that are common to tonsillitis are also found in peritonsillar abscesses, although peritonsillar abscesses may have a greater incidence of anaerobic bacteria.

11. Are there typical signs and symptoms of peritonsillar abscess?

Patients with peritonsillar abscess often have a history of a sore throat for 3–7 days, fever, dysphagia, odynophagia, trismus, and a "hot potato" or muffled voice. Airway obstruction is uncommon. Examination reveals an inflamed oropharynx with an infected, swollen tonsil. The peritonsillar area is also inflamed and swollen, displacing the soft palate and uvula away from the midline. Occasionally, fluctuance may be demonstrated on palpation.

12. How is quinsy managed properly?

Either needle aspiration or incision with drainage is necessary. These procedures can often be done in the office or emergency room. After drainage, broad-spectrum antibiotics such as amoxicillin/clavulanate or clindamycin are recommended. A tonsillectomy is best performed after complete resolution of the infection but may be necessary before this time if incision and drainage are inadequate.

13. Which conditions are associated with adenotonsillar hypertrophy?

Quinsy

Retro- or peripharyngeal abscess

Cervical lymphadenitis

Rhinitis

Paranasal sinusitis

Olfactory disorders

Otitis media

Impairments of speech and hearing

Abnormalities of dentition

Fetor oris

Failure to thrive

14. What are the definite indications for tonsillectomy?

Obstructive sleep apnea or cor pulmonale

Malignancy or suspected malignancy

Tonsillitis resulting in febrile convulsions

Persistent or recurrent tonsillar hemorrhage

15. What are some proposed indications for an elective tonsillectomy?

Recurrent acute or chronic tonsillitis

Peritonsillar abscess

Recurrent sore throats

Recurrent upper respiratory tract infections

Cervical adenitis

Tonsillolithiasis

Eating or swallowing disorders

Orofacial and dental abnormalities

Halitosis

16. What are some proposed indications for an adenoidectomy?

Recurrent or chronic middle ear disease

Obstructive adenoid hypertrophy

Sleep apnea

Obligate mouth breathing or snoring

Recurrent acute or chronic adenoiditis

17. After how may episodes of tonsillitis should a patient be considered for surgery?

7 infections in 1 year (not necessarily streptococcus-positive infections)

5 infections/year for 2 consecutive years

3 infections/ year for 3 consecutive years

> 2 weeks missed from school or work in any 1 year

18. On examination, you see a bifid uvula. Is it safe to proceed with adenotonsillectomy?

The presence of a bifid uvula has been associated with various disorders of the soft palate. **Submucous cleft** is the most common of these disorders. Adenotonsillectomy with a submucous cleft leads to a higher incidence of **velopharyngeal insufficiency**. Careful evaluation of the palate should be done prior to tonsillectomy and adenoidectomy in any patient, but special attention should be given to patients with a bifid uvula. If a submucous cleft is encountered, a "superior" adenoidectomy should be done. This adaptation leaves some bulk in the posterior pharyngeal wall, which provides adequate velopharyngeal closure after surgery.

19. Why does velopharyngeal insufficiency occur after adenoidectomy?

Velopharyngeal insufficiency (VPI) occurs when there is incomplete closure of the soft palate against the posterior pharyngeal wall. This is manifest by hypernasal speech and nasopharyngeal regurgitation. In children, adenoid tissue significantly adds to the bulk of the posterior pharyngeal wall. The soft palate abuts against this wall during speech and swallowing. An adenoidectomy reduces this bulk and can lead to incomplete closure, resulting in VPI. Different studies show the incidence of VPI after adenoidectomy to range from 1/1500 to 1/10,000 in normal patients. The incidence of VPI in patients with palatal disorders, such as submucous cleft, is much higher.

20. When is a tonsillectomy and adenoidectomy contraindicated?

Blood dyscrasias (leukemias, purpuras, hemophilia, etc.)

Uncontrolled systemic diseases (diabetes, heart disease, etc.)

Cleft palate

Acute infections

21. What are the complications of tonsillectomy and adenoidectomy?
Airway obstruction   Pain
Bleeding (up to 7-10 days after procedure)   Weight loss
Pulmonary edema (especially after relief of obstruction)   Death
Velopharyngeal insufficiency

22. Can tonsils and adenoids grow back?
If not all of the lymphoid tissue is removed during a tonsillectomy and adenoidectomy, the residual tissue may hypertrophy and again cause symptoms.

23. How is postoperative bleeding managed?
Postoperative bleeding generally occurs either soon after the procedure, while the patient is still in the hospital, or several days after the procedure when the eschar sloughs off the tonsillar fossae. Frequently, the bleeding stops spontaneously and requires only a period of observation. Many recommend overnight admission, but some cases can be adequately handled in the office or emergency room if the bleeding point is easily identifiable and the patient is cooperative. In many cases, patients with refractory bleeding should be taken back to the operating room.

24. What does the postoperative management of adenotonsillectomy involve?
Pain is always an issue, especially in adults. Therefore, good pain control is a necessity. In addition, oral antibiotics have been shown to decrease postoperative pain. Patients should be warned of the possibility of postoperative bleeding and given explicit instructions should bleeding occur. For the first few days, a liquid diet is suggested; this may be advanced slowly to a soft food diet. Patients should not participate in heavy activity for 2 weeks after the procedure. Although tonsillectomies and adenoidectomies are commonly performed as outpatient surgeries, it is wise to admit patients with complicated cases, especially if the procedure is done to relieve an obstruction. Many of these patients require continuous-pulse oximetry, often in an intensive care facility.

CONTROVERSIES

25. Is it safe to perform an adenotonsillectomy as an outpatient procedure for uncomplicated patients?
Those who advocate that this procedure be performed on an outpatient basis feel that it is more cost-effective. They also cite a low incidence of major postoperative complications. In opposition, others argue that an adenotonsillectomy is a major surgery fraught with serious postoperative complications; these complications are best handled in the inpatient setting.

26. How old should the patient be before undergoing adenotonsillectomy?
There is no set age, but several studies show an increased incidence of complications with children < 3 years of age. When indicated, tonsillectomy and adenoidectomy (T&A) are viable options for this age group, but both parents and physicians need to be aware of the increased complication rate. Patients in this age group are probably not candidates for routine outpatient surgery.

27. What is the role of antibiotic and steroid administration following T&A?
Several studies show earlier recovery, less postoperative pain, and fewer complications with the use of antibiotics and steroids following T&A. Other studies show no significant difference. Advocates of their use state minimal adverse effects in the face of potential benefits. Opponents cite unnecessary costs and development of resistant bacterial strains.

BIBLIOGRAPHY

1. Brook I, Hirokowa R: Treatment of patients with a history of recurrent tonsillitis due to group A beta-hemolytic streptococci. Clin Pediatr 24:331, 1985.
2. Catlin FI, Grimes WJ: The effect of steroid therapy on recovery from tonsillectomy in children. Arch Otolaryngol Head Neck Surg 117:649, 1991.

3. Goeringer GC, Vidic B: The embryogenesis and anatomy of Waldeyer's ring. Otolaryngol Clin North Am 20:207, 1987.
4. Grandis JR, et al: The efficacy of perioperative antibiotic therapy on recovery following tonsillectomy in adults: Randomized double-blind placebo-controlled trial. Otolaryngol Head Neck Surg 106:137, 1992.
5. Kielmovitch IH, et al: Microbiology of obstructive tonsillar hypertrophy and recurrent tonsillitis. Arch Otolaryngol Head Neck Surg 115:721, 1989.
6. Nicklaus PJ, Herzon FS, Steinle EW: Short stay outpatient tonsillectomy. Arch Otolaryngol Head Neck Surg 121:521, 1995.
7. Paradise JL: Tonsillectomy and adenoidectomy. In Bluestone CD, Stool SE (eds): Pediatric Otolaryngology, 2nd ed. Philadelphia, W.B. Saunders, 1990.
8. Potsic WP, et al: Relief of upper airway obstruction by adenotonsillectomy. Otolaryngol Head Neck Surg 94:476, 1986.
9. Richtsmeier WJ, Shikhani AH: The physiology and immunology of the pharyngeal lymphoid tissue. Otolaryngol Clin North Am 20:219, 1987.
10. Rothschild MA, Catalano P, Biller HF: Ambulatory pediatric tonsillectomy and the identification of high-risk subgroups. Otolaryngol Head Neck Surg 110:203, 1994.
11. Telian SA, et al: The effect of antibiotic therapy on recovery after tonsillectomy in children. Arch Otolaryngol Head Neck Surg 112:610, 1986.
12. Volk MS: The effect of preoperative steroids on tonsillectomy patients. Otolaryngol Head Neck Surg 109:726, 1993.

67. CONGENITAL MALFORMATIONS

Michelle R. Kuntz, M.S., and Kenny H. Chan, M.D.

1. How does the differential diagnosis of a congenital neck mass differ with its location?

Site	Characteristics
Lateral neck	
Branchial anomalies	Anterior to sternomastoid muscle
Lymphangioma	Thin-walled multiloculated cysts on ultrasound
External laryngoceles	Air-filled, compressed
Midline	
Thyroglossal duct cyst	Elevates with swelling
Plunging ranula	Midline or just off, cystic and extends to floor of mouth
Dermoid	Usually submental, somewhat compressible
Thymic cyst	Usually lower in neck
Teratoma	Neonate with airway obstruction
Entire neck	
Lymphangioma	Thin-walled, multiloculated cysts on ultrasound
Invasive hemangioma	Localized, swelling, most common in trapezius, scalene, and sternomastoid muscles

Adapted from May M: Neck masses in children: Diagnosis and treatment. Pediatr Ann 5:8, 1976.

2. How does a branchial fistula form? A branchial cyst? A branchial sinus?

The branchial apparatus consists of five mesodermal arches. On the external wall, these arches are lined with ectodermal grooves or clefts; on the internal wall, they are lined with endoderm pouches. Each arch contains a cartilaginous portion, an artery, nerve, and musculature that begins to develop in the fourth week. As the structures within each arch proliferate, a cervical sinus is formed. The cervical sinus eventually becomes obliterated by the growth of the surrounding structures. Of all of the branchial arches, the second arch is the most commonly malformed. A **branchial fistula** is caused by the persistence of a sinus external opening. A

branchial cyst occurs when the cervical sinus remains patent and the external opening is obliterated. A **branchial sinus** is open into the skin or lumen of the foregut and ends blindly in the deep tissues of the neck.

3. What are the possible complications of a lymphangioma?

Cervical lymphangiomas, also known as **cystic hygromas,** do not usually produce symptoms, although the cosmetic deformity is often of concern. Large lymphangiomas in the anterior neck can cause **airway** or pharyngeal **compression.** These cystic spaces can also become infected, forming an **abscess. Hemorrhage** into the cyst may also occur. A lymphangioma often presents when it becomes associated with infection or hemorrhage.

4. Why does a thyroglossal duct cyst move on swallowing?

A thyroglossal duct cyst is a remnant of the thyroid gland's descent from the foramen cecum, at the base of the tongue, to the pretracheal space. Because of the close proximity to the hyoid bone superiorly and the attachment to the thyroid gland inferiorly, the lesion moves during swallowing. Thyroglossal duct cysts are the most common anterior midline neck masses in children. These masses must be removed because they have the potential for neoplastic transformation.

5. Compare a teratoma and a dermoid cyst.

Both are anomalies involving pluripotential embryonal cells. Teratomas are composed of all three germ layers and are much larger than dermoid cysts. Dermoid cysts are composed of ectoderm and mesoderm and tend to occur along the lines of embryonic fusion (midline). Dermoid cysts characteristically have an adipose matrix that appears "cheesy." Dermoid cysts do not exclusively occur in the neck.

6. Name the six types of tracheoesophageal fistulas.

1. Isolated esophageal atresia without fistula (6–7%)
2. Esophageal atresia with proximal tracheoesophageal fistula (1%)
3. Esophageal atresia with distal tracheoesophageal fistula (86%)
4. Esophageal atresia with proximal and distal tracheoesophageal fistula (1–5%)
5. Tracheoesophageal fistula without atresia (5%), also called H-type
6. Esophageal stenosis without fistula (1%)

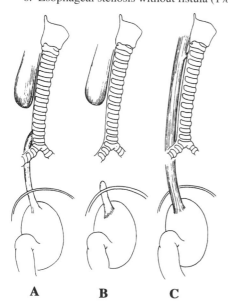

Esophageal atresia. *A,* The most common form of esophageal atresia (85%) consists of a dilated proximal esophageal pouch and a connection of the distal esophagus to the carina of the trachea. *B,* Pure esophageal atresia. *C,* Fistula of the H-type without atresia. (From Coran AG (ed): Surgery of the Neonate. Boston, Little, Brown, 1978, p 46, with permission.)

A   B   C

In cases of atresia, the presentation is usually the inability to swallow, excess salivation, and episodes of coughing and cyanosis in the first few days of life. The presentation depends on the severity of the atresia. The H-type often present later with recurrent problems with pneumonia, coughing when fed, or abdominal distention.

7. Which is the most common malformation associated with the supraglottis?

Of the structures in the upper aerodigestive tract, the larynx is the most commonly affected with anomalies. Affecting the supraglottis, laryngomalacia is a congenital flaccid larynx that is diagnosed by high-pitched stridor. The problem is usually self-limited and treatment is unnecessary.

8. What are the most common malformations of the glottis?

The glottis may be affected by **unilateral vocal cord paralysis**, usually a self-limited condition. When **bilateral vocal cord paralysis** occurs, a thorough workup should be performed to rule out other concurrent malformations (i.e., Arnold-Chiari syndrome). **Webs** usually affect the anterior part of the glottis and cause aphonia. **Posterior clefts** are rare but occur because the tracheoesophageal septum fails to develop.

9. What are the two most common malformations of the subglottis?

Congenital stenosis of the subglottis is generally secondary to a deformed cricoid cartilage. Stenosis is defined by an anteroposterior diameter of < 4 mm in the newborn. A **hemangioma** of the subglottic area usually presents in the third or fourth week of life. Spontaneous regression of these lesions can occur. When the lesion is obstructing the airway, it must be surgically removed.

10. What are the two groups of tracheal malformations? What causes them?

Intrinsic malformations are caused by maldevelopment of the trachea. Some examples of intrinsic malformations include tracheal agenesis, stenosis (hypoplasia), tracheomalacia, tracheomegaly, and tracheal diverticula.

Extrinsic malformations are secondary to compression of the airway from the structures that surround it. Extrinsic malformations are less common (10% of cases). Causes include vascular (i.e., innominate artery compression or other aberrant malformations, such as a double aortic arch or aberrant right subclavian artery), masses in the neck and mediastinum, and an enlarged thyroid.

11. Describe the common congenital malformations of the auricle.

The most common malformations of the auricle are microtia, preauricular cysts, and canal atresia. **Microtia** is hypoplasia of the external ear. It can be associated with or without **atresia** of the external auditory canal. It may be present as an isolated deformity or may be accompanied by hemifacial or bilateral facial microsomia. There are three types of microtia. In grade I, the auricle is misshapen, but the landmarks are recognizable. In grade II, the auricle is hook-shaped or looks like a question mark. In grade III, only one or two protuberances mark the position of the lobule. Current therapy for microtia is reconstructive surgery using an autologous rib graft for the framework in a multistage operation.

A **preauricular cyst** is a remnant of the first branchial or pharyngeal groove. Surgical excision is required when the cyst becomes infected.

12. Explain the anomalies of the first branchial groove.

The first branchial groove gives rise to the external auditory canal (EAC). Anomalies are divided into aplasia, atresia, stenosis, and duplication of the EAC. **Aplasia** occurs when the first branchial groove does not develop. The groove usually persists as a tract. **Atresia** anomalies occur when the EAC is present but the lumen is not. The lumen is blocked by bone, fibrous tissue, or both. **Stenosis** occurs when the lumen is narrowed which occurs in varying degrees of severity. **Duplication** occurs when the EAC develops normally and the tract persists from the canal to the skin of the neck.

13. What are the common congenital malformations of the nose?
Choanal atresia
Dermoid cysts
Nasal gliomas and encephaloceles

14. How do gliomas and encephaloceles differ?
Both gliomas and encephaloceles are ectodermal neural tissue of the brain that has remained in the nasal cavity or nasopharynx following embryologic development. Encephaloceles are herniated glial tissue that always maintain the communication with the CSF. They are differentiated from gliomas by the presence of a defect in the cranium that allows for the herniation to occur. Unlike encephaloceles, gliomas are not always connected to the CSF.

15. What is the CHARGE association?
Choanal atresia is the most common nasal anomaly. Atresia of the nares can be unilateral or bilateral, bony or membranous, and complete or incomplete. Bilateral atresia is a serious life-threatening airway emergency. Most choanal atresia occurs along with other anomalies, hence the CHARGE association:

C = Coloboma
H = Heart disease
A = Atresia, choanal
R = Retarded development of the CNS
G = Genital hypoplasia
E = Ear anomalies or deafness

16. How do cup ear deformities and prominent ear deformities differ?
A **cup ear deformity** is a congenital malformation of the auricle in which the upper and middle portions are abnormal and the lower portion is normal. The upper portion is bent forward and downward. The middle portion is generally large and at a 90° angle from the skull. It can be present in various degrees of severity. In a **prominent ear deformity**, the child has protruding ears. Measured from the mastoid to the ear, an angle of > 40° or a distance of > 20 mm characteristically exists. Both cup ear and prominent ear deformities can be improved with reconstructive surgery.

CONTROVERSIES

17. Is preoperative imaging required before removing a midline anterior neck mass?
An ectopic thyroid can be the only functioning thyroid tissue present in a patient. It can also mimic a thyroglossal duct cyst. Injudicious removal of an ectopic thyroid may result in permanent thyroid replacement therapy for a patient. Therefore, ongoing controversy revolves around obtaining a preoperative radionuclide scan and/or a sonogram of the neck before operative intervention.

18. Explain the two theories for congenital cholesteatoma formation.
Theory 1—The more commonly approved theory states that an ectodermal cell rest remains behind the tympanic membrane in the postnatal period. Proliferation of these cell rests results in the formation of a cholesteatoma (cyst-like mass that is filled with desquamating debris).

Theory 2—Most children with cholesteatoma have had otitis media with an effusion. This theory states that the cholesteatoma is the result of metaplasia secondary to middle ear inflammation.

BIBLIOGRAPHY

1. Austin DF: Congenital malformations of the ear. In Ballenger JJ (ed): Diseases of the Nose, Throat, Ears, Head, and Neck, 14th ed. Philadelphia, Lea & Febiger, 1991, pp 1172–1174.
2. Barricade J: Pediatric plastic and reconstructive surgery of the head and neck. In Bluestone CD, Stool SE (eds): Pediatric Otolaryngology. Philadelphia, W. B. Saunders, 1990, p 699.

3. Belenky WM: Nasal obstruction with rhinorrhea. In Bluestone CD, Stool SE (eds): Pediatric Otolaryngology. Philadelphia, W. B. Saunders, 1990, p 662.
4. Bordley JE, Brookhouser PE, Gabriel FT Jr: Neck. In Ear, Nose, and Throat Disorders in Children. New York, Raven Press, 1986, pp 383–388.
5. Cotton RT, Reilly JS: Stridor and airway obstruction. In Bluestone CD, Stool SE (eds): Pediatric Otolaryngology. Philadelphia, W. B. Saunders, 1990, p 1098.
6. Healy GB: Congenital anomalies of the aerodigestive tract. In Bailey BJ (ed): Head and Neck Surgery–Otolaryngology. Philadelphia, J. B. Lippincott, 1993, pp 848–860.
7. Janusz B: Congenital malformations of the nose. In Cummings CW, et al (eds): Otolaryngology–Head and Neck Surgery. St. Louis, Mosby, 1986, pp 2865–2875.
8. Karmody CS: Developmental anomalies of the neck. In Bluestone CD, Stool SE (eds): Pediatric Otolaryngology. Philadelphia, W. B. Saunders, 1990, pp 1308–1309.
9. Lambert PR: Congenital aural atresia. In Bailey BJ (ed): Head and Neck Surgery–Otolaryngology. Philadelphia, J. B. Lippincott, 1993, pp 1579–1590.
10. May M: Neck masses in children: Diagnosis and treatment. Pediatr Ann 5:8, 1976.
11. Radkowski D, et al: Thyroglossal duct remnants: Preoperative evaluations and management. Arch Otolaryngol Head Neck Surg 117:1378–1381, 1991.
12. Pincus RL: Congenital neck masses and cysts. In Bailey BJ (ed): Head and Neck Surgery–Otolaryngology. Philadelphia, J. B. Lippincott, 1993, pp 754–759.
13. Sessions RB, Hudkins C: Congenital anomalies of the nose. In Bailey BJ (ed): Head and Neck Surgery–Otolaryngology. Philadelphia, J. B. Lippincott, 1993, pp 793–800.
14. Spector JG, Anderson K: Tracheostenosis. In Cummings CW, et al (eds): Otolaryngology–Head and Neck Surgery. St. Louis, Mosby, 1986, pp 2436–2441.
15. Stool SE, Eavey RD: Tracheotomy. In Bluestone CD, Stool SE (eds): Pediatric Otolaryngology. Philadelphia, W. B. Saunders, 1990, p 1229.

68. GENETIC ISSUES IN OTOLARYNGOLOGY

Katie J. Hanson, M.S., and Anne L. Matthews, R.N., Ph.D.

1. What are the major inheritance patterns for single gene disorders?

Autosomal dominant (AD): If one parent carries a gene coding for such a disorder, the risk to the offspring is 50%.

Autosomal recessive: These disorders imply a 25% risk for children of two carrier parents.

X-linked recessive: The abnormal gene is carried on the X chromosome. Most X-linked disorders are recessive, implying a risk to the offspring of an unaffected "carrier" female. If a woman is a carrier, 50% of her sons will be affected and 50% of her daughters will be carriers. Men with X-linked recessive conditions can pass the trait only to their daughters, making all of their daughters obligate carriers. The sons of men with X-linked recessive conditions are not at risk.

X-linked dominant: These conditions are rare. In these instances, both males and females are clinically affected. Females are affected because the affected gene on the abnormal X chromosome is dominant over the corresponding gene on the normal X chromosome. Both daughters and sons of women with X-linked dominant traits will have a 50% chance of inheriting the abnormal gene, thus being affected. Affected men will only pass the trait to their daughters, but in every case, their daughter will also be affected.

2. Which factors complicate the identification of an autosomal dominant pedigree in a family history?

Expressivity and penetrance. Ideally, a classic dominant inheritance pattern reflects a specific phenotype or feature throughout a family history. In reality, dominant genes often lead to a variation in **phenotypic expression**. **Decreased penetrance** is also common with dominant genes, so that a carrier of a dominant gene may not have any detectable phenotypic expression. Lastly, **new mutations** are commonly associated with autosomal dominant disorders. In these cases, a person is considered to have a new mutation if they are affected with a dominant disorder despite a negative family history. With each pregnancy, the individual who is affected by the mutation has a 50% risk of transmitting the abnormal gene to their offspring.

3. One class of genetic inheritance, multifactorial, is often responsible for isolated congenital malformations such as cleft lip or palate. What does this mean?

Many common disorders run in families, but they are not associated with single-gene, chromosomal, or teratogenic factors. Because these traits are caused by many factors, both genetic and environmental, they are known as multifactorial. Multifactorial disorders recur within families, but they do not show any specific recognizable pattern of inheritance. A geneticist can estimate the approximate heritability, or the importance of genetic factors in a given trait and recurrence risks. The empiric risk to first-degree relatives, as determined by family studies, is approximately the square root of the population risk. As expected, the recurrence risk is greater when > 1 family member is affected. Similarly, the more severe the malformation, the greater the recurrence risk. In many multifactorial traits, one sex is more frequently affected for reasons that are not always understood. For example, a trait may be more commonly seen in males than females. If a female exhibits the trait, her offspring have a greater chance of inheriting it.

4. What are the indications for obtaining cytogenetic studies?

Reasonable criteria for obtaining cytogenetic studies would be the presence of two major malformations or a single malformation with two or more minor malformations. In addition, whenever developmental delay and/or mental retardation is also present, cytogenetic studies should be considered.

Minor Anomalies	Major Malformations and Disabilities
High-arched palate	Growth retardation
Cleft uvula	Mental retardation
Hypertelorism	Motor delay
Abnormal slant of palpebral fissures	Congenital heart defects
Micrognathia	Spina bifida
Clinodactyly	Genitourinary malformations
Hernia	Deafness
Pectus excavatum/carinatum	Microcephaly
Large auricles	Cleft lip/ palate
Short neck	Absent or hypoplastic ears
Synophrys	Renal anomalies
Abnormal dermatoglyphics	Eye anomalies

Bordloy JE, Brookhouser PE, Tucker GF: Ear, nose, and throat disorders in children. New York, Raven Press, 1986, p 108.

5. Cleft lip or palate can be associated with other birth defects or abnormalities. What percentage are associated with a genetic syndrome?

When a child with a cleft is encountered, a genetic evaluation should be conducted. It is important to ensure that the defect is isolated and not part of a syndrome. One percent of cleft lip and/or palate defects are associated with a genetic syndrome. In contrast, 8% of cleft palates without cleft lips are associated with genetic syndromes.

6. If the brain, eyes, heart, or limbs are involved in a child with a cleft, which syndrome should be considered?

Cleft lip is associated with genetic conditions such as Van der Woude syndrome (AD), chromosomal abnormalities, and in utero teratogenic environmental exposures. Cleft palate alone is more likely to be associated with genetic syndromes. These conditions include Stickler syndrome (AD), Treacher Collins syndrome (AD), Pierre Robin sequence (sporadic), and chromosome 22q deletions.

7. If a cleft lip and/or palate is determined to be an isolated condition, what is the recurrence risk when the same parents desire to have a second child? Is the risk changed if the cleft is unilateral or bilateral?

The recurrence risk for an isolated cleft lip or a cleft lip in association with a cleft palate is about 4%. An isolated cleft lip with or without a cleft palate has many features of a classic multi-factorial threshold trait. More severe expression of the trait is associated with a higher recurrence risk. For example, a bilateral cleft has a higher recurrence rate than a unilateral cleft. A cleft lip and palate has a higher recurrence rate than a cleft lip alone. About 60–80% of those affected by cleft lip and/or palate are males, so therefore the recurrence risk is slightly increased if the affected child is a female.

8. What is Pierre Robin sequence?

Pierre Robin sequence occurs in about 1 in 30,000 births and affects both males and females equally. Although its inheritance is most likely multifactorial, it can occur as part of a syndrome. The initiating defect of Pierre Robin sequence may be hypoplasia of the mandibular area prior to 9 weeks' gestation. This hypoplasia restrains the tongue posteriorly, thus impairing closure of the posterior palatal shelves at the midline. Cardinal features of this sequence include striking micrognathia, glossoptosis, and cleft palate. Newborns with Pierre Robin are at risk of apnea due to an obstructed airway.

9. What is choanal atresia?

Embryologically, the bucconasal membrane ruptures at the seventh week of gestation. If this rupture fails to occur, the primitive nasal cavity does not communicate with the pharynx, resulting in choanal atresia. The incidence of this malformation is 1 in 5000 live births. Choanal atresia affects females to males in a 2:1 ratio. In 90% of cases, the defect is a bony atresia, with the remaining 10% being membranous. Although this disorder is usually unilateral and diagnosed later in life, bilateral atresia is usually recognized in the neonatal period. Because newborns are obligate nose breathers, those affected by a bilateral atresia exhibit cyanosis.

10. Which embryologic branchial arches contribute to external ear development?

Congenital malformations of the auricle and external ear are related to developmental defects of the first and second branchial arches and to lesions of the branchial groove. The groove joins with endoderm of the first pharyngeal pouch to form the external auditory canal.

11. Embryologically, how does congenital lop or cup ear malformation occur?

Lop or cup ear defect represents one of the most common malformations of the external ear. With an incidence of 1 in 1000 births, it is inherited as an autosomal dominant trait. In this disorder, hypoplasia of the superior one-third of the auricle causes a downward folding and deficiency of the superior aspect of the helix. Most of the auricle originates from the second branchial arch. The tragus and a small part of the helix arise from the first branchial arch. If the antihelix fails to unfold between the 12th and 16th weeks of development, a protruding helix persists, resulting in lop or cup ear.

The mildest form of this defect may be the result of intrauterine constraint and will resolve in the first year of life. Otherwise, the lop/cup ear can be surgically corrected in severe cases. Among these cases have been a few reports of nonsyndromic lop/cup ear defects that are seen as an autosomal dominant trait in families. Rarely, the lop or cup ear is associated with a genetic syndrome.

12. Do auricular tags lend significance to any otolaryngologic or genetic concern?

Auricular appendages or tags are common, mild malformations that are usually located just anterior to the auricle near the tragus. Auricular tags often follow a line of predilection where the first and second branchial arches join. Generally, this mild malformation is an isolated finding, not part of a syndrome. However, children with disorders such as oculo-auriculo-vertebral spectrum commonly have auricular tags. Taken as a whole, one author reported that approximately 2% of individuals with auricular tags have some associated syndrome. Another author reported that among neonates who had an isolated ear tag, 13% had some sensorineural hearing loss. Therefore, some suggest screening for hearing loss in all children with this finding.

13. What are the most common causes of prenatal congenital hearing loss? Perinatal hearing loss? Postnatal hearing loss?

A common **prenatal** cause of hearing loss is intrauterine infection. Low birthweight and microcephaly are often associated with such infections. In these cases, an ophthalmologic evaluation may reveal chorioretinitis. **Perinatal** causes of hearing loss may be due to hypoxia, hyperbilirubinemia, infection, and ototoxic drugs. A sloping high-frequency hearing loss is suggestive of a perinatal etiology. The major **postnatal** cause of severe to profound sensorineural deafness is bacterial meningitis.

14. What is the incidence of hearing loss in children due to genetic factors?

Recent studies estimate that 68% of childhood hearing loss is due to genetic factors. About 20–25% of these cases are due to identifiable environmental causes, either prenatal or postnatal, and 25–30% are sporadic with unknown etiologies.

15. How often is genetic hearing loss due to autosomal recessive inheritance? Autosomal dominant? X-linked?

Most authors attribute 75–80% of genetic deafness to autosomal recessive genes and 18–20% to autosomal dominant genes. The remainder of cases are classified as X-linked or chromosomal disorders.

16. Twenty percent of children with a congenital sensorineural hearing loss have subtle or severe abnormalities of the inner ear. Describe the most common autosomal inner ear dysmorphologies.

Scheibe aplasia is the most common of the inherited inner ear anomalies. It is usually inherited in an autosomal recessive pattern and may also be seen in association with Usher syndrome. Although the bony labyrinth, utricles, and semicircular canals are normal, a membranous cochlea-saccular aplasia is characteristic.

Michael aplasia is inherited in an autosomal dominant manner. Although this aplasia has a wide phenotypic spectrum, it is usually characterized by complete developmental failure of the inner ear. Typically, Michael aplasia is associated with a normally developed middle ear and external auditory canal.

Mondini aplasia is believed to be autosomal dominant in transmission. It is characterized by incomplete development of the bony or membranous labyrinth. The cochlea may be represented by a single curve, while the vestibule and semicircular canals may be abnormally wide or completely absent. Hearing may be unaffected, or complete hearing loss may be present.

Alexander aplasia is associated with an abnormal cochlear duct. The basal coil and its adjacent ganglion cells are the most affected. Patients with an Alexander aplasia have a high-frequency hearing loss.

17. In many cases of hereditary hearing loss, accompanying abnormalities are seen in other body systems. Which other systems deserve a complete evaluation?

The integument, eyes, nervous system, skeletal system, endocrine system, and urinary system.

18. Most genetic deafness in childhood is attributed to autosomal recessive genes, and about half of them are associated with recognizable genetic syndromes. Which syndromes should be considered?

Usher syndrome is an autosomal recessive disorder characterized by sensorineural hearing loss and retinitis pigmentosa. **Pendred syndrome** is characterized by profound congenital sensorineural hearing loss and goiter. Individuals demonstrate a partial failure of iodine organification. About half of these individuals are euthyroid; the remainder are hypothyroid. Pendred syndrome probably accounts for at least 5% of cases of congenital hearing loss.

19. If a family history reveals an autosomal dominant hearing loss, which genetic syndromes should be considered? Which systems should be evaluated in each?

Waardenburg syndrome is one of the more readily recognizable hearing loss syndromes. It is seen in at least 2–5% of those affected with congenital hearing loss. Affected individuals have variable degrees of telecanthus, synophorus, heterochromatic irides, white forelock, early graying, and some degree of hearing loss. There are two types of Waardenburg syndrome. A greater percentage of individuals with type II show hearing loss (50% of affected individuals). Only about 20% of those with type I have hearing loss.

Stickler syndrome, also called progressive arthro-ophthalmopathy, is characterized by micrognathia, cleft palate, high myopia with retinal detachment and cataracts, joint hypermobility, and early adult arthritis. Progressive sensorineural high-frequency hearing loss is seen in many cases. More infrequently, conductive hearing loss is reported.

Branchio-oto-renal syndrome involves branchial characteristics, including ear pits and tags, cervical fistulae, and renal involvement. Hearing loss may be sensorineural, conductive, or mixed. As many as 2% of deaf children have this syndrome.

Treacher Collins syndrome, or mandibulofacial dysostosis, is a craniofacial disorder. Manifestations include microtia, aural meatal atresia, and conductive hearing loss. Sensorineural hearing loss and vestibular dysfunction may also be present. Facial features include malar hypoplasia with underdevelopment of zygomatic arches resulting in down-turned palpebral fissures, coloboma of lower lids, and a hypoplastic mandible.

Neurofibromatosis (NF) is a neurocutaneous disorder. Bilateral acoustic neuromas are found in 95% of patients with NF type II. NF type I is associated with cutaneous findings, including café-au-lait spots and cutaneous and plexiform neurofibromas; rarely, it is associated with unilateral acoustic neuromas. However, patients with both types of NF should receive audiologic evaluation.

20. If a child of two hearing patients has a sporadic hearing loss, what is the recurrence risk for later children?

Unexplained or sporadic hearing loss recurs 10–16 % of the time.

21. If two hearing parents have two hearing-impaired children, what is the recurrence risk? What if one hearing-impaired parent has one hearing-impaired child?

The recurrence risk given to hearing parents of two hearing-impaired children increases to 25%. If a family has one hearing-impaired parent and one hearing-impaired child, the risk ranges from negligible (if the case is nongenetic or a very rare recessive disorder) to 50% (if the parent is affected by an autosomal dominant syndrome).

22. Which factor complicates a family pedigree of otosclerosis?

Otosclerosis is most likely inherited in an autosomal dominant fashion and involves delayed-onset conductive or mixed hearing impairment. However, because of decreased penetrance, only 40% of gene carriers actually demonstrate otosclerosis.

23. What otolaryngologic problems exist for individuals with craniosynostosis?

Individuals with craniosynostosis syndromes are at risk for having high arched or cleft palate, deviated septum, low-set malformed ears, and hearing loss. Syndromes to consider include Apert, Crouzon, Pfeiffer, Saethre-Chotzen, Jackson-Weiss, and Carpenter.

24. Chromosomal abnormalities increase a child's risk for otolaryngologic problems. Which particular chromosomal defects have otolaryngologic considerations?

Patients with trisomy 21, trisomy 13, cri du chat (5p–), Wolf-Hirschhorn (4p–), and deletion of the long arm of chromosome 18 (18q–). Trisomy 13 and Wolf-Hirschhorn are associated with cleft lips with or without cleft palates. The typical, mewing cry described in infants with cri du chat syndrome is ascribed to abnormal laryngeal development. In patients with 4p deletion, the endolarynx is narrow and diamond-shaped with a persistent interarythroid cleft. Individuals with 18q– are at risk for narrow or atretic ear canals, contributing to frequent otitis media and deafness.

25. Are there otolaryngologic considerations in evaluating a child with Down syndrome?
Children with Down syndrome are at increased risk for upper respiratory tract infections. Due to eustachian tube dysfunction, they are also susceptible to frequent otitis media. Because they often have significant middle ear anomalies, they are predisposed to mixed hearing losses. The assessment of audiologic function is essential because significant hearing losses in young children affect all aspects of development. Because of their narrow nasopharynx, narrow oropharyngeal airway, and macroglossia, these children are susceptible to upper airway obstruction. Over 50% of Down syndrome patients have obstructive sleep apnea.

26. Why is an otolaryngologist likely to evaluate a patient with cystic fibrosis?
The children often have severe and chronic pansinusitis. Ten percent develop obstructive nasal polyposis which is usually refractory to medical or surgical management.

BIBLIOGRAPHY

1. Balantyne J, Martin MC, Martin A: Hereditary deafness. In Deafness. London, Whurn Publishers, 1993.
2. Beighton, Sellars: Genetics and Otology. New York, Churchill Livingstone, 1982.
3. Brookhauser PE: Genetic hearing loss. In Bailey BJ (ed): Head and Neck Surgery–Otolaryngology. Philadelphia, J.B. Lippincott, 1993.
4. Bluestone CD, Stool SE (eds): Pediatric Otolaryngology, 3rd ed. Philadelphia, W.B. Saunders, 1990.
5. Crockett DM, Seibert RW, Brumstead RM: Cleft lip and palate: The primary deformity. In Bailey BJ (ed): Head and Neck Surgery–Otolaryngology. Philadelphia, J.B. Lippincott, 1993.
6. Gorlin RJ, Toriello HV, Cohen MM Jr: Hereditary Hearing Loss and Its Syndromes. New York, Oxford University Press, 1995.
7. Gorlin RJ, Cohen MM Jr, Levin LS: Syndromes of the Head and Neck, 3r ed. New York, Oxford University Press, 1990.
8. Jones KL: Smith's Recognizable Patterns of Human Malformation, 7th ed. Philadelphia, W.B. Saunders, 1988.
9. Thompson MW, McInnes RR, Willard HF: Thompson and Thompson Genetics in Medicine, 5th ed. Philadelphia. W.B. Saunders, 1991.

69. CLEFT LIP AND PALATE

David A. Hendrick, M.D.

1. Who treats clefts?
Clefts are surgically repaired by otolaryngologists and plastic surgeons trained in pediatric facial plastic surgery. However, the treatment is not purely surgical, and children with clefts should be treated by a team that includes reconstructive surgeons, dentists, pediatricians, otologists, speech pathologists, audiologists, psychologists/psychiatrists, nutritionists, and geneticists.

2. What is the incidence of cleft lip or palate? Do race or sex predilections exist?
Cleft lip or palate is second only to clubfoot when considering frequencies of congenital malformations. The overall incidence of cleft lip (with or without cleft palate) is 1/1000 newborns, while the overall incidence of cleft palate (alone) is 1/2000 newborns. Asians and Native Americans have the highest rate of clefts (3.6/1000), while blacks have the lowest (0.3/1000). Males have more cleft lips (with or without cleft palate) than females by a 2:1 ratio. In contrast, females have more isolated cleft palates than males by a 2:1 ratio. Among clefts, 45% involve the lip, alveolus, and palate; 25% involve only the lip (with or without the alveolus); and 30% involve only the palate.

3. Do clefts demonstrate any inheritance patterns?
Clefts may be related to a known teratogenic insult or part of a recognized malformation syndrome. Others are transmitted with incomplete penetrance in a multifactorial nonmendelian pattern. Therefore, genetic counseling for families with nonsyndromic clefts can be complex.

Cleft recurrence in a family ranges from 2–17%, depending on the number of affected parents and siblings.

4. Embryologically, when do cleft lips and/or palates develop?

The upper lip, nose, and palate form in two phases. Anterior to the incisive foramen, the upper lip, nose, and premaxilla develop during the second month of gestation. Posterior to the incisive foramen, the palate develops during the third month.

5. What is the primary palate? The secondary palate?

The primary and secondary palates are separated by the incisive foramen. The **primary palate** consists of the lip, alveolar arch, and palate anterior to the incisive foramen (the premaxilla). The **secondary palate** consists of the soft palate and hard palate posterior to the incisive foramen.

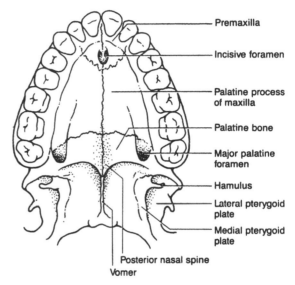

Basic anatomy and divisions of the palate. (From Randall P, LaRossa D: Cleft palate. In McCarthy JG (ed): Plastic Surgery. Philadelphia, W.B. Saunders, 1990, p 2726, with permission.)

6. What is a complete cleft lip? An incomplete cleft lip?

A **complete** cleft lip includes a cleft of the entire lip and the underlying premaxilla, or alveolar arch. An **incomplete** cleft lip only involves the lip.

7. What is a Simonart's band?

In the case of a severe incomplete cleft lip, this thin remnant of tissue, or "band," in the floor of the nasal vestibule bridges the medial and lateral lip elements together across the cleft.

8. What is a submucous cleft?

In a child with a submucous cleft, the musculature of the palate is deficient. However, the palate looks intact because the overlying oral and nasal mucosa is present. A **zona pellucida**, or bluish midline streak on the soft palate, is the result of the muscular diastasis. A submucous cleft is characterized by a bifid uvula and loss of the posterior nasal spine. A notch may be present in the posterior hard palate. A child with a submucous cleft has difficulties with speech because the soft palate is unable to function normally.

9. Describe the initial priorities for managing a newborn with a cleft.

The initial priorities are **feeding assistance** for the infant and **counseling** for the family. Infants must develop adequate suction around a nipple and need frequent rests and burping as they often swallow much air. Special nipples can bypass or occlude the cleft, bulb syringes can eliminate the need for suckling, and a palatal prostheses can occlude an extremely wide cleft palate.

10. What kinds of problems can an otolaryngologist expect to encounter with the cleft palate patient?

Aside from the feeding problems and the cleft repairs, the otolaryngologist can expect to deal with eustachian tube dysfunction and velopharyngeal dysfunction.

Eustachian tube dysfunction is secondary to the hypoplastic levator and tensor veli palatini muscles which control the eustachian tube. Eustachian tube dysfunction can lead to chronic otitis media, possible formation of cholesteatomas later in life (in 7% of cleft palate cases), conductive hearing deficits, and associated speech delays. With increasing age, eustachian tube function will usually normalize.

Velopharyngeal dysfunction is due to deficiencies in the palatal and pharyngeal musculature and/or inadequate palatal length. Velopharyngeal dysfunction can lead to speech articulation difficulties and potential **velopharyngeal insufficiency** (VPI). VPI is characterized by hypernasal speech and nasal regurgitation of food and liquids. Note that these problems are inherent to cleft palate and are *not* associated with isolated cleft lips.

11. Aside from cleft repair, what interventions should the otolaryngologist consider?

Pressure equalization tube placement   Audiologic monitoring
Otitis media management   Speech therapy coordination
Cholesteatoma management   VPI surgery

12. When should cleft lips be repaired?

Cleft lips are generally repaired at 10–14 weeks of age. Using the "rule of 10's," clefts may be repaired when the infant is > 10 weeks, weighs > 10 pounds, and has a hemoglobin of 10 gm/dl.

13. When should cleft palates be repaired?

Timing for palate repair is a balance between establishing speech development and minimizing adverse effects on the growing palate and occlusal relationships. Most centers prefer to repair cleft palates between 10–18 months of age, the age at which articulate speech skills are beginning to develop. In contrast, some centers wait until 18–24 months of age, after eruption of the first molars.

14. Name the muscular deficiencies associated with cleft lip and palate.

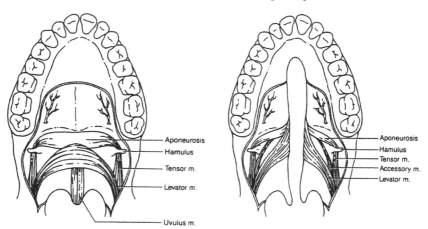

Normal Palate   **Cleft Palate**

Musculature of the normal and cleft soft palate. Not illustrated are the palatopharyngeus muscle (comprises the posterior tonsillar pillar) and the palatoglossus muscle (comprises the anterior tonsillar pillar). (From Randall P, LaRossa D: Cleft palate. In McCarthy JG (ed): Plastic Surgery. Philadelphia, W.B. Saunders, 1990, pp 2728, 2730, with permission.)

In a cleft lip, the orbicularis oris muscle is deficient at the cleft. Muscle fibers tend to follow the cleft up into the base of the nose and must be dissected out to be reapproximated across the cleft. In a cleft palate, the (1) levator veli palatini muscle, (2) tensor veli palatini, (3) uvular muscle, (4) palatopharyngeus muscle, and (5) palatoglossus muscle normally have midline raphes and are therefore all deficient at the palate's cleft. Muscle fibers normally form a muscular "sling" across the soft palate but, in clefts, tend to have abnormal insertions into the posterior margin of the hard palate. Reconstruction of this muscular "sling" is critical to functional success after palatoplasty.

15. Describe the Millard repair.

The Millard repair is the most popular method of cleft lip repair and involves a "rotation advancement" technique. The philtrum of the lip is rotated downward as a flap, and the lateral lip segment is advanced across the cleft and into the space left behind by the central lip segment. Unlike other methods, the final suture line of the Millard repair closely recreates the philtrum of the lip.

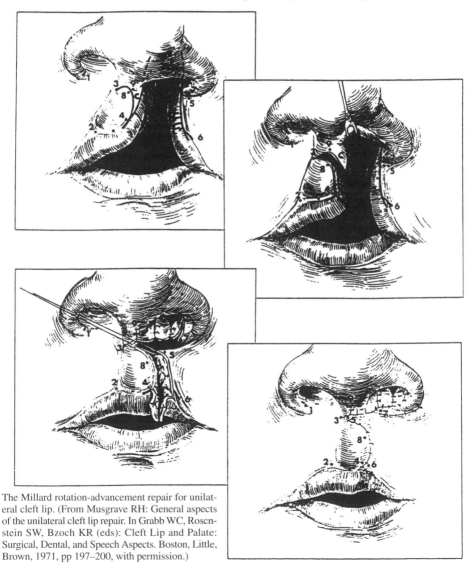

The Millard rotation-advancement repair for unilateral cleft lip. (From Musgrave RH: General aspects of the unilateral cleft lip repair. In Grabb WC, Rosenstein SW, Bzoch KR (eds): Cleft Lip and Palate: Surgical, Dental, and Speech Aspects. Boston, Little, Brown, 1971, pp 197–200, with permission.)

16. What are some other methods of cleft lip repair?
- Lip adhesion (Randall-Graham)—less commonly performed today
- Straight-line repair (Rose-Thompson)—very limited applications
- Rectangular flap repair (LeMesurier)—not as aesthetic as Z-plasty flap methods
- Triangular flap repairs (including Skoog, Bardach, and Tennison-Randall repairs)—all variations on Z-plasty techniques; best for wide cleft lip defects.

17. Describe the critical elements or goals of successful cleft lip repairs.
Correct alignment of cupid's bow
Correct approximation of the orbicularis oris muscle
Symmetric reconstruction of the lip vermilion
Creation of a nasal floor and vestibular sill
Symmetric placement of the nasal alar bases and columella

18. What are the methods of cleft palate repair?
The **V–Y pushback** (Oxford method) and **two-flap palatoplasties** are the most commonly used techniques for repairing incomplete and complete clefts of the palate, respectively. The essential difference between these two methods is whether or not the anterior premaxilla mucoperiosteum is included with the posterior-based pedicled flaps. Of these two methods, only the V–Y pushback provides additional palate length, and only the two-flap technique provides adequate closure of the cleft alveolus, thereby defining their favored roles. Other methods of palatoplasty include:

Four-flap palatoplasty—essentially converts a more complete cleft palate into a shorter incomplete cleft case in order to take advantage of the V–Y pushback technique for palatal lengthening. The mucoperiosteum of the anterior hard palate is raised as two anteriorly based flaps, which are then reapproximated across the anterior cleft. A standard V–Y pushback is then performed using the two remaining posterior-based flaps.

Von Langenbeck palatoplasty—basically a precursor to the two-flap technique in which the flaps are bipedicled both posterior and anterior. Rarely used except perhaps for clefts of the soft palate only.

Schweckendiek's primary veloplasty—a less extensive version of the Von Langenbeck technique designed to close only the soft palate as part of a staged approach. Rarely used now.

Furlow palatoplasty—an "opposing Z-plasty" technique for closing and elongating the soft palate where oppositely oriented Z-plasties are employed to close the nasal and oral mucosal surfaces. The muscle sling can be reconstructed by retaining and reorienting the muscle fibers with the appropriate flaps of the Z-plasties.

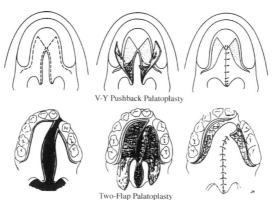

V-Y Pushback Palatoplasty

Two-Flap Palatoplasty

The V-Y pushback and two-flap palatoplasties. (From Randall P, LaRossa D: Cleft palate. In McCarthy JG (ed): Plastic Surgery. Philadelphia, W.B. Saunders, 1990, p 2744, with permission; and from Bumsted RM: The Management of Cleft Lip and Palate. Rochester, MN, American Academy of Otolaryngology, 1980, pp 34, 37, with permission.)

19. Discuss the goals and critical elements of successful cleft palate repairs.
- Separation of the nasal and oral cavities through closure of both mucosal surfaces
- Construction of a water-tight, air-tight velopharyngeal valve
- Preservation of facial growth
- Good development of aesthetic dentition and functional occlusion

In addition to the above basic goals, most surgeons believe that reconstruction of the muscular sling of the soft palate is essential for good functional results of the repair.

20. What are the most common postoperative complications of cleft palate repair?

Hypernasal speech is the most common complication following cleft palate repair, occurring in up to 30% of the cases. **Oral-nasal fistulas** are the second most common complication and occur in 10–21% of cleft palate repairs. These fistulas typically occur at either end of the hard palate (i.e., at the anterior alveolus or at the junction of the soft and hard palate).

21. Which "secondary procedures" are associated with cleft lip and palate surgery?

Secondary procedures are those following the initial repairs of the cleft lip and palate. Besides revisions of the lip and palate, procedures are often necessary to address velopharyngeal insufficiency, alveolar clefts, and nasal deformities.

22. How is velopharyngeal incompetence (VPI) managed?

The deficiency should be assessed with various diagnostic tools, including speech articulation tests, cinefluoroscopy, lateral neck x-rays, manometry, and nasopharyngoscopy. **Speech therapy** should begin with parental counseling when the child is 6 months old, and individual child therapy should begin when the child is about 4 years of age. **Dental prosthesis** may improve palatal lift. About 20–25% of VPI cases may need **surgery**. Methods include secondary palatal lengthening (e.g., Furlow palatoplasty), pharyngeal augmentation (narrow the anteroposterior diameter of the nasopharynx using soft tissue or implants), and pharyngeal flaps (convert the incompetent nasopharynx into two lateral "ports"). Pharyngeal flaps require good lateral pharyngeal wall motion for functional success.

23. What are the rhinoplasty concerns in the surgical management of the cleft lip patient?

Most patients will have a nasal deformity that becomes more apparent and severe with age. Classically, the cleft nose deformity involves:

Shortened columella with its base angled to the noncleft side

Nasal spine deviation to the noncleft side with a similar deflection of the caudal septum toward the noncleft side and a compensatory hypertrophy of the cleft side inferior turbinate

Medial crura of lower lateral cartilage collapsed inferomedially on the cleft side

Lateral crura of lower lateral cartilage collapsed and buckled on the cleft side. Generally it will be weaker and longer than the noncleft lower lateral cartilage.

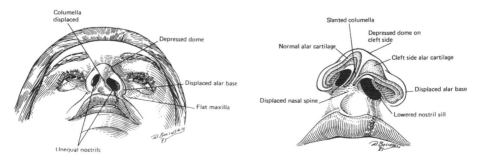

The cleft nose. (From Smith HW: The Atlas of Cleft Lip and Cleft Palate Surgery. New York, Grune & Stratton, 1983, pp 290, 293, with permission.)

Deflection of the nasal tip toward the cleft side due to the above deficiencies
Relative stenosis of the nasal valve on the cleft side
Hypoplastic maxilla on the cleft side, causing lateralization of the alar base and widening of the nare
Possible deviation of the bony nasal pyramids toward the cleft side
Broad nasal dorsum
Thick skin over the nasal tip

CONTROVERSIES

24. How is the cleft alveolus surgically managed?
Ultimately, the cleft alveolus must be structurally reconstructed to provide for alveolar arch integrity and for tooth eruption or support at the cleft. Traditionally, this reconstruction requires placement of bone grafts harvested from the iliac crest, rib, or cranium. Cancellous bone from the iliac crest has been favored by most surgeons, although many others prefer cortical or corticocancellous onlay grafts from the rib or cranium.

The timing of repair has been controversial, with most centers performing "secondary" grafting prior to canine eruption during the stage of mixed dentition (9–12 years of age). Some centers continue to perform "primary" grafting in early childhood at the time of cleft lip repair.

25. In a child with a cleft, when should the nasal tip deformities be repaired?
Partial correction of the nasal deformities is accomplished at the time of primary lip repair by reconstructing the nasal sill, straightening or lengthening the columella, and placing the alar base in a more symmetric position. The timing for nasal tip rhinoplasty is controversial, with some surgeons attempting repairs at the time of primary lip repair and others waiting until 6–10 years of age. More complete rhinoplasty is deferred until facial growth is nearly complete, at approximately 14–18 years of age.

BIBLIOGRAPHY

1. Bumsted RM: The Management of Cleft Lip and Palate. Rochester, MN, American Academy of Otolaryngology, 1980.
2. Cotton RT, Meyer CM: Cleft lip and palate. In Lee KJ (ed): Essential Otolaryngology–Head & Neck Surgery, 6th ed. Norwalk, CT, Appleton & Lange, 1995, pp 275–288.
3. Crocket DM, Seibert RW, Bumsted RM: Cleft lip and palate. In Bailey B (ed): Head and Neck Surgery–Otolaryngology. Philadelphia, J.B. Lippincott, 1993, pp 816–831.
4. Seibert RW, Bumsted RM: Cleft lip and palate. In Cummings CW, et al (eds): Otolaryngology–Head and Neck Surgery. St. Louis, Mosby, 1993, pp 1128–1164.
5. Willet JM, Lee KJ: Otolaryngology: 630 Questions & Answers. Norwalk, CT, Appleton & Lange, 1995.

X. Related Specialties

70. TASTE AND SMELL

Miriam R.I. Linschoten, Ph.D., Pamela M. Eller, M.S., and Anne K. Stark, M.D.

1. What are taste papillae??
Papillae are specialized structures that are involved in taste. Three of the four types of papillae contain taste buds.

1. The **fungiform papillae** are located on the anterior two-thirds of the tongue. Each fungiform papilla contains 0–18 taste buds. Fungiform taste buds contribute about 750 taste buds to the oral cavity.

2. Several **foliate papillae** are located on the posterior lateral surface of the tongue. These papillae consist of a series of clefts containing as many as 1300 taste buds.

3. The **circumvallate papillae** are located on the posterior dorsal tongue. Humans have 8–12 circumvallate papillae arranged in an inverted V-form. The total number of circumvallate taste buds is about 2400, which is roughly half the total number of buds in the oral cavity.

4. The **filiform papillae** are distributed over the entire dorsal surface of the tongue. These structures contain no taste buds but help in sustaining tastants on the surface of the tongue.

2. Describe the topographic map of taste.
There is no topographic map of taste. All four basic tastes—sweet, salty, sour, and bitter—are perceived on all loci with taste receptors. On the tongue, taste buds are situated in papillae. The soft palate, larynx, pharynx, and epiglottis contain extrapapillar taste buds situated within the epithelium.

3. How are taste buds innervated?
The lingual taste buds are innervated by three cranial nerves (CN). The chorda tympani branch of the facial nerve (CN VII) supplies the taste buds in all the fungiform papillae and some buds in the foliate papillae. The remaining foliate taste buds receive innervation from the lingual branch of the glossopharyngeal nerve (CN IX). This last branch also provides innervation to the circumvallate papillae. The vagus nerve (CN X) innervates buds in the epiglottis and larynx.

The three cranial nerves—the facial, glossopharyngeal, and vagus—have their first central relay in the nucleus of the solitary tract in the brainstem medulla. The brainstem gustatory relay mediates ingestive and food rejection behavior. From the nucleus of the solitary tract, the axon projections reach the ventroposteromedial nucleus in the thalamus. From the thalamus, the pathway travels to the gustatory cortex. Presumably, all projections are mainly ipsilateral.

4. What is the role of the trigeminal nerve in taste and smell disorders?
The trigeminal nerve (CN V) provides most of the sensory innervation of the face. In addition to responding to mechanical, proprioceptive, and nociceptive stimuli, the trigeminal nerve fibers of the nose, oral cavity, and eye are sensitive to chemical stimuli. This is considered part of the **common chemical sense** and serves as a protective mechanism to warn of the presence of potentially dangerous chemicals. Trigeminal chemoreception is not a simple sensory system. Stimulation of trigeminal chemoreceptors modulates perception of subsequent or concurrent chemical stimuli. Although loss of trigeminal sense has not been documented, it is important clinically to verify the function of this protective sense, especially in patients with other chemosensory dysfunction.

5. Define anosmia. Hyposmia.

These terms describe different types of olfactory dysfunction. **Anosmia** is the inability to qualitatively detect an olfactory sensation. Total anosmia is the complete inability to detect olfactory sensation, while partial anosmia is the inability to detect some, but not all, odorants. Along the same lines, total **hyposmia** is a decreased sensitivity to all odorants, while partial hyposmia is a decreased sensitivity to some odorants.

6. What is dysosmia? Olfactory agnosia?

Dysosmia may be either a distortion in the perception of an odor (**parosmia**) or the perception of an odor when no olfactory stimulus is present (**phantosmia**). **Olfactory agnosia** is the inability to classify or identify an odorant verbally even though the patient may find it recognizable.

7. What is dysgeusia?

An alteration in normal taste perception.

8. What are the major causes of smell disorders?

1. **Nasal and paranasal sinus disease** often is accompanied by diminished olfactory acuity for several likely reasons. Obstruction of the nasal passages results in restriction of airflow to the olfactory neuroepithelium, presumably altering the ability to smell. In many cases, excess mucus from diseased cells will convey an obnoxious odor which is detected only by the patient.

2. **Upper respiratory tract infections** should be considered if the anosmia or hyposmia is sudden in onset.

3. **Head trauma**, with or without loss of consciousness, can result in anosmia. It is usually bilateral and permanent, although some variations have been reported.

4. **Inhalation of volatile chemicals** has been implicated in anosmia and hyposmia. Presumably, these toxic fumes cause direct damage to the olfactory receptor cells.

9. Which diseases are associated with smell disorders?

Neurodegenerative diseases	Systemic diseases
Alzheimer's disease	Diabetes mellitus
Parkinson's disease	Graves' disease
Myotrophic lateral sclerosis	Other thyroid disease
Familial dysautonomia	Arthritis and related autoimmune diseases
Multiple sclerosis	Psychiatric disorders
Myasthenia gravis	Inherited disorders (e.g., Kallmann's syndrome)
Temporal lobe epilepsy	

10. What is Kallmann's syndrome?

Kallmann's syndrome, transmitted in an autosomal dominant pattern with variable penetrance, consists of congenital hypogonadotropic eunuchoidism and anosmia. This syndrome illustrates the probable association of smell and sexual development. Some of these patients have shown agenesis of the olfactory bulbs and stalks, incomplete development of the hypothalamus, or no olfactory epithelium in the olfactory cleft. Patients with Kallmann's syndrome also have a high incidence of renal abnormalities, cryptorchidism, deafness, diabetes, and midline facial deformities.

11. What are the major causes of taste disorders?

Pure taste disorders are not as well-documented as smell disorders. However, viral infections and head trauma have been reported to result in dysgeusias. Many drugs lead to taste dysfunction.

12. How often do patients who suffer head trauma subsequently have a taste or smell disorder?

Review of the literature reveals numerous case reports detailing loss of smell following head trauma. In summary, 5% of all head trauma victims suffer from anosmia. Dysgeusia in head trauma is rare, but well-documented reports indicate that it occurs in 0.4% of all cases.

13. Which diseases are associated with taste disorders?

Loss or distortion of taste is less prevalent than loss of smell. However, taste disorders may be debilitating. Taste pathways may be interrupted by lesions such as acoustic neuromas. Bell's palsy may also lead to taste dysfunction. Taste alteration during radiation therapy and chemotherapy have been well-documented. Epilepsy, psychiatric disorders, hypothyroidism, and diabetes are also reported to have secondary taste symptoms.

14. What is burning mouth syndrome (BMS)?

BMS is an intraoral pain disorder that occurs despite a clinically normal appearance of the oral mucosa. The tongue tip, anterior hard palate, and oral lower lip are most frequently affected. For most patients, the burning pain starts midmorning or early afternoon and is followed by dry mouth, dysgeusia, and thirst. Most patients diagnosed with BMS are postmenopausal women. The etiology is still unclear. The dysgeusia involves either a persistent taste or an alteration in taste perception. The persistent taste is most commonly described as bitter and/or metallic in quality. Complaints of altered tastes include all taste qualities—sour and bitter taste stronger than normal, sweet tastes weaker, and salt tastes either stronger or weaker.

15. Can a mouthwash cause a taste disorder?

Yes. Antibacterial mouthrinses containing chlorhexidine or hexetidine might induce disorders ranging from persistent taste loss to transient selective losses for one or two qualities. Both agents are also associated with dysgeusia.

16. Describe the taste and smell effects of cardiovascular drugs.

Angiotensin-converting enzyme inhibitors, especially **captopril** and **enalapril**, have been reported to affect both taste and smell function. Although estimates vary, as many as 20% of patients using captopril develop a loss of taste or smell. Captopril may also lead to sweet, salty, and metallic phantogeusias. These side effects often resolve when captopril is discontinued, although a persistent taste change may linger for over a year. Nine percent of patients taking nifedipine report hyposmia, while others report a sweet, salty, or metallic phantogeusia.

17. Do other drugs commonly affect taste and smell?

Acetazolamide, used to treat glaucoma and mountain sickness, almost always causes a mild bitter taste when patients drink carbonated beverages. This effect resolves within 48 hours after the drug is discontinued. Antiprotozoals commonly affect taste and smell. Specifically, **metronidazole and pentamidine**, both parenteral and inhaled forms, induce hypogeusia and metallic phantogeusia. About one-third of patients taking the antirheumatic drug **penicillamine** develop hypogeusia or dysgeusia. Over 10% of patients treated with **gold** for rheumatoid arthritis develop a dysgeusia that may precede stomatitis. Several antithyroid drugs have been associated with taste and smell disorders, especially **carbimazole, thiamazole,** and **methimazole**. The antidepressants **imipramine, clomipramine,** and **lithium carbonate** are also implicated in taste and smell disorders. **Bromocriptine**, an antiparkison drug, may cause phantosmias in 9% of patients, and **levodopa** may cause dysosmia, bitter phantosmia, or hypogeusia in 20–40% of patients. **Felbanate**, an anticonvulsant, causes dysgeusia in 6% of patients.

18. In your evaluation of a patient, what are the key questions to be asked in your history?

1. Questions which differentiate between taste and smell disorders (Are you able to taste salty, sweet, sour, and bitter substances? Can you smell flowers or cooking odors?)

2. Questions that address the duration and onset (gradual or sudden) of the disorder as well as events concurring with the disorder.

3. Questions about current and past history of diseases, trauma, surgeries, and medications.

19. How do you differentiate between a taste and a smell disorder?

Most patients presenting with a smell disorder complain that they are unable to taste. This phenomenon is mainly a question of language and definition. One has to appreciate the distinction and overlap between taste, smell, and flavor. **Taste** refers to the sensations arising from the taste receptors and is most commonly described as sweetness, saltiness, sourness, and bitterness. **Smell** refers to the sensations arising from the olfactory receptors. There are many different smell qualities for which no satisfactory classification exists. **Flavor** is the combined sensation of taste, smell, temperature, texture, and pungency.

A patient with nasal obstruction will have a decreased sense of smell, and therefore the flavor of foods will change. Questions to help make the distinction are: Are you able to taste the sweetness of sugar? The saltiness of pretzels? The sourness of a lemon? The bitterness of black coffee? Some confusion between sour and bitter is fairly common and does not indicate a taste problem. Perfumes, Vicks rub, and cleaning agents (such as ammonia and bleach) have a trigeminal component, and the ability to "smell" these does not warrant a functional sense of smell.

20. How do you proceed with the workup?

You may wish to refer the patient to a taste and smell center for psychophysical testing. The most common clinical tests examine the ability to detect and identify odorants and tastants. Testing should be unilateral as well as bilateral. For taste testing, differences in the sensitivity or suprathreshold sensation might exist between the two halves of the tongue. Differences may also exist between the anterior and posterior parts on one side of the tongue. To evaluate dysgeusias, topical anesthesia can be helpful in determining the site of origin. Blood tests may indicate that the disorder is the result of hyponatremia, liver disease, or kidney disease. If you suspect that the patient's symptoms are the result of chronic sinus infections, a sinus CT may be indicated. If the patient has other neural symptoms, an MRI may be necessary to evaluate for brain lesions.

21. Both sinus disease and upper respiratory infections may lead to taste and smell complaints. How are the etiologies differentiated?

The primary distinction revolves around the time of onset. Although patients with sinus disease may detect occasional "whiffs" of odor, overall they report a slowly deteriorating sense of smell. In contrast, patients with a URI can often report the exact day when their sense of smell became impaired.

22. How do you categorize the loss of olfactory and gustatory sensitivity?

Anatomic categories for losses include transport losses, sensory losses, and neural losses.

Transport losses result from conditions which interfere with the accessibility of the receptor cells. For olfaction, this may involve swollen nasal mucosa or structural obstructions, such as neoplasms, polyps, or a deviated septum. In gustation, transport losses are caused by bacterial colonization of the taste pores, oral inflammation, or xerostomia.

Sensory losses are the result of injuries to the receptor cells. Olfactory sensory loss may occur with viral infections, exposure to toxic chemicals or antiproliferative drugs, and radiation to the head and neck. Gustatory sensory loss is caused by drugs that affect cell turnover, radiation therapy, viral infections, and endocrine disorders.

Neural losses are caused by damaged peripheral and central pathways. In olfaction, neural losses occur with neoplasms of the anterior cranial fossa, head trauma, neurosurgical procedures, and neurotoxic substances. Kallmann's syndrome also leads to neural olfactory loss. Neural gustatory losses stem from neoplasms, head trauma, and damage to the afferent nerves with dental and otologic procedures.

23. Does the psyche play any role in taste and smell disorders?

Depressed persons may exhibit chemosensory dysfunction. When compared with normal controls, depressed patients often exhibit hypogeusia. In contrast, depression does not lead to hyposmia. A recent study found that patients with chemosensory distortions or hallucinations (dysgeusia and dysosmia) had significantly higher scores on the Beck Depression Inventory. The same study found a close relationship between dysgeusia and antidepressant use. However, the clinician must distinguish between the effects of the medication and the effects of the underlying condition. Burning mouth syndrome may also be related to affective disorders such as depression; however, the clinician must be cautious in interpreting these complaints as purely psychogenic. Conversely, a patient who suffers from a taste or smell disorder may become depressed. Because taste and smell play an important role in one's sense of safety and pleasure, distortions often affect general well-being.

BIBLIOGRAPHY

1. Doty RL: Handbook of Olfaction and Gustation. New York, Marcel Dekker, 1995.
2. Getchell TV, et al: Smell and Taste in Health and Disease. New York, Raven Press, 1991.
3. Henkin RI: Drug-induced taste and smell disorders. Drug Saf 11:318–377, 1994.
4. Jafek BW, et al: Congenital anosmia. Ear Nose Throat J 69:331, 1990.
5. Jafek BW, et al: Post-traumatic anosmia: Ultrastructural correlates. Arch Neurol 46:300–304, 1989.
6. Leopold DA: Physiology of olfaction. In Cummings CW, et al (eds): Otolaryngology–Head and Neck Surgery. St. Louis, Mosby, 1993, pp 640–664.
7. Norgren R: Gustatory system. In Paxinos G (ed): The Human Nervous System. New York, Academic Press, 1990, pp.845–861.

71. ALLERGY AND IMMUNOLOGY

Monique L. McCray, Betty Luce, B.S.N., M.A., and William H. Wilson, M.D.

1. What is the primary function of the immune system?

The immune system differentiates self from non-self. While recognizing and protecting self components, it identifies and eliminates any element that is foreign to the body. This function is carried out by cells (macrophages, monocytes, mast cells, lymphocytes, neutrophils, eosinophils, basophils) and the molecules that they produce (immunoglobulins, lymphokines, interleukins, interferons).

2. How does the immune system function in the allergic condition?

IgE is the immunoglobulin associated with the **type I** or **immediate hypersensitivity** reaction. IgE-sensitized mast cells, most abundant in the respiratory and gastrointestinal mucosa and in the skin, mistakenly recognize normally innocuous allergens such as pollen, food, or mold as foreign. When cell-bound IgE antibody is exposed to allergen, mediators such as histamine and platelet-activating factor are released which, in turn, produce acute inflammation.

3. Describe the sequence of events after an allergen is exposed to IgE and mast cells.

IgE binds by its Fc receptor to mast cells and basophils. When two adjacent, cell-bound IgE molecules of identical specificity are bridged by an antigen, the two receptor molecules are brought into close proximity. This disturbance of membrane structures causes an influx of calcium ions into the cells, precipitating the exocytosis of granule contents with the release of preformed mediators (histamine, heparin, and proteolytic enzymes). These mediators then induce the synthesis of newly formed mediators from membrane-bound phospholipids, which ultimately results in the production of prostaglandins, leukotrienes, and platelet-activating factor.

4. The serum half-life of IgE is about 2.5 days. After passive sensitization to an allergen, why does an individual maintain long-term hyperreactivity to that allergen?

Cell binding of IgE molecules by their Fc fragment extends their half-life and reduces degradation. Mast cells can remain sensitized for as long as 12 weeks after passive sensitization with atopic serum containing IgE. These mast cells degranulate on repeated exposure to an allergen, causing immediate hypersensitivity reactions.

5. Who were Prausnitz and Kustner?

Prausnitz and Kustner first described the allergic reaction in 1921. They showed that the serum factor from one individual with an allergic skin response could cause the same allergic response in the skin of a normal individual. Forty-five years later, Ishizaka defined the antibody as IgE.

6. Are children of allergic parents at risk for developing allergies as well?

Fifty percent of children with two allergic parents will develop an allergy. The incidence decreases to 30% with one allergic parent. The mode of inheritance of high levels of IgE is not yet known. A family history of allergic disease is important to obtain whenever a patient is evaluated for allergic diathesis.

7. What is atopy?

Atopy describes the clinical incidence of asthma, urticaria, hay fever, and eczema in patients with a hereditary predisposition to hypersensitivity.

8. Is a positive skin test necessary to verify allergic disease?

No. Approximately 30% of those tested will produce a measurable response to common allergens. An IgE-mediated response suggests the presence of allergic disease and must be verified by associated clinical symptoms.

9. Does a negative skin test prove the absence of allergic diathesis?

No. Allergy should be considered as a diagnosis when a physical complaint of seasonal or perennial nasal allergy, asthma, food sensitivity, headache, or eczematoid dermatitis is offered. A family history of allergy is a strong indicator of possible allergic diathesis. The absence of an immediate positive IgE skin test suggests that the allergy is mediated by an alternative hypersensitivity reaction.

10. Describe the four types of hypersensitivity reactions.

Type I (immediate hypersensitivity) is an IgE-mediated hypersensitivity reaction to normally innocuous inhalants, molds, foods, or chemicals. Inflammatory mediators are released by IgE-sensitized mast cells, producing an acute inflammatory response. Symptoms may range from rhinitis to anaphylaxis.

Type II (autoimmunity) involves the formation of antibodies to self. A foreign antigen may cross-react with a normal body element, or a previously sequestered self-antigen may be released, as is the case with orchitis following mumps. Other cases may involve a deficiency or the depletion of suppressor T cells. Goodpasture disease, myasthenia gravis, and rheumatic heart disease are examples of pathology related to type II hypersensitivity.

Type III (immune complexes) are activated when antibody forms a soluble complex with antigen, which then deposits and precipitates in the basement membranes of blood vessels with considerable plasma outflow. These complexes activate complement, which initiates a characteristic neutrophil inflammatory response. The blood vessel walls and adjacent tissues are subsequently damaged by the inflammation. Affected vessels commonly line serosal surfaces, such as peritoneum and pleura, joints, kidneys and skin. Type III hypersensitivity is implicated in systemic lupus erythematosus, rheumatoid arthritis, and serum sickness.

Type IV (delayed-type hypersensitivity) is basically an overenthusiastic T-cell-mediated immune response. Attracted macrophages do not recognize self from non-self and consequently destroy adjacent normal cells as well as infected cells. Tuberculosis is an example of pathology caused by type IV hypersensitivity.

11. Which foods are most commonly associated with type I, III, or IV hypersensitivity reactions?

Foods most commonly eaten are associated with hypersensitivity. Wheat, corn, eggs, cow's milk, sugar, soy, yeast, cola, and chocolate are frequently implicated as a cause of atopic symptoms.

Hypersensitivity is a function of frequency of exposure. Allergy to a specific food is often masked as a craving or an addiction, whereby the patient perceives that the food increases his or her sense of well-being. This belief results in the food being ingested several times each day, on a daily basis.

12. What is meant by a "threshold allergic response"?

Many individuals are predisposed to allergy but never experience allergic symptoms. Exposure to their allergens never reaches the *threshold* or concentration level that would be associated with an allergic response. This threshold may be reached by overwhelming exposure to a single allergen or by the cumulative effects of several. This explains why a change in environment may cause symptoms in one who has never previously experienced an active allergic response. Conversely, an environmental change may eliminate allergic symptoms in some patients.

13. How does stress affect the required threshold for an allergic response?

Stress may be a major excitant of an allergic response in a susceptible individual. Stress may effectively lower the threshold needed to provoke allergic response. Stressors may be physical (viral or bacterial infection), environmental (polluted air), or emotional. Removal of the stress factor may cause the symptoms to abate and the threshold to normalize.

14. What is RAST?

RAST stands for **radioallergosorbent test**, of which there are two types: Phadebas RAST and Fadal-Nalebuff RAST. This test determines the degree of sensitivity for an allergen by measuring the specific IgE for each. The test uses a radioactive isotope (iodine-125)-labeled paper disc. The results are measured using a gamma-counter or the calorimetric enzyme method. Although the Phadebas RAST has been the standard, today more laboratories are using the Fadal-Nalebuff method, which can be used to calculate the initial starting dose of immunotherapy.

15. What is immunotherapy?

Immunotherapy is a method by which an atopic individual's allergic responses are attenuated by hyposensitization to specific allergens. Using the skin endpoint titration technique or the RAST, the relieving dose of an injected allergen is tailored to the specific tolerance of the patient. Symptomatic relief is safely, rapidly, and efficiently obtainable with these techniques, which are quantitative as well as qualitative.

16. How does immunotherapy work to hyposensitize an individual to an allergen?

If IgE is to activate and multiply, there must be an excess of helper T-cell activity and a deficiency of suppressor T-cells. Immunotherapy increases the number of suppressor T-cells in relation to IgE helper T-cells. Less IgE is produced and fewer mast cells are sensitized. Immunotherapy also produces IgG-blocking antibodies with an affinity for receptors on mast cells. A mast cell cannot become sensitized when its receptors are saturated with IgG.

17. What is seasonal allergic rhinitis? What is the standard medical treatment for this condition?

Tree, grass, and weed pollens in their seasons may cause allergic rhinitis symptoms in susceptible individuals. Symptomatic relief may be afforded by oral antihistamines or steroid or Nasochrome nasal sprays. Saline nasal lavages may facilitate ciliary action to clear nasal secretions and wash away allergens, and have the disadvantage of also removing the protective coating of secretory IgA. Immunotherapy may offer relief to those whose symptoms are not adequately controlled with medication or local applications.

18. What is perennial allergic rhinitis? What is the standard medical treatment for this condition?

Perennial symptoms may be caused by a hypersensitivity to ingested and inhalant molds, dust, foods, and chemicals. Perennial symptoms are unlikely to respond to nonspecific measures.

Identification of the antigen(s) may be determined by an exhaustive history, skin testing, or in vitro methods (RAST). Avoidance of the antigenic substance is the best treatment. Extensive investigation and effort may be necessary to identify and remove environmental contaminants such as mold. Elimination of dietary antigens requires an educational program to aid patients in total removal of offending foods from the diet. Hyposensitization with antigen extracts (immunotherapy) may help to decrease symptoms.

19. A patient presents with nasal allergy symptoms but has a negative allergy workup. What is the proper management?

These patients are commonly diagnosed as having vasomotor rhinitis. Efforts to identify an offending allergen must be redoubled. An individual with acute or chronic infection and/or antihistamines or steroids in the system may have negative skin tests, resulting in this misdiagnosis. Skin tests must be observed 48 hours after testing to detect delayed type IV T-cell responses. Negative skin tests in atopic individuals strongly suggest non-IgE-mediated food hypersensitivities. Alteration by surgery should be considered as a last resort if airway obstruction continues.

20. Define anaphylactic shock.

Anaphylactic shock is an acute IgE-mediated allergic reaction in a sensitized person. Clinical manifestations may be immediate or delayed and include pruritus, urticaria, angioedema, hypotension, respiratory distress (secondary to laryngeal edema, laryngospasm, or bronchospasm), abdominal pain, and shock. Death is primarily due to airway obstruction. Anaphylaxis may be caused by Hymenoptera stings, food products such as peanuts, nonsteroidal anti-inflammatory drugs, salicylates, penicillin and its derivatives, and local anesthetics.

21. A patient presents with an acute anaphylactic reaction. What is the proper management?

Airway management is always the first priority. If it is not possible to ventilate the patient, intubation is indicated and ventilation should begin with 100% oxygen. If laryngeal edema is unresponsive to epinephrine and intubation is also unsuccessful, surgical airway management may be indicated. **Hypotension** should be treated with epinephrine, glucagon, volume expansion with crystalloid or colloid, followed by titration to blood pressure and urine output. Resistant **bronchospasm** should be treated with inhaled β-agonists such as metaproterenol or albuterol. Aminophylline is indicated as a second-line drug. Antihistamines do not have an immediate effect, but may shorten the duration of the acute reaction. Glucocorticoids (hydrocortisone, methylprednisolone) have no therapeutic effect in the setting of an acute anaphylactic reaction, as their peak effect occurs at 6–12 hours. They may, however, prevent recurrence or relapse of severe reactions.

22. How does one recognize nonacute upper airway obstruction?

Partial or incomplete obstruction may be difficult to recognize, as the symptoms may be attributed to other causes. Symptoms of partial obstruction may be present only when the patient is in the supine position. Consequently, obstruction tends to occur at night and the resulting symptoms are not immediately identifiable as related to airway obstruction. Complaints of a dry throat on waking, fatigue, or loud snoring may indicate partial airway obstruction. These symptoms must be differentiated from those commonly seen in allergic patients.

23. What are the otologic manifestations of allergy?

Allergic otitis externa must be differentiated from canal infections, which are usually treated with antibiotic-steroid drops. The most common infecting agent is *Pseudomonas*, which may be treated with ciprofloxacin. Allergic otitis may be dry and scaly, or moist. A fungal hypersensitivity is commonly implicated. Control of dietary and inhalant fungal derivatives as well as a program of specific hyposensitization supplemented by antifungal medication may be necessary to control allergic otitis media.

Recurrent acute otitis media with chronic middle ear effusion in children is frequently caused by a food allergy and may be often associated with a history of colic in infancy. Commonly eaten foods, particularly cow's milk, corn, soy, and fruit juice, are most often implicated. If middle ear effusion persists, tympanostomy tubes should be inserted to prevent infection. Preservation of hearing, normal development of speech, and prevention of chronic mastoiditis are primary therapeutic goals. Politzerization or myringostomy with needle aspiration is indicated before tubes are placed.

Inner ear symptoms such as vertigo, tinnitus, and fluctuating hearing loss (Meniere's disease) are known to be caused by allergy in 26% of cases. Control of allergies is essential to prevent permanent hearing loss.

24. What causes nasal and sinus polyps?

Allergy and infection cause nasal and sinus polyps. Polyps that obstruct the airway and sinus ostia require surgical removal, although deposteroids, decongestants, and beclomethasone sprays may temporarily relieve symptoms. Polyps are commonly seen in triad with asthma and aspirin allergy. Obstruction due to polyps may be the cause of chronic sinus infection. Because of mucolytic enzymes and transport problems, laboratory growth is not always obtained from nasal cultures. Sinus irrigation and cytology examinations may be necessary for diagnosis.

BIBLIOGRAPHY

1. Dixon HS, Dixon BJ: Otolaryngic allergy. In Common Problems of the Head and Neck Region. Philadelphia, W.B. Saunders, 1992, pp 9–25.
2. Houck JH: Immunology. In Lee KJ (ed): Essential Otolarygology. Norwalk, CT, Appleton & Lange, 1995, pp 289–318.
3. King WP: Allergic disorders in the otolaryngologic practice. Otolaryngol Clin North Am 18:677–690, 1985.
4. Majchel AM, Naclerio RM: Allergy and immunology. In Bailey BJ (ed): Head and Neck Surgery–Otolaryngology. Philadelphia, J.B. Lippincott, 1993, pp 71–82.
5. Richtsmeier WJ: Basic allergy and immunology. In Cummings CW, et al (eds): Otolaryngology–Head and Neck Surgery. St. Louis, Mosby, 1993, pp 243–276.

72. RADIOLOGY OF THE HEAD AND NECK

Caroline L. Hollingsworth, M.D., David Rubinstein, M.D., and B. Burton Putegnat, M.D.

1. What are the major advantages and disadvantages of MRI in head and neck imaging?

Advantages
1. Multiple pulse sequences can be used to characterize lesions
2. Multiplanar imaging without reconstructing images
3. Demonstration of arteries and veins without contrast
4. No use of ionizing radiation
5. Direct imaging of bone marrow

Disadvantages
1. Imaging studies take significantly more time than CT; claustrophobia may interfere with exam
2. More sensitive to patient motion (e.g., swallowing) than CT
3. Contraindicated in patients with pacemakers, some aneurysm clips, cochlear implants, neurostimulators, and other metallic foreign bodies
4. Does not delineate cortical and trabecular bone detail as well as CT
5. Higher cost than CT

2. What structures are located in the parapharyngeal space? Why is this space important radiographically?

The parapharyngeal space runs from the skull base to the hyoid bone and is just deep to the pharyngeal mucosa and superficial to the carotid sheath. Inferiorly, it communicates openly with the submandibular space. The parapharyngeal space contains relatively few structures (fat, the mandibular branch of the facial nerve, pterygoid venous plexus, and branches of the ascending pharyngeal artery). Although a rare source of primary pathology, this space is extremely important as a radiographic landmark because the fat makes it readily visible on MR and CT images of the suprahyoid neck. Due to its central anatomic position, the origin of pathologic processes within the deep fascial spaces of the neck can be identified by the specific displacement pattern of the parapharyngeal space. The parapharyngeal space may provide a path for pathology to extend superiorly to the skull base.

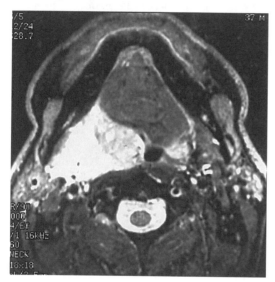

T2-weighted MRI of the suprahyoid neck depicts a homogeneously hyperintense mass with its center in the parapharyngeal space. The right carotid sheath is displaced posterolaterally. (Courtesy of Gregory Chaljub, M.D., Department of Radiology, University of Texas Medical Branch at Galveston.)

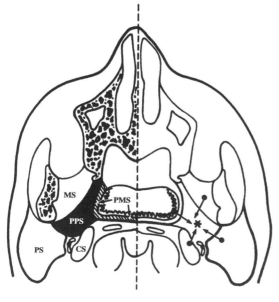

Axial view of the midnasopharynx illustrates the parapharyngeal space, carotid space, masticator space, pharyngeal mucosal space, and parotid space as well as the displacement pattern typical of a mass located in one of these spaces. (From Harnsberger HRic: Handbook of Head and Neck Imaging, 2nd ed. St. Louis, Mosby, 1995, p 18, with permission).

3. What is the most common benign tumor of the parapharyngeal space?
   Pleomorphic adenomas of ectopic salivary gland tissue are the most frequently encountered benign tumors of the parapharyngeal space. It is important to determine whether the
tumor actually originates from the deep lobe of the parotid gland because the surgical
approaches differ. A tumor that originates in the deep lobe may be accessible with a trans-
parotid approach, which presents less risk to the facial nerve than an oral or submandibular
approach.

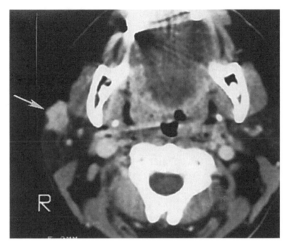

Axial CT of a pleomorphic adenoma
(white arrow) located in the superficial
lobe of the right parotid gland. (Courtesy
of Gregory Chaljub, M.D., Department
of Radiology, University of Texas Medical Branch at Galveston.)

4. Describe the location, contents, and anatomic relations of the masticator space.
   The masticator space runs anterolateral to the parapharyngeal space from the temporal
fossa to the mandible. Important structures contained within this space include the muscles of
mastication (masseter, temporalis, and medial and lateral pterygoid) as well as the third portion
of the fifth cranial nerve. The majority of masses in the masticator space originate from an
infection secondary to dental carries or dental extraction. Neoplasm or infection may spread
to the skull base by tracking along the mandibular division of the trigeminal nerve or temporalis muscle.

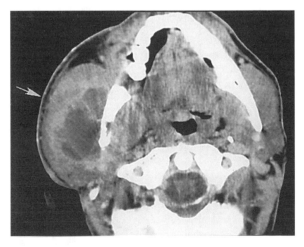

Axial CT of an abscess (white arrow) located in the masticator space. (Courtesy of Faustino Guinto, M.D.,
Department of Radiology, University of Texas Medical Branch at Galveston.)

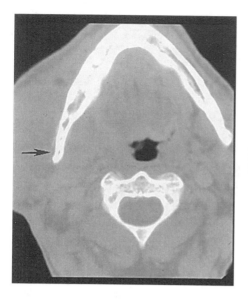

Axial CT with bone windows shows bone destruction associated with osteomyelitis (black arrow) of the mandible secondary to an abscess. (Courtesy of Faustino Guinto, M.D., Department of Radiology, University of Texas Medical Branch at Galveston.)

5. When a lesion is localized to the carotid space, what are the most common entities in the differential diagnosis?

The borders of the carotid space are the jugular and carotid foramina superiorly, the deep lobe of the parotid laterally, the retropharyngeal space medially, and the aortic arch inferiorly. This space is surrounded by a tough fascia formed from the three layers of the deep cervical fascia. Since this space communicates intracranially via the jugular foramen, it provides the opportunity for intracranial and extracranial spread of disease. To formulate a differential diagnosis, one must know the contents of the space. The contents include important vascular (common carotid artery and internal jugular vein), neural (cranial nerves IX–XII and sympathetic plexus), and lymphatic structures (deep cervical chain, including the jugulodigastric or sentinel node). Paraganglioma, schwannoma, and nodal metastasis from a squamous cell carcinoma are the most common lesions found within the carotid space.

Right carotid space schwannoma (white arrow) on axial contrast-enhanced CT. (Courtesy of Faustino Guinto, M.D., Department of Radiology, University of Texas Medical Branch at Galveston.)

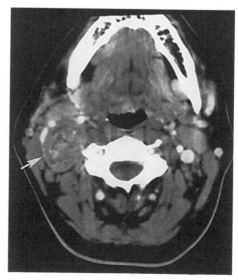

6. Describe the characteristic appearance of a paraganglioma on CT and MRI.
   MRI of a paraganglioma reveals a heterogeneous tubular mass in the carotid space, jugular foramen, or middle ear characterized by multiple areas of low intensity that represent flow voids. On CT, a paraganglioma characteristically appears as an intensely enhancing mass. Paraganglioma produce irregular, permeative bony changes around the jugular foramen, whereas schwannomas, another lesion found in the jugular foramen, produce regular, smooth, scalloped changes. Carotid body tumors separate the internal and external carotid arteries.

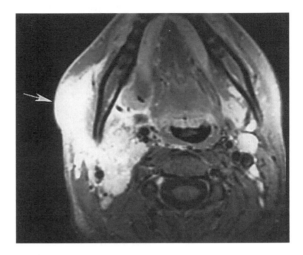

Enhanced fat-saturated T1-weighted MRI depicts a paraganglioma (white arrow) on the right involving the parapharyngeal and masticator spaces inferiorly. (Courtesy of Gregory Chaljub, M.D., Department of Radiology, University of Texas Medical Branch at Galveston.)

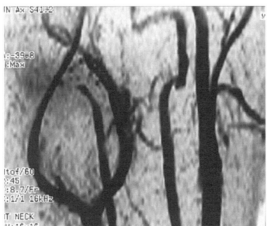

Magnetic resonance angiogram (MRA) shows increased separation of the right internal and external carotid arteries secondary to a paraganglioma located at the carotid bifurcation. (Courtesy of Gregory Chaljub, M.D., Department of Radiology at the University of Texas Medical Branch at Galveston.)

7. What is the most appropriate imaging technique for evaluating a suspected abscess of the head and neck?
   Both MRI and CT can be used to evaluate an abscess for the presence of osteomyelitis. CT has the advantages of being faster and more economical. On CT, an abscess usually appears to have a thick wall surrounded by inflammatory changes. These changes are usually characterized by enhanced soft tissue with or without septations.

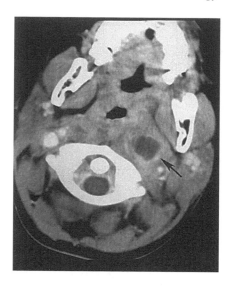

Contrast-enhanced axial CT demonstrates an abscess (black arrow) with a hypodense center and peripheral enhancement. (Courtesy of Susan John, M.D., Department of Radiology, University of Texas Medical Branch at Galveston.)

8. Which clinical conditions may mimic a retropharyngeal space abscess on radiologic evaluation?

Fluid that has collected in the retropharyngeal space, for whatever reason, often appears radiologically identical to a retropharyngeal abscess. Such a collection may be due to various causes, including surgery or venous obstruction from superior vena cava syndrome. In addition, internal jugular thrombosis causing transudation of fluid into the retropharyngeal space or distal lymphatic obstruction that impairs drainage from the retropharyngeal space may also mimic an abscess on radiologic evaluation.

9. Describe the clinical presentation and radiologic appearance of branchial cleft cysts.

Ninety-five percent of branchial cleft abnormalities are derived from the second branchial cleft. In children, the usual presentation is a submandibular mass that may be associated with a sinus tract opening just above the clavicle. In young adults, the appearance of a submandibular mass is often preceded by viral infection or trauma. Ultrasound, often performed in pediatric cases, typically shows a well-circumscribed, hypoechoic lesion. Sectional imaging often shows a simple cystic mass at the angle of the mandible along the anterior margin of the sternocleidomastoid muscle. The cyst characteristically displaces the carotid space posteromedially, the sternocleidomastoid muscle posterolaterally, and the submandibular gland anteromedially. It is

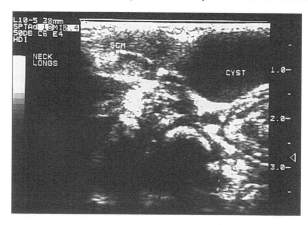

Ultrasound of a second branchial cleft cyst at the anterior border of the sternocleidomastoid (SCM). (Courtesy of Susan John, M.D., Department of Radiology, University of Texas Medical Branch at Galveston.)

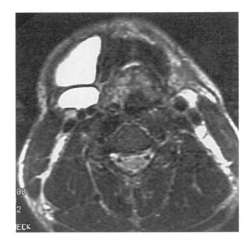

T2-weighted axial MRI of a second branchial cleft cyst at the anterior margin of the right sternocleido-mastoid. (Courtesy of Gregory Chaljub, M.D., Department of Radiology, University of Texas Medical Branch at Galveston.)

important to image a suspected branchial cleft cyst to differentiate it from jugulodigastric node adenopathy, which may present similarly.

10. What are the usual locations of thyroglossal duct cysts?

Thyroglossal duct cysts may be found anywhere along the course of the duct. The duct arises from the foramen cecum in the posterior tongue and extends inferiorly through the muscle of the tongue and the mylohyoid muscle at the floor of the mouth into the anterior neck to the normal position of the thyroid gland posterior to the strap muscles. Most cysts occur below the level of the hyoid bone and in the midline. The cysts may be imbedded in the strap muscles. They rarely contain carcinomas but may become infected.

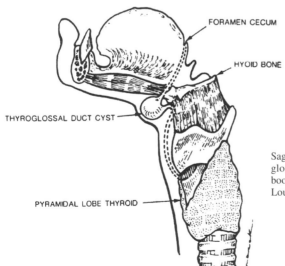

Sagittal view of the migration tract of a thyroglossal duct cyst. Harnsberger HRic: Handbook of Head and Neck Imaging, 2nd ed. St. Louis, Mosby, 1995, p 206, with permission).

11. Discuss the application of CT and MRI in the evaluation of a neck mass that is suspected to be malignant.

Although a thorough clinical examination is fundamental in the evaluation of a neck mass, radiologic imaging is often essential for diagnosis. CT or MRI can determine precise anatomic relationships, presence of an occult primary that has led to cervical metastases, and the solid or cystic nature of the mass. MRI is most helpful in defining the extent of neoplastic infiltration. Discrete lesions are well demonstrated by both modalities. CT is faster and more helpful with patients who have trouble holding still or controlling their secretions. The MRI or CT should be performed before biopsy to avoid confusion due to changes created by the biopsy.

12. What characteristics of a lymph node on CT or MRI suggest malignancy?

The characteristics of a lymph node that suggest malignancy include the presence of central necrosis, ill-defined margins indicating extracapsular spread to adjacent tissues, and size. Nodes in the parotid or retropharyngeal chains are classified as malignant if their maximum diameter is ≥ 1.0 cm. There is less consensus in the case of nodes in the spinal accessory, deep cervical, or submandibular groups. Many authorities believe that in these chains, only nodes ≥ 1.5 cm should be called malignant. Others maintain that the increase in specificity is not worth the decrease in sensitivity and that all nodes ≥ 1.0 cm should be considered malignant. In the presence of a known malignancy, nodes with central necrosis (with central low attenuation by enhanced CT or central low intensity by T1-weighted, contrast-enhanced MRI) are considered to be malignant regardless of their size. Similarly, nodes with ill-defined margins are considered malignant with extranodal spread of neoplasm.

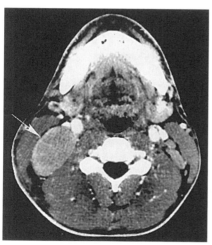

Axial CT of an enlarged lymph node (white arrow) in the right jugular chain. (Courtesy of Faustino Guinto, M.D., Department of Radiology, University of Texas Medical Branch at Galveston.)

13. Can neoplastic invasion of the carotid artery be accurately determined radiologically?

No imaging modality can determine neoplastic invasion of the carotid artery with 100% accuracy. Demonstration of fat between the artery and neoplasm by any modality indicates that the artery is not involved. The likelihood of involvement of the artery increases with increased circumferential contact of the neoplasm with the artery. The wall of the carotid artery can be seen only with ultrasound, but even this modality is not 100% accurate in determining invasion of the artery by an adjacent neoplasm. The wall may appear affected when it is not. MRI and CT demonstrate the lumen of the artery and adjacent structures but not the arterial wall. Consequently, both modalities only estimate the likelihood of invasion by the degree of circumferential contact. Angiography can demonstrate only the lumen of the artery and is the least sensitive method for determining invasion of the wall.

14. Why are both CT and MRI indicated in the evaluation of suspected rhabdomyosarcoma?

Rhabdomyosarcoma is the most common soft tissue sarcoma and the second most common solid tumor in children. Both CT and MRI are important in the evaluation because treatment decisions are made based on bone involvement and exact extent of soft tissue spread. Bone destruction,

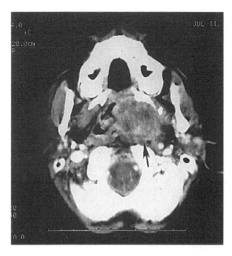

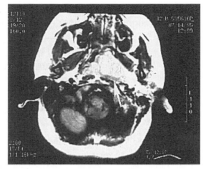

Rhabdomyosarcoma (white arrow) demonstrated on MRI. (Courtesy of Susan John, M.D., Department of Radiology, University of Texas Medical Branch at Galveston.)

Rhabdomyosarcoma (black arrow) with bone destruction (white arrow) demonstrated on CT. (Courtesy of Susan John, M.D., Department of Radiology, University of Texas Medical Branch at Galveston.

a common feature of rhabdomyosarcomas, is best demonstrated by CT. The margins of the neoplasm, including intracranial spread, are best demonstrated by MRI.

15. What are the important radiologic findings in evaluating a cholesteatoma before surgery?

The radiologist must make several important observations when assisting in the preoperative evaluation of a cholesteatoma. The relationship of a cholesteatoma to the facial nerve must be established to determine the risk of injury to this structure. Extension of the lesion into the sinus tympani should be evaluated radiographically because it is an area that cannot be visualized during surgery (mastoid approach). The status of the tegmen tympani (intact or not) helps to predict complications involving the temporal lobe. The relationship of the lesion to the membranous labyrinth helps to establish the risk of fistula formation postoperatively. The location of the lesion relative to the ossicles also helps with surgical planning.

16. How are congenital anomalies of the ear best defined?

Because the middle and external ear arise from different structures than the inner ear, congenital anomalies affect either the external ear (with possible involvement of the middle ear) or the inner ear. The structures of the external and middle ear consist mainly of bone and air-filled spaces. Air and bone are well differentiated from each other by CT, but both appear black on MRI. As a result, CT is the best modality to demonstrate stenosis or atresia of the external canal, possible involvement of the middle ear cavity and the ossicles, and the location of the descending portion of the facial nerve in its bony canal. The membranous labyrinth of the inner ear is filled with fluid and can be imaged by MRI. The membranous labyrinth is surrounded by the bony labyrinth, which can be imaged by CT. Because CT allows better spatial resolution than MRI, the structures of the inner ear are better defined by CT. The resolution of MRI is improving, however, and new techniques allow sections ≤ 1 mm. MRI may provide better or complementary data in the future.

17. How are vascular anomalies that cause pulsitile tinnitus best evaluated?

Although angiography and MRI can demonstrate the course of the internal carotid artery and the jugular vein, CT best demonstrates the relationship of these vessels to the middle ear. CT determines whether the lateral margin of the carotid canal is intact and demonstrates the aberrant carotid artery in the middle ear. Similarly, CT determines whether the bony covering of the jugular bulb is intact and demonstrates any portion of the jugular vein in the middle ear. Correct identification of these anomalies is important to prevent a disastrous biopsy of misplaced but otherwise normal vessels.

18. What is the most common location of neoplasms in the posterior fossa?

In the posterior fossa, the cerebellopontine angle is the most common location of neoplasms. Although approximately 90% of primary neoplasms in the cerebellopontine angle are acoustic neuromas, other lesions must be considered. Meningiomas, epidermoid tumors, and facial nerve schwannomas account for approximately 5% of the remaining primary tumors. Other primary tumors are rare in this location.

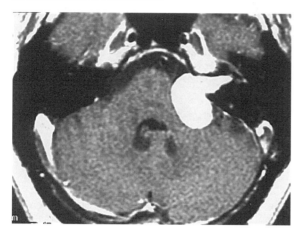

T2-weighted axial MRI of an acoustic neuroma located in the left cerebellopontine angle with extension into the internal auditory canal. (Courtesy of Gregory Chaljub, M.D., Department of Radiology, University of Texas Medical Branch at Galveston.)

19. What is the appropriate radiologic evaluation of a patient with a history of trauma to the temporal bone?

Once the patient's circulatory and respiratory status is stable, radiologic studies should include a high resolution CT to evaluate the skull base for fractures. When evaluation of the vasculature is clinically indicated, angiography best demonstrates the luminal anatomy, but MRI and MRA may be sufficient to characterize vascular injuries.

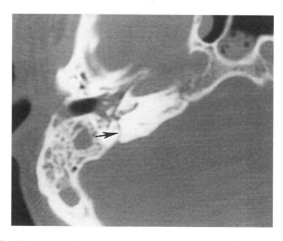

Unenhanced axial CT (with bone windows) shows a right petrous fracture (black arrow) extending from the posterior portion of the petrous pyramid to the bony labyrinth. (Courtesy of Gregory Chaljub, M.D., Department of Radiology, University of Texas Medical Branch at Galveston.)

20. Describe the appropriate radiologic evaluation of a patient with cerebrospinal fluid (CSF) rhinorrhea.

CT or MR of the skull base should be performed. If the initial study does not show an abnormality that could cause a CSF leak but demonstrates possible CSF in the paranasal sinus or mastoid air cells, a CT cisternogram may be helpful. For this study, contrast is injected intrathecally by a lumbar puncture. The patient's head is lowered below the level of the lumbar spine to move the contrast into the head. The presence of contrast in air cells indicates a CSF leak. CT best demonstrates fractures, but MRI best demonstrates skull base anomalies such as encephaloceles.

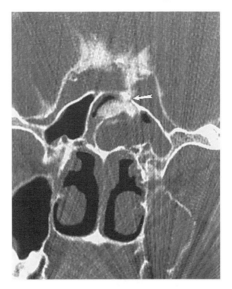

CT cysternogram with a CSF leak into the posterior ethmoid and sphenoid sinuses secondary to a fracture (white arrow) through the right planum sphenoidale and left carotid sulcus. (Courtesy of Gregory Chaljub, M.D., Department of Radiology, University of Texas Medical Branch at Galveston.)

21. Discuss radiologic imaging of the paranasal sinuses.

Although the sinuses have traditionally been evaluated with plain films, CT offers superior imaging and is now the gold standard. The presence of air-fluid levels without history of recent trauma or lavage is evidence of an acute inflammatory condition. Mucoperiosteal thickening in the absence of air-fluid levels may indicate either acute or chronic disease. Severe unilateral sinusitis may result from a bacterial or fungal process. It may also represent sinuses obstructed by inverted papilloma, polyp, or another lesion. Fungal causes, most commonly *Aspergillus*, should be considered when a hyperdense area (thought to represent calcium, iron, and manganese) is seen in the context of chronic sinusitis.

22. What is the significance of incidental ethmoid or sphenoid sinusitis in a patient who has had a CT for an unrelated condition?

The majority of patients with incidental ethmoid sinus abnormalities have localized disease involving only a few of the air cells. The demonstrated mucosal thickening may indicate the presence of granulation tissue, acutely or chronically edematous mucosa, or a clinically silent ethmoid sinusitis. In most patients, particularly adults, this finding has little clinical significance. It has been reported that approximately 10% of patients undergoing CT of the head for other reasons are found to have ethmoid sinus disease. However, incidentally discovered sphenoid sinusitis is much less common. Because of the anatomic location and proximity to neurovascular structures, neurologic and optic complications are found in up to 25% of patients with severe sphenoid sinusitis.

23. Which imaging modality is best for evaluating a nontraumatic brachial plexopathy?

MRI is the modality of choice because of its ability to acquire images in multiple planes. Coronal and parasagittal images best demonstrate the anatomy of the brachial plexus and the surrounding structures. CT demonstrates the area only in axial images. In addition, intravenous contrast is necessary to delineate blood vessels with CT but not with MRI. CT images obtained at or below the level of the shoulders may be degraded by beam-hardening artifact.

24. What radiographic findings confirm the diagnosis of epiglottitis?

In an equivocal presentation of epiglottitis, lateral neck radiographs are a useful diagnostic tool. The patient must be accompanied by a physician who is capable of securing the airway in the event of rapid respiratory decompensation. Important signs of epiglottitis include a swollen epiglottis, arytenoid prominence, and aryepiglottic folds. This constellation creates the classic "thumb-print" sign. Air trapping secondary to airway obstruction may lead to dilatation of the hypopharynx.

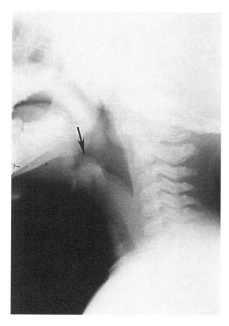

Lateral neck radiograph of a patient with a swollen epiglottis and the classic "thumb-print" sign indicative of epiglottitis. (Courtesy of Susan John, M.D., Department of Radiology, University of Texas Medical Branch at Galveston.)

25. What is the role of radiology in the diagnosis and treatment of juvenile angiofibromas?

Both CT and MRI can demonstrate the nasopharyngeal mass, which may indent the posterior margin of the maxillary sinus, involve the infratemporal fossa, or extend into the nasal cavity. CT best demonstrates bone destruction if the skull base is involved, but MRI best shows the involvement of the cavernous sinus or other intracranial structures. Angiography also demonstrates the extent of this benign but invasive vascular neoplasm but does not define its exact relationship to surrounding structures. Angiography provides a road map of the feeding vessels for preoperative intra-arterial embolization of the neoplasm.

ACKNOWLEDGMENT

Special thanks to members of the Department of Radiology at the University of Texas Medical Branch at Galveston for their support and guidance.

BIBLIOGRAPHY

1. Cohan M: Imaging of Children with Cancer. St.Louis, Mosby, 1992.
2. Cummings CW, et al (eds): Otolaryngology–Head and Neck Surgery. St. Louis, Mosby, 1993.
3. Diger KB, Maxner CE, Crawford S, Yuh WTC: Significance of CT and MR findings in sphenoid sinus disease. AJNR 10:603, 1989.

4. Duvoisin B, Agrifoglio A: Presence of ethmoid sinus abnormalities on brain CT of asymptomatic adults. AJNR10:599, 1989.
5. Gooding GAW, Langman AW, Dillon WP, Kaplan MJ: Malignant carotid artery invasion: Sonographic detection. Radiology 171:435–438, 1989.
6. Gritzmann N, Grasl MC, Helmer M, Steiner E: Invasion of the carotid artery and jugular vein by lymph node metastases: Detection with sonography. AJR 154:411–414, 1989.
7. Harnsberger HRic: Handbook of Head and Neck Imaging, 2nd ed. St. Louis, Mosby, 1995.
8. Lee KJ (ed): Essential Otolaryngology–Head and Neck Surgery. East Norwalk, CT, Appleton & Lange, 1995.
9. Shockley WW, Pillsbury HC III: The Neck: Diagnosis and Surgery. St. Louis, Mosby, 1994.
10. Som PM, Bergeron RT (eds): Head and Neck Imaging, 2nd ed. St. Louis, Mosby, 1991.
11. Yousem DM, Hatabu H, Hurst RW, et al: Carotid artery invasion by head and neck masses: Prediction with MR imaging. Radiology 195:715–720, 1995.
12. Zeifer A: Sinus imaging. In Bailey BF, et al (eds): Head and Neck Surgery–Otolaryngology. Philadelphia, J.B. Lippincott, 1993.

73. ANESTHESIA IN OTOLARYNGOLOGY

Kathryn Beauchamp, M.D., and Matthew Flaherty, M.D.

1. What premedications are appropriate for the otolaryngology patient?

Medications such as benzodiazepines and barbiturates provide sedation and relief of anxiety preoperatively. Opioids can be given to provide analgesia. Undesirable reflexes, such as salivation or increase in vagal tone, can be prevented with anticholinergics. Postoperative nausea and vomiting can be better controlled with the use of preoperative antiemetics (droperidol and ondansetron) and by providing gastric emptying with metoclopramide or intraoperative gastric suction.

2. What causes malignant hyperthermia (MH)?

MH is an inherited membrane defect that occurs primarily in skeletal muscle. When these patients are exposed to triggering drugs (e.g., potent inhalation anesthetics and succinylcholine), calcium is released at an enhanced rate from the sarcoplasmic reticulum. The excess calcium overwhelms the ATPase pump responsible for returning calcium from the mycoplasm to the sarcoplasmic reticulum, and a hypermetabolic state results. This decreases the amount of ATP available to the cell. Without ATP, the actin–myosin crossbridge cannot detach and muscle remains contracted, resulting in rigidity. MH is inherited in an autosomal dominant fashion and has a highly variable clinical presentation. This may indicate that multiple genes play a role. Current research is focusing on chromosomal analysis and DNA linkages. Mortality due to MH is currently 5–20%.

3. How does malignant hyperthermia present?

MH is primarily a clinical diagnosis. Signs and symptoms are related to the hypermetabolism of skeletal muscle and generally include tachycardia, trismus, muscle rigidity, hyperventilation, cyanosis, sweating, unstable blood pressure, and increased temperature. Laboratory tests commonly show hypercarbia, hyperkalemia, respiratory and metabolic acidosis, hypoxia, myoglobinuria, and an increased creatine kinase (often > 20,000 IU).

4. Why is malignant hyperthermia important to the otolaryngologist?

Although susceptible patients may not experience MH with every anesthetic exposure, it is important for the otolaryngologist to recognize who is at risk. The overall incidence is generally about 1 in 40,000 anesthetics in adults and 1 in 10,000–15,000 in children. It is rarely seen in children under 3 years of age. Patients who are considered to be at higher risk are those with a myopathy such as Duchenne's muscular dystrophy, those with a family history of MH, and those with a history of a questionable reaction to anesthesia.

5. How is the malignant hyperthermia managed?

When the diagnosis of MH is made, all triggers must be stopped immediately. The surgical procedure must be stopped as soon as possible. The following mnemonic is attributed to Zuckerberg:

Some	Stop all triggering agents, go to 100% oxygen
Hot	Hyperventilate
Dude	Dantrolene, 2.5 mg/kg immediately
Better	Bicarbonate sodium, 1 mEq/kg to start
GIve	Glucose, 0.5 gm/kg; Insulin, 0.15 U/kg
Iced	IV fluids, cooling blanket
Fluids	Fluid output; Furosemide, mannitol as needed
fasT	Tachycardia, be prepared to treat ventricular tachycardia

6. Describe local anesthetics.

Local anesthetics block sodium channels which results in an inability of the cell to achieve threshold potential. A propagated action potential fails to develop and therefore conduction is blocked. Structurally, local anesthetics consist of an aromatic moiety with a substituted amine. The linkage between the two is either an ester or an amine. The linkage tends to create a number of clinical similarities; therefore, local anesthetics are grouped into either the ester or amide group. Amides are often metabolized in the liver and esters in the plasma (by pseudo-cholinesterase). Ester local anesthetics may cause allergic reactions since they are metabolized to *para*-aminobenzoic acid (PABA). Amide local anesthetics rarely cause allergic reactions.

All amide local anesthetics have two *i*'s in their names: lidocaine, bupivacaine, mepivacaine, etidocaine, and prilocaine. Ester local anesthetics have one *i*: tetracaine, cocaine, chloroprocaine, and procaine.

7. Which is affected first by local anesthetics—pain or motor information?

Pain is usually affected before motor activity. Small, myelinated nerves are blocked before small unmyelinated or large nerves. Pain fibers are the smaller A-delta (myelinated) and C fibers (unmyelinated).

8. Which local anesthetic is unique (almost) to otolaryngology?

Cocaine is one of the local anesthetics used almost exclusively in otolaryngology. Its unique advantage is vasoconstriction, which other local anesthetics lack. In fact, lidocaine is a vasodilator and is often prepared with epinephrine. Cocaine is used topically on mucosal surfaces, providing anesthesia and vasoconstriction to provide a bloodless surgical field.

9. What are the toxic doses of the local anesthetics?

LOCAL ANESTHETIC	MAXIMUM DOSE
Procaine	6.0 mg/kg
Chloroprocaine	11.0 mg/kg
Tetracaine	1.4 mg/kg
Lidocaine	5.0 mg/kg
Mepivacaine	4.0 mg/kg
Bupivacaine	2.5 mg/kg
Etidocaine	4.0 mg/kg

10. What is the toxic dose of cocaine?

2–4 mg/kg. Cocaine was the first known drug to have local anesthetic action and is still used routinely by > 90% of otolaryngologists for topical anesthesia to facilitate nasal surgery. Cocaine can sensitize the myocardium to arrhythmias, especially in association with epinephrine and halothane.

11. How is the airway best secured during an ENT procedure in the mouth?

If the procedure is minor and lateral in the mouth, endotracheal tubes may be used and moved if necessary. Specialized endotracheal tubes called **RAE tubes** are formed with a sharp bend to angle the tube past the chin and out of the surgeon's exposure to the mouth. RAE tubes are used for tonsillectomies. Occasionally, the endotracheal tube will obstruct the surgical field, or the jaws will be wired shut during the case, and in these cases, the endotracheal tube is passed via the nostril to the nasopharynx and then into the trachea.

12. Why must nitrous oxide be used carefully when performing surgery in the middle ear?

Nitrous oxide is 34 times more soluble than nitrogen and therefore will enter an air-filled cavity rapidly, resulting in **increased pressure**. This situation can be problematic in the case of ear surgery, where pathology may limit normal venting of the middle ear via the eustachian tube. To avoid complications, nitrous oxide is not commonly used during middle ear surgery. However, if it is used, it should be discontinued 15 minutes or more before surgical closure of the middle ear cavity.

13. Discuss the unique anesthetic considerations during laser surgery.

It is important for the patient to be protected from inadvertent **laser exposure** and to prevent **laser-related fires**. The perioperative site should be draped with wet towels. All personnel in the operating room, as well as the patient, should wear protective eyewear. Nitrous oxide should be avoided because it supports combustion, and the inspired oxygen concentration is lowered to the lowest acceptable oxygen saturation, usually guided by the pulse oximeter.

Because laser surgery in the airway is often in close proximity to the endotracheal (ET) tube, the possibility of **airway fire** exists. Specialized ET tubes for laser surgery are designed to resist laser ignition, although even these tubes are occasionally ignited. The smoke of a burning ET tube contains a variety of toxic chemicals. When a tube is ignited, regardless of the type, it must be removed immediately. If tracheal tissue continues to burn, it should be irrigated with saline solution. Reintubation should follow quickly since the airway may rapidly become edematous in response to thermal and chemical injury. The ET tube cuff is the thinnest and most easily ignited part of the tube. The cuff is often filled with saline or water when laser surgery is planned, and when laser energy strikes the cuff, it will puncture and the fluid may extinguish a potential fire. Methylene blue dye also may be used to color the fluid, alerting the surgeon to a punctured cuff if blue dye is seen leaking into the surgical field. Airway fires may be avoided by performing surgery without an ET tube. For example, laser surgery is often accomplished via a ventilating bronchoscope, which has no flammable components.

14. What are the special anesthesia considerations during endoscopy?

During endoscopy, access to the patient's airway must be shared between the otolaryngologist and anesthesiologist. This must be done in a way that oxygenation and ventilation are adequately maintained. If using an endotracheal tube, it can be positioned to the left in the patient's mouth, allowing the otolaryngologist access to the right side. Alternative methods of oxygenation may be used, such as a ventilating bronchoscope or laryngoscope. Topical anesthetics may facilitate these procedures, as will the use of anticholinergics to control secretions. It is important to remember that patients undergoing these procedures may have significant airway pathology, and attention to airway maintenance is the priority.

15. Are there special considerations in patients with malignancies of the head and neck?

A high degree of suspicion must be maintained for a difficult airway. Approximately 50% of the tracheal lumen may be obstructed before a patient experiences any symptoms. However, once a patient is under general anesthesia, a mass in or around the trachea may become more apparent. Often, when muscle relaxants are administered, the muscles of the airway lose tone and a tumor may suddenly obstruct the airway. Alternative methods of airway management, such as an awake tracheostomy or awake fiberoptic intubation, may be indicated.

Additionally, these patients may have hepatic damage from extensive alcohol abuse. Coagulopathy associated with liver disease may contribute to extensive airway bleeding. Some patients may have had radiation therapy, leading to epiglottic fibrosis or laryngeal edema. Smoking history is associated with malignancy, increased secretions, and chronic obstructive pulmonary disease.

16. What are the unique considerations in thyroid surgery?

Hyperthyroid patients should be rendered euthyroid and continue their medications through the morning of surgery. Tracheomalacia may develop in response to encroachment of an enlarged thyroid. Careful preoperative examination of the airway should seek to identify potential airway difficulties. To avoid hemodynamic instability, you should use medications that stimulate the sympathetic nervous system with caution, and an appropriate depth of anesthesia should be maintained to prevent an exaggerated sympathetic response. Muscle relaxants that provide cardiovascular stability, such as vecuronium, are preferred.

17. When is intubation indicated?

- Protection of the airway from secretions, bleeding, or aspiration of gastric contents
- Positive pressure ventilation when spontaneous ventilation fails or during the use of muscle relaxants
- Providing an airway when infected tissues, hematoma, tumor, or edema threaten obstruction

18. How can endotracheal tube placement be confirmed?

- Direct visualization of the tube in glottic opening
- Presence of carbon dioxide in exhaled gas
- Symmetric bilateral chest movement with manual ventilation
- Presence of bilateral breath sounds with auscultation
- Absence of air movement during epigastric auscultation
- Maintenance of arterial oxygen saturation
- Reservoir bag movement during spontaneous ventilation
- Condensation of water vapor in the tube lumen during exhalation

19. How can a difficult airway be recognized prior to surgery?

The **Mallampati classification** evaluates the patient according to the relative size and position of the tongue to the palate. Class I and II airways are usually manageable with conventional laryngoscopy. Class III and IV airways predict higher incidences of difficulty when intubating by conventional laryngoscopy. Inability to extend the head, a small mouth, limited mouth opening, prominent upper incisors, and any distorting airway pathology can all lead to a difficult airway and require special attention and planning.

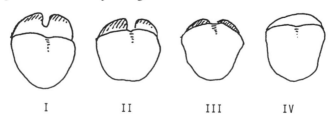

I   II   III   IV

The Mallampati classification of posterior pharyngeal visualization. In class I and II airways, the uvula is completely or partially seen, respectively. In class III and IV airways, the base of the uvula or soft palate only may be seen, respectively.

20. How much epinephrine is contained in each milliliter of 1:200,000 solution?

Epinephrine 1:200,000 is frequently added to local anesthetic solutions and contains 5 µg/ml. At a concentration of 2 µg/kg, patients receiving halothane anesthesia may begin to have ventricular ectopy.

21. A patient with Down syndrome is scheduled for tonsillectomy. Are there special concerns regarding the airway?

Down syndrome is associated with **macroglossia** and **atlantoaxial instability**. Preoperative assessment should always include airway examination. Patients may have no preoperative cervical spine symptoms and still suffer intraoperative cervical spine and spinal cord damage if the neck is flexed or extended beyond its normal range of motion. Radiologic exam prior to surgery is occasionally indicated depending on the degree of head extension and flexion planned intraoperatively.

22. What are the more common acid-base disorders seen in the postoperative period?

- **Respiratory acidosis** is very common secondary to residual anesthetics and neuromuscular blocking agents, which blunt the response to rising $PaCO_2$.
- **Metabolic acidosis** may occur when surgical blood loss or third-space losses are underappreciated and volume resuscitation is inadequate.
- **Respiratory alkalosis** is also common due to pain or anxiety.

23. Name the most common coagulopathy seen after massive transfusion.

Blood transfusion of > 1 blood volume is considered massive transfusion. The most common coagulopathy that develops is **dilutional thrombocytopenia**. Stored red blood cells contain almost no active platelets. When transfusion volumes approach the patient's entire blood volume, the original platelets are either lost or diluted.

24. What are the potential causes of intraoperative tachycardia?

Tachycardia during general anesthesia may be secondary to hypoxia, and this is always checked first. Next are cardiac arrhythmias, ventricular tachycardias, and supraventricular tachycardias. Secondary causes include hypercarbia, pain, fever, sepsis, malignant hyperthermia, and thyrotoxicosis. Drugs such as atropine, glucopyrrolate, catecholamines, isoflurane, pancuronium, and cocaine all can cause tachycardia.

CONTROVERSIES

25. Should a child with a minor upper respiratory infection (URI) undergo general anesthesia?

Yes: Although URIs can increase the risk of perioperative respiratory complications, in the absence of fever and productive cough, most children will experience minimal intraoperative and postoperative difficulties. Procedures such as typanostomy and tubes may alleviate infections and improve patient comfort. It is difficult to define when the upper respiratory irritation associated with an infection has subsided, but the mucosa usually returns to normal within 8 weeks. Many children will have a new URI within this time period, further extending the delay in surgery.

No: URIs increase the irritability of the airway and lead to increased bronchospasm, laryngospasm, and desaturation. Pulmonary aspiration, negative pressure pulmonary edema, and aggravated postoperative respiratory infection can arise from these airway reflexes and their treatment. Prolonged hospitalization and morbidity may result from anesthesia during acute infection and recovery.

26. Masseter muscle rigidity occurs in a child during anesthetic induction for elective surgery. Do you proceed with surgery or stop and reschedule?

Stop: Masseter muscle rigidity (MMR) is an early sign of malignant hyperthermia (MH). Frequently, if the triggering anesthetic is stopped, the patient will recover without further symptoms. Continuing the inhaled anesthetic may lead to MH within 10–20 minutes. Instead of continuing with surgery, time is better spent preparing for the treatment of MH. The child can return for elective surgery with a nontriggering anesthetic.

Proceed: MMR is common in children, and as many as 1 in 100 children receiving halothane and succinylcholine will have MMR to some degree, lasting 2–3 minutes. MMR is usually easily overcome after that time. MH is rare (1 in 10,000–15,000 anesthetics in children). It is unlikely then that the MMR will develop into MH. The anesthetic could be changed to a nontriggering type at this time, and the surgery could proceed.

BIBLIOGRAPHY

1. Andrews JJ: Anesthesia systems. In Barash PG, Cullen BF, Stoetling RK (eds): Clinical Anesthesia. Philadelphia, J.B. Lippincott, 1989, pp 516–522.
2. Bridenbaugh P, Cruz M, Helton SH: Anesthesia for otolaryngologic procedures. In Paparella MM, Shumrick D, Gluckman J, Meyerhoff W (eds): Otolaryngology, 3rd ed. Philadelphia, W.B. Saunders, 1991, pp 2949–2970.
3. Brown A: Anesthesia. In Cummings CW, et al (eds): Otolaryngology–Head and Neck Surgery, 2nd ed. St. Louis, Mosby, 1993, pp 214–242.
4. Campell JP, et al: Comparison of the vasoconstrictive and anesthetic effects of intranasally applied cocaine versus xylometazoline/lidocaine solution. Otolaryngol Head Neck Surg 107:697–700, 1992.
5. Davidson JK, Eckhardt WF, Perese DA: Clinical Anesthesia Procedures of the Massachusetts General Hospital, 4th ed. Boston, Little, Brown and Company, 1993.
6. Feinstein R, Owens WD: Anesthesia for ENT. In Barash PG, Cullen BF, Stoetling RK (eds): Clinical Anesthesia. Philadelphia, J.B. Lippincott, 1989, pp 1067–1078.
7. Gal TJ: Monitoring the function of the respiratory system. In Lake CL: Clinical Monitoring. Philadelphia, W.B. Saunders, 1990, pp 315–341.
8. Kaus SJ, Rockoff MA: Malignant hyperthermia. Pediatr Clin North Am 41:221-237, 1994.
9. Stoetling RK, Miller RD: Basics of Anesthesia, 2nd ed. New York, Churchill Livingstone, 1989.
10. Vender JS, Gilbert HC: Blood gas monitoring. In Blitt CD, Hines RL (eds): Monitoring in Anesthesia and Critical Care Medicine, 3rd ed. New York, Churchill Livingstone, 1995, pp 407–421.
11. Tzabar Y: Intra-operative tracheal obstruction by tumour fragments. Anaesthesia 50:250, 1995.
12. Zuckerberg A: A hot mnemonic for the treatment of malignant hyperthermia. Anesth Analg 77:1135–1138, 1993.

74. THE EYE AND ORBIT

David M. Kleinman, M.D., David W. Johnson, M.D., and Jon M. Braverman, M.D.

1. What is an afferent pupillary deficit?

An afferent pupillary deficit is a condition due to disease along the afferent (incoming light signal) pathway, in which the pupillary response to direct light stimulation in the abnormal eye is sluggish as compared to the uninvolved eye. This phenomenon is also called a **relative afferent pupillary deficit** (RAPD) because the pupillary responses are being compared. It can be graded from mild (1+) to severe (4+). Another frequently used term to describe this condition is the **Marcus Gunn pupil**.

2. What are the causes of an RAPD?

An RAPD can be caused by optic nerve disease (ischemia, trauma, infection, inflammation, tumor, glaucoma) and severe retinal problems (large retinal detachments, infections, central retinal artery or vein occlusions). Media opacities such as a cataract or a corneal scar will not cause an RAPD.

3. How do you test for an RAPD in the setting of injury to the iris constrictor mechanism?

The iris sphincter or its innervation can be damaged during blunt or penetrating ocular trauma, and this problem can interfere with the direct pupillary light response in the injured eye. In this situation, careful attention must be applied to the consensual pupillary response when light is presented to the injured eye during the swinging flashlight test. In low ambient light, a bright test light is passed back and forth between both eyes as the direct and consensual reflexes are noted and compared. If an RAPD is present in the injured eye, the consensual pupillary response in the healthy eye is diminished as compared to its response to direct light stimulation. Thus, the status of the retina and optic nerve can be established in the setting where one eye has a pupil that does not react due to trauma.

4. Name the four basic ocular emergencies and describe their immediate treatments.

Chemical burn: Following chemical exposure, the eye must be irrigated with normal saline administered in large quantities as soon as possible.

Acute glaucoma: Symptoms include eye pain, blurred vision, headache, and nausea or vomiting. On examination, the eye is red, the pupil is generally partially dilated, and corneal haze is seen. Initial management involves topical β-blockers and oral carbonic anhydrase inhibitor (i.e., acetazolamide, 500 mg po). Intravenous acetazolamide or osmotic agents (i.e., mannitol) are used in severe cases.

Central retinal artery occlusion: This condition is diagnosed in the setting of acute unilateral painless loss of vision. An RAPD is present, and on funduscopic examination, the retina appears pale, except for a cherry red spot in the center of the macula (posterior retina). Ocular massage can be administered in an attempt to dislodge the central retinal artery emboli and facilitate their transfer downstream in the retinal circulation. Anterior chamber paracentesis, oral carbonic anhydrase inhibitors, and/or inspired carbogen (95% O_2/5% CO_2, to dilate the retinal arterioles) may be used to treat this condition as well.

Ruptured globe: This is suspected in the setting of periocular trauma (especially penetrating) with subconjunctival hemorrhage, decreased vision, and a shallowed or deepened anterior chamber; sometimes, obvious scleral or corneal lacerations are seen. An eye shield should be placed to protect the eye and broad-spectrum intravenous antibiotics (i.e., a cephalosporin and aminoglycoside) are administered. Additional emergent care includes tetanus toxoid, if applicable, and antiemetics, if needed.

Emergent ophthalmologic consultation is indicated in all of these situations.

5. How should orbital injuries be evaluated by nonophthalmologist examiners?

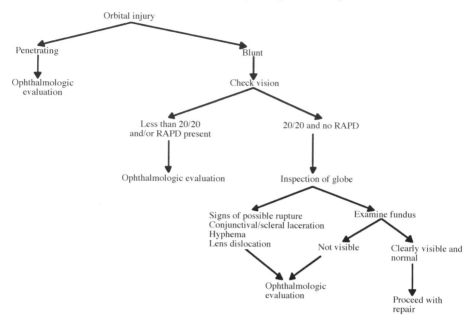

Steps in the evaluation of orbital injuries by nonophthalmologists. (Adapted from Weisman RA, Savino PJ: Management of patients with facial trauma and associated ocular/orbital injuries. Otolaryngol Clin North Am 24:50, 1991.)

6. What is a hyphema? How is it managed?

A hyphema is defined as blood in the anterior chamber of the eye. Trauma is the most frequent cause, and the blood arises from tears in iris vessels. The extent of a hyphema can range from very small, requiring a slit lamp for diagnosis, to large, filling the whole anterior chamber with blood. Management is controversial, but generally some form of steroid (or aminocaproic acid) is given to decrease the risk of secondary bleeding. Additionally, the pupil is dilated pharmacologically, the eye is protected with a shield, and patients must avoid platelet inhibitors such as aspirin or aspirin products. Bedrest with head elevation is recommended. Close ophthalmologic followup is also recommended, as the incidence of rebleeding is greatest during the first week following the injury.

7. What is traumatic optic neuropathy?

Traumatic optic neuropathy (TON) is the result of indirect traumatic injury to the optic nerve. Direct penetrating injuries of the optic nerve are excluded, but compression from edema or orbital bone fragments is included in the definition of this condition. Visual loss and an RAPD are necessary to make this diagnosis, and other ocular injuries should not be sufficient to account for the findings. The mechanisms that cause TON are multiple and not mutually exclusive. They include tears or shear injuries of the optic nerve, bone fractures of the optic canal injuring the nerve, and vascular compromise, inflammation, and/or hematomas involving the optic nerve. The condition is either instantaneous or delayed (primary or secondary TON), and secondary injury has a better prognosis as its effects may be somewhat reversible.

8. What are blowout fractures? What are the indications for their surgical repair?

Orbital blowout fractures are fractures in one or more of the walls of the orbit. They occur when direct blunt trauma to the globe increases intraorbital pressure, causing these thin bones to "blow out." The orbital floor and medial wall are most frequently involved.

The generally accepted indications for repair of these fractures include symptomatic diplopia with extraocular muscle entrapment demonstrated by forced duction testing and CT, early enophthalmos of 3 mm or more, a large orbital wall defect (usually defined as 50%) likely to cause late enophthalmos, or significant hypo-ophthalmos.

9. Can findings on plain films suggest the diagnosis of a blowout fracture?

While plain films are not the study of choice to evaluate the orbits, they are frequently obtained in the emergency department in the setting of facial trauma, and familiarity with the findings associated with blowout fractures can be helpful. Common radiographic signs include fragmentation of the orbital floor, depression of bony fragments of the floor, the "teardrop sign" (prolapse of orbital tissue into the maxillary sinus), and medial orbital wall fractures. Associated findings include air-fluid levels in or opacification of the maxillary sinus, opacification of the ethmoid sinus, orbital rim fractures, and air in the orbit.

10. Which radiologic studies are necessary for the appropriate evaluation of orbital fractures?

CT thin cuts (~3 mm) of the orbit, with axial and coronal views, provide the best detail of the bony anatomy and are the studies of choice.

11. Are there contraindications for surgery on blowout fractures?

Contraindications include hyphema, retinal tears, and globe perforation. These conditions can be aggravated by surgical exploration of the orbit, and repair of the fracture should be delayed. Additionally, if a patient has only one seeing eye, diplopia will not be a problem; the risk of enophthalmos should be accepted to prevent a rare but potential surgical complication that would result in a patient losing all vision. Furthermore, a blowout fracture should not be repaired in patients who are too medically unstable to safely undergo general anesthesia.

12. What are the possible complications of surgical repair of an orbital blowout fracture?

Orbital cellulitis
Persistent or late enophthalmos
Extrusion of the implant
Optic nerve injury with vision loss
Injury to the neurovascular bundle along the orbital floor causing infraorbital hypesthesia
Retrobulbar hemorrhage
Oculomotor nerve palsy
Ectropion or skin traction from the incision
Extraocular muscle injury

13. How does a retrobulbar hemorrhage present? What other disease entities are in the differential diagnosis in the setting of head trauma?

A retrobulbar hemorrhage in the setting of trauma presents with symptoms of pain and decreased vision. Signs include proptosis, resistance to retropulsion, subconjunctival hemorrhage extending posteriorly, elevated intraocular pressure, afferent pupillary deficit, and restriction of extraocular motility. Intraocular pressure should be monitored closely; occasionally a lateral canthotomy and lateral tendon cantholysis must be performed to relieve some of the pressure on the globe. Orbital cellulitis, globe rupture, and carotid cavernous fistula are in the differential diagnosis.

14. What clinical findings differentiate preseptal from postseptal (or orbital) cellulitis? When should imaging be obtained?

In the setting of eyelid edema and erythema, chemosis (conjunctival edema), decreased visual acuity, restriction of extraocular movements, and proptosis all point toward orbital involvement and are indications for intravenous antibiotics and CT imaging. Thin cut coronal and axial views are most helpful. MRI is indicated when CNS manifestations are present.

15. How is orbital cellulitis staged?

Stage 1 Preseptal (periorbital) cellulitis: Inflammation anterior to the orbital septum, with edema, erythema, warmth, and tenderness; one or both eyelids may be involved.

Stage 2 Subperiosteal abscess: Preseptal cellulitis present, as well as an abscess between the bony wall of the orbit and the periorbita; clinically, chemosis, asymmetric proptosis, extraocular muscle restriction, and decreased vision may be present.

Stage 3 Orbital cellulitis: Inflammation within the retrobulbar contents of the orbit, but enclosed by the periorbita; clinical findings include marked preseptal cellulitis, chemosis, proptosis (generally axial), ophthalmoplegia, and decreased vision.

Stage 4 Orbital abscess: Orbital cellulitis and abscess in the retrobulbar tissue; the findings are those of orbital cellulitis, but with more severe proptosis and visual loss.

Stage 5 Cavernous sinus thrombosis: Inflammation within the cavernous sinus in addition to the findings of orbital cellulitis; this condition may become bilateral; CN III, IV, and VI palsies are present, episcleral venous dilation occurs; meningitis may be present.

Adapted from: Moloney JR, Badham NJ, McRae A: The acute orbit: Preseptal (periorbital) cellulitis, subperiosteal abscess and orbital cellulitis due to sinusitis. J Laryngol Otol Suppl 12:1, 1987.

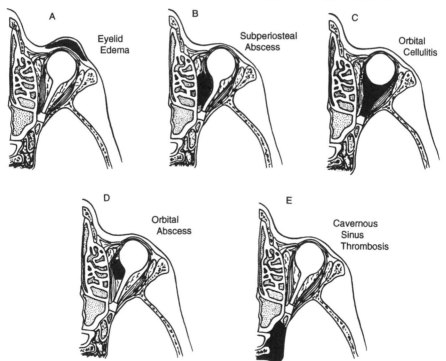

Stages of orbital cellulitis. (From Stankiewicz JA, Newell DJ, Park AH: Complications of inflammatory diseases of the sinuses. Otolaryngol Clin North Am 26:641, 1993, with permission.)

16. How are periorbital and orbital cellulitis treated?

The patient with **periorbital cellulitis** can generally be treated on an outpatient basis with oral antibiotics and warm compresses to the inflamed area three times daily. Conjunctivitis is treated if present. Incision and drainage of any face or lid abscess are indicated. Patients who appear noncompliant, toxic, fail to respond, or are < 5 years of age will need hospitalization and IV antibiotics. The patient is followed daily until improvement is noted.

The patient with **orbital cellulitis** is hospitalized. Broad-spectrum intravenous antibiotics are initiated, nasal decongestant spray is administered as needed, and erythromycin ointment is applied three times daily if corneal exposure from proptosis is present. The patient is re-evaluated frequently. Surgical drainage of the sinuses is indicated urgently if visual acuity decreases, if the patient's condition deteriorates over 24 hours, or if it fails to improve over 48–72 hours. Repeat imaging may be necessary. Exploration and drainage of subperiosteal or orbital abscesses are indicated.

17. What are the etiologies of orbital cellulitis?

Sinusitis is the cause of orbital cellulitis 70–80% of the time. The ethmoids are most commonly involved. Other causes include cutaneous infections (from lacerations, abrasions, or impetigo), penetrating trauma, lacrimal infection, odontogenic sources, or dental or mid-facial surgery.

18. Why is orbital cellulitis in a diabetic concerning?

Infection with mucormycosis should be considered in any diabetic with orbital cellulitis. Rhinocerebral mucormycosis is a fungal disease that spreads rapidly from the paranasal sinuses and orbit to the brain; untreated, it is fatal. This infection is most likely to be seen in a patient with diabetic ketoacidosis. The diagnosis should also be considered in immunocompromised patients, in patients receiving steroid or antibiotic therapy, and in patients with severe burns or malignancies who demonstrate orbital or periorbital inflammation. Appropriate treatment includes correcting the underlying disorder, antifungal therapy, and debridment.

19. What are the possible complications of orbital cellulitis?

Retrobulbar abscess	Elevated intraocular pressure
Cavernous sinus thrombosis	Central retinal artery or vein occlusion
Ophthalmoplegia	Optic neuritis
Orbital apex syndrome	Endophthalmitis
Permanent cranial nerve dysfunction	Meningitis
Variable degrees of visual loss	Death

20. How does the anatomy of the orbit predispose to the spread of infection from the sinuses?

The thin walls of the orbit and their close proximity to the sinuses facilitate spread in complicated sinusitis. The lamina papyracea is exceptionally thin and fragile; it forms the lateral wall of the ethmoid labyrinth and a significant portion of the medial wall of the orbit. Additionally, the venous system of the orbit predisposes to hematogenous spread of infection to the orbit. The veins around and within the orbit, including the superior and inferior ophthalmic veins, form a diffuse network of interconnected valveless branches, and the direction of blood flow depends on local pressure gradients. Thus, communication between the nose, ethmoids, face, orbit and cavernous sinus exists.

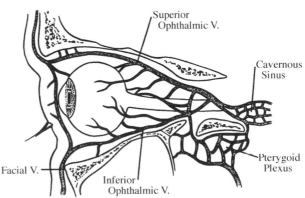

The venous network around the face, orbit, and cavernous sinus. (From Stankiewicz JA, Newell DJ, Park AH: Complications of inflammatory diseases of the sinuses. Otolaryngol Clin North Am 26: 640, 1993, with permission.)

21. What is the orbital septum?

The orbital septum is a thin fibrous membrane that arises from the periorbita of the orbital rim and extends into the eyelids. It lies between the orbicularis muscle and the tarsus of the lids. The superior orbital septum blends at the superior tarsus with the levator palpebrae superior is aponeurosis. The inferior orbital septum blends with the inferior tarsal plate. Laterally and medially, the orbital septum forms the lateral and medial palpebral ligaments, respectively. This membrane acts as a barrier between the eyelids and orbit.

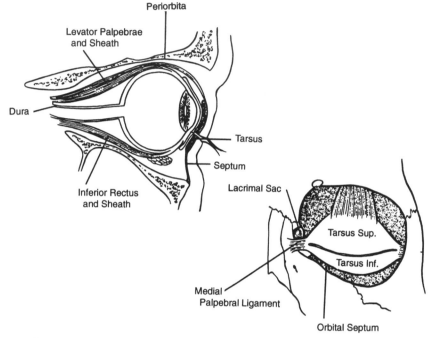

Anatomy of the orbital septum. (From Stankiewicz JA, Newell DJ, Park AH: Complications of inflammatory diseases of the sinuses. Otolaryngol Clin North Am 26:642, 1993, with permission.)

22. How does a patient with retinal detachment present?

Symptoms suggesting retinal detachment include scotoma (blind area in the visual field—the patient may describe a "curtain" in his or her vision), photopsia (flashes of light), floaters, and blurred vision. Clinical signs may include an afferent pupillary deficit and a decreased red reflex. Retinal detachments are not always seen with the direct ophthalmoscope, and referral to an ophthalmologist is indicated.

23. What are the special concerns in the evaluation of eyelid lacerations?

When lid lacerations extend medially, the lacrimal drainage system can be injured. This injury may be difficult to diagnose initially because lid edema can obscure adequate visualization of the canaliculus, lacrimal duct, or sac. Knowledge of the anatomy of the lacrimal drainage system and the location and mechanism of the laceration will play the major role in determining whether to probe the lacrimal drainage system prior to repairing the laceration.

24. Why are eye problems in children so concerning?

The visual system in humans develops from birth to age 8 or 9. Any eye problem that interferes with sight in one eye in this age group can potentially cause **amblyopia** (reduction of vision due to arrested CNS development). Thus, problems such as congenital media opacities, strabismus, ptosis, and unilateral refractive errors need close ophthalmologic management.

25. When is a third nerve palsy worrisome? Why?

A third nerve palsy is concerning when the pupil is involved because a posterior communicating artery aneurysm is a common etiology. Emergent CT or MRI is indicated, and cerebral angiography is frequently necessary as well. Pupil-sparing third nerve palsies generally have a microvascular etiology (i.e., diabetes), but imaging is necessary in certain subsets of patients.

26. What are the ocular complications of AIDS?

Molluscum contagiosum of the lids and face	CMV retinitis
Kaposi's sarcoma of the lids	Acute retinal necrosis
Microsporidia keratitis	Progressive outer retinal necrosis
Nonspecific iritis	Orbital lymphoma
Herpes zoster ophthalmicus	Neuro-ophthalmic disorders of
HIV retinopathy	multiple etiologies

27. What is the differential diagnosis for a red eye?

Conjunctivitis	Corneal abrasion
Blepharitis	Iritis
Episcleritis	Acute angle closure glaucoma
Scleritis	Subconjunctival hemorrhage
Inflamed pinguecula or pterygium	Dry eye syndrome
Corneal or conjunctival foreign body	

28. What are the ocular concerns with Stevens-Johnson syndrome?

Stevens-Johnson syndrome can have severe ocular manifestations, and care needs to be taken when managing these patients. Conjunctival scarring (symblepharon), dry eyes, corneal neovascularization, corneal scarring, corneal ulcers, corneal perforation, and endophthalmitis have been known to occur secondary to this condition.

29. Which findings point toward a malignancy in an eyelid lesion?

Lid lesions that grow rapidly, destroy the lash line, interfere with the meibomian orifices, ulcerate, cause inflammation, or recur after excision are more likely to be malignant. Benign and malignant tumors of the eyelids can have similar appearances, and biopsy is generally necessary to establish a diagnosis.

30. Discuss the treatments for the ocular complications of facial nerve palsy.

Exposure keratitis, which can be very severe, is the main concern in patients with a facial nerve palsy, as this cranial nerve innervates muscles that close the eye. Treatment for mild exposure problems entails the frequent use of artificial tears. If the artificial tears are being used more frequently than four times daily, preservative-free solutions should be used. Lubricating ointment should be applied at night, but the eye also may be taped shut at night. For cases not responding to these measures where regeneration of the nerve is expected, a moisture chamber can be worn around the eye, temporary plugging of the puncta can be performed, or temporary external eyelid weights can be used. In more severe or permanent cases, a gold weight or eyelid spring can be placed in the upper lid to help it close, or a tarsorrhaphy (lid suturing procedure) can be performed. Artificial tears are utilized adjunctively with the latter procedures.

CONTROVERSIES

31. How is traumatic optic neuropathy (TON) managed?

When inflammation and edema of the nerve itself are the most likely etiologies, management of this condition becomes controversial. Although spontaneous improvement in patients with TON is well documented, most ophthalmologists will treat these injuries with intravenous corticosteroids. The doses vary, however, from conventional doses of dexamethasone or methylprednisolone to megadoses of methylprednisolone at spinal cord injury levels. Optic canal decompression has been utilized for the treatment of this condition as well. The timing of surgery is also controversial, but patients are usually started first on IV corticosteroids, and if the condition worsens or does not improve within a few days, then decompression surgery may be recommended. Surgical decompression of the optic canal is not performed at all medical centers in the United States. There are no randomized controlled studies comparing the various therapies.

32. How long after the injury should a blowout fracture of the orbit be repaired?
The best timing for repair of blowout fractures is undecided. The controversy stems from the fact that documented improvement in diplopia does occur sometimes months after the injury and that suspected late enophthalmos frequently does not manifest. Most surgeons propose operating within 1–2 weeks, however, if any of the usual indications are present (see Question 8). A minority of surgeons will wait up to 6 months before operating for diplopia or cosmetically unacceptable enophthalmos. Nowadays, some surgeons recommend operating within 7 days, sometimes within 24 hours, to reduce scarring and fibrosis and to allow the orbital contents to heal in a normal-volume orbit.

BIBLIOGRAPHY

1. Berestka JS, Rizzo JF: Controversy in the management of traumatic optic neuropathy. Int Ophthalmol Clin 34:87, 1994.
2. Bhattacharyya AK, Deshpande AR, Nayak SR, et al: Rhinocerebral mucormycosis: An unusual case presentation. J Laryngol Otol 106:48, 1992.
3. Cullom RD, Chang B, Friedberg MA, Rapuano CJ: The Wills Eye Manual: Office and Emergency Room Diagnosis and Treatment of Eye Disease, 2nd ed. Philadelphia, J.B. Lippincott, 1994.
4. Dutton JJ: Atlas of Clinical and Surgical Orbital Anatomy. Philadelphia, W.B. Saunders, 1994.
5. Dutton JJ, Manson PN, Iliff N, Putterman AM: Management of blow-out fractures of the orbital floor. Surv Ophthalmol 35:279, 1991.
6. Mathog RH: Management of orbital blow out fractures. Otolaryngol Clin North Am 24:79, 1991.
7. Moloney JR, Badham NJ, McRae A: The acute orbit: Preseptal (periorbital) cellulitis, subperiosteal abscess and orbital cellulitis due to sinusitis. J Laryngol Otol Suppl 12:1, 1987.
8. O'Hare TH: Blow out fractures: A review. J Emerg Med 9:253, 1991.
9. Osguthorpe JD, Hochman M: Inflammatory sinus disease affecting the orbit. Otolaryngol Clin North Am 26:657, 1993.
10. Schramm VL, Curtain HD, Kennerdell JS: Evaluation of orbital cellulitis and results of treatment. Laryngoscope 92:732, 1982.
11. Stankiewicz JA, Newell DJ, Park AH: Complications of inflammatory diseases of the sinuses. Otolaryngol Clin North Am 26:639, 1993.
12. Steinsapir KD, Goldberg RA: Traumatic optic neuropathy. Surv Ophthalmol 38:487, 1994.
13. Vaughan DG, Asbury T, Riordan-Eva P: General Ophthalmology, 14th ed. Norwalk, CT, Appleton & Lange, 1995.
14. Weisman RA, Savino PJ: Management of patients with facial trauma and associated ocular/orbital injuries. Otolaryngol Clin North Am 24:37, 1991.

75. COST-EFFECTIVE OTOLARYNGOLOGY

Arlen D. Meyers, M.D., M.B.A.

1. What does cost-effective otolaryngology mean?
Practicing cost-effective otolaryngology means using as few resources as possible to achieve a desired outcome or to get maximum benefit from an expenditure of resources.

2. How are costs defined?
Health care costs can be divided into direct and indirect components. **Direct costs** are the values of goods and services used to detect, treat, and rehabilitate individuals with a disease or

impairment. **Indirect costs** include those used to administer the health care system (e.g. administration, insurance transactions). There are several other ways to measure costs, including average costs, marginal costs, fixed costs, and variable costs. Accounting for the true "cost" of a given treatment or service can be extremely difficult.

3. How are benefits defined?

The outcome of a given treatment can be measured in several ways. **Cost minimization** assumes a given outcome and seeks methods for achieving this outcome at lesser costs. **Cost-effectiveness** analysis expresses the outcome in units that can be measured objectively, such as measures of disability or 5-year survival. **Cost-benefit** analysis converts the costs and benefits into dollars. **Cost-utility** analysis expresses the denominator as the worth of a change in health status. The most commonly used unit for this measurement is **quality-adjusted life-years** (QALY).

4. What features of otolaryngology affect cost-effective practice?

Several features of otolaryngology have important implications for cost-effective practice:
1. Otolaryngologists represent only 1.5% of all physicians in the United States.
2. Many other specialists care for patients with otolaryngology complaints.
3. Otolaryngology concentrates on the pediatric and geriatric age groups, with the care of the geriatric patient being three times as costly as that of the younger patient.
4. Otolaryngology is primarily an office- and ambulatory-based specialty.
5. Medications constitute an important part of patient management in otolaryngology.
6. Approximately 1 in 30 patients seen by otolaryngologists requires an operation.

5. Where is there potential to save money in otolaryngology?

The 20 most common otolaryngology procedures account for 87% of all otolaryngology operations performed in the United States. These are relatively low-cost, high-volume procedures. Unfortunately, the precise indications for several of these operations are unclear (e.g., tonsillectomy, sinus surgery, septoplasty, and bilateral myringotomy with tubes). Managed care and capitation have forced a reevaluation of the necessity for many of these procedures, with an emphasis on refining indications, documenting outcome, and reducing costs.

6. How can otolaryngologists use fewer resources to achieve a given result?

Altering certain practice patterns offers the most potential for optimizing the use of resources.
• Eliminating unnecessary tests and office visits
• Determining appropriate place of care
• Prescribing appropriate medications, particularly antibiotics
• Using appropriate prehospitalization and postdischarge ancillary services to minimize length of stay
• Basing therapeutic decisions on data rather than anecdote.

7. How can the costs of ambulatory surgery be reduced?

1. Surgeons should not routinely order unnecessary preoperative lab tests. Frequently, ASA class I patients only need a preoperative hematocrit. Routine studies to screen for clotting disorders, EKGs in patients < 50 years old, chest x-rays, routine pregnancy tests, and routine preoperative urinalyses are not cost-effective.
2. The use of perioperative medications should be strictly monitored and limited to those with proven effectiveness.
3. Quality improvement programs should be in place to identify adverse trends, such as postoperative infections, hospital readmission following ambulatory surgery, and drug reactions.

8. When should prophylactic antibiotics be used in otolaryngologic surgery?

Prophylactic antibiotics are indicated in patients undergoing **clean contaminated** head and neck surgery. Patients having clean salivary gland surgery, thyroid surgery, most ear surgery, trauma surgery, and cosmetic procedures do not benefit from prophylactic antibiotics. When prophylactic antibiotics are administered, they should be given preoperatively and for 24–48 hours postoperatively at the appropriate dose.

9. When should you order sinus x-rays in patients with nasal and sinus complaints?

Routine x-rays of the paranasal sinuses have limited sensitivity and specificity when compared to CT scans. They are of some value in monitoring the progress of an air-fluid level of the maxillary sinus during treatment. In general, however, a limited coronal CT scan of the sinuses without contrast administration is the image of choice for diagnosing sinusitis.

10. When should you take a culture of the ear, nose, or throat?

Cultures of the ear canal, nasal cavity, and nasopharynx are usually not helpful in managing infections of those regions. Situations in which sinus aspiration or tympanocentesis may be helpful include:

Failure of the patient to respond to medical management

Outright or impending infectious complication

Suspicion of a resistant organism causing infection

11. Which antibiotic should be used to treat acute otitis and sinusitis?

Amoxicillin is still the initial drug of choice (sulfa in penicillin-allergic patients). Clinicians should be aware of emerging resistant strains of *Haemophilus* and *Pneumococcus*, however, and may need to adjust the antibiotics according to the clinical response of the patient.

12. Do all patients with squamous cell cancer of the head and neck need staging panendoscopy?

Probably not. Although there are not enough data to say for sure yet, patients with lesions of the anterior floor of the mouth can probably be staged adequately with fiberoptic laryngoscopy in the office and an MRI. The MRI is used to look for second primaries and metastatic lymph nodes.

13. When should a patient with ENT problems be referred to an otolaryngologist?

The American Academy of Otolaryngology–Head and Neck Surgery has published referral guidelines for primary care practitioners covering the most common ENT ambulatory problems. Request a copy at One Prince Street, Alexandria, VA 22314, or fax (703) 683-5100.

CONTROVERSY

14. Can primary care practitioners take care of ambulatory otolaryngologic problems more cost-effectively than specialists and still maintain quality of care?

The data are insufficient to say. Studies in the past have looked at specific diseases in an attempt to determine if primary care or specialty care is more cost-effective in these situations. However, until we get a better handle on how to measure general health quality, account for comorbidity, and define the outcomes, we will not have an accurate answer.

BIBLIOGRAPHY

1. Meyers A, Eiseman B: Cost Effective Otolaryngology. Philadelphia, B.C. Decker, 1990.
2. Rutkow I: The twenty most common otolaryngology procedures. Arch Otolaryngol Head Neck Surg 112:873–876, 1986.

XI. Critical Care Issues

76. FLUID AND ELECTROLYTE MANAGEMENT

Anne K. Stark, M.D.

1. Water composes what percentage of the human body?

Total body water (TBW) ranges from 50–70%. Women tend to possess a higher relative adipose content and less total body water. A kilogram of water is approximately equivalent to 1 liter. Therefore, a 70-kg man is composed of about 42 liters of water.

2. How is this water distributed?

Total body water is distributed into three functional compartments—the intracellular, extracellular, and interstitial spaces. The intracellular compartment is the largest, accounting for 30–40% of total body weight. The intravascular and plasma compartments combine to form the extracellular fraction, contributing 5%. The interstitial compartment contributes the remaining 15%.

3. What three factors should be considered when estimating fluid needs?

Therapy should be directed toward maintaining or correcting three facets of fluid needs. Maintenance therapy replaces sensible and insensible fluid losses that occur with normal body functioning. Replacement therapy is secondly aimed at correcting previous deficits such as losses associated with trauma. Finally, replacement therapy is estimated for ongoing losses associated with the underlying disease process.

4. How do you calculate maintenance fluids?

The following formula can be used in adults or children and is based on weight. This formula calculates maintenance need in ml/day.

$$0–10 \text{ kg} = 100 \text{ ml/kg}$$
$$11–20 \text{ kg} = 1000 \text{ ml} + (50 \text{ ml/kg for every kg over 10)}$$
$$> 20 \text{ kg} = 1500 \text{ ml} + (20 \text{ ml/kg for every kg over 20)}$$

For example, a 12-kg child would need a maintenance of 1000 ml + (50 ml × 2 kg) = 1100 ml/day.

Applying the **4, 2, 1 rule** is perhaps an easier way to calculate fluid requirements. This formula calculates maintenance need in ml/hr.

$$0–10 \text{ kg} = 4 \text{ ml/kg}$$
$$11–20 \text{ kg} = 40 \text{ ml} + (2 \text{ ml/kg for every kg over 10)}$$
$$> 20 \text{ kg} = 60 \text{ ml} + (1 \text{ ml/kg for every kg over 20)}$$

For example, a 70-kg man needs a maintenance of 60 ml + (1 ml × 50 kg) = 110 ml/hr.

To maintain obligatory **sodium** losses from urine, feces, and sweat, healthy adults need 1–2 mEq Na/kg/day and children need 1 mEq Na/kg/day. To maintain obligatory **potassium** losses, a healthy adult also needs 0.5–1.0 mEq K/kg/day. An appropriate maintenance regimen in a healthy adult would be 2500 ml of 0.45% NaCl with 5% dextrose and 20 mEq KCl/L. A previously healthy patient may need calcium, magnesium, phosphorus, vitamin, and protein replacement after 1 week of parenteral therapy.

5. What are colloids and when are they indicated?

Albumin and hetastarch (Hespan) are two commonly used colloids, also referred to as volume expanders. They are often used to treat previous fluid deficits. These substances have a high molecular weight and are unable to rapidly pass capillary membranes. They are, theoretically, confined to the vascular space, where they exert a high osmotic force. This pressure retains fluid in the blood vessels. Blood products can also be used as efficient colloids. Keeping in mind that all colloids are extremely expensive, they should be used only in situations where intravascular replenishment is critical. Crystalloids can also effectively increase the intravascular volume but cannot maintain the high intravascular osmotic pressure. Therefore, crystalloids require as much as four times the volume of colloids to achieve equivalent hemodynamic effects.

6. How do you administer albumin?

Albumin is usually administered in a 25% solution. For every 100 ml of 25% albumin solution, the plasma volume will expand approximately 500 ml.

7. What are the electrolyte compositions of commonly used IV fluids?

	Na^+ (mEq/L)	K^+ (mEq/L)	Cl^- (mEq/L)	HCO_3^- (mEq/L)	Ca^{2+} (mEq/L)	pH	Calories (Cal/L)
Extracellular fluid	142	4	103	27	5	7.4	—
NS	154	—	154	—	—	5.0	—
$^1/_2$ NS	77	—	77	—	—	—	—
D_5W	—	—	—	—	—	—	170
D_5NS	154	—	154	—	—	5	170
D_5W $^1/_2$ NS	77	—	77	—	—	—	170
Ringer's lactate	130	4	109	28	3	6.5	—
Hespan	154	—	154	—	—	—	—
25% albumin	130–160	0.25	130–160	—	—	—	—

NS, normal saline; D_5W, dextrose 5% in water.

8. How do you calculate plasma osmolality?

Plasma Osm = $(2 \times Na)$ + glucose/18 + BUN/2.8

9. How can you best assess of daily fluctuations in fluid status?

Changes in fluid status are best assessed through diligent input, output, and daily weight records.

10. What is the minimum acceptable urinary output in a postoperative patient?

30 ml/hr (0.5 ml/kg/hr). Lower flows suggest hypovolemia or a decrease in intravascular volume.

11. What are the most reliable clinical indicators of hypovolemia?

Tachycardia, orthostasis, decreased pulse pressure, and decreased urine output are the most sensitive and reliable clinical indicators of hypovolemia. Systolic blood pressure is a late and insensitive indicator, usually remaining stable until 20–30% of blood volume is lost.

12. Name four sources of ongoing fluid loss.

Loss of body fluid is one of the most common sources of ongoing volume deficit. Nasogastric suctioning is best replaced with D_5W $^1/_2$ NS with 20 mEq KCl/L. The potassium concentration may need to be increased if the deficit persists. Fluid deficits caused by diarrhea are replaced with Ringer's lactate with the possible addition of 10 mEq KCl/L. **Fever** significantly contributes to insensible fluid loss, causing 2–2.5 ml/kg/day loss for each degree above 37°C. Excessive fever replacement is best accomplished with D_5W ¼ NS with 5 mEq KCl/L. Other potential sources of ongoing fluid losses are **third spacing** and **burns**.

13. Describe "third spacing."

Third spacing refers to a situation in which fluid is drawn from the vascular space, accumulating in tissues and hollow visceral spaces. This sequestered fluid becomes nonfunctional, unable to participate in transport processes. Third spacing leads to a functional volume depletion. Attempts to restore the intracellular and extracellular fluid deficits only lead to further "third space" fluid accumulation. This situation is seen in surgical patients with hemorrhagic shock, ischemic injury, postoperative wounds, bowel obstruction, infection, trauma, burns, and peritonitis.

14. What is the relationship between blood glucose and serum sodium?

For each 100 mg/dl that the blood glucose level is above 100 mg/dl, the serum sodium is reduced by 1.6 mEq/L. This is a condition known as **pseudohyponatremia**.

15. What are the symptoms of severe hyponatremia? What happens if the hyponatremia is corrected too quickly?

Hyponatremia usually does not produce symptoms until the concentrations drop to 120–125 mEq/L. These levels may produce neurologic symptoms, such as confusion, lethargy, nausea, vomiting, seizures, and coma.

Overly vigorous correction of hyponatremia may lead to a situation in which the brain is surrounded by a hypertonic plasma, dehydrating surrounding tissue. This condition is known as **osmotic demyelination syndrome** or **central pontine myelinosis**. A symptomatic sodium deficit therefore should be corrected no faster than 2 mEq/L/hr and should not exceed 12 mEq/L/day. The correction maneuvers should cease if the patient becomes asymptomatic or if the serum levels reach 120–125 mEq/L.

16. What are the two most common causes of hypernatremia in the critical care setting?

In the ICU, hypernatremia is usually caused by the iatrogenic administration of salts with insufficient water. Diabetes insipidus may also lead to hypernatremia.

17. You believe that your patient has developed a hypovolemic hypernatremia. How should you correct this disturbance?

First, correct the volume status with lactated Ringer's or isotonic saline, and then correct any remaining sodium abnormality with 0.2% saline or 5% dextrose in water. You can calculate the patient's water deficit with the following formula.

$$\text{Water deficit (liters)} = 0.6 \times \text{weight (kg)} \times \left[\frac{\text{serum Na} - 140}{\text{serum Na}}\right]$$

18. Describe the EKG changes associated with hyperkalemia and hypokalemia.

The heart is the first organ to reflect changes in potassium concentration. EKGs are therefore important tools in guiding therapy. Increasing serum potassium levels will lead to peaked T waves followed by a prolonged PR interval, absent P waves, prolonged QRS-T, and finally, sine waves. Decreasing potassium levels lead to flattened T waves, followed by the appearance of U waves and, finally, depressed ST segments with flat or inverted T waves and prominent U waves.

19. How does catabolism in the postoperative period affect potassium.

In the postoperative period, catabolism often leads to an increase in the serum potassium levels. For this reason, it is important to monitor the potassium concentration carefully, ensuring that it is not iatrogenically overcorrected when calculating maintenance requirements.

BIBLIOGRAPHY

1. Bowyer MW: Fluid therapy. In Parsons PW, Weiner-Kronish JP (eds): Critical Care Secrets. Philadelphia, Hanley & Belfus, 1992, pp 24-26.
2. Bridges EW: Fluids and electrolytes in surgical patients. In Bailey BJ (eds): Head and Neck Surgery–Otolaryngology. Philadelphia, J.B. Lippincott, 1993, pp 2373–2385.
3. Humphreys MH: Fluid and electrolyte management. In Way LW (eds): Current Surgical Diagnosis and Treatment. Norwalk, CT, Appleton & Lange, 1988, pp 128–135.
4. Pemberton LB, Pemberton DK: Treatment of Water, Electrolyte, and Acid-Base Disorders in the Surgical Patient. New York, McGraw-Hill, 1994.
5. Wilson RF: Fluid and electrolyte problems. In Critical Care Manual—Applied Physiology and Principles of Therapy. Philadelphia, F.A. Davis, 1992, pp 651–714.

77. ACID-BASE DISTURBANCES

Anne K. Stark, M.D.

1. What is a respiratory acidosis? How is it diagnosed?

A respiratory acidosis is characterized by an increased blood PCO_2 in combination with a decreased blood pH. In an **acute respiratory acidosis**, carbon dioxide retention results in an increase in blood PCO_2. For each 10-mmHg rise in PCO_2, the plasma bicarbonate level increases by approximately 1 mEq/L, while the blood pH decreases by 0.08. After 2–5 days of **chronic respiratory acidosis**, renal compensation will result. The kidneys increase their hydrogen ion secretion and bicarbonate production in the distal nephron, leading to an increased plasma bicarbonate level. Subsequently, for each 10-mmHg rise in PCO_2, the plasma bicarbonate level increases by 3–4 mEq/L, while the blood pH decreases by 0.03.

2. A 63-year-old patient with subglottic cancer who has refused treatment now presents to the emergency department with extreme shortness of breath. This patient is probably experiencing what acid-base disorder?

Respiratory acidosis, due to severe chronic obstruction with inadequate ventilation. Because more carbon dioxide is produced metabolically than is excreted, hypoventilation leads to an accumulation of this product.

3. What are other common causes of respiratory acidosis?

In addition to chronic obstruction, there are many other etiologies of respiratory acidosis. The alveolar–arterial mismatch of pulmonary disease in its late stages is associated with carbon dioxide retention. A respiratory acidosis may also be the result of physical limitations, as seen in neuromuscular and thoracic cage disorders. Likewise, primary CNS dysfunction or drug-induced neurologic depression may lead to reduced ventilation and carbon dioxide retention.

Causes of Respiratory Acidosis

1. Airway obstruction
   Foreign body
   Severe bronchospasm
   Laryngospasm
2. Thoracic cage disorders
   Pneumothorax
   Flail chest
   Kyphoscoliosis

3. Defects in peripheral nervous system
   Amyotrophic lateral sclerosis
   Poliomyelitis
   Guillain-Barré syndrome
   Botulism
   Tetanus
   Organophosphate poisoning
   Spinal cord injury

(Continued on following page)

Causes of Respiratory Acidosis (Cont'd)

4. Depression of respirtory system	5. Defects in muscles of respiration
Anesthesia	Myasthenia gravis
Narcotics	Muscular dystrophy
Sedatives	Hypokalemia
Vertebral artery embolism or thrombosis	6. Failure of mechanical ventilator
Increased intracranial pressure	

Adapted from Ferry FF: Acid-base disturbances. In Ferry FF (ed): Practical Guide to the Care of the Medical Patient. St. Louis, Mosby-Year Book, 1991, pp 128–135.

4. Describe the clinical features of a respiratory acidosis.

Because cerebral blood flow is regulated by PCO_2, a respiratory acidosis may be associated with an increascd flow and CSF pressure. A patient may therefore experience symptoms of generalized CNS depression. The acidemia associated with a respiratory acidosis may also lead to cardiac disorders. The heart may display reduced output, resulting in pulmonary hypertension. Subsequently, vital organs may become critically and inadequately perfused.

5. How do you treat a respiratory acidosis?

Treatment involves identifying the underlying cause and restoring adequate ventilation. This may require relieving the obstruction, muscle dysfunction, or pulmonary status. In cases of drug-induced respiratory acidosis, the offending agent should be cleared from the patient's system. In serious cases of respiratory compromise, when the blood PCO_2 increases to 60 mmHg, assisted ventilation may be indicated. However, when a patient is placed on a ventilator, the rapid correction of a chronic respiratory acidosis can be dangerous. The previously compensated respiratory acidosis may be quickly converted into a severe metabolic alkalosis.

6. What is a respiratory alkalosis? How is it diagnosed?

This imbalance is characterized by a decreased blood PCO_2 in combination with an increased blood pH. In **acute respiratory alkalosis,** for each 10-mmHg decrease in blood PCO_2, the plasma bicarbonate level decreases by 2 mEq/L, while the blood pH increases by 0.08. Within hours, the distal nephron begins to compensate, leading to a decrease in hydrogen ion secretion and plasma bicarbonate. In **chronic respiratory alkalosis**, for each 10-mmHg decrease in blood PCO_2, the plasma bicarbonate level decreases by 5-6 mEq/L, while the blood pH increases by 0.02.

7. What are the clinical features of a respiratory alkalosis?

Respiratory alkalosis is usually associated with alkalemia and, in an acute situation, may lead to several organ system disorders. In the CNS system, the disturbance may lead to anxiety, progressing to obtundation and possibly coma. In the neuromuscular system, an acute alkalemia may produce a tetany-like syndrome. A mild alkalemia may stimulate the heart, while a severe alkalemia (pH > 7.7) will depress cardiac function.

8. What are common causes of a respiratory alkalosis?

Anxiety is the most common cause of respiratory alkalosis. Any drug that stimulates respiratory drive will also lead to this disturbance. Aspirin intoxication initially stimulates the respiratory center, leading to a respiratory alkalosis. This disturbance may be seen in combination with a metabolic acidosis from the salicylate overload itself. Any disorder associated with hypoxia or space-occupying lesion in the lungs may increase the respiratory rate, thus leading to a respiratory alkalosis. CNS lesions such as cerebrovascular accidents, tumors, infections, or trauma may also stimulate the respiratory system. Although the mechanism is unknown, early manifestations of gram-negative septicemia include respiratory stimulation leading to a respiratory alkalosis. Throughout pregnancy, ventilation is also stimulated.

Common Causes of Respiratory Alkalosis

1. Hypoxemia	4. CNS disorders
Pneumonia	Tumor cerebrovascular accident
Atelectasis	Trauma
High-altitude living	Infections
2. Drugs	5. Psychogenic hyperventilation
Salicylates	Anxiety
Xanthines	Hysteria
Progesterone	6. Gram-negative sepsis
Epinephrine	7. Hyponatremia
Thyroxine	8. Sudden recovery from metabolic acidosis
Nicotine	9. Assisted ventilation
3. Hepatic encephalopathy	10. Pregnancy

Adapted from Ferry FF: Acid-base disturbances. In Ferry FF (ed): Practical Guide to the Care of the Medical Patient. St. Louis, Mosby-Year Book, 1991, pp 128–135.

9. A 55-year-old man was previously treated for an esophageal carcinoma. He returns to your clinic with recurrence. He is cachetic, having been unable to eat for over a month. What acid-base disturbance will this man probably demonstrate?

A severe tumor obstruction of the upper digestive tract is preventing this patient from obtaining adequate nutrition. He is probably in a state of starvation, leading to a metabolic acidosis with an increased anion gap.

10. What is a metabolic acidosis? How is it diagnosed?

A metabolic acidosis characterized by a decrease in blood pH in combination with a decrease in plasma bicarbonate concentration. It may be due to a loss of bicarbonate or a gain in acid. In a pure metabolic acidosis, the PCO_2 is 1.5 times the bicarbonate concentration plus 8 mmHg ($\pm$ 2 mmHg).

11. What is meant by an anion gap and how is it calculated?

An anion gap represents the difference between the plasma cations and anions. It reflects the concentration of anions that are present in the serum but are not routinely evaluated. It is usually calculated by subtracting the chloride and bicarbonate from the sodium concentration.

$$\text{Anion gap} = [Na^+] - ([Cl^-] + [HCO_3^-])$$

This "gap" is composed of negatively charged plasma proteins and normally averages 12 ($\pm$3) mEq/L. Because of its plasma-buffering capacity, the bicarbonate concentration is reduced by titration in the presence of excess acid salts. The accompanying anion, which maintains electroneutrality in the face of the reduced bicarbonate, is not routinely measured in an electrolyte profile. With unchanged sodium and chloride concentrations, the reduced bicarbonate will lead to an increased anion "gap."

12. How do anion gap and non-anion gap metabolic acidosis differ?

An anion gap acidosis is caused by the addition of an acid to the extracellular fluid, while a non-anion gap acidosis is usually caused by loss of bicarbonate. Examples of acid addition leading to an anion gap acidosis include diabetic ketoacidosis, uremic acidosis, and lactic acidosis. Sources of bicarbonate loss leading to a non-anion gap acidosis include diarrhea and urine loss with renal tubular acidosis. Therefore, when evaluating an anion gap acidosis, one should consider possible sources of acid gain. When evaluating a non-anion gap acidosis, one should consider possible sources of bicarbonate loss.

13. Describe the clinical features of a metabolic acidosis.

The clinical features of a metabolic acidosis are usually related to the underlying condition until the acidosis becomes severe. Cardiac function may deteriorate at a pH < 7.2. Hypotension may also result, as acidosis is associated with vascular cathecholamine resistance and decreased vasoconstriction. The patient may exhibit Kussmaul's respirations as he or she increases ventilation in response to the falling serum pH.

14. Name the common causes of a metabolic acidosis with an increased anion gap.
1. Lactic acidosis (see Question 18)
2. Ketoacidosis
    Diabetes mellitus
    Ethanol intoxication
    Starvation
3. Uremia
4. Ingestion of toxins
    Paraldehyde
    Methanol
    Salicylate
    Ethylene glycol
5. High-fat diet (mild)

Adapted from Ferry FF: Acid-base disturbances. In Ferry FF (ed): Practical Guide to the Care of the Medical Patient. St. Louis, Mosby-Year Book, 1991, pp 128–135.

15. Metabolic acidosis with a normal anion gap?
1. Renal tubular acidosis
2. Intestinal loss of bicarbonate
    Diarrhea
    Pancreatic fistula
3. Carbonic anhydrase inhibitors (acetazolamide)
4. Dilutional acidosis (resulting from rapid infusion of HCO_3-free isotonic saline)
5. Ingestion of exogenous acids
    Ammonium chloride
    Methionine
    Cystine
    Calcium chloride
6. Ileostomy
7. Ureterosigmoidostomy
8. Drugs
    Amiloride
    Triamterine
    Spironolactone
    Beta-blockers

Adapted from Ferry FF: Acid-base disturbances. In Ferry FF (ed): Practical Guide to the Care of the Medical Patient. St. Louis, Mosby-Year Book, 1991, pp 128–135.

16. How is metabolic acidosis treated?
Treatment revolves around identification and correction of the underlying disorder. If the pH drops to 7.2, the situation becomes life-threatening. At this point, $NaHCO_3$ administration is advised. "Overshoot alkalosis" is a side effect of overaggressive $NaHCO_3$ therapy. Therefore, only half of the bicarbonate deficit should be corrected over 12 hours and the bicarbonate level should be corrected only to 15 mEq/L. To calculate the required amount of bicarbonate, remember that HCO_3^- occupies a space that accounts for about 50% of the body's weight. For example, the amount of HCO_3^- needed to raise the plasma level from 6 mEq to 14 mEq is 8 mEq/L $\times$ 0.5 $\times$ kg of body weight. This calculation is an approximation, necessitating repeated measurement of blood gases and electrolyte panels with therapy. Following $NaHCO_3$ therapy, hypernatremia and fluid overload may be concerns, especially in patients with renal failure or congestive heart failure.

17. What causes a decreased anion gap?
An anion gap < 12 mEq/L is also abnormal and associated with specific disorders. Unmeasured cations such as K^+, Ca^{2+}, and Mg^{2+} and the introduction of foreign cations such as lithium will decrease the anion gap. A patient may have a decreased anion gap because of a loss of unmeasured anions or a gain in unmeasured cations. Serum hypoalbumemia is an example of a loss in unmeasured anions. Plasma cell dyscrasias may increase the concentration of cationic immunoglobulins, also leading to a decreased anion gap.

18. What conditions cause lactic acidosis?

1. Tissue hypoxia
   Shock (hypovolemic, cardiogenic, endotoxic)
   Respiratory failure (asphyxia)
   Severe congestive heart failure
   Severe anemia
   Carbon monoxide or cyanide poisoning
2. Associated with systemic disorders
   Neoplastic diseases (leukemia, lymphoma)
   Liver or renal failure
   Sepsis
   Diabetes mellitus
   Seizure activity
   Abnormal intestinal flora (D-lactic acidosis)
   Alkalosis
3. Secondary to drugs or toxins
   Salicylates
   Ethanol, methanol, ethylene
   glycol
   Fructose, sorbitol
   Biguanides (phenformin)
   Isoniazid
   Streptozocin
4. Hereditary disorders
   G6PD deficiency and others

Adapted from Ferry FF: Acid-base disturbances. In Ferry FF (ed): Practical Guide to the Care of the Medical Patient. St. Louis, Mosby-Year Book, 1991, pp 128–135.

19. What is a metabolic alkalosis? How are the two types differentiated?

A metabolic alkalosis is characterized by an increased blood pH in combination with an increased plasma bicarbonate concentration. Metabolic alkalosis is divided into two types based on urinary chloride levels. In the chloride-responsive form, the urinary chloride level is < 15 mEq/L, reflecting extracellular fluid depletion. Fluid depletion due to vomiting is an example of a chloride-responsive metabolic alkalosis. In the chloride-unresponsive form, the urinary chloride level is > 15 mEq/L, reflecting *no* extracellular volume contraction. Diuretic use may lead to a chloride-unresponsive metabolic alkalosis.

20. What are common causes of a metabolic alkalosis?

The increased bicarbonate levels may originate endogenously (e.g., stomach or kidney) or exogenously (e.g., administration of bicarbonate or other alkali). A metabolic alkalosis may also originate from a loss of acid, as seen in vomiting.

Causes of Metabolic Alkalosis

1. **Chloride-responsive**
   Vomiting
   Nasogastric suction
   Diuretics
   Post-hypercapnic alkalosis
   Stool losses (laxative abuse, cystic fibrosis, villous adenoma)
   Massive blood transfusions
   Exogenous alkali administration
2. **Chloride-resistant**
   Hyperadrenocorticoid states (Cushing's syndrome, primary hyperaldosteronism, secondary mineralocorticoidism [licorice, chewing tobacco])
   Hypomagnesemia
   Hypokalemia
   Bartter's syndrome

Adapted from Ferry FF: Acid-base disturbances. In Ferry FF (ed): Practical Guide to the Care of the Medical Patient. St. Louis, Mosby-Year Book, 1991, pp 128–135.

21. Which is the most common primary acid-base disorder seen in surgical patients? What three factors usually lead to this state?

Metabolic alkalosis is the most common acid-base disturbance in surgical patients. Because of an accumulation of bicarbonate in the plasma, the hydrogen concentration is decreased. The pathogenesis involves three primary factors. Many surgical patients experience not only (1) volume depletion, but also (2) potassium depletion. It is not unusual for surgical patients to experience (3) a loss of gastric secretions which are rich in hydrochloric acid. These three factors may lead to a subsequent metabolic alkalosis.

22. How is a metabolic alkalosis treated?
    Treatment revolves around rehydration with correction of the hypokalemia. In chloride-resistant forms, the underlying etiology should be determined and corrected.

BIBLIOGRAPHY

1. Bridges EW: Fluids and electrolytes in surgical patients. In Bailey BJ (ed): Head and Neck Surgery–Otolaryngology. Philadelphia, J.B. Lippincott, 1993, pp 2373–2385.
2. Ferry FF: Acid-base disturbances. In Ferry FF (cd): Practical Guide to the Care of the Medical Patient. St. Louis, Mosby-Year Book, 1991, pp 128–135.
3. Goldfarb S, Ziyadeh FN: Renal diseases and fluid and electrolyte disorders. In Meyers AR (ed): Medicine. Philadelphia, Harwal Publishing, 1994, pp 298–304.
4. Humphreys MH: Fluid and electrolyte management. In Way LW (eds): Current Surgical Diagnosis and Treatment. Norwalk, CT, Appleton & Lange, 1988, pp 136–139.
5. Wesson DE, Prabhakar S, Zollo AJ: Acid/base and electrolyte secrets. In Zollo AJ (ed): Medical Secrets. Philadelphia, Hanley & Belfus, 1991.
6. Wilson RF: Acid-base problems. In Critical Care Manual—Applied Physiology and Principles of Therapy. Philadelphia, F.A. Davis, 1992, pp 651–714.

78. NUTRITIONAL ASSESSMENT AND THERAPY

Anne K. Stark, M.D.

1. How is nutritional status evaluated?
    Nutritional status is best evaluated with an initial history and physical exam. Muscle atrophy and edema suggest malnutrition. Anthropometric measurements, although imprecise, may be used to estimate nutritional loss. The triceps skinfold thickness estimates body fat, while the midarm muscle circumference estimates skeletal muscle mass. Indirect calorimetry is used in the critical patient to estimate caloric expenditure.

2. How is basal metabolic rate (BMR) calculated?
    The BMR is the resting energy requirement (kcal/kg/day) and can be calculated with the **Harris-Benedict equation**. This equation, based on body surface area, calculates the daily energy expenditure in healthy resting adults. This formula must be modified depending on the severity of the patient's condition. For example, in a patient with a fever, the BMR increases 13% for each °C of temperature elevation. In general, the basal caloric need for a nonstressed person at bedrest is 25–35 kcal/kg/day. Most hospitalized patients require 35–45 kcal/kg/day. Postoperative patients and those with multiple trauma, sepsis, or extensive burns have a significantly increased metabolism, requiring 50–70 kcal/kg/day.

$$\text{Women (kcal/day):} \quad 655 + (9.60 \times W) + (1.8 \times H) - (4.7 \times A)$$
$$\text{Men (kcal/day):} \quad 66 + (13.7 \times W) + (5.0 \times H) - (6.8 \times A)$$

where W is actual or usual weight (kg), H is height (cm), and A is age (years).

3. What is the daily protein requirement in a surgical patient?
    The average 70-kg man uses approximately 70 gm of **protein** per day. The surgical patient may require increased protein intake, necessitating 1.0–1.5 gm/kg/day. Increased requirements occur with

excessive gastrointestinal losses, such as diarrhea, nasogastric suction, or exudation. Skin processes such as exfoliative diseases, burns, and draining wounds may also increase protein requirements.

Nitrogen balance may be calculated with the following formula:

$$\text{Nitrogen balance (gm/d)} = \frac{\text{protein intake (gm/d)}}{6.25} - [\text{UUN (gm/d)} + 4]$$

where UUN is urine urea nitrogen.

If a patient has a negative nitrogen balance, the patient is experiencing increase protein catabolism and could benefit from nutritional therapy. Patients with renal failure or hepatic cirrhosis may have impaired nitrogen excretion or metabolism, and in these cases, protein administration should be approached carefully.

4. What is the daily fat requirement?

It is possible that caloric requirements cannot be met by protein and carbohydrate administration alone. In these cases, fat administration is indicated. Fat is administered parenterally as long-chain fatty acids, often linolenic acid (50–60%), in combination with linoleic, oleic, palmitic, and stearic acids. Fat administration is initiated at 0.5 gm/kg/day. If serum triglycerides remain at reasonable levels, and additional calories are required, this therapy may be increased 0.5 gm/kg every 1–2 days to a maximum of 2.5 gm/kg/day.

5. Define enteral nutrition.

Enteral nutrition is the administration of nutrients through the existing and functional gastrointestinal tract. This therapy may be supplemental to an oral diet, or it may fulfill all caloric, protein, and hydration requirements.

6. When is enteral nutrition indicated?

- Any patient with a functional GI tract who is unable to fulfill his or her nutritional requirements for > 4 days
- A patient who has unintentionally lost > 10% of normal body weight
- Patients suffering severe protein malnutrition (kwashiorkor) or severe protein-calorie malnutrition (marasmus)
- Some postoperative patients, malnourished cancer chemotherapy or radiation patients, trauma patients, and bone marrow transplant candidates

7. Are there potential complications to enteral nutrition?

The two main complications are **aspiration pneumonia** and **diarrhea**. To avoid aspiration, feedings may need to be changed from large-volume boluses to small-volume continuous feedings. In patients at high risk for aspiration, the feedings may be directed into the jejunum. To prevent diarrhea, hyperosmolar or bolus feedings should be avoided. Bacterial overgrowth in the solution may also lead to diarrhea.

8. A severely malnourished patient with esophageal cancer needs nutritional therapy. He is alert and cooperative. What type of therapy should you initiate?

This patient is probably unable to benefit from an oral regimen. A nasogastric tube should be placed distal to the lesion, and enteral therapy may be initiated. Alternatively, a gastric feeding tube may be placed either endoscopically or via an open approach, in anticipation of long-term enteral therapy.

9. What is parenteral nutrition?

Parental nutrition is the administration of all calories and nutrients through a peripheral or central intravenous line. Patients requiring total parental nutrition (TPN) are usually critically ill patients who are unable to fulfill caloric, protein, and hydration requirements. Patients who do not have a functional GI system are also candidates for TPN. However, if a patient has a functional gut, enteral nutrition is usually superior to TPN.

10. What should a TPN prescription include?

Daily requirements of water, calories (dextrose, lipid, etc.), protein (amino acids), vitamins, minerals, and essential fatty acids.

11. How is TPN delivered?

Central lines are superior, as they allow for the administration of a high-concentration, low-volume, 25–45% dextrose solution. **Peripheral catheters** only permit a 5–15% solution and therefore require a higher volume.

12. When is parenteral nutrition indicated?

Total parental nutrition is designed to maintain nutrient balance, restore depleted nutrients, and rest the GI tract. This therapy is often used when protein and calorie depletion is severe or when the course of the illness is predicted to deplete the nutritional status of the patient. Bowel rest with parental nutrition is often indicated in Crohn's disease, inflammatory colitis, and severe pancreatitis. When evaluating a patient for nutritional supplementation, the enteral route should always be considered initially. The parental route may increase cost and morbidity. In addition, parenteral nutrition cannot provide a diet that is as complete as enteral nutrition.

13. Which vitamin deficiency is the most commonly seen with TPN?

Because it is omitted from the daily multivitamin preparation, patients may become vitamin K deficient.

14. A critically ill patient on mechanical ventilation is receiving a parenteral formula that is approximately 50% carbohydrate and 50% lipid emulsion. Why such a high fat content?

Fat oxidation produces one-third less CO_2 than glucose oxidation. Therefore, a patient in respiratory failure would benefit from this solution because it provides adequate calorie content without producing hypercapnia.

15. What is a respiratory quotient (RQ)? How is it measured?

RQ is the ratio of carbon dioxide production to oxygen consumption. A normal RQ is between 0.8–0.9. This value may be measured in the ICU with a metabolic cart, which utilizes a closed-circuit, indirect calorimetric method. Caloric needs are subsequently based on this ratio. The RQ may be manipulated by changing carbohydrate and fat concentrations in the TPN formula.

16. Name the eight trace elements. When should they be included in the TPN prescription?

Zinc	Manganese	Iron
Copper	Chromium	Cobalt
Selenium	Iodine	

Zinc, copper, selenium, manganese, chromium, and iodine should be administered daily, although manganese and copper should be withheld in patients with liver disease. Two milligrams of iron should be administered daily. Vitamin B12 (cynanocobalamin), usually administered with the daily multivitamin, fulfills the cobalt requirement. Additional zinc (5–15 mg/day) may be indicated if the patient is experiencing excessive gastrointestinal losses.

17. Explain the other metabolic complications of TPN.

1. Acidosis is common and alkalosis is occasionally seen.

2. Hyperglycemia and hyperosmolarity may occur within the first few days of therapy. Hyperglycemia should be treated with regular insulin IM or SC, with subsequent insulin added directly into the TPN bottles. Insulin should be initiated at 5–10 U/L of 25% dextrose. A glucose of > 200 mg/dl can lead to diuresis and inhibition of WBC function.

3. Hypoglycemia may result with the abrupt cessation of TPN, especially if insulin has been supplemented. A severe hypoglycemia can be treated with 10% D/W IV. To prevent hypoglycemia, taper TPN cessation over 48 hours.

4. Electrolytes imbalances are often corrected by the addition or elimination in subsequent TPN bags.

5. An elevation of blood urea nitrogen (BUN) commonly occurs with the initiation of TPN. If the BUN increases to 75 mg/dl, then modification of the regimen is indicated.

6. If a malnourished patient is unable to increase his or her minute ventilation, TPN may cause hypercapnia. Because CO_2 production is greater with carbohydrate metabolism than with fat metabolism, carbohydrate administration should be reduced or substituted with fat.

7. Vitamin K deficiencies should be considered, as this vitamin is not included in the standard multivitamin regimen. Deficiencies should be identified and corrected in subsequent TPN bags.

8. After extensive TPN, trace minerals such as copper, manganese, iodine, molybdenum, and selenium, may become deficient.

9. Patients may experience a wide array of lipid reactions. Immediate reactions include dyspnea, cyanosis, cutaneous reactions, nausea, vomiting, flushing, fever, and dizziness. Delayed reactions include hepatomegaly, jaundice, splenomegaly, thrombocytopenia, and leukopenia.

10. TPN administration also may cause liver dysfunction, gallbladder disease, and metabolic bone disease.

18. Name the three nonmetabolic complications of TPN.

1. Placement of a central catheter may induce pneumothorax, arrhythmia, and air emboli. The subclavian, carotid, superior vena cava, and thoracic duct may be punctured with placement.

2. Venous thrombosis may be a late complication of central line placement. Low-dose heparin administration to the TPN bag may reduce this risk.

3. With TPN comes the risk of catheter infection.

19. You initiate TPN for a critically ill patient. What lab tests should be monitored and how often?

A full electrolyte panel should be drawn on initiation of TPN administration. This panel should include Na, K, Cl, HCO_3, glucose, BUN, creatinine, PO_4, Mg, albumin, calcium, liver function tests, and a complete blood count with a differential. Intake, output, and weight should be monitored daily. Electrolytes and glucose should be monitored daily for 3 days until the values stabilize. At this point, these values may be checked every 3–4 days. Albumin and liver function tests should be evaluated every 10–14 days. Trigylceride levels should be evaluated closely if lipid emulsion is being administered.

20. An ICU patient who is receiving TPN via a central venous catheter has developed a fever. How should you manage the situation?

Perform a physical exam with emphasis on isolating the etiology of the fever. This exam includes evaluation of the access site for signs of infection. Chest x-rays, peripheral blood smears, and urine cultures should also be obtained. Some recommend removing the catheter over a guidewire, culturing the catheter tip, and placing a new catheter over this guidewire. Others would suggest placing a new line. In any case, obvious purulence at the catheter site or hypotension with suspected sepsis should prompt catheter removal. A new access site should be considered at this point.

BIBLIOGRAPHY

1. Albeit JM, Way LW: Surgical metabolism and nutrition. In Way LW (ed): Current Surgical Diagnosis and Treatment. Norwalk, CT, Appleton & Lange, 1988, pp 141–145.
2. Campagna AC: Enteral nutrition in the critically ill patient. In Parsons PE, Wiener-Kronish JP (eds): Critical Care Secrets. Philadelphia, Hanley & Belfus, 1992, pp 27–30.
3. Campagna AC: Parenteral nutrition in the critically ill patient. In Parsons PE, Wiener-Kronish JP (eds): Critical Care Secrets. Philadelphia, Hanley & Belfus, 1992, pp 30–34.
4. Clouse RE: Nutritional therapy. In Dunagen WC (ed): Manual of Medical Therapeutics. Boston, Little, Brown, 1989, pp 35–51.
5. Moritz MJ: Principles of surgical physiology. In Jarrel BE, Carabasi RA (eds): Surgery. Philadelphia, Harwal Publishing, 1991, pp 3–31.

79. BLOOD PRODUCTS AND COAGULATION

Chitra Rajagopalan, M.D.

1. Which blood components are commonly available in a hospital blood bank?

Most blood banks have packed red blood cells (RBCs), fresh frozen plasma, platelets, and cryoprecipitate readily available for transfusion. Other products, such as whole blood and antithrombin III, may be available from the local blood center.

2. Define the terms "type and screen" and "type and crossmatch."

Type and screen refers to a process of determining a patient's ABO and Rh blood type and screening the patient's serum for the presence of unexpected antibodies directed against RBC antigens. **Type and crossmatch** refers to performing a type and screen *and* selecting compatible donor units by doing a major crossmatch (patient's serum and donor red cells).

3. How do you decide whether to request "type and screen" or "type and crossmatch"?

Request a **type and screen** for surgical procedures that have minimal blood loss intraoperatively, e.g., septoplasty. If you encounter an unexpected bleeding problem in the operating room, crossmatched compatible blood can be available within 10–20 minutes.

Request a **type and crossmatch** when there is a high probability of perioperative blood loss or the patient has a history of a bleeding disorder. When crossmatched blood is requested, compatible units are selected, labeled with the patient's name, and separated from the general blood bank inventory.

4. What is a maximum surgical blood order schedule (MSBOS)?

Every hospital blood bank has a list of commonly performed surgical procedures and the median numbers of units transfused for those procedures. The MSBOS is established as a collaborative document between the hospital blood bank and the surgeons, and is used routinely in determining the number of units of blood that will be required for a surgical procedure. The MSBOS are guidelines, and some patients with a history of a bleeding disorder will need additional units to be set up prior to surgery.

Surgical Procedure	Units
Branchial cleft cyst	T&S
Glossectomy	2
Laryngectomy	2
Radical neck dissection	4
Mandibulectomy	2
Ethmoidectomy	T&S
Mastoidectomy	T&S
Septoplasty/rhinoplasty	T&S
Maxillectomy	2
Tongue dissection	4
Vascular tumor resection (e.g., angiofibroma)	6
Myringotomy	—

* Units refers to the number of crossmatched units that should be requested.
  T&S = type and screen only; — = no T&S or crossmatch required.

5. When should you request autologous units for your patients?

When a patient donates a unit of blood for himself or herself, it is termed **autologous blood**. These units are reserved for the same donor/patient and are usually discarded if not used. If the patient has bacteremia or metastatic tumor, autologous blood will not be collected. The MSBOS can be used to decide which patients qualify for this procedure and on the number of autologous units that will be needed.

6. What types of autologous blood components can you request?

Autologous blood is traditionally prepared as a unit of packed RBCs. Whole blood, platelets, cryoprecipitate, or fresh frozen plasma may be ordered as special requests.

7. What is directed blood?

When a patient's family members or friends donate a unit of blood for the patient, it is termed **directed blood**. All directed blood units are subject to the same screening tests as homologous units. Directed blood collected from family members is irradiated to eliminate the risk of graft versus host disease. If the patient is not transfused with these directed units, the units can be given to another patient (unlike autologous blood units).

8. What is fibrin glue?

Fibrin glue, or fibrin adhesive, consists of two components: human fibrinogen solution and thrombin solution. The adhesive serves to provide fixation of tissues and hemostasis. To eliminate the risk of disease transmission by this product, many surgeons request autologous cryoprecipitate.

9. Which routine screening tests are performed on homologous blood donors?
1. Hepatitis B surface antigen
2. Hepatitis B core antibody
3. Screening test for syphilis (rapid plasma reagin test)
4. Hepatitis C antibody
5. HIV types 1 and 2 antibody
6. Human T-cell leukemia virus (HTLV I/II) antibody
7. Cytomegalovirus (CMV) antibody (special circumstances)

These tests are performed on every unit of homologous blood collected in the United States. Screening of donor blood for elevated levels of the liver enzyme alanine aminotransferase (ALT, or SGPT) as a surrogate test for hepatitis C is no longer a requirement.

10. What are the risks of HIV 1, HTLV 1, HBV, and HCV to patients?

In a recently published report, the risk of transmission of AIDS and hepatitis is:

HIV 1	1 in 225,000 units
HTLV 1	1 in 50,000 units
Hepatitis B	1 in 200,000 units
Hepatitis C	1 in 3,300 units

When obtaining an informed consent for a blood transfusion, the above data must be discussed with the patient.

11. How is compatibility determined for various blood components?

Whenever possible, only compatible components are issued for transfusion. The following tests are performed to determine the compatibility of the blood components.

Component	ABO Type Only	ABO and Rh Type	Crossmatch
Packed RBCs	—	Yes	Yes
Fresh frozen plasma	Yes	—	—*
Platelets	—	Yes	—*
Cryoprecipitate	Yes	—	—*

* Platelets, fresh frozen plasma, and cryoprecipitate do not require a crossmatch.

12. Which is the most common transfusion reaction?

Fortunately, the most common type of transfusion reaction is a **febrile nonhemolytic transfusion reaction**. This reaction is most often due to antibodies directed against WBC antigens. Because fever is also an early sign of a **hemolytic** transfusion reaction, it should not be ignored. After the blood bank has confirmed the compatibility status of the unit implicated in the reaction, you can resume the transfusions. The unit in question, however, is discarded after the serologic workup. It is recommended that patients with previous febrile nonhemolytic transfusion reactions be premedicated with antipyretics such as acetaminophen (*not* aspirin) 30 minutes before their transfusions and be given leukodepleted blood products.

13. How do you recognize a transfusion reaction in an anesthetized patient?

Some clues to recognizing a transfusion reaction in the OR are:
Fall in blood pressure
Pink urine
Unexplained bleeding
Oozing from IV sites
Shock
This situation is tricky, and several factors in the OR mask the detection of a transfusion reaction. Your anesthesiologist is aware of this entity and can help.

14. Your patient develops a fever during the transfusion of a unit of autologous blood. What do you consider in your differential diagnosis?

It is rare to encounter a transfusion reaction with autologous blood transfusions. However, if faced with this situation, you should consider these possibilities:
1. Bacterial contamination of the unit
    Patient with transient bacteremia during donation
    Improper storage/transportation
2. Mislabeled unit
    During collection
    On release from the blood bank
If the patient has an underlying infection or is on chemotherapy, the fever may be unrelated to the transfusion.

15. A patient in your outpatient clinic tells you that during a tooth extraction several years ago, he had extensive bleeding. What laboratory tests should you request for the initial workup?

The following tests will assist you in identifying most, but not all, hemostatic defects:
Peripheral smear
Platelet count
Prothrombin time (PT)
Activated partial thromboplastin time (aPTT)
Bleeding time
Fibrinogen level
The usefulness of the bleeding time test has been questioned by many coagulationists due to the variables associated with performing the procedure. However, it is currently the only screening test available to assess primary hemostasis.

BIBLIOGRAPHY

1. Alving BM, Weinstein MJ, Finlayson JS, et al: Fibrin sealant. Transfusion 35:783–790, 1995.
2. Dodd RY: The risk of transfusion-transmitted infection [editorial]. N Engl J Med 327:419–421, 1992
3. Gibble JW, Ness PM: Fibrin glue: The perfect operative sealant? Transfusion 30:741–747, 1990.
4. Harker LA, Slichter SJ: The bleeding time as a screening test for evaluation of platelet function. N Engl J Med 287:155–157, 1978.

5. Infectious disease testing for blood transfusions: NIH Consensus Statement, 1995 Jan 9–11. 13(1):1–27, 1995.
6. Vamvakas EC, Taswell HF: Mortality after blood transfusion. Transfus Med Rev 8:267–280, 1994.
7. Welch HG, Meehan KR, Goodnough LT: Prudent strategies for elective red cell transfusion. Ann Intern Med 116:393–402, 1992.
8. Zuck TF, Thomson RA, Schreiber GB, et al: The retrovirus epidemiology donor study (REDS): Rationale and methods. Transfusion 35:944–951, 1995.

80. WOUND HEALING AND DEHISCENCE

Cara Hyman Dawson

1. Describe the three physiologic phases of wound healing.

1. The **substrate phase** occurs during the first 4 days. This phase involves the acute inflammatory response, with neutrophils predominating in the first 24–48 hours. In the third day, the neutrophils are replaced by macrophages, which remove dead tissue and prepare the tissue for new capillary growth.

2. The **proliferative phase** occurs over the next 4–5 weeks and involves the migration of fibroblasts and capillaries into the wound. Wound strength begins to increase during this phase.

3. The **maturation phase**, the final phase, involves the maturation of collagen for increased strength.

2. How much strength can wounds regain?

Wounds reach a maximum of 80% of the strength of the original structures over many years.

3. Which is the predominant type of collagen in wounds?

Collagen is synthesized by fibroblasts. **Type III** collagen predominates in early wound healing but is replaced by **type I** collagen.

4. What agents are required for collagen synthesis?

Ferrous iron, oxygen, ascorbic acid (vitamin C), and α-keto-glutarate.

5. Describe the three types of wound closure.

• **First intention healing** (primary healing)—The edges of the wound are immediately reapproximated after injury.

• **Second intention healing** (secondary healing)—The wound edges are left unopposed, allowing the wound to heal spontaneously through production of granulation tissue, wound contraction, and epithelialization.

• **Third intention healing** (delayed primary closure)—The wound is allowed to heal spontaneously for days to weeks and is then actively closed.

6. What is granulation tissue?

Granulation tissue consists of inflammatory cells, i.e., macrophages, fibroblasts, new collagen, and new blood vessels. It is the red, granular, moist tissue that is characteristic of secondary healing.

7. How do you determine whether the wound should be closed?

All wounds contain bacteria, but several factors affect the degree of contamination of each wound, including blood supply to the wound, amount of necrotic debris, local wound care requirements, and the use of systemic or topical antibiotics. Most wounds can tolerate up to 10,000 organisms/gm of tissue and still be closed successfully. However, any wound infected with streptococci should not be closed.

8. What factors impair wound healing?

Increased age
Severe malnutrition
Poor vascularity
Anti-inflammatory drugs
Inadequate oxygen levels

9. Describe the best way to cleanse a wound to reduce the risk of infection.

All necrotic tissue must be sharply debrided. Any blood clots, debris, and foreign bodies are then removed. The wound should be maximally irrigated with a physiologic saline solution.

10. Should prophylactic antibiotics be given to every patient with a wound?

No. Antibiotics are of little benefit for clean wounds and are considered to be therapeutic in grossly contaminated wounds. Prophylactic antibiotics are most effective when they are used to prevent infection in **clean contaminated wounds**. Clean contaminated wounds occur when the wound is associated with a nonsterile body cavity, but spillage is minimal. When such a wound is anticipated, antibiotics should be given just hours before surgery or during surgery.

11. What are the clinical signs of an infected wound?

Inflammation and infection are identified by the cardinal signs of redness, heat, swelling, and pain. These are easily remembered in Latin as *rubor, calor, tumor,* and *dolor*, respectively.

12. How do you treat an infected wound?

Most importantly, infected wounds should be opened and drained. Frequent dressing changes, every 4 hours, and topical antibiotics, such as mafenide acetate or silver sulfadiazine, may help to reduce the infection.

13. What is wound dehiscence?

Wound dehiscence occurs when infection spreads throughout the layers of the wound, causing the wound to break down. This usually occurs 7–10 days postoperatively.

14. When should skin grafts be used?

Skin grafts may be used to cover large wounds that are covered by healthy granulation tissue. The graft is placed over the wound and becomes vascularized from the underlying tissue. The graft can be a **split-thickness skin graft**, which includes the epidermis and part of the dermis. Split-thickness skin grafts are more commonly used because they vascularize rapidly. A **full-thickness skin graft** includes the epidermis and all of the dermis.

15. How do a hypertrophic scar and a keloid differ?

Both are caused by excess collagen synthesis during wound repair and are more common in darker-skinned patients and young patients. **Hypertrophic scars** are confined to the wound area and usually stabilize by 3 months. **Keloids** invade adjacent normal tissue and may continue to grow even after 6 months. Keloids commonly occur on the earlobes, mandible, and anterior neck.

16. Is there any available treatment to reduce these scars?

Treatment is difficult because excised scars may recur. Steroid injections into the scar or following excision may improve the cosmetic result. Radiation therapy has also been attempted.

17. Describe the most appropriate method to repair a wound on the face.

Because the face is a non-pressure-bearing area, a wound closure strip may be used if the wound edges can be exactly approximated. If exact apposition is not possible, nonabsorbable fine (5.0 or 6.0) suture should be used and then removed in 3–5 days due to the vascular nature of the face.

BIBLIOGRAPHY

1. Gibson FB, Perkins SW: Dynamics of wound healing. In Bailey BJ (ed): Head and Neck Surgery–
   Otolaryngology. Philadelphia, J.B. Lippincott, 1993, pp 187–197.
2. Hunt TK, Mueller RV: Wound healing. In Way LW (ed): Current Surgical Diagnosis and Treatment.
   Norwalk, CT, Appleton & Lange, 1994, pp 80–93.
3. Montz MJ: Principles of surgical physiology. In Jarrell BE, Carabasi RA (eds): Surgery: The National
   Medical Series for Independent Study, 2nd ed. Philadelphia, Harwal Publishing, 1991, pp 3–30.
4. Robson MC, Raine T, Smith DJ: Wounds and wound healing. In Lawrence PF (ed): Essentials of General
   Surgery. Baltimore, Williams & Wilkins, 1992, pp 119–125.

81. TRACHEOTOMY

Anne K. Stark, M.D.

1. What are the indications for a tracheotomy?

The most critical indication for a tracheotomy is **airway obstruction**. Causes of airway obstruction include large tumors, congenital anomalies, severe maxillofacial trauma, and inflammatory swelling of the neck. A tracheotomy is also indicated if a patient is in need of long-term **ventilatory support**. Tracheotomies facilitate suctioning of excessive **airway secretions** and contribute to the **prevention of aspiration**.

2. How does a tracheotomy differ from a tracheostomy?

A tracheotomy is a temporary alternative airway, while a tracheostomy is a permanent or semipermanent tracheocutaneous fistula. In practice, the two terms are often used interchangeably.

3. How is an elective tracheotomy performed?

The first incision is made horizontally, midway between the sternal notch and cricoid cartilage. This incision is continued down through the skin, subcutaneous tissue, and platysma. At this point, the surgeon separates the sternohyoid and sternothyroid muscle pairs ("strap muscles") with a midline vertical dissection. These muscles are pulled to either side with retractors, thus revealing the isthmus of the thyroid gland. The isthmus is transected vertically, and each side is suture-ligated. A cricoid hook is placed between the cricoid cartilage and the first tracheal ring and is used to pull the trachea superiorly while the tracheal incision is placed.

4. What is the best method of entering the trachea?

Some surgeons feel that an inferior-based flap, also known as the **Björk flap**, is the safest entry. With this method, the anterior portion of either the second or third tracheal ring is sutured to the inferior skin margin. This method protects against accidental decannulation and makes reinsertion of the tube easy if accidental displacement does occur. The Björk flap poses the threat of a subsequent tracheocutaneous fistula, and therefore it should not be used in cases of temporary tracheotomy or in children. Other surgeons prefer to enter the trachea with a vertical incision, and still others prefer to remove a square centimeter section of one tracheal ring.

5. Your medical student feels that because you have created an enterocutaneous fistula with the introduction of the tracheotomy, prophylactic antibiotics are indicated. What is your response?

Experience has shown that the tracheotomy is always colonized with bacteria. The use of prophylactic antibiotics, however, will only result in colonization with resistant organisms.

6. How is a tracheotomy performed in a child?

The pediatric tracheotomy is performed in a similar fashion to the adult procedure. However, the trachea is almost always entered with a simple vertical incision into the second and third tracheal rings.

7. What are stay sutures?

Stay sutures are advised in pediatric tracheotomies. A suture is placed on either side of the vertical tracheal incision. These sutures help to reguide the tube into the trachea if it is accidentally displaced.

8. Where should an elective tracheotomy be performed?

The surgeon is often most comfortable in the setting of the operating room, where all of the instrumentation, proper lighting, and familiar nursing staff are available. The surgeon must consider the patient's status, keeping in mind the potential hazards of transport. In some cases, tracheotomies should be performed in the ICU if the room can safely and efficiently accommodate the procedure.

9. What is the significance of tube cuff pressure?

Cuff pressures should not exceed **25 mmHg**, or the approximate capillary perfusion pressure. If the cuff pressure exceeds the perfusion pressure, mucosal ischemia, followed by tracheal stenosis, may result.

10. How do you determine the proper tracheotomy tube size?

The outer diameter of the tracheotomy tube should be approximately two-thirds the diameter of the trachea at the insertion site. Although a smaller caliber tube may decrease the risk of tracheal stenosis, it may increase the risk of mucosal ischemia, as high cuff pressures are necessary to keep the tube aligned. In addition, a small tube may cause difficulties with tracheal care, airway suctioning, ventilation, and fiberoptic bronchoscopy. In contrast, tubes that are too large prevent adequate cuff inflation. This may lead to mucosal abrasion by the rigid tube. An insufficient seal poses an aspiration risk.

11. What are the intraoperative complications of a tracheotomy?

1. Violation of the cupula of the lung may result in **pneumothorax** or **pneumomediastinum**. For this reason, postoperative orders following tracheotomies must include a chest x-ray.

2. A **tracheoesophageal fistula** may result if the posterior membranous tracheal wall is lacerated. The surgeon can prevent this complication by opening the trachea against a protective cannula, such as an endotracheal tube. Should a posterior tracheal laceration occur, immediate repair is necessary to avoid mediastinitis or pneumothorax.

3. The **recurrent laryngeal nerve**, running in the tracheoesophageal groove, should not be severed with careful midline dissections.

4. Great vessels of the neck also necessitate the need for careful dissection. Reports of intraoperative **hemorrhage** range from 1–37%. Even minor bleeding may become critical if it obscures the identification of the trachea.

12. What are the early postoperative complications of a tracheotomy?

1. **Mucous plugging** is the most common complication in the early postoperative period. For this reason, meticulous tracheotomy care must begin immediately after surgery. Frequent sterile saline washes followed by suctioning often prevent most plugging problems. Humidification may also be of value.

2. **Tube displacement** may be a problem, especially in the pediatric population. The child's undeveloped soft neck tissue is at special risk in the presence of the soft pliable pediatric tube.

3. **Respiratory arrest** may result in patients who receive a tracheotomy after they have labored with partial airway obstruction for some time. Prior to the procedure, hypoxia maintains

their drive to breathe. A tracheotomy may suddenly eliminate this hypoxic drive, thus leading to the arrest.

4. A patient presenting with frothy sputum immediately following tracheotomy may be suffering from **postobstructive pulmonary edema**. This phenomenon may also occur immediately postoperatively in patients who have labored with airway obstruction for a significant time. Prior to the procedure, these patients exhibit extremely negative intrathoracic pressures during inspiration and extremely positive pressures during expiration. The introduction of the tracheotomy causes a sudden loss of these aberrant pressures, subsequently leading to an increase in venous return and thus a hydrostatic pressure gradient across the alveolar membrane.

13. And the late postoperative complications of tracheotomy?

1. **Tracheal stenosis** is the most common late complication and may occur at the level of the stoma, cuff, or tube tip.

2. Bleeding at the tracheotomy site within the first 48 hours probably originates from the incision. Patients who continue to bleed 48 hours after surgery should be evaluated for a **tracheal-innominate fistula**. This serious complication commonly occurs because the tracheotomy has been improperly placed below the third tracheal ring. At this level, the tracheotomy tip may erode the tracheal wall. Erosions from a high cuff pressure, tube torsion, and infection can also lead to fistula formation.

14. When should a fenestrated tracheotomy tube be used?

Fenestrated tracheotomy tubes promote spontaneous speech in patients who are being weaned from mechanical ventilation or are spontaneously breathing. These tubes have multiple small holes, or fenestrations, on their greater curvature. When the inner cannula is removed, patients can occlude the stomal port and speak through their native airway. In patients who are not at risk for aspiration, the cuff may be deflated to improve natural laryngeal airflow.

15. What is the role of one-way tracheotomy valves?

One way valves, such as the Passy-Muir valve, are placed on the stomal port of a fenestrated tube and are used to promote speech. These one-way valves allow the passage of air through the tracheotomy tube during inspiration, but close during expiration. They guide expiratory airflow through the fenestration and natural upper airway, thus promoting speech.

16. It is your first day of internship in the ICU. You are concerned about a patient's tracheotomy and want to discuss it with the ENT resident on call. What five things should you know before approaching the resident?

1. *What is the tracheotomy brand?* Brands vary in size, pliability, shape, and material. Residents become familiar with the specific properties and limitations of each brand. Knowing this information can help the resident give you better suggestions about the specific tracheotomy's care.

2. *Does the tracheotomy have an inner cannula?* Plugging can easily be managed if the cannula is properly cleaned. If no cannula is present, however, and the tracheotomy is plugged, the resident may need to evaluate the situation personally.

3. *Is the tracheotomy tube fenestrated?* A fenestrated tracheotomy has a hole in the tube, allowing potential communication between the upper and lower airway.

4. *Does the tracheotomy have a cuff?* Cuff status is important when evaluating leaks and aspiration risks.

5. *What is the tube size?* Narrow tubes may be troublesome when cleaning, as they tend to plug easily. The tube diameter must also be considered when evaluating airway pressures.

17. What is a tracheal button?

Tracheal buttons are used to assist in weaning from the tracheotomy tube. This plastic tube maintains the stomal patency, as its distal end opens into the anterior tracheal wall.

18. Which type of nutrition is used in a patient who has received a tracheotomy in the ICU?

The addition of a tracheotomy in a critically ill patient opens the option for oral nutrition, an option unavailable to the translaryngeally intubated patient. A tracheotomy may, however, interfere with swallowing function, and tube feedings may predispose to aspiration. With appropriate precautions, tube feeding can usually enhance alimentary nutrition and present several advantages over parental nutrition. Oral feeding is less expensive than parental nutrition. It also ameliorates the risk of central line sepsis. Tube feedings promote the intestinal mucosal barrier, protecting the patient against endogenous sepsis. Enteral feeding in the presence of a tracheotomy may be associated with several complications, however, including aspiration pneumonia, mucosal ulceration, tracheoesophageal fistula, and purulent sinusitis.

19. A patient is believed to need a tracheotomy after evaluation for obstructive sleep apnea. What type of tracheotomy is recommended?

Once a patient is thoroughly evaluated with an extensive polysomnograph, and it is believed that the occlusive problem could benefit from a tracheotomy, management is often with a fenestrated tube. During the waking hours, the tube is plugged, allowing for a functioning voice. At night, the patient unplugs the tube to facilitate respiration.

20. When should a cricothyrotomy be used?

There are three situations in which a cricothyrotomy is recommended:

1. In **emergency situations**, it is often the preferable method to secure the airway. The cricothyroid membrane is usually easily palpable at the skin surface, and very little dissection is necessary to access this portion of the airway.

2. It may also be used for **palliative treatment**. For example, a terminally ill patient may require respiratory hygiene.

3. It is indicated in the presence of **anatomic variations** that prevent the standard tracheotomy. These situations are rare.

21. When is the cricothyrotomy not recommend?

There are three situations in which the cricothyrotomy is *not* indicated:

1. Pediatric patients
2. Presence of laryngeal infection or inflammation
3. Endotracheal tube already in place for > 1 week.

22. How is a cricothyrotomy performed?

The right-handed surgeon stands on the patient's right side. The thyroid cartilage should be secured with the right hand, while the left index finger locates the cricothyroid membrane 2–3 cm below the thyroid notch. This membrane is located 1.5–2 cm below the vocal cords, averaging 10 mm in height. With the scalpel in the right hand, a quick stab is placed through the overlying skin and directly through the cricothyroid membrane. When the knife blade has pierced the membrane, the knife handle is inserted into the subglottic space and twisted vertically, thus enlarging the access for tube placement.

CONTROVERSY

23. Should a cricothyrotomy be used as a definitive long-term airway?

Some surgeons have reported favorable results, but most surgeons reserve the cricothyrotomy for emergency situations, converting the access to a standard tracheotomy if a surgical airway is to be needed for > 3–5 days. Most feel that this conversion decreases the risk of subglottic stenosis.

BIBLIOGRAPHY

1. Applebaum EL, Wenig BL: Indications for and techniques of tracheotomy. Clin Chest Med 12:545–553, 1991.
2. Carrau RL, Myers EN: Early complication of tracheotomy. Clin Chest Med 12: 589–595, 1991.
3. Esses BA, Jafek BW: Cricothyroidotomy: A decade of experience in Denver. Ann Otol Rhinol Laryngol 96:519, 1987.
4. Godwin HC: Special critical care considerations in tracheostomy management. Clin Chest Med 12:573–583, 1991.
5. Heffner JE (ed):Airway management in the critically ill patient. Clin Chest Med 12:415–630, 1991.
6. Heffner JE: Medical indications for tracheotomy. Chest 96:186–190, 1989.
7. Heffner JE: Tracheotomy. In Parsons PE, Wiener-Kronish JP (eds): Critical Care Secrets. Philadelphia, Hanley & Belfus, 1992, pp 49–52.
8. Johnson JT, Rood SR, Stool SE, et al: Tracheotomy: A Self-Instructional Package form the Committee on Continuing Education in Otolaryngology. Washington, DC, American Academy of Otolaryngology–Head and Neck Surgery Foundation, 1988.
9. Weissler MC: Tracheotomy and intubation. In Bailey BJ (ed): Head and Neck Surgery–Otolaryngology. Philadelphia, J.B. Lippincott, 1993, pp 711–724.

82. MECHANICAL VENTILATION

Michael F. Spafford, M.D., Catherine P. Winslow, M.D., and Joel H. Witter, M.D.

1. What are indications for mechanical ventilation?

Airway protection, inefficient gas exchange (hypoxia), or respiratory pump failure (hypoventilation) are all potential indicators for mechanical ventilation. Any patient with a compromised airway should be intubated. Hypoxia which is refractory to noninvasive treatments is almost always an indication for mechanical ventilation. Hypoventilation must be interpreted in light of the patient's clinical situation (i.e., in general, PCO_2 > 50 mmHg would indicate a need for ventilatory assistance, while a patient with chronic obstructive pulmonary disease may live with a PCO_2 of 80 mmHg).

2. What are the types of ventilator modes? How does one decide which is appropriate for a given patient?

Pressure-cycled: These ventilator settings deliver a pre-set pressure. The tidal volume is variable. (Tidal volume and inspiratory time are related to compliance.)

1. **Pressure-support ventilation (PSV):** This setting delivers breath to pre-set pressure, regardless of volume, and is generally supplied for 90% of the duration of the breath. Tidal volume and flow rate are not set by the ventilator. This mode is good for difficult-to-wean patients because the work of breathing is decreased. However, the pressure must be adjusted to ensure an adequate tidal volume.
2. **Pressure-control ventilation (PCV):** This setting is similar to PSV but delivers pressure throughout the entire breath. It is often used with inverse-ratio ventilation (IRV). IRV prolongs ventilatory time and minimizes alveolar collapse, but patients are at an increased risk for barotrauma.

Volume-cycled: These ventilator settings deliver a pre-set volume. The pressure is variable.

1. **Synchronized intermittent mechanical ventilation (SIMV):** The machine delivers breaths at a pre-set tidal volume and rate per minute regardless of patient effort. Nonetheless, the breaths can be synchronized with patient effort. The patient must generate his or her own tidal volume for additional breaths. This setting is good for weaning but requires more respiratory effort than assisted-controlled ventilation.

2. **Assisted-controlled ventilation (AC):** Each patient-initiated breath is "assisted" by the ventilator to the set tidal volume. In addition, the ventilator initiates "backup" or "control" breaths if the patient is breathing more slowly than the set rate. This setting is good for "resting" patients as it minimizes the work of breathing, but it is difficult to wean patients in this mode and hyperventilation is possible.

3. **How are starting parameters for the volume-controlled ventilator determined?**

Tidal volume	10–12 ml/kg (in general, about 700–900 ml for an adult)
Rate	10–15 breaths/min, dependent on mode
O$_2$ concentration (FiO$_2$)	Start at 100% and wean rapidly if able
PEEP	0–5 cm H$_2$O
Minute volume	8–10 liters/min.

4. **What are potential complications of mechanical ventilation?**

Hypoxia, severe hyperventilation or hypoventilation, infection, elevated intracranial pressure, sodium and water retention, barotrauma (such as pneumothorax), alveolar damage, decreased cardiac output, and atrophy of respiratory muscles. Also, oxygen toxicity and endotracheal tube complications may occur. Nutritional status should be monitored closely and supplemented if necessary.

5. **What type of monitoring is appropriate for patients on mechanical ventilation?**

An arterial blood gas (ABG) should be checked at regular intervals (every 15–30 minutes) and ventilator adjustments made until desired blood gas levels are reached and the patient is stable. An ABG should then be checked every morning while the patient is on the ventilator or if the clinical condition changes. Airway pressures should be monitored to prevent barotrauma. Continuous pulse oximetry should be monitored, and vital signs should be followed closely. Intake and output are monitored to prevent pulmonary edema. A chest x-ray should be obtained immediately after intubation and at least once a week thereafter. Remember that changes such as tachycardia, hypotension and agitation may be the result of improper ventilator settings.

6. **How can positive-pressure ventilation cause hypotension?**

Positive-pressure ventilation causes hypotension by decreasing cardiac output. Increased intrathoracic pressure generated by the ventilator decreases venous return, elevates pulmonary vascular resistance, and decreases ventricular compliance and filling. All of these effects can decrease cardiac output and blood pressure. Other potential causes of postintubation hypotension include vasovagal episode, barotrauma (i.e., auto-PEEP or pneumothorax), medications such as narcotics or benzodiazepines, or relief of stress with a drop in catecholamines.

7. **What is PEEP? What are the hazards of PEEP?**

PEEP is **positive end-expiratory pressure**. It can help prevent atelectasis by redistributing alveolar H$_2$O into the perivascular space. It can also be used to treat hypoxia by recruiting more lung units and decreasing intrapulmonary shunting. However, it does not decrease extravascular pulmonary H$_2$O, it can decrease cardiac output, and it can cause barotrauma (*see* Question 8).

8. **What is auto-PEEP? How is it detected?**

Auto, or intrinsic, PEEP, is positive distal airway pressure at end-exhalation in the absence of mechanically supplied pressure. It is typically found in patients with chronic obstructive pulmonary disease who require a prolonged expiratory time due to air-trapping in the distal airways. If not anticipated, this situation can cause barotrauma at normal ventilator settings. It is detected by occluding the expiratory port of the circuit at the end of expiration in a relaxed patient. The pressure in the lungs is approximately equal to that in the circuit. The level of auto-PEEP will be displayed on the circuit. Its presence may also cause the patient to have difficulty in triggering the ventilator.

9. How do you wean a patient from the ventilator?

There are several commonly used methods:

1. The patient may be weaned on IMV by simply decreasing the rate of intervals (once the patient is stable on an FiO_2 of 40% and a PEEP of 5) and monitoring the patient's tolerance. If the patient does well on a rate of 2, parameters and an ABG are evaluated.

2. A T-piece can deliver oxygen with the patient still intubated but receiving no additional mechanical support, if the patient's tolerance is questionable.

3. A pressure support wean is advocated for the difficult-to-wean patient. The pressure support is decreased at regular intervals, again closely following the patient's tolerance. The patient may be weaned for several hour intervals throughout the day, and "rested" at a higher pressure support (or AC) at night. If the patient is stable on a pressure support of < 5mmHg, he or she is probably ready to extubate.

10. What parameters predict a successful wean?

Some commonly used weaning parameters are as follows:

Tidal volume	> 5ml/kg
Respiratory rate	< 20 breaths/min
Negative inspiratory pressure (NIF)	more negative than –30 cm H_2O
Vital capacity	> 10 ml/kg
Minute volume	< 12 liters/min
FiO_2	< 40%

A ratio of respiratory frequency/tidal volume of < 100 is an excellent predictor of a successful wean. The patient should be awake and cooperative at the time of extubation.

11. What factors in mechanical ventilation affect the PO_2? The PCO_2?

The PO_2 is affected by FiO_2 and PEEP. The PCO_2 is affected by respiratory frequency and tidal volume.

12. How should you evaluate the ventilated hypoxic patient?

Clinical evaluation, including vital signs and physical exam, are mandatory. ABGs should be obtained, as well as a chest x-ray and EKG if clinically indicated. The exam should focus on ruling out pulmonary edema (fluid overload); pneumothorax, atelectasis, or pneumonia (abnormal breath sounds); mucous plug (hypercarbia); cardiovascular inadequacy (vital signs); pulmonary edema (tachycardia); or a disruption in the system (tube disconnection). The FiO_2 should be increased, and consideration should be given to increasing PEEP. Continuous pulse oximetry should be correlated to ABGs, and both should be followed closely until the patient is stable.

13. What is barotrauma? Who is at risk?

Barotrauma results from overdistension and rupture of the airways and alveoli under positive pressure. Many complications, such as subcutaneous emphysema, pneumothorax, and systemic air emboli, can ensue. If peak airway pressure is < 50 cm H_2O, the risk of barotrauma is negligible. The risk of barotrauma increases rapidly after this point, with an incidence approaching 50% at pressures > 70 mm H_2O.

14. Why are ventilated patients at an increased risk for infection?

The risk for nosocomial pneumonia may approach 5% per day in mechanically ventilated patients, although the risk appears to fall with long-term ventilation. Causes include disruption of mucociliary clearance, presence of a foreign body (the endotracheal tube), and aspiration of oropharyngeal or gastric contents.

15. What is biPAP? How may it be useful in preventing intubation?

BiPAP provides both inspiratory and expiratory positive airway pressure (PAP). It is similar to measuring PS/PEEP. The inspiratory PAP given is a function of PCO_2, and the expiratory PAP is a function of PO_2. A standard starting parameter for biPAP would be 8/4, which provides 8 cm O_2 during inspiration and 4 cm O_2 on expiration. In patients who are nose-breathers and are able to tolerate the machine, it may provide enough positive pressure to reverse borderline hypoxia.

16. Describe the pathophysiology of injury from long-term intubation.

Capillary perfusion pressure is the most important factor in intubation injury. If the pressure of the endotracheal tube is greater than mucosal capillary pressure, ischemia occurs, followed by irritation, congestion, edema, and ulceration. The mucociliary flow is interrupted, causing stasis of secretions and infection. If the tube continues to exert pressure, progressive ulceration causes perichondritis, chondritis, and then necrosis involving the cricoid cartilage and cricoarytenoid joints. The healing process then begins, as granulation tissue proliferates at the edges of the ulcer. This healing by secondary intention may continue even after removal of the endotracheal tube, resulting in deposition of new collagen. With maturation of the wound, firm scar tissue is left in the airway which contracts with time, causing such lesions as subglottic and posterior glottic stenosis.

17. How can laryngeal injury from intubation and mechanical ventilation be minimized?

The smallest tube that allows adequate ventilation should be chosen. In children, uncuffed endotracheal tubes should be used that allow a leak with 20 cm H_2O ventilation pressure. In adults, low-pressure high-volume cuffs should be used and should only contain the minimum volume needed to occlude the airway. In addition, tube motion can cause mucosal trauma. It can be minimized by adequate stabilization of the tube. Some have argued that a nasotracheal tube is better stabilized by the tissues of the nasopharynx and nose than an orotracheal tube. The ventilator tubing should be suspended to protect the patient from the shearing motion of the mechanical ventilator. Excessive patient movement and coughing can be minimized by adequate sedation and proper suctioning technique. Infection may also complicate the pathophysiology, and antibiotics may be indicated. Gastroesophageal reflux aggravates the local intubation injury and may be exacerbated by the presence of a nasogastric tube. Finally, and most importantly, limiting the duration of intubation is the most important way to minimize laryngeal injury.

18. What parts of the larynx are most at risk in long-term intubation?

Endotracheal tubes lie in and exert pressure on the posterior larynx. Most damage is expected in three sites.
1. The medial surfaces of the arytenoid cartilages, cricoarytenoid joints, and vocal processes
2. The posterior glottis and interarytenoid region
3. The inner surface of the cricoid cartilage in the subglottis

The narrowest part of the airway is also at risk. In children, the narrowest part of the airway is the subglottis at the level of the cricoid, and in adults, it is the glottis at the level of the true vocal cords.

19. Discuss the common injuries from long-term endotracheal intubation.

1. An **intubation granuloma** is a rounded, pedunculated mass arising from the vocal process and medial surface of the arytenoid, causing symptoms that range from dysphonia to airway obstruction.

2. An **interarytenoid adhesion** is a transverse fibrous bridge that tethers the vocal cords together, leaving a small posterior and larger anterior airway with partial obstruction.

3. **Posterior glottic stenosis** represents transverse scar tissue between the arytenoids at the glottic level, which may extend downward into the subglottic region.

4. **Subglottic stenosis** is a narrowing of the area below the vocal cords and above the inferior margin of the cricoid cartilage sufficient to cause respiratory compromise. Complete obstruction can occur at any of these levels.

5. **Ductal retention cysts** result from irritation and obstruction of mucous glands in the subglottic region. These can become quite large and obstructive up to months after extubation.

6. **Vocal cord paralysis**, most often unilateral, is thought to result from endotracheal tube compression of the recurrent laryngeal nerve between the arytenoid and laryngeal cartilages.

7. **Dislocation of the arytenoid cartilage**, most commonly on the left (most intubations are right-handed), may present as hoarseness and odynophagia after extubation.

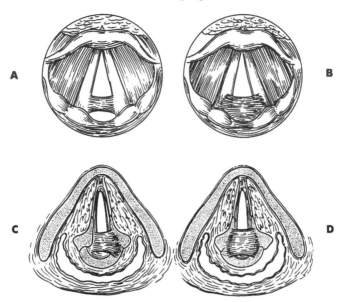

Posterior glottic stenosis. *A,* Interarytenoid adhesion with mucosally lined tract posteriorly. *B,* Posterior commissure and interarytenoid scar without mucosally lined tract posteriorly. *C,* Posterior commissure scar extending into right cricoarytenoid joint. *D,* Posterior commissure scar extending into both cricoarytenoid joints (From Cummings CW, et al (eds): Otolaryngology–Head and Neck Surgery, 2nd ed. St. Louis, Mosby-Year Book, 1993, p 1986, with permission.)

20. What is the common factor in most long-term intubation laryngeal injuries?

These complications are most commonly associated with failure to regenerate mucosa after extubation, with the persistence of granulation tissue and healing by secondary intention.

21. Which patients are most at risk for permanent laryngeal damage from intubation and mechanical ventilation?

Certain groups of patients are at risk for laryngeal damage even with a short-duration intubation:

Unconscious head-injury patients allowed to remain intubated for long periods

Children cared for in an adult setting in whom large, rubber, or cuffed tubes were used

Patients with prolonged intubation followed by tracheotomy (bacterial colonization occurs in an already-traumatized airway)

Patients with serious and/or multisystem disease with poor cardiac output or other organ failure

Infants with congenital subglottic stenosis

Low-birthweight premature infants who undergo prolonged or repeated intubation

Pediatric patients intubated for croup (acute laryngotracheitis)

Patients with injured or otherwise abnormal larynges

22. How is endotracheal tube size chosen?

The smallest tube that provides adequate ventilation should be chosen. In adults, the upper limit of size is generally 7.0–8.0 mm inside diameter in males and 6.0–7.0 mm in females. For neonates, 2.5–3.0-mm tubes are generally chosen, and 3.0–3.5-mm tubes are used for ages 3–9 months. For children 1 year of age or more, the formula [age in years + 16]/4 predicts the correct size tube in over 95% of children. In emergencies, or when history is lacking, a tube is chosen that is approximately the width of the fifth (pinkie) fingernail, a method that predicts the correct tube size in 91% of children.

CONTROVERSIES

23. How long can an adult be safely endotracheally intubated?

There is no definite safe time limit for endotracheal intubation. One study reported severe injury after 17 hours of intubation in adults. Several studies have shown that 7–10 days of intubation is acceptable, after which the incidence of laryngotracheal complications increases. Other authorities advocate intubation for no longer than 5–7 days without endoscopic evaluation of the airway.

24. How long can a child be safely endotracheally intubated?

This decision is also controversial, and the duration varies with the age of the patient. Most authorities agree that neonates with properly sized, uncuffed endotracheal tubes and skilled neonatal intensive care can be intubated for extensive periods (weeks to months) with a low incidence of complications. It is thought that the laryngeal cartilages in infants may mold and yield to pressure more than those of older children and adults. However, duration of intubation remains the chief risk factor for long-term complications.

BIBLIOGRAPHY

1. Benjamin BR: Prolonged intubation injuries of the larynx: Endoscopic diagnosis, classification, and treatment. Ann Otol Rhinol Laryngol Suppl 160:1–15, 1993.
2. Corbridge TC, Hall JB: Techniques of ventilating patients with obstructive pulmonary disease. J Crit Ill 9:1027–1036, 1994.
3. Cotton RT, Zalzal GH: Glottic and subglottic stenosis. In Cummings CW, et al (eds): Otolaryngology–Head and Neck Surgery, 2nd ed. St. Louis, Mosby-Year Book, 1993, pp 1981–2000.
4. Einarsson O, Rochester CL, Rosenbaum S: Airway management in respiratory emergencies. Clin Chest Med 15:13–34, 1994.
5. Esteban A, et. al: A comparison of four methods of weaning patients from mechanical ventilation. N Engl J Med 332:345–350, 1995.
6. Gurevitch MJ: Pressure-controlled inverse ratio ventilation: What have we learned? Chest 104:664–665, 1993.
7. Holcroft JW, Wisner DH: Shock and acute pulmonary failure in surgical patients. In Way LW (ed): Surgical Diagnosis and Treatment. East Norwalk, CT, Lange, 1994, pp 195–202.
8. King BR, Baker MD, et al: Endotracheal tube selection in children: A comparison of four different methods. Ann Emerg Med 22:530–534, 1993.
9. Rappaport SH, et al: Randomized prospective trial of pressure limited versus volume-controlled ventilation in severe respiratory failure. Crit Care Med 22:22–32, 1994.
10. Schuster DP: A physiologic approach to initiating, maintaining and withdrawing mechanical ventilatory support during acute respiratory failure. Am J Med 88:268–278, 1990.
11. Stoelting RK, Miller RD: Critical care medicine. In Stoelting RK (ed): Basics of Anesthesia. New York, Churchill Livingstone, 1989, pp 449–456.
12. Tobin MJ: Mechanical ventilation. N Engl J Med 330:1056–1060, 1994.
13. Tobin MJ, Yang K: Weaning from mechanical ventilation. Crit Care Clin 6:725–746, 1990.
14. Weissler MC: Tracheotomy and intubation. In Bailey BJ (ed): Head and Neck Surgery–Otolaryngology. Philadelphia, J.B. Lippincott, 1993.

83. CARDIOPULMONARY RESUSCITATION AND ADVANCED CARDIAC LIFE SUPPORT

Terry G. Murphy, R.N., C.C.R.N., M.S.

1. What are the common causes of cardiac arrest?

In infants and children, most cardiac arrests are preceded by respiratory compromise and hypoxia. For adults, the etiology is usually myocardial ischemia, which results in decreased contractility and electrical instability.

2. What are the ABCD's of treating a patient in cardiac arrest?

When you are first on the scene of an unconscious patient, assess responsiveness, call for assistance, and do the **primary survey**:

A—Open the **airway**, either with a head-tilt chin-lift maneuver or, if cervical spine injury is suspected, with a jaw thrust.

B—Assess **breathing**. If the patient is apneic, ventilate with an oropharyngeal airway and bag-mask apparatus.

C—Assess **circulation** and begin chest compressions if carotid artery pulse (or brachial pulse in infants) is absent.

D—**Defibrillate** appropriate patients as soon as possible. If a defibrillator is available immediately, D takes priority over ABC.

3. What is the secondary survey?

Once the primary survey is completed, ABCD stands for:

A—**Airway** management with endotracheal intubation.

B—**Breathing** assessment via verification of endotracheal tube placement.

C—**Circulation**. Continue CPR and establish IV access.

D—**Differential diagnosis**. Assess patient history and clinical presentation to identify possible causes of the arrest and reversibility of the patient's condition.

4. How does CPR differ for infants, children, and adults?

Age	Breaths/ Minute	Chest Compressions/ Minute	Compression Depth	Hand Placement
Infants < 1 yr	20	> 100	0.5–1 in	2 fingers. 1 finger-width below horizontal nipple line
Children 1–8 yrs	20	100	1–1.5 in	Heel of 1 hand. Lower half of sternum 2 finger-breadths above xiphoid
Children > 8 yrs, adults	> 8–12	80–100	1.5–2 in	Same as for children, but with 2 hands with interlocking fingers

5. What are the potential complications of CPR?

Survivors must be assessed for possible complications and treated promptly.

• Skin injury: chest burns, abrasions, contusions
• Intrathoracic trauma: rib or sternal fractures, barotrauma, pulmonary embolus, pneumothorax, hemothorax
• Cardiac trauma: tamponade, contusion, pericarditis
• Airway injury: oral trauma, tracheal trauma, aspiration
• Abdominal injury: gastric perforation, splenic or hepatic laceration

6. How can complications of CPR be prevented?

While some complications cannot be avoided, especially in a patient with brittle bones, many can be avoided with proper hand placement for chest compressions and flawless techniques. The physician in charge of managing a cardiac arrest should frequently reassess the quality of CPR, as should other members of the team. If the provider is fatigued and his or her technique is deteriorating, another team member should take over the chest compressions.

7. What is adequate CPR?

The presence of:
• Palpable femoral and carotid pulses with compressions
• Chest movement, no air leak, and bilateral breath sounds with bag-mask or endotracheal tube ventilation.
• End-tidal CO_2 >10 mmHg. This has been correlated with cardiac output, perfusion pressure, and successful outcome in experimental animal models.

8. Who should be defibrillated?

Only patients with ventricular fibrillation or pulseless ventricular tachycardia should be defibrillated. Patients with stable ventricular tachycardia should be monitored and treated pharmacologically. Patients with ventricular tachycardia and a pulse who have hypotension, chest pain, dyspnea, or other signs or symptoms of hypoperfusion should be treated emergently with synchronized cardioversion.

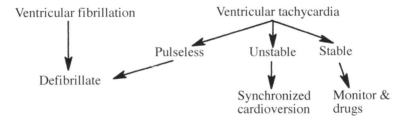

9. What is the procedure for emergent defibrillation?

  1. All defibrillation situations are emergent!
  2. Confirm dysrhythmia and pulselessness.
  3. Charge machine to 200 joules.
  4. While charging the defibrillator, apply conductive gel pads to chest at right sternal border and cardiac apex.
  5. When the defibrillator is charged, apply paddles firmly to sternum and apex over the gel pads.
  6. State firmly, "all clear," and look around to confirm team members are not touching the patient or bed.
  7. Press both paddle discharge buttons simultaneously.
  8. Recharge to 200–300 J and assess rhythm and pulse. If unchanged, defibrillate immediately.
  9. Recharge to 360 J and assess again. If unchanged, defibrillate immediately.
  10. If the rhythm at any point converts to a viable rhythm, assess pulse and blood pressure and do **not** defibrillate.

10. What are common errors in defibrillation?

  1. Waiting too long to charge the defibrillator. It takes up to 11 sec to charge the machine. If the charge is not needed, i.e ., the patient's rhythm changes, the paddles can be returned to the defibrillator holders or turned off.
  2. Improper paddle placement.

3. Insufficient paddle pressure on the chest. Less than 25 lbs of pressure per paddle results in patient burns and electrical arcing when discharged.

4. Not doing verbal and visual "all clear."

5. Having the synchronized button on for defibrillation, which results in the machine not discharging on command.

11. How does synchronized cardioversion differ from defibrillation?

Synchronized cardioversion is a timed discharge of electricity that occurs at the peak of the R wave in the ventricular complex, thus preventing the dangerous R-on-T phenomenon which can precipitate lethal ventricular dysrhythmia. In **defibrillation**, the discharge occurs as soon as the discharge buttons are depressed, and thus it is not timed with the cardiac cycle.

Synchronized cardioversion is reserved for patients with unstable tachycardia with a pulse, while defibrillation is used for patients with ventricular dysrhythmias without a pulse. Common rhythms responsive to synchronized cardioversion include unstable ventricular tachycardia, paroxysmal supraventricular tachycardia, supraventricular tachycardia with aberrancy, atrial flutter, and uncontrolled atrial fibrillation.

12. Describe the procedure of synchronized cardioversion.

1. Energy levels for supraventricular dysrhythmias begin at 50 J, with doubling of the energy level on successive attempts. For ventricular tachycardia, start with 100 J, then 200, 300, and 360 if rhythm is refractory to lower levels.

2. The patient may be conscious with unstable tachycardias. If so, consider IV sedation or anesthesia support if immediately available.

3. The defibrillator/cardioverter monitor leads must be attached to the patient and display a rhythm with prominent R waves of greater amplitude than T waves.

4. The "synch" button must be on. Assess proper function by visualizing the heavy green line "synch" markers superimposed on every R wave marching across the monitor.

5. After "all clear," keep the discharge buttons depressed until the discharge is appreciated. It may take a few seconds, unlike the immediate discharge of defibrillation.

6. The "synch" mode must be reset after each discharge. Most machines default to the unsynchronized defibrillation mode after each discharge.

13. What is asystole?

Literally, asystole is the absence of electrical activity and mechanical contraction as demonstrated by a flat line on the EKG tracing. It is confirmed by verifying the following:

1. The patient is pulseless and apneic.
2. Monitor leads are connected to the patient.
3. Asystole must be confirmed in two leads.

14. What is the differential diagnosis of asystole?

The following causes must be considered quickly:

Hypoxia
Hypokalemia
Hyperkalemia
Acidosis
Hypothermia
Drug overdose
Deterioration of another rhythm, such as ventricular fibrillation or severe bradycardia

15. When is transcutaneous pacing used in treating cardiac arrest?

Transcutaneous pacing (TCP) is considered a first-line therapy in the treatment of asystole, along with CPR, epinephrine, atropine, and treatment of specific causes. TCP should also be instituted for symptomatic bradycardiac rhythms unresponsive to IV atropine. There is no role for TCP in asymptomatic patients.

16. What is PEA?

Pulseless electrical activity (PEA) is the absence of pulse and blood pressure in a patient with a viable electrical rhythm. It was formerly known as **electromechanical dissociation**. It is a very disconcerting scenario with a very high mortality (90–100%) unless its etiology can be quickly ascertained and corrected. The differential diagnosis includes:

Cardiac tamponade	Hypoxia	Hyperkalemia
Massive pulmonary embolism	Hypovolemia	Tension pneumothorax
Acidosis	Hypothermia	Massive acute myocardial infarction

Drug overdose (tricyclic antidepressants, β-blockers, calcium channel blockers)

17. What are the signs of cardiac tamponade?

The cardinal signs are known as **Beck's triad**:
• Jugular venous distention
• Muffled heart sounds
• Hypotension

18. Describe the drug classification system for Advanced Cardiac Life Support (ACLS) as defined by the American Heart Association.

Class I	Acceptable, definitely effective, generally considered a first-line agent
Class IIa	Acceptable, probably effective
Class IIb	Acceptable, possibly effective
Class III	Not indicated, may be harmful

In this system, a drug can have different recommendations depending on the patient situation. For example, sodium bicarbonate ($NaHCO_3$) is Class I for severe hyperkalemia; Class IIa to alkalinize urine in drug overdose or to treat a known metabolic acidosis; Class IIb in a continued long arrest in an intubated patient; Class III for hypoxic acidemia.

19. Name the four most common Class I drugs in the management of cardiac arrest.

1. Oxygen for all symptomatic patients, stable and unstable
2. Epinephrine for ventricular fibrillation, asystole, and PEA
3. Atropine for symptomatic bradycardia and for asystole
4. Lidocaine for stable ventricular tachycardia and for wide QRS tachycardia of unknown origin

20. What resuscitation medications can be given down the endotracheal tube?

Think of the mnemonic **NAVEL**. Note that doses are generally 2–2.5 times those given by the IV route for adults. Be sure to dilute endotracheal drugs in 10 ml of normal saline.

N	Naloxone
A	Atropine
V	Valium
E	Epinephrine
L	Lidocaine

21. Which laboratory tests should be drawn during a prolonged cardiac arrest?

ABGs, Chem 7, magnesium, and calcium can document acidosis, hypoxemia, and electrolyte imbalance and guide treatment. The bottom line is **consider the cause**! If bleeding is suspected, a hematocrit and red-top tube for type and crossmatch should be drawn. Cardiac enzymes are not accurate in the acute phase during cardiac massage and so should be deferred until the postresuscitation phase of management, when they can be trended with serial measurements.

22. How long must a patient be resuscitated in refractory cardiac arrest?

1. Asystole most often represents a confirmation of death. If pacing, medications, and intubation do not serve to restore the patient to a viable rhythm, termination of efforts should be considered.

2. If a patient is responding to interventions, the resuscitation should continue.

3. The probability of defibrillating a patient back to a viable rhythm decreases from 2–10% with each passing minute.

4. Certain special circumstances, such as hypothermia and cold-water drowning, require prolonged resuscitation and special procedures, even in a seemingly refractory patient.

23. Must CPR be done on every hospitalized patient sustaining cardiac arrest?

CPR should not be performed if there are written orders for "do not resuscitate" (DNR) or written advance directives outlining resuscitation restrictions on the chart. If there is any doubt, a vigorous resuscitation effort must be done. There is no legal justification for a "slow code." All physicians should discuss code status with their hospitalized patients to prevent futile or inappropriate resuscitation.

24. What is the success rate of CPR?

The likelihood of survival decreases with each minute of cardiac arrest. Even the best CPR yields a cardiac output only 30% of normal. Basic CPR alone merely slows the decline of decreasing survivability. If a patient in ventricular fibrillation or ventricular tachycardia can be defibrillated immediately, as might occur in an ICU or cath lab, survival can be 70–80% or more. Generally, patients < 70 years old have a 16.2% survival until discharge, while those > 70 years old have a 12.4% chance according to one large study. If cardiac arrest occurs during an acute illness in the hospital, survival to discharge declines to 10–17%. For aged patients with chronic illness, in-hospital cardiac arrest survival rates are 0–5%. Finally, of all survivors, half sustain permanent neurologic injury.

25. What about postresuscitation management?

The most important goal in the 30 minutes following successful resuscitation is to optimize oxygenation and perfusion to limit brain injury. Specific actions include:
• Perform ABGs, chest x-ray, EKG, and cardiac enzymes
• Support blood pressure to a normal or slightly elevated level with fluids or vasopressors
• Elevate the head of the bed to promote cerebral venous drainage
• Treat dysrhythmias
• Prevent/treat fever
• Diagnose the precipitating cause of the arrest and any complications of CPR.

CONTROVERSIES

26. What is the role of high-dose epinephrine?

For: In 1992, the American Heart Association adopted for ACLS an alternative to the 1 mg IV every 5 minutes dosage in certain algorithms, and instead offered moderate or high-dose epinephrine (0.1 mg/kg IV every 3–5 minutes) as Class IIb choices. Increased survival has been demonstrated in children. Physiologically, epinephrine increases systemic vascular resistance, perfusion pressure, coronary and cerebral blood flow, and electrical activity in the myocardium.

Against: High-dose epinephrine has never statistically been shown to improve survival until discharge in adults. In patients with coronary artery disease, it may actually do more harm than good, as increases in myocardial oxygen demand are not met with supply.

27. Do alternative CPR techniques have any role?

Several new techniques—such as interposed abdominal counterpulsation (IAC) CPR, active compression/decompression (ACD) CPR, and the CPR vest—have shown improved blood pressure in small studies with improved survival at 24 hours. However, the American Heart Association has not approved these methods, and further research with larger studies is warranted.

BIBLIOGRAPHY

 1. Cummins RO (ed): Textbook of ACLS. Dallas, American Heart Association, 1994.
 2. Frank SE: High dose epinephrine in CPR: Are we missing the question? Crit Care Med 22:2030–2031, 1994.
 3. Gonzalez ER, Ornato JP: The dose of epinephrine during CPR in humans: What should it be? DICP 2(5):
    773–777, 1991.
 4. Idris AH: Reassessing the need for ventilation during CPR. Ann Emerg Med 27:569–575, 1996.
 5. Jones J, Fletter B: Complications after CPR. Am J Emerg Med 12:687–688, 1994.
 6. Murphy DJ, Burrows D, Santilli S, et al: The influence of the probability of survival on patients' prefer-
    ences regarding CPR. N Engl J Med 330:545–549, 1994.
 7. O'Neil BJ, Wilson RF: The controversies in CPR on high-dose epinephrine still continue. Crit Care Med
    22:194–195, 1994.
 8. Ornato JP, Peberdy MA: The mystery of bradyasystole during cardiac arrest. Ann Emerg Med 27:576–
    587, 1996.
 9. Sack JB, Kesselbrenner MB: Hemodynamics, survival benefits, and complications of interposed abdom-
    inal compression during CPR. Acad Emerg Med 1:490–497, 1994.
10. Sanders AB: Cardiopulmonary resuscitation. Acad Emerg Med 1:136–139, 1994.
11. Schneider AP, Nelson DJ, Brown DD: In-hospital CPR: A 30 year review. J Am Board Fam Pract 6:91–101,
    1993.
12. Sommers MS: Potential for injury: Trauma after CPR. Heart Lung 20:287–293, 1991.
13. Tuchschmidt JA, Mecher CE: Predictors of outcome from critical illness, shock, and CPR. Crit Care Clin
    10:179–195, 1994.
14. Tucker KJ, Galli F, Savitt MA, et al: Active compression-decompression resuscitation: Effect on resusci-
    tation success after in-hospital cardiac arrest. J Am Coll Cardiol 24:201–209, 1994.

84. SHOCK

Gregory J. Martin

1. Define shock.
   Shock is an acute, generalized, inadequate perfusion of critical organs. The ischemia and resultant hypoxia of shock causes cell, tissue, and organ damage and can lead to death unless it is
promptly and adequately treated.

2. What are the four categories of shock?
   1. **Hypovolemic shock**, the most common, is caused by a loss of intravascular fluid but not
necessarily total body fluid. Hemorrhagic shock is the most common subtype of hypovolemic shock.
   2. **Septic shock** develops as a result of the systemic effects of infection. Such infections are
usually bacterial or fungal.
   3. **Cardiogenic shock** is most commonly caused by reduced cardiac output, leading to inadequate oxygen delivery.
   4. **Neurogenic shock** is commonly seen in trauma and describes hypotension secondary to
CNS dysfunction.

3. List some of the causes of hypovolemic shock.
   Hemorrhage, protracted diarrhea and/or vomiting, burns, trauma, nephrotic syndrome, and
malnutrition. In burns and trauma, fluid is lost to injured tissues. In nephrotic syndrome and malnutrition, there is a loss of intravascular oncotic pressure.

4. How does the body respond to hypovolemic shock?
   Decreased intravascular fluid causes decreased venous return and, therefore, decreased cardiac output. Decreased cardiac output causes decreased systemic arterial pressure, which in turn
causes increased sympathetic output (via the carotid baroreceptor reflex). In addition to increasing

heart rate and contractility, the release of norepinepherine and epinepherine causes arteriole and venule vasoconstriction. The pituitary releases antidiuretic hormone, and the kidney, in response to inadequate perfusion, activates the renin-angiotensin axis. All of this is aimed at increasing intravascular volume and systemic arterial pressure. If the cause of the hypovolemic shock is hemorrhagic, then there will also be a decrease in hemoglobin and oxygen-carrying capacity, an increase in anaerobic activity and lactic acid, and a decrease in pH.

5. How is hypovolemic shock diagnosed?

Diagnosis of shock should be obtained by an overall assessment of tissue perfusion. Signs of hypovolemic shock include postural hypotension, cutaneous vasoconstriction, collapse of neck veins, concentrated urine, oliguria, tachycardia, tachypnea, and decreased core temperature. Patients also frequently present with nausea and vomiting. Depending on the degree of hypovolemic shock, the patient may complain of feeling cold or thirsty. With more severe hypovolemia, the patient may be restless, confused, agitated, obtunded, or even comatose.

6. Based on this information, what simple steps should be taken to help confirm hypovolemic shock?

1. *Take a blood pressure reading while the patient is supine.* If it is low or decreases by over 10 mmHg while the patient is sitting, be suspicious, especially if it remains lower for several minutes.

2. *Look at and feel the skin.* Is it cold, clammy, and/or pale? Are subcutaneous veins visible? Is capillary refill noticeably slow?

3. *Look for collapsed neck veins.* This sign will give you an idea of the central venous pressure. While the patient's head, neck, and torso are elevated at 30°, the neck veins should be distended to about 4 cm above the manubrium.

4. *Collect a urine sample.* Insert a Foley catheter if needed. Normal urine osmolality is 500–850 mosm/kg. Follow by measuring *urine output* to see if the patient is oliguric.

5. *Check the patient's pulse and respiratory rate.* With hypovolemic shock, the pulse is often weak and thready. Tachycardia and tachypnea are also common findings but are relatively nonspecific and should not be considered confirmatory in themselves.

7. Summarize the different degrees of severity of hypovolemic shock.

Clinical Classifications of Hypovolemia

SEVERITY OF HYPOVOLEMIA	DEFICIT OF BLOOD VOLUME	PATHOPHYSIOLOGY	MANIFESTATIONS
Mild	< 20%	Decreased perfusion of organs that withstand ischemia well (skin, fat, skeletal muscle, bone).	Patient complains of feeling cold. Postural changes in BP and pulse. Pale, cool, clammy skin. Flat neck veins. Concentrated urine.
Moderate	20–40%	Decreased perfusion of organs that withstand ischemia poorly (pancreas, spleen, kidneys).	Patient complains of being thirsty. Occasionally, low BP and rapid pulse in supine position. Oliguria.
Severe	> 40%	Decreased perfusion of brain and heart.	Patient is restless, agitated, confused, obtunded, or "drunk." Low BP and sometimes rapid, weak, irregular pulse. Deep breaths at rapid rate. Cardiac arrest.

Adapted from Holcroft JW, Wisner DH, Ways LW: Current Surgical Diagnosis and Treatment. Norwalk, CT, Appleton & Lange, 1994, p 187, with permission. BP = blood pressure.

8. In general, how should you go about treating hypovolemic shock?

Remember the **ABCs** of life support—**A**irway, **B**reathing, **C**irculation. With hypovolemic shock, the clinician should remember **ABCIC**—**A**irway, **B**reathing, **C**irculation, and **I**ntravenous **C**rystalloid.

9. Summarize the steps taken in ABCIC.

A   In the case of hemorrhage, especially by trauma, establish an airway if necessary.
B   If the patient is breathing well, supplemental nasal oxygen is usually sufficient.
C   External hemorrhage should be controlled.
IC An intravenous catheter should then be established for sufficient fluid access. For mild hypovolemia, use a percutaneously placed venous catheter. For more severe hypovolemia, large-bore intravenous needles placed by venous cutdown (e.g., saphenous veins) should be used. Crystalloid solution approximating the sodium concentration of plasma (e.g., lactated Ringer's injection) should be used for initial resuscitation.

10. How much crystalloid should be used?

The severity of shock should determine the rate and amount of fluid given. In severe shock, 2 liters of crystalloid should be given as quickly as possible, and a third liter should be infused over the following 10 minutes. Less severe shock requires less crystalloid.

11. Should blood or blood products be used to correct hypovolemic shock?

Usually no, unless the hypovolemic shock state is caused by hemorrhage. Even with hemorrhage, blood should be withheld until bleeding is controlled to minimize the loss of transfused blood cells. Patients who remain unstable after the initial crystalloid infusion present an exception.

12. How much blood should be given for hemorrhagic shock victims?

In young patients with normal coronary arteries, the hematocrit level should be brought into the mid 20s. In older patients, the hematocrit should be brought into the low to mid 30s, depending on their state of health.

13. What is septic shock?

Septic shock is shock that develops as a result of the systemic effects of **infection**, usually bacterial or fungal. It is the second most common type of shock in surgical patients.

14. Name the two stages of septic shock.

Early or "warm," and late or "cold."

15. Describe the clinical features in the two stages of septic shock.

In general, patients in **early, "warm" septic shock** have a low systolic blood pressure, normal pulse pressure and stroke volume, and normal to high cardiac output. They tend to be vasodilated with low systemic vascular resistance. Consequently, the skin is often warm, flushed, and dry. Often a marked tachycardia and tachypnea is present. Oxygen delivery is good, but oxygen consumption is reduced. An arterial blood gas shows a moderate respiratory alkalosis with a comparatively small change in bicarbonate.

Late, "cold" sepsis includes the impairment of organ function. Intravascular volume is depleted by increasing capillary permeability and cell dysfunction. The cardiac index (a measure of cardiac output versus body surface area) falls below normal. Bicarbonate levels decrease. Lactate levels increase, and the pH decreases. Vasoconstriction occurs in response to depleted intravascular volume, resulting in cold, clammy, and cyanotic skin. The patient often becomes lethargic and confused. Death often ensues.

16. What are the primary pathogens responsible for septic shock?

Pseudomonas aeruginosa, Klebsiella, Serratia, and *Bacteroides* are the primary pathogens. All of these are gram-negative, endotoxin-producing bacilli—hence the term **gram-negative**

endotoxic shock. Some gram-positive organisms, including pneumococci and streptococci, also have been associated with septic shock.

17. How do you treat a patient who has septic shock?

First, eradicate the pathogen with antibiotics. If an abscess or empyema is present, drain it surgically. Second, try to restore intravascular volume. Packed red cells remain in the intravascular space and increase oncotic pressure. If the cardiac index is low, inotropes may be used. Norepinepherine may be used to raise systemic vascular resistance. In addition, mechanical ventilation may also be used. Treating septic shock is a complex process, and the vast majority of patients who develop septic shock die despite the best medical management.

18. Define cardiogenic shock.

Cardiogenic shock is an underperfusion of critical organs due to pump failure. Strictly speaking, cardiogenic shock occurs when cardiac output falls to a level where cardiac index is < 1.8 (normal is 2.8–4.2).

19. How do you distinguish cardiogenic shock from congestive heart failure and other kinds of shock?

In congestive heart failure, there is normal to increased systemic arterial pressure. In cardiogenic shock, the reduction in cardiac function produces hypotension. Vasodilation in patients with septic and neurogenic shock produces warm extremities. In cardiogenic shock, systemic vascular resistance is increased, producing cool extremities. Hypovolemic shock is far more common than cardiogenic shock and is not the result of an acute, major insult to cardiac function.

20. What are the etiologies of cardiogenic shock?

Etiologies of Cardiogenic Shock

Ischemic heart disease
    Acute myocardial infarction, usually anteroseptal
    Rupture of ventricular septal defect
    Papillary muscle rupture
    Ventricular aneurysm

Valvular heart disease
    Acute mitral or aortic insufficiency
    Severe aortic stenosis

Arrhythmias
    Supraventricular
    Ventricular

Trauma
    Tension pneumothorax
    Pericardial tamponade, may include nontraumatic causes
    Cardiac contusion

From Lawrence PF: Essentials of General Surgery, 2nd ed. Baltimore, Williams & Wilkins, 1992, p 1; with permission.

21. What is the main goal in the treatment of cardiogenic shock?

To improve cardiac function without significantly increasing the metabolic demands on the heart.

22. Describe some of the defining characteristics of neurogenic shock.

Neurogenic shock is defined as hypotension secondary to CNS dysfunction. This type of shock most commonly results from trauma. Cardiac output and oxygen delivery are normal or possibly elevated. Often, there is a disruption of the sympathetic nervous system. Acid-base status, renal function indices, and hemoglobin levels are usually unaffected.

23. How does the prognosis differ for the various categories of shock?
The prognosis varies depending on the type of shock, its duration, and the age and health of the individual. For example, 80% of young healthy individuals with **hypovolemic shock** survive with appropriate medical treatment. However, even with the best medical care, both **cardiogenic shock** from extensive myocardial infarction and gram-negative **septic shock** have mortality rates of 70–80%. Prognosis for **neurogenic shock** depends on the severity of the trauma.

24. Outline the common signs and symptoms that help to distinguish the four categories of shock.

A Comparison of the Common Clinical Manifestations in the Different Categories of Shock

	HYPOVOLEMIC	SEPTIC	CARDIOGENIC	NEUROGENIC
Vascular resistance	↑	↓ (early) ↑ (late)	↑	↓
Heart rate	↑	↑	↑	↓
Respiratory rate	↑	↑	↑	↓ (variable)
Skin changes	Cold, clammy	Warm (flushed early) Cold (clammy late)	Cold, clammy	Warm
Neck veins	Flat	Flat (late)	Distended	Flat
Acidosis/alkalosis	Metabolic acidosis	Respiratory alkalosis (early) Metabolic alkalosis (late)	Metabolic acidosis	Metabolic acidosis
Cardiac index	↓	Normal to ↑ (early) ↓ (late)	↓	↓

25. A 60-year-old woman underwent endoscopic and open surgery for chronic sinusitis. Postoperatively she was placed on cephalexin and prednisone, and packing was removed on postop day 5, with no evidence of infection at time of surgical debridement. Three weeks later, the patient returned with a sudden onset of sore throat, fever, vomiting, and abdominal rash. She experienced a syncopal episode in the emergency department. After hospital admission for possible sepsis, CT scan revealed clouding of the sinuses. Sinus cultures grew *Staphylococcus aureus*. What is the diagnosis?
Toxic shock syndrome. Toxic shock has been reported after several cases of nasal or sinus surgery. The normal nose is often colonized with *S. aureus*. With surgery, the bacteria have access to traumatized mucosa. Bacterial growth is then supported by postoperative packing, which establishes a closed environment in which toxins may accumulate.

Toxic shock is a potentially life-threatening syndrome caused by the toxins of *S. aureus*. A fatality rate as high as 10% has been reported. Toxic shock syndrome has four major disease characteristics:

1. Fever > 38.9°C (102°F)
2. Diffuse macular rash
3. Skin desquamation of the palms and soles occurring 1–2 weeks after the onset of illness
4. Hypotension

CONTROVERSIES

26. What fluids should be administered when resuscitating a shock victim?
The primary noncontroversial treatment for shock includes oxygen, adequate venous access for fluids, and appropriate emergency stabilizing procedures. However, some disagree in what

fluids should be used for resuscitation of shock victims. For example, some still consider albumin-containing solutions (other than blood) to be good volume-expanders for hypovolemic shock. However, today, it is generally accepted that albumin solutions do not retain fluids in the vascular space during shock. With the amount of vasodilation and vascular permeability associated with endotoxic shock, the effectiveness of colloids such as dextran and hetastarch has been questioned. Generally, crystalloid is preferred to raise intravascular volume. The one colloid exception is red cells, which are large enough to remain in the intravascular space. In addition, red cells increase the amount of hemoglobin available.

27. Name some controversial drugs which are utilized in shock management.
    The variety of drugs available for the treatment of shock includes inotropes, vasodilators, antibiotics, diuretics, and chronotropic agents. Each drug has beneficial effects and side effects. For example, inotropes, such as dopamine and dobutamine, can be effective when used in cardiogenic shock, as they increase cardiac output. However, these inotropes also place mechanical strain on the heart, increase vasoconstriction, and can increase heart rate sharply. Therefore, it is generally recommended that these inotropes be given only to closely monitored ICU patients and that these drugs be used cautiously and in small doses. Norepinepherine, a vasoconstrictor and an inotrope, can be used in the late stage of septic shock to raise blood pressure and systemic vascular resistance. However, the added increase in vascular resistance can result in necrosis of the ears and fingertips.

BIBLIOGRAPHY

1. Holcroft JW, Wisner DH, Ways LW: Current Surgical Diagnosis and Treatment. Norwalk, CT, Appleton & Lange, 1994.
2. Johnson LE: Edema, Congestion, and Shock [Videodisc]. Washington, DC, National Library of Medicine, 1988.
3. Kumar V, Cotran RS, Robbins SL: Basic Pathology. Philadelphia, W.B. Saunders, 1992.
4. Lawrence PF: Essentials of General Surgery, 2nd ed. New York, Williams & Wilkins, 1992.
5. Merli GJ, Weitz HH: Medical Management of the Surgical Patient. Philadelphia, W.B. Saunders, 1992.
6. Miller W, Stankiewicz JA: Delayed toxic shock syndrome in sinus surgery. Otolaryngol Head Neck Surg 111(1):121–123, 1994.
7. Wotkyns RS: Shock. In Abernathy C (ed): Surgical Secrets. Philadelphia, Hanley & Belfus, 1986, pp 22–26.

85. FEVER IN THE CRITICAL CARE PATIENT

John W. Hollingsworth, M.D.

1. Why are we concerned with fever?
    Fever is a common complaint of patients who are seeking medical care. The causes of fever are extensive and can range from a simple problem requiring reassurance to a problem necessitating ICU admission. Fever occurs in 29–36% of medical inpatients. Medical inpatients who develop fever have a 13% mortality rate, while those who remain afebrile have a 3% mortality rate.

2. How is fever defined?
    Fever is a symptom. A "set-point" increase in the hypothalamic thermoregulatory center causes an elevation of the body temperature above the normal circadian variation. Elevated temperature accompanies many illnesses and is a valuable marker of disease activity. Normal body temperature is 37°C (98.6°F) and has a normal circadian variation of 0.5–1.0°C with the peak in the late afternoon. Quantitatively, fever is a temperature > 37.8°C (100°F) orally or 38.2°C (100.8°F) rectally. In humans, fever does not usually exceed 41.1°C.

Fever must be distinguished from **hyperthermia**, an elevation in temperature that is not associated with a change in the hypothalamic thermoregulatory "set-point." Hyperthermia, which potentially has a higher risk of mortality, must be treated more aggressively.

3. What are some causes of hyperthermia?

Hyperthermia may be due to an **increased heat production**, as seen in exercise-induced hyperthermia, thyrotoxicosis, malignant hyperthermia, pheochromocytoma, and neuroleptic malignant syndrome. It may also be due to a **decreased heat loss**, as seen with heat stroke, drug-induced fever, autonomic dysfunction, dehydration, occlusive dressing, and excessive clothing. **Hypothalamic disorders**, such as infections (granulomatous disease), tumors, trauma, vascular accidents, and drug-induced disorders (i.e., phenothiazine toxicity), may also result in hyperthermia.

4. What subjective symptoms are associated with fever?

Myalgia	Anorexia	Somnolence	Piloerection
Arthralgia	Low back pain	Chills	Sweats

5. How does your body control thermoregulation and cause fever?

Endogenous pyrogens (EP) are produced, released into the circulation, reach the anterior hypothalamus via the arterial system, and penetrate the blood-brain barrier in the region of the organum vasculosum laminae terminalis. This penetration stimulates the release of arachidonic acid from the endothelial lining of this specialized cluster of neurons. The arachidonic acid is rapidly metabolized into prostaglandin E_2. Prostaglandin modulates the hypothalamic thermoregulatory centers by increasing cAMP levels, which subsequently increase the normal thermic set-point. Mediated by sympathetic efferents, this alteration induces peripheral vasoconstriction, shivering, and behavioral changes such as posturing and seeking warm environments. Continuing until the warmer blood reaches the hypothalamus and matches the new set-point, this process will continue until the concentration of EP falls or EP-induced prostaglandin synthesis is blocked by antipyretics.

6. What are the differences between exogenous and endogenous pyrogens?

Pyrogens are substances that cause fever. **Exogenous pyrogens** are microbes, microbial products, or toxins. Gram-negative bacteria have lipopolysaccharide endotoxins in their outer membrane, while gram-positive bacteria have lipoteichoic acid, peptidoglycans, various exotoxins, and enterotoxins which induce fever. Exogenous pyrogens cause fever by inducing the release of endogenous pyrogens. **Endogenous pyrogens** include interleukin-1, tumor necrosis factor, interleukin-6, and interferon-alpha (i.e., cytokines). They are produced by many cells and typically act locally, initiating autocrine and paracrine effects.

7. What are the protective mechanisms of fever?

Despite extensive study into the pathophysiology of fever, it remains unclear whether fever is a defense mechanism that enhances survival or a harmful response that accompanies injury or stress. The beneficial role of fever during infection has not been established but is strongly speculated. There are three basic protective mechanisms of fever. (1) The growth and virulence of several bacteria species are impaired by increases in temperature (e.g., pneumococcus), while other organisms cannot survive with fever (e.g., gonococcus). (2) Fever causes increased phagocytic and bactericidal polymorphonuclear leukocyte activity and increased cytotoxic lymphocytic activity. (3) Because of the inhibition of RNA, DNA, and protein synthesis, fever has adverse effects on many types of tumor cells. Although no human clinical studies support the benefit of fever, strong speculation about the beneficial effects of fever exist. Therefore, a fever should not be routinely suppressed.

8. How does fever affect the body?

Besides the protective mechanisms, fever increases metabolism. Each 1°C increase results in a 10-13% increase in oxygen consumption. Increased metabolic demands may place a burden on the cardiovascular system, precipitating **cardiac failure** or **ischemia**. Increased muscle catabolism can lead to a **negative nitrogen balance** and **loss of body weight**. There is a 10–15% increase in **insensible water loss** for each 1°C elevation (8% per °F). This loss often requires an additional 500 ml or more of salt-free water per day in febrile patients. **Caloric requirements** are increased in a febrile patient. Fever can decrease **mental acuity**, leading to delirium and stupor. Some febrile children are prone to **seizures**.

9. When do you treat a fever?

Treatment should be reserved for patients in extreme discomfort or patients at high risk. High-risk patients include children at risk of febrile seizures, pregnant women, patients with cardiac or pulmonary insufficiency, and patients with impaired cerebral function. Although they can improve patient comfort, antipyretics are often used without a therapeutic rationale. Hyperpyrexia (fever ≥ 41.0°C) is clearly an exception, as both antipyretics and physical cooling are necessary.

10. What do you use to treat a fever?

Antipyretics include nonsteroidal anti-inflammatory drugs (NSAIDs), acetaminophen, and glucocorticoids. There are also some endogenous antipyretics, including arginine vasopressin, adrenocorticotropin, α-melanocyte-stimulating hormone, and cortisol-releasing hormone. **NSAIDs** are antipyretic, analgesic, and anti-inflammatory. They act both centrally and peripherally by inhibiting cyclooxygenase (prostaglandin synthetase). Side effects include GI irritation, reversible inhibition of platelet aggregation, transaminase elevations, and potential renal toxicity. **Aspirin** causes irreversible inhibition of platelet aggregation and should be avoided in children because of the risk of Reye's syndrome. **Acetaminophen** acts centrally as an antipyretic and is also an analgesic. It is potentially hepatotoxic and should be used carefully in patients with hepatic insufficiency. **Glucocorticoids** are potent antipyretics with potent immunosuppressive and antiphagocytic effects. This limits their use to febrile states in which inflammation is the major pathogenic factor (e.g., bacterial meningitis, tuberculosis, pericarditis, vasculitis).

11. How do you treat hyperthermia?

Once again, we must distinguish fever from hyperthermia. If the patient has hyperthermia, or an increase in core temperature without an increase in the hypothalamic set-point, treatment is definitely indicated. Heat stroke and malignant hyperthermia are medical emergencies. Treatment with conventional antipyretics (aspirin, NSAIDs, steroids) is *not* effective, and hyperthermia must be treated by other means. Hypothermic (cooling) blankets, though requiring careful monitoring, may be helpful. However, they should be discontinued when the temperature drops below 39.0°C. Ice baths are reserved for extreme cases of hyperthermia.

12. How do you begin an evaluation of fever in the ICU?

The evaluation of the febrile ICU patient requires a meticulous and thoughtful approach to ensure that the cause of the fever is identified accurately and treated appropriately. The causes of fever can be broadly divided into two categories, **infectious** and **noninfectious**. One must elicit a thorough history and perform a complete physical exam. Initial investigation should be directed toward finding an infectious etiology. Laboratory studies may include a complete blood count with differential, blood cultures, sputum cultures, sputum KOH and Gram stain, urinalysis, blood chemistries, and antibody titers. Pertinent radiologic studies may include chest x-ray, CT, ultrasound, or indium scan. Other diagnostic procedures include endotracheal aspirate, bronchoalveolar lavage, bronchoscopy, and biopsy. A haphazard approach to the febrile patient in the ICU is very inefficient and expensive. Diagnostic modalities should be chosen according to each individual patient. If no source of infection can be found, the possibility of noninfectious causes of fever should be considered.

13. List the noninfectious causes of fever. Which are the most common?

The most common causes of noninfectious fever are neoplasias, CNS disease, myocardial infarction, drug reactions, procedures, and alcohol withdrawal.

Noninfectious Causes of Fever in the ICU

Neoplasia	Metabolic/endocrine	Gastrointestinal
CNS	Drug withdrawal	Pancreatitis
Hemorrhage	Hyperthyroidism	Cholecystitis
Nonhemorrhagic infarct	Adrenal insufficiency	Inflammatory bowel disease
Seizures	Heat stroke	Ischemic colitis
Cardiovascular	Malignant hyperthermia	Nonviral hepatitis
Myocardial infarction	**Hematologic**	**Inflammatory**
Dressler's syndrome	Deep venous thrombosis	Collagen vascular disease
Dissecting aortic aneurysm	Pulmonary embolism	Intramuscular injections
Pericarditis	Hemorrhage (GI, retroperi-	Vasculitis
Miscellaneous	toneal)	Gout/pseudogout
Drug fever	Sickle cell disease	**Other**
Procedure-related		Postoperative
Atelectasis		Intramuscular injections
Burns		

14. Which drugs can cause fever?

Drug fever, largely a diagnosis of exclusion, is relatively uncommon. Drugs have been documented to be the cause of 2–6% of fevers on internal medicine services. Drug fever is most likely an immunologic phenomenon in which the formation of immune complexes is thought to stimulate the release of endogenous pyrogen. Antibiotics, particularly β-lactams, are the class of drugs most commonly associated with fever. α-Methyldopa, quinidine, procainamide, and diphenylhydantoin are also commonly implicated.

15. Can hemorrhage cause fever?

Yes, fever can occur as the result of hemorrhage. CNS hemorrhage, in particular subarachnoid hemorrhage, can occur as a result of a variety of disease processes and is a potentially unrecognized source of fever.

16. Do procedures cause fever in the absence of infection?

Yes. Repeated intramuscular injections can cause fever. This is especially important to remember in the ICU setting, where patients undergo many different procedures. Bronchoscopy with transbronchial needle aspiration also has been shown to cause fever in the absence of infection.

17. What is the most common etiology of fever?

Infection is probably the most common cause of fever. There are four major sites of nosocomial infections. In order of frequency, these infections include urinary tract infections, surgical wound infections, pneumonia, and bacteremia. Many factors influence the risk of nosocomial infection in ICU patients, including underlying diseases, severity of illness, type of ICU, duration of ICU stay, and use of invasive devices and procedures.

Infectious Causes of Fever

Respiratory	Cardiovascular	Gastrointestinal
Pneumonia	Endocarditis	Viral hepatitis
Empyema	Pacemaker infection	Colitis due to drugs
Sinusitis	Infection of intravascular devices	Biliary infection
Tracheobronchitis	Local infections	Abdominal abscess
Miscellaneous	Catheter-related sepsis	Diverticulitis
Sepsis	**Procedure-related**	**Renal**
Meningitis	Wound infection	Urinary tract infection
Septic arthritis	**Skin infections**	Pyelonephritis
	Cellulitis	
	Decubitus ulcer	

18. On postop day 3 after a modified radical neck dissection, a 62-year-old man develops a new-onset fever to 38.8°C. He looks diaphoretic and pale but is alert. A nasogastric tube and ventilator are in place, and a Foley catheter and IV line are in place without signs of infection. The neck incisions have mild serosanguineous drainage without swelling, warmth, or tenderness. Chest exam reveals diffuse crackles and decreased breath sounds with dullness to percussion over the right lower lobe. Over the past 24 hours, the settings on the ventilator have been changed several times. What is the etiology of this patient's fever?

Ventilator-associated pneumonia is the most likely diagnosis. This diagnosis refers to a bacterial pneumonia developing in patients with acute respiratory failure who have received mechanical ventilation for at least 48 hours. The diagnosis is strongly suggested by fever, changes on physical exam and chest radiographs, leukocytosis, purulent tracheobronchial secretions, and positive tracheal aspirate on Gram stain and culture. Definitive diagnosis revolves around invasive tests, such as bronchoalveolar lavage, protected specimen brush, or bronchoscopy. *Streptococcus pneumoniae* is the most likely pathogen in this patient because a lobar pneumonia is present. Nosocomial pneumonias most commonly affect the right lower lobe. *Pseudomonas aeruginosa* is common in ventilator-associated pneumonia and should be considered; it is usually a bilateral bronchopneumonia, but lobar consolidation is occasionally seen.

19. Can intravascular lines cause fever?

Intravascular devices are well-documented causes of sepsis, and therefore attention should be focused on the presence of phlebitis and infection of IV lines. Risk factors for such infections include the degree of asepsis when the IV was inserted, endothelial damage produced during insertion of large-bore needles, and length of time the line is left in place. Nosocomial septicemia in patients with intravascular devices is usually caused by *Staphylococcus aureus*, coagulase-negative *Staphylococcus*, aerobic gram-negative bacilli, or enterococci. Diagnosis should be based on clinical suspicion with multiple blood cultures and catheter culture for confirmation.

20. What are the most common causes of postoperative fever? When would you expect each to occur?

To remember the most common causes of postoperative fever, think of the **5 Ws**:

Wind—pulmonary atelectasis. This condition usually accounts for fever within the first 48 hours postoperatively. Important exceptions include soft tissue infection, leakage of bowel anastomosis, and aspiration pneumonia.

Water—urinary tract infections. UTIs are highly suspected on postop day 2–3.

Wound—an incision infection, commonly occurring around postop day 3–5. Inspect and palpate the wound edges for evidence of inflammation or drainage. Culture any drainage. Treatment includes facilitating drainage, surgical debridement, and antibiotics.

Walk—deep venous thrombosis (DVT) or intravascular lines. Fever associated with infection of intravascular devices should be suspected around postop day 3–4. Inspect for thrombophlebitis and suppurative phlebitis. *Staphylococcus aureus* or *S. epidermidis* are the most common pathogens. Fever secondary to DVT or pulmonary embolism should be considered around postop day 7–10 but can occur anytime.

Wonder drugs—drug-induced fever. These can cause fever at anytime and are usually a diagnosis of exclusion.

21. What is an FUO?

Classically, **fever of unknown origin** (FUO) is defined as a documented fever > 38.3°C (101°F) that lasts 3 weeks and defies diagnosis after intensive medical investigation. Recently, however, this definition has been challenged with the advent of nosocomial FUO, neutropenic FUO, and AIDS FUO.

22. List the most common etiologies of FUO.

Infectious (39%)   **Neoplastic** (17%)   **Miscellaneous** (16%)
   Endocarditis   Lymphoma/leukemia   Pulmonary embolus
   Abdominal abscess   Carcinoma   Sarcoidosis
   Hepatobiliary   Miscellaneous   Hypersensitivity
   Mycobacterial
   Brucellosis   **Collagen/vascular** (18%)
   Bone/joint   Systemic lupus erythematous
   Meningitis, bacterial   Rheumatoid arthritis
   Viral disease   Miscellaneous
   Miscellaneous

CONTROVERSY

23. Can atelectasis cause postoperative fever?

Almost every surgical textbook states that atelectasis is the most common cause of postoperative fever in the first 48 hours, but many physicians challenge this theory. Because pulmonary atelectasis is common postoperatively, physicians may assume that fever is the result of atelectasis, but unfortunately, no data support that theory. In fact, there is evidence that fever occurring in patients with atelectasis indicates concurrent pulmonary infection. Two groups of investigators induced atelectasis in animals, and neither group was able to demonstrate the occurrence of fever with atelectasis unless there was coexisting pulmonary infection. Two more recent prospective clinical studies have also weakened the link between atelectasis and postop fever. The first study included 100 patients scheduled for elective abdominal surgery: 31% developed atelectasis, and 18% developed fever. Of those who had a fever, 4 patients had atelectasis and 14 did not. There was no significant association between atelectasis and fever. Another recent study looked at 100 postop cardiac surgery patients. In this group, the daily incidence of atelectasis increased from 43 to 69 to 79%. However, the incidence of fever (> 38.0°C) fell from 37 to 21 to 17%. When fever was defined as temperature $\geq$ 38.5°C, the daily incidence fell from 14 to 3 to 1%. Using chi-squared analysis, no association could be found between fever and the amount of atelectasis. These studies contradict common textbook dogma.

ACKNOWLEDGMENT

Special thanks to faculty at University of Texas Medical Branch in Galveston, including B. Baily, M.D. (Chair, Department of Otolaryngology) and M. Boyars, M.D. (Department of Pulmonary Medicine), for review of this chapter prior to submission.

BIBLIOGRAPHY

1. Bailey BJ (ed): Head and Neck Surgery–Otolaryngology. Philadelphia, J.B. Lippincott, 1993.
2. Berkow R: The Merck Manual, 16th ed. Rahway, NJ, Merck Research Laboratories, 1992.
3. Beckman CRB: Obstetrics and Gynecology. Baltimore, Williams & Wilkins, 1992, pp 211–215.
4. Borman KE: Occult fever in surgical intensive care unit patients is seldom caused by sinusitis. Am J Surg 164:412–416, 1992.
5. Clarke DE, Kimelman J, Raffin TA: The evaluation of fever in the intensive care unit. Chest 100: 213–220, 1991.
6. Durack DT: Fever of unknown origin—reexamined and redefined. Curr Clin Topics Infect Dis 11:35–51, 1991.
7. Engoren M: Lack of association between atelectasis and fever. Chest 107:81–84, 1995.
8. George DL: Epidemiology of nosocomial pneumonia in the ICU patient. Clin Chest Med 16:29–44, 1995.
9. Isaac B, et al: Unexplained Fever. Boca Raton, FL, CRC Press, 1991.
10. Isselbacher AB, et al (eds): Harrison's Principles of Internal Medicine, 13th ed. New York, McGraw-Hill, 1994.
11. Jarvis WR, et al: Nosocomial infection rates in adult and pediatric intensive care units in the U.S. National Nosocomial Infection Surveillance System. Am J Med 91(3B):185S–191S, 1991.
12. Kelly W: Essentials of Internal Medicine. Philadelphia, J.B. Lippincott, 1994.

13. Koutlas T, et al: The Mont Reid Surgical Handbook, 3rd ed. St. Louis, Mosby, 1994. pp 124–125.
14. Lawrence PF: Essentials of General Surgery, 2nd ed. Baltimore, Williams & Wilkins, 1992.
15. Mackowiak PA: Fever—Basic Mechanisms and Management. New York, Raven Press, 1991.
16. Mackowiak PA, LeMaistre CF: Drug fever: A critical appraisal of conventional concepts. Ann Intern Med 106:728–733, 1987.
17. Meduri GU: Diagnosis and differential diagnosis of ventilator associated pneumonia. Clin Chest Med 16:61–93, 1995.
18. Nelson S, et al: Pathophysiology of pneumonia. Clin Chest Med 16(1):1–12, 1995.
19. Perez-Aispuro I, et al: A reconsideration of postoperative fever due to pulmonary atelectasis. Gac Med Mex 127:27–30, 1991.
20. Schonbaum E, et. al: International Encyclopedia of Pharmacology and Therapeutics: Sect. 132. Thermo-regulation: Pathology, Pharmacology, and Therapy. New York, Pergamon Press, 1991.
21. Semel JD: Fever associated with repeated intramuscular injections of analgesics. Rev Infect Dis 8:68–72,1986.
22. Witte MC, et al: Incidence of fever and bacteremia following transbronchial needle aspiration. Chest 89:85–87, 1986.

XII. Conclusion

86. MINUTIAE IN OTOLARYNGOLOGY
(Things You Shouldn't Really Be Expected to Know, But Will Really Impress the Attending on Rounds or in Conferences)

Bruce W. Jafek, M.D., and Anne K. Stark, M.D.

1. How did otolaryngology originate?

The specialty of otolaryngology is a product of the 20th century amalgamation of two specialties having quite different origins, otology and laryngology. Otologists ("aurists") trace their origins to the mid-19th century efforts of Toynbee, Wilde, von Tröltsch, and Politzer. Laryngology had a more specific birthdate, September 1854, when Manuel Garcia first visualized the human larynx with a mirror. Türck and Czermak popularized the new discipline of laryngology. As laryngologists herniated upward into the airway via the larynx, and otologists probed deeper into the ear via the eustachian tube, the two disciplines met a unifying organ, the nose, and the specialty of otorhinolaryngology, shortened by some to otolaryngology, was born.

2. Where was the first chair of otology located?

The first chair of otology was created at the University at Vienna, and the first otology clinic was also founded there in 1873. Billroth, the great general surgeon, supported the creation of the chair noting, "It is desirable to give this small and yet not unimportant subject a place in the curriculum of the universities." Billroth characterized otology as a "difficult and thankless" discipline. Josef Gruber and Adam Politzer were codirectors.

3. Where was the first chair of laryngology located?

Vienna, also.

4. Was the first laryngology clinic in Vienna, too?

No. In 1863, Morell Mackenzie, the great English laryngologist, opened The Metropolitan Free Dispensary for Diseases of the Throat and Loss of Voice in London, beating the Viennese in this area. But Morell wasn't always so great. More about that to follow later.

5. Why do otolaryngologists wear head mirrors?

The use of the head mirror dates to the time of Bozzini, who used the mirror to visualize his larynx. John Avery, a London surgeon, mounted a curved mirror on his head and used a candle as his light-source. Garcia, a Spaniard, put the two together.

6. Whose larynx did Garcia first visualize?

Through a complex series of mirrors and a candle, this Spanish musician was able to realize his lifelong dream (so the story goes), as he reflected light onto his own larynx and visualized the reflected image.

7. What was the early understanding of the function of the ear?

Probably the most interesting superstition about the ear's function was that it served as the female organ of generation. This thought originated from the belief that the Virgin Mary's conception was caused by the breath of the Holy Ghost into her ear, a legend often illustrated by medieval artists. Similar legends existed in Mongolian, Indian, and Persian mythology. Male and female fertility legends apparently commingled, as the practice of cutting off thieves' ears originated as a means of rendering them sterile. This idea was based on Hippocratic belief that the passage of semen took place from the head, where it was generated, via the veins behind the ear, and ultimately to the genitalia. Pliny located the seat of the memory to the ear, while Noury felt that the seat of Nemesis, the goddess of retribution, was behind the right ear.

8. Who are the patron saints of otolaryngology?

Throughout history, many died from severe nosebleeds. Others sought protection in St. Fiacre, the patron saint of epistaxis. St. Blaise is not only the patron saint of wild animals, winds, and storms, but is also the patron saint of the throat, goiter, and whooping cough. This Christian physician became a saint by removing a fishbone from a patient's throat. On February 3, Roman Catholic churches still celebrate the feast of St. Blaise with the "blessing of the throat."

9. If in Morocco on March 25th, what ritual might you witness?

Moroccans have traditionally collected rainwater on March 25th. Moroccan history recounts that this ritual was performed yearly to ward off all diseases of the ear and nose.

10. What happened on July 18, 1856?

Trick question. Nothing of significance in the field of otolaryngology that I know of. Otolaryngology attendings and residents are occasionally guilty of a "trick question," as are members of other disciplines.

11. Who did the first tracheotomy?

Galen credited Asclepiades of Bithynia (2nd century AD) with the origin of this operation. The term *trachea* was not introduced until the 16th century. At this time, a tracheotomy was performed only in the direst of emergencies. Nearly another century passed before it came into common acceptance.

12. When was the myringotomy introduced?

The myringotomy was probably first naturally introduced when the first caveman (or cave child) suffered acute otitis media, as their tympanic membrane may have perforated spontaneously. But Thomas Willis (better known for his description of the arteries of the base of the brain, the circle of Willis, and cofounder of the Royal Society of England), Antonio Valsalva (also better known for his description of the maneuver to inflate the middle ear via the Eustachian tube, originally used to try to rid the middle ear of pus), and William Cheselden all perforated the tympanic membrane of dogs to see if their hearing diminished. Sir Astley Paston Cooper, however, popularized the procedure in London in the early 1800s as "an operation for the removal of a particular species of deafness." He even described the special trochar and cannula that he used.

13. Who described the eustachian tube?

(Hint: It was not Gabriele Falloppio. That was a different tube.) Another Italian, Bartolomeo Eustachio, one of the great pioneers of otology, was one of the foremost anatomists of his era (the 1500s), possibly greater than Falloppio. Personal physician to the Pope, Eustachio made his greatest contribution in providing a precise description of the tubular structure that bears his name. He also recognized the functional nature of the tube. Incidentally, Eustachio also discovered the stapes in the course of his anatomic investigations.

14. For whom is the organ of Corti named?

Getting a little easier. Marquis Alfonso Corti (1822–1888) was a well-known Italian histologist whose microscopic observations of this organ made a major contribution to Helmholtz's "resonance" theory—i.e., that vibration of the basilar membrane is a factor in hearing.

15. What otolaryngologic disease contributed to George Washington's death?

The answer remains a matter of debate and might be quinsy (peritonsillar abscess or peritonsillitis), bacteremia, or the inappropriate attempts of an early surgeon. However, it is known that Washington had a severe sore throat with fever and was treated by blood-letting, a form of therapy to release the "evil humors" (early barber-surgeons marked their offices with a red and white-striped pole, representing the soiled bandages from blood-letting). Shortly thereafter, he died, possibly of any of the above. Otolaryngologists like to tell stories of surgical misadventures by members of other disciplines.

16. Which American presidents had cancer?

Two had cancer of the head and neck region, Ulysses S. Grant (cancer of the tongue base) and Grover Cleveland (maxilla, or hard palate). Ronald Reagan had colon cancer. Some also think Franklin D. Roosevelt may have had a melanoma above his eyebrow (which may have metastasized intracranially and bled, leading to his "stroke"), but that was never verified.

17. Tell me more about Grant's cancer.

In early 1884, 7 years after the completion of his Presidency, Grant noted the onset of a sore throat, especially when eating peaches, "of which he was fond." Then 62 years old and a stubborn man, Grant delayed seeking medical advice. However, at the insistence of his wife, he was examined by a physician named Da Costa. Grant was spending the summer with his family in Long Beach, New Jersey, and was advised to see his personal physician, Dr. Fordyce Barker, on his return to New York. As Dr. Barker was vacationing in Europe at the time, Grant received no additional evaluation until October. When Barker examined the ex-president 12 weeks later, he referred him immediately to Dr. John H. Douglas. Dr. Douglas was a leading "throat specialist" of the day. On October 22, 1884, Douglas described a lesion of the right tonsil with a small neck node (today classified as a T1N1M0, Stage 3 tumor) of "epithelial" origin. To Grant, Douglas characterized the tumor as "serious . . . sometimes capable of being cured."

Grant was both a heavy smoker, preferring cigars, and a heavy drinker, predisposing him to squamous cell carcinoma of the oral cavity. This tonsillar lesion was initially treated with a combination of cessation of smoking, topical iodoform, salt-water gargles, dilute carbolic acid gargle, and 4% topical cocaine solution applied topically for pain relief. These measures did not slow the tumor growth and by December, it had spread extensively to involve the tongue base and palate.

A biopsy was obtained in February 1885, suggesting a tumor that would today be diagnosed as squamous cell carcinoma. The pathologic examination was done with a new instrument, a microscope, regarded as a toy at the time. Radical excision, involving a resection of the lateral tongue, lateral palate, and involved upper cervical nodes, was considered via a lateral mandibulotomy, but "in the best interests of the distinguished patient, the surgeons did not feel inclined to recommend the procedure." It was felt that the surgery "did not offer a guarantee of complete tumor removal" (but what cancer operation does?) and that there was a "risk to life by the severe shock to a constitution already much enfeebled." Clearly, the surgeons of the time "blinked," but in their defense, it must be remembered that general anesthesia was only 41 years old and modern techniques of sterility, blood transfusion, and antibiotics were unknown. The patient likely would have died of the surgery, and the surgeons probably made a wise choice.

As Grant's tumor advanced, he developed apprehensions that he might choke to death in his sleep and slept sitting up (and as little as possible to avoid choking). He undertook the completion of writing his memoirs, both to justify his decisions as well as to try to recoup some of his financial losses. During the latter part of his illness, he was unable to speak and his gasping breathing and gurgling could be heard for some distance.

On June 16, 1885, Grant was moved to Mount McGregor, New York, a small village outside of Saratoga known for its fresh mountain air. He died there 5 weeks later, completing his memoirs 3 days before his death.

18. How about Grover Cleveland?

Grover Cleveland, the only President of the United States who served two different disconnected terms, was a large bull of a man. Shortly after his second inauguration, in 1893, he was found to have a sore area of ulceration in the roof of his mouth. Biopsies were nondiagnostic (the science of pathology was yet in its infancy!), but a friend of the President and an eminent surgeon, Dr. Joseph Bryant, concluded, "Were it in my mouth, I would have it removed at once." This was not simply accomplished, as 1893 was a year of economic crisis and Cleveland was regarded as the leader to give the country stability and leadership during this crisis. His medical condition was therefore concealed, lest it should cause panic.

On the evening of June 30, 1893, Cleveland boarded a yacht, the Oneida, heading out of New York's East River into Buzzard's Bay. On board were Drs. W.W. Keen (Professor of Neurosurgery at Jefferson Medical College and an eminent neurosurgeon), Ferdinand Hasbrouck (a dentist and anesthesiologist of note), Edward Janeway (a prominent New York physician), Robert O'Reilly, and J.F. Erdman. All were sworn to secrecy.

On July 1, 1893, an intraoral partial maxillectomy was performed in the yacht's saloon, which had been converted into an operating room. Bone was removed from the bicuspid region on the left side as far back as the palatine bone, carefully avoiding external incisions. The tumor was gelatinous in nature, suggesting a sarcoma. The procedure took 1.5 hours, with blood loss of 168 cc. The Oneida returned to port on July 5, and the public was told that the President had caught a cold, suffered a toothache, and had required an extraction. He was subsequently fitted with a maxillary obturator made of vulcanized rubber. Cleveland served out his entire term and died, apparently tumor-free, in 1908 of unrelated causes.

The operation was not concealed for long. Rumors and leaks continued to surface until 1917, when Keen released the story to the *Saturday Evening Post*. Mystery, however, continued to surround the diagnosis. Dr. William M. Welch, of Johns Hopkins, was said to have confirmed the initial diagnosis of sarcoma. By 1917, Keen felt that the diagnosis was carcinoma. Others subsequently questioned the diagnosis of malignancy, in view of the President's "cure," and raised the possibility of ameloblastoma, a benign salivary mixed tumor, and even necrotizing sialometaplasia or a syphilitic gumma. The specimen remained in the Mutter Museum of the College of Physicians of Philadelphia until 1980, when a definitive examination revealed verrucous carcinoma, partially accounting for the good prognosis.

19. Had Grant and Cleveland lived today, how might they have fared?

Renehan offers a comprehensive discussion of how Grant's and Cleveland's tumors might have been handled today. Cleveland's might have been handled with the laser, and certainly the prosthetic rehabilitation would have been superior. But the result—apparent cure and NED at death—could not have been improved upon. Grant, on the other hand, would have been the beneficiary of a number of major advances in the field and could have expected a greater than 50% five-year survival rate for his T1N1M0, Stage 3 tonsillar fossa tumor.

20. What famous German leader died of laryngeal cancer?

Crown Prince Frederick ascended the German throne as Frederick III but lived only 99 days in this position, dying on June 15, 1888. Many feel that his young successor was heavily influenced by the militant Bismark, contributing to Germany's provocation of World War I. The management of this famous patient has been repeatedly analyzed but briefly recounted. Frederick had an English wife who encouraged his evaluation by the most noted laryngologist of the time, Morell Mackenzie of England. Mackenzie simply missed the diagnosis, thinking that he was observing a syphilitic gumma. A biopsy was initially misread by the best-known pathologist of the time, Virchow (although it must be admitted that pathology and pathologic diagnosis was in its infancy) and treatment was delayed. By the time the proper diagnosis was made, laryngectomy was impossible (although laryngectomy was also in its infancy, having first been performed by Billroth 5 years previously), and only a palliative tracheotomy was performed. It should also be admitted that few surgeons even considered a laryngectomy. Who would want to be remembered as the surgeon whose royal patient died under the knife? Mackenzie was subsequently criticized and censured by the Royal Society of Surgeons and the British Medical Association and forced to resign from the Royal College of Physicians.

21. What otolaryngologist received a Nobel Prize?

Gyorgy von Békésy, a Hungarian, won the Nobel Prize in 1947 for developing the semiautomatic audiometer. This advancement produced threshold measurements which were valuable in the differentiation of conductive and sensorineural hearing loss.

22. Is all of this historical stuff really important?

Walter Howarth, a rhinologist, observed, "We are so much preoccupied nowadays with the problems of the present and the future that our debt to the past is sometimes apt to be overlooked. We are, in fact, inclined to take our present state of knowledge for granted, and when we think of the generations which have preceded our own, we are apt to do so with a sense of superiority and of pity for their mistakes, rather than with a sense of humanity and of admiration for their achievement."

23. Who are some of the 20th century gurus of otolaryngology?

This is a toughie, because many friends will be overlooked (my apologies to them and my assurances that they will be in the second edition!). Carl Olof Nylén developed the operating microscope, and Jack Urban perfected the binocular operating microscope and its many attachments, allowing microscopic surgery to evolve. Sourdille and Lempert pioneered surgery for otosclerosis, but Sam Rosen and John Shea simplified it to surgery of the stapes. Howard House and Harold Schuknecht developed the stapes prosthesis. Zöllner and Wullstein developed tympanoplasty, now facilitated with a variety of prostheses, via several (e.g., trans-canal, canal-up, canal-down) approaches. Bill House reported a number of procedures around the skull base, founding neuro-otology. Blair Simmons did much of the early American work on the cochlear implant, along with Bill House. Otitis media was relieved by Beverly Armstrong's collar button tube, although the indications for placement remain subject to debate (and if you ask who "she" is, you probably don't know that *he* published his results in 1954, either). Mosher and Cottle are two of the best-known older rhinologists, while the development of the Hopkins rod endoscope has allowed the development of transnasal functional endoscopic surgery by Messerklinger, Stammberger, and Wigand. Jacques Joseph is the best-known early plastic surgeon of the nose, with recent contributions by Goldman, Anderson, and Tardy. McCullough and Tardy have popularized facial plastic surgery within the field of otolaryngology. A number of otolaryngologists contributed to the evolution of the modern endoscope, especially the development of distal, fiberoptic lighting and fiberscopes. The treatment of head and neck cancer recognizes John Conley, John Loré, John Kirchner, and Joseph Ogura as three of its guiding lights, while Paul Ward trained a number of the leading educators of the field, building on the tradition founded by John Lindsey and Cesar Fernandez, of the University of Chicago. Blom and Singer pioneered the tracheoesophageal puncture and valved prosthesis for surgical voice rehabilitation after laryngectomy.

I apologize again to many friends, colleagues, and mentors who have contributed mightily to the development of the field of otolaryngology and whose names I have omitted. Next edition...

24. Who was Bruce W. Jafek, and what did he do?

Bruce W. Jafek wrote this chapter and helped to edit this book. And that's the last question and final answer for which we'll hold you responsible. Thanks for reading *ENT Secrets*, and thanks for your curiosity about the interesting and challenging field of otolaryngology! P.S.: Anne Stark is a resident in otolaryngology at the University of Colorado School of Medicine.

BIBLIOGRAPHY

1. Brooks JJ, Enterline HT, Aponte GE: The final diagnosis of President Cleveland's lesion. Trans Stud Coll Physician Phila 2(1), 1980.
2. Keen WW: The surgical operations on President Cleveland in 1893. Saturday Evening Post (Sept 22):24–25, 1917.
3. Renehan A: The oral tumours of two American presidents: What if they were alive today? J R Soc Med 88:377–383, 1995.
4. Weir N: Otolaryngology: An Illustrated History. London, Butterworths, 1990.

INDEX

Page numbers in **boldface type** indicate complete chapters.

ABCs (airway, breathing, circulation)
  of epistaxis management, 287
  of life support, 415
ABCDs (airway, breathing, circulation,
    defibrillate/differential diagnosis), of cardiac
    arrest management, 408
ABCICs (airway, breathing, circulation, intravenous
    crystalloids), of hypovolemic shock
    management, 415
Abducens nerve, in temporal bone fractures, 316
Abscess
  abdominal, 423
  cerebral, 101
  epidural, 101
  of head and neck, 162, 358
  lymphangioma-related, 330
  of masticator space, 356
  of nasal septum, 292–293
  orbital, 293, 374
  peritonsillar (quinsy), 142, 326–327, 427
  retrobulbar, 375
  of retropharyngeal space, 142, 358
  subdural, 101
  subperiosteal, 374
Accessory ostium, 95
Acetaminophen, as fever therapy, 420
Acetazolamide, taste effects of, 347
Achalasia, 135
Acid-base disturbances, **384–389**
  postoperative, 369
Acid ingestion, as esophageal injury cause, 132
Acidosis
  lactic, 387, 388
  metabolic, 386–387
    postoperative, 369
  respiratory, 384–385
    postoperative, 369
  total parenteral nutrition-related, 391
Acinic cell carcinoma, 189
Acoustic analysis, for laryngeal function analysis,
    171
Acoustic gain, 29
Acoustic nerve, anatomy of, 138
Acoustic reflex, 19
Acquired immunodeficiency syndrome (AIDS)
  dementia of, 153
  fever of unknown origin associated with, 422
  indicator diseases of, 153
  Kaposi's sarcoma associated with, 236
  otolaryngologic manifestations of, **153–158**
    benign lymphoepithelial cysts, 157
    facial paralysis, 125
    hairy leukoplakia, 155
    ocular manifestations, 377
    oral candidiasis, 155
    otitis media, 154–155
    periodontal disease, 155

Acquired immunodeficiency syndrome (AIDS) (*cont.*)
  otolaryngologic manifestations of (*cont.*)
    Ramsay Hunt syndrome, 155
    sinusitis, 105, 155, 156–157
Acquired immunodeficiency syndrome patients,
    survival time of, 154
Activated partial thromboplastin time (aPTT), 395
Acyclovir, 163
Addison's disease, 121
Adenitis, cervical, as tonsillectomy indication, 327
Adenocarcinoma
  esophageal, 217
  laryngeal, 208
  of salivary glands, 189
  sinonasal, 205
    occupational exposure-related, 206
  thyroid
    follicular, 223
    papillary, 222
Adenoid cystic carcinoma
  esophageal, 217
  laryngeal, 208
  of salivary glands, 189, 195
  sinonasal, 205
  tracheal, 214
Adenoidectomy, 42, 327, 328
Adenoids
  function of, 326
  post-adenoidectomy regrowth of, 328
Adenoma
  bronchial, 180
  follicular thyroid, 222
  parathyroid, 186
  pleomorphic parapharyngeal, 355, 356
  of salivary glands, 189
Adenomatoid odontogenic tumors, 200, 203
Adenopathy, in HIV-infected patients, 156
Adenotonsillar disease, 326
Adenotonsillectomy, 328
Adenovirus, as tonsillitis causal organism, 326
Adnexa, neoplasms of, 236
Adrenal insufficiency, as fever cause, 421
Advanced cardiac life support, **408–413**
Aerodynamic ability, of laryngeal function, 171
Afferent pupillary deficit, 371
African Americans, esophageal cancer in, 218
Agger nasi cells, 95
Aging, of skin, 251–252
Agnosia, olfactory, 346
Aguilar's classification system, for external ear
    malformations, 269
Air-bone gap, 16–17
Air pressure, above sea-level, 62
Air travel, as ear injury cause, 62–64, 65–67
Airway
  artificial, 298, 299
  difficult, presurgical identification of, 368, 369

Airway (cont.)
  excessive secretions from, 398
  intubation-related injury to, 405
  laser surgery-related fires in, 367
  narrowest area of, 405
  stents for, 302
  surgical, in upper-airway obstruction, 298
Airway management
  in head and neck cancer patients, 368
  in thyroid surgery patients, 368
  in trauma patients, 283–284
Airway obstruction
  anaphylactic shock-related, 353
  deep neck space infection-related, 141, 142
  esophageal cancer-related, 218
  LeFort fracture-related, 310
  neck penetrating trauma-related, 295
  pediatric, **321–325**
  as respiratory acidosis cause, 384
  as tracheostomy indication, 398
  upper, **296–302**
    differential diagnosis of, 296
    signs and symptoms of, 297
Airway protection, during swallowing, 131–132
Alar cartilage, volume reduction of, 259
Albumin solution, 382
Alcohol use
  as esophageal cancer cause, 218
  as esophageal dysmotility cause, 134
  as laryngeal cancer cause, 208–209
  as obstructive sleep apnea cause, 146, 147
  as oral cancer cause, 195
Alkalemia, 385
Alkalosis
  as lactic acidosis cause, 388
  metabolic, 388–389
  "overshoot", 387
  respiratory, 385–386
    postoperative, 369
Allen, Woody, 261
Allergy and allergic reactions, **350–354**
  chemotherapy-related, 242
  immunology of, 350–352
  as otolaryngology specialty, 1, 2
  as rhinitis cause, 86, 87, 88
  as sinusitis cause, 97
  sinusitis management in, 69
  threshold, 352
Allografts, in rhinoplasties, 261
Allopurinol, interaction with theophylline, 165
Alopecia
  chemotherapy-related, 242
  radiation therapy-related, 239
  rhytidectomy-related, 279
Alport's syndrome, 26, 202
Alveolar nerve, inferior, course of, 304
Alveolar process fractures, 302, 303
Alveolus, cleft, 342, 343
Alzheimer's disease, 346
Amantadine, as influenza A treatment, 163
Ambient pressure changes, as ear pain cause, 62
Amblyopia, in children, 376

Ambulatory surgery, cost reduction of, 379
Ameloblastic carcinoma, 203
  differentiated from ameloblastoma, 202
Ameloblastoma, 194, 200, 201–202, 203
  differentiated from ameloblastic carcinoma, 202
American Academy of Ophthalmology and
  Otolaryngology, 1
American Academy of Otolaryngology-Head and
  Neck Surgery, referral guidelines of, 380
American Board of Medical Specialties, 2
American Board of Otolaryngology-Head and Neck
  Surgery, 2
American Heart Association, Advanced Cardiac
  Life Support guidelines of, 411, 412
American Joint Committee on Cancer, laryngeal
  cancer staging system of, 210
American Thoracic Society, lymph node mapping
  scheme of, 183
American Tinnitus Association, 61
Amides, as local anesthetics, 366
Amikacin, ototoxicity of, 55
Amiloride, as metabolic acidosis cause, 387
Aminoglycosides, 161
  ototoxicity of, 26, 55, 59
Ammonium chloride, as metabolic acidosis cause,
  387
Amoxicillin, 161, 162, 380
Amoxicillin clavulanate potassium, use with
  anterior packs, 288
Amphotericin B, 163, 168
Ampicillin, interaction with oral contraceptives, 166
Anaerobic bacterial infections, antibiotic therapy
  for, 159, 160, 161
Anastomosis, of traumatic facial nerve injuries, 71
"Andy Gump" deformities, 250
Anemia, as epistaxis cause, 287
Anesthesia, **365–370**
  for bronchoscopy, 177
  for laryngoscopy, 169, 170, 171, 172
  as respiratory acidosis cause, 385
  for rhinoplasty, 254
  as tinnitus cause, 59, 60
  as transfusion reaction cause, 395
Aneurysm
  of cerebellopontine angle, 74
  of posterior communicating artery, 377
  of superior mediastinum, 186
  of thoracic aorta, as esophagoscopy
    contraindication, 174
Angina, Ludwig's, 142, 296, 297
Angioedema, 297
Angiofibroma, juvenile nasopharyngeal, 196, 205,
  228, 286, 324, 365
Angiography
  for neck trauma evaluation, 294, 295
  for temporal bone penetrating trauma evaluation,
    317
Angiotensin-converting enzyme inhibitors, 59, 347
Angle classification, of occlusion, 304
Angle fractures, mandibular, 302, 303, 306
Anion gap, metabolic acidosis-related, 386, 387
Anosmia, 346

Antacids, as gastroesophageal reflux therapy, 167
Anterior commissure glottic cancer, 213
Anterior cricoid split technique, 325
Anterior packs, 288, 289
Anthropometric measurements, for nutritional status evaluation, 389
Antibacterial drops, as external auditory canal treatment, 167
Antibiotic(s). *See also* specific antibiotics
    β-lactam, 160, 421
    as tinnitus cause, 59
    use in upper airway obstruction, 299
Antibiotic prophylaxis
    indications for, 379–380
    for meningitis, 320
    in surgical patients, 163–164
    for wound infections, 397
Antibiotic therapy, **158–164**. *See also* specific antibiotics
    in adenoidectomy patients, 328
    administration route determination in, 159
    use with anterior packs, 288
    for deep space neck infections, 143
    as fever cause, 421
    in mandibular fracture management, 305, 308
    in nasal fracture management, 293
    ototoxicity of, 165
    for septal abscesses, 292
    for septic shock, 416, 418
    for sinusitis, 102–103
    in tonsillectomy patients, 328
Antidepressants
    as temporomandibular disorder pain therapy, 117
    as tinnitus cause, 59
Antihistamines
    action mechanisms of, 176
    as rhinitis therapy, 88
    sedating effects of, 165
    as tinnitus cause, 59
Antihypertensives, side effects of, 48, 118
Anti-inflammatory drops, as external auditory canal treatment, 167
Antimalarials, as tinnitus cause, 59
Antiprotozoals, taste and smell effects of, 347–348
Antipsychotics, as xerostomia cause, 118
Antipyretics, 420
Antithyroid drugs, taste and smell effects of, 348
Antiviral agents, 163
Antrostomy, maxillary, 110
Anxiety
    evaluation of, 48–49
    as respiratory alkalosis cause, 385
Anxiolytics
    preoperative administration of, 365
    as tinnitus cause, 59
Aorta, as esophageal landmark, 173
Aortic arch
    double, 186
    mediastinoscopy-related injury to, 184
Apert syndrome, 337
Aphonia, 150
    hysterical, 152

Aplasia, types of, 331, 336
Aretaeus of Cappadocia, 55
Armstrong, Beverly, 429
Arnold's nerve, 62
Arrhythmias, cardiac
    as cardiogenic shock cause, 416
    intraoperative, 369
Arterial blood gas (ABG) monitoring
    in mechanical ventilation patients, 403
    in upper airway obstruction patients, 298
Arteries. *See also* specific arteries
    as nasal vascular supply, 79
Arteriosclerosis, as epistaxis cause, 286, 287
Arteriovenous malformations, as tinnitus cause, 58
Arteritis, temporal, 99
Arthritis
    as olfactory disorders cause, 346
    rheumatoid, as fever of unknown origin cause, 423
Arthrography, for temporomandibular disease evaluation, 116
Arthroscopy, temporomandibular, 117
Arthrotomy, temporomandibular, 117
Arytenoid cartilage
    contact granuloma of, 152
    dislocation of, 323, 406
Asclepiades of Bithynia, 426
Aspergillus infections, of paranasal sinuses, 364
Asphyxia, neonatal, as hearing loss cause, 21
Aspiration. *See also* Fine-needle aspiration biopsy
    of maxillary sinuses, 99
    of pulmonary lesions and lymph nodes, prior to biopsy, 183–184
    tracheotomy and, 398, 401
Aspirin
    as epistaxis cause, 287
    as fever therapy, 420
    as respiratory alkalosis cause, 385
Assisted-controlled ventilation, 403
Assistive listening devices (ALDs), 32
Asystole, 410, 411
Atelectasis
    bronchoscopic evaluation of, 178–179
    as fever cause, 421, 422, 423
Atlantoaxial instability, Down syndrome-related, 369
Atopy, 350
Atresia
    choanal, 322, 332, 335
    congenital aural, 36, 71–72, 76, 331
    esophageal, 173, 330, 331
    of first branchial groove, 331
Atretic plate, 71
Atropine
    in cardiopulmonary resuscitation, 411
    as intraoperative tachycardia cause, 369
Audiogram, definition of, 14
Audiometer, semiautomatic, 429
Audiometry
    for acoustic neuroma evaluation, 73
    behavioral, 20
    for conductive hearing loss evaluation, 22

Audiometry (*cont.*)
  for facial nerve paralysis evaluation, 127
  otosclerosis-related cochlear reserve and, 46
  in pediatric patients, 20
  play, 20
  speech, 20
Auditory brainstem response (ABR), 19–20, 73
  in children, 20
  in sudden sensorineural hearing loss, 28
Auditory canal
  cultures of, 380
  external
    anatomy of, 9
    foreign bodies in, 58, 61
    neoplasms of, 68
    in temporal bone trauma, 316, 319
  internal, anatomy of, 72
  physical volume test of, 18
Auditory nerve
  traumatic injury to, 28
  tumors of, 13
Auricle
  anatomy of, 34
  congenital malformations of, 331
  frostbite to, 35
  neoplasms of, 68
  perichondritis of, 34–35
  reconstruction of, 273
  reduction of, 272
Auricular nerve, greater, rhytidectomy-related
    injury to, 277, 278, 279
Auricular tags, 335–336
Auriculotemporal nerve, 62
Aurists, 425
Autoimmune disease
  as dizziness cause, 48
  as facial paralysis cause, 125
Autoimmunity, 351
Autosomal dominant disorders, 333–334
hearing loss as, 336, 337
Autosomal recessive disorders, 333
hearing loss as, 336
Avery, John, 325
AVPU mnemonic, for neurologic status, 285
Axonotmesis, 124–125
Azithromycin, 160
Azoles, as candidiasis therapy, 163
Aztreonam, 160, 161–162

Bacampicillin, interaction with oral contraceptives,
    166
Bacterial infections
  as dizziness cause, 48
  sinusitis as, 96–97, 98–99
  of wounds, 396
Bacteroides infections
  antibiotic therapy for, 160, 161
  deep space neck infections as, 141
  otitis media as, 40
  as septic shock cause, 415–416
  sinusitis as, 97
  tonsillitis as, 326

Balance disorders
  skull-base surgery-related, 75
  surgical procedures for, 69–70
Barbiturates, for preoperative sedation, 365
Barium swallow
  for esophageal cancer evaluation, 218–219
  for tracheal tumor evaluation, 215
Barker, Fordyce, 427
Barotitis media, 65
Barotrauma
  diving-related, 62
  of external ear, 63
  of inner ear, 66–67
  mechanical ventilation-related, 403, 404
  of middle ear, 62, 66
  as peripheral vestibular system lesion cause, 48
  as sensorineural hearing loss cause, 28
  as sinusitis cause, 97
Barrett's esophagus, 219
Bartter's syndrome, 388
Basal cell carcinoma
  of auricle, 68
  risk factors for, 230
  staging and grading systems for, 232–233
Basal cell nevus syndrome, 194, 201
Basal metabolic rate (BMR), calculation of, 389
Basal nevus carcinoma, 230
Basilar membrane
  resonance theory of, 427
  rupture of, 27
Battle's sign, 316
Beck's triad, 411
Bee and wasp stings, as anaphylactic shock cause,
    352–353
Behavior modification, as obstructive sleep apnea
    therapy, 147
Behçet's disease, 27, 57
Békésy, Gyorgy von, 11, 429
Belladonna alkaloids, as xerostomia cause, 118
Bell's palsy, 36, 70–71, 125, 127, 130, 347
Bell's phenomenon, 263
Benzodiazepines
  as preoperative sedation, 365
  as temporomandibular disorder pain therapy,
    116–117
Bernoulli effect, 84
Beta-blockers, adverse effects of, 59, 387
Betel nut, 194
Bicarbonate therapy, for metabolic acidosis, 387
Billroth, Theodore, 425
Biofeedback, as tinnitus therapy, 61
Biopsy. *See also* Fine-needle aspiration biopsy
  bronchoscopic, 179
  of lymph nodes, in HIV-infected patients, 156
  for melanoma evaluation, 234
  nasal, for Wegener's granulomatosis evaluation,
    83–84
  of neck mass, 196
  open, for jaw swelling evaluation, 203
  of supraclavicular fat pad, 186
  translobar lung, 180
  of vocal cords, 170

biPAP (inspiratory/expiratory positive airway pressure), 405
Bite appliance, for temporomandibular disorder pain management, 116
Björk flap, 398
Bleeding time test, 395
Bleomycin, 241, 242
Blepharitis, 377
Blepharochalasis, 262
Blepharoplasty, 253, **262–268**
Blepharospasm, essential, 129
Blood banks, 393
Blood glucose, relationship to serum sodium, 383
Blood loss
    classes of, 284
    epistaxis-related, 287
Blood transfusion
    autologous, 394, 395
    blood products for, **393–396**
    coagulopathy associated with, 369
    directed, 394
    hemolytic and nonhemolytic reactions to, 395
    for hemorrhagic shock management, 284
    homologous, screening tests for, 394
    HIV infection transmission by, 153, 394
    as hypovolemic shock treatment, 415
    as metabolic alkalosis cause, 388
Blood typing, 393
    in trauma patients, 284
Blood urea nitrogen (BUN), in total parenteral nutrition patients, 392
Blowout fractures, 311, 312, 314, 372–373
    teardrop sign of, 312, 373
    timing of repair of, 378
Blunt trauma, to neck, 295
Board certification, of otolaryngologist-head and neck surgeons, 1
Body fractures, mandibular, 302, 303, 304, 306
Body weight, fever-related loss of, 419–420
Bone, blood supply to, 249
Bone cyst, traumatic, of jaw, 200
Bone grafts, 245, 246
Bordetella pertussis infection, 160
Botulinum-A toxin, 167
Bovie-assisted glossectomy, 147
Bovie-assisted uvulopalatoplasty, 148
Bowen's disease, 232
Boyle's law, 62
Brachial plexus, imaging of, 364
Brachytherapy, 238
Brainstem tumors, 56
Branchial arches, embryologic, in external ear development, 335
Branchial cleft cyst, 329–330, 358–359
Branchial fistula, 329
Branchial groove, first, congenital malformations of, 331
Brancial sinus, 330
Branchio-oto-renal syndrome, 337
Breastfeeding, maternal-fetal HIV transmission during, 153
Breathlessness, bronchoscopic evaluation of, 178–179

Breslow thickness, of malignant melanoma, 234
British Medical Association, 429
Bronchi
    embryologic development of, 176
    eparterial, 178
    functions of, 176
Bronchial arteries, as tracheal blood supply source, 214
Bronchiectasis, as keratitis obturans cause, 35
Bronchoesophagology, 1
Bronchoscopy, **176–180**
    closed, 177
    for endotracheal tumor removal, 215
    as fever cause, 421
    fiberoptic, use in nasotracheal intubation, 300
    flexible versus rigid, 180
    open, 177
    rigid
        for tracheal tumor evaluation, 215
        versus flexible, 180
    for upper airway obstruction evaluation, 297–298
Bronchospasm, anaphylactic shock-related, 353
Bryant, Joseph, 428
Buccal mucosa, examination of, 5
Bulimia, as salivary gland enlargement cause, 138
Bullet wounds, to neck, 294
Bullous myringitis, 39
Bupivacaine, 366, 367
Burning mouth syndrome, 347, 349
Burns
    as fever cause, 421
    as fluid loss cause, 383
    ocular, 371
    of upper airway, 298
Buttress system, of midface, 309

Calcium channel blockers, as tinnitus cause, 59
Calcium chloride, as metabolic acidosis cause, 387
Calculi, of salivary glands, 139
Caldwell-Luc procedure, 110, 111, 201, 290
Caloric requirements, of febrile patients, 420
Caloric responses, normal, 52
Calorimetry, indirect, 389
Canalithiasis, 57
Canal squeeze, 63
Cancer. See also specific cancers
    as epistaxis cause, 286
    as facial paralysis cause, 125, 129
    as fever cause, 420, 421, 423
    as lactic acidosis cause, 388
Candidiasis
    antibiotic therapy for, 163
    azole therapy for, 163
    esophageal, 153, 155
    in HIV-infected patients, 155
    oral, 119, 120, 155
Capillary perfusion pressure, in intubation injury, 405
Captopril, taste and smell effects of, 347
Carbimazole, taste and smell effects of, 348
Carbonic anhydrase inhibitors, as metabolic acidosis cause, 387

Carboplatin, 241, 242
Cardiac arrest, cardiopulmonary resuscitation in, **408–413**
Cardiac pain, differentiated from esophageal pain, 135
Cardiopulmonary resuscitation (CPR), **408–413**
Cardioversion, synchronized, differentiated from defibrillation, 410
Carhart notch, 46
Caries. *See* Dental caries
Carlens, Eric, 181
Carotid artery
    aneurysm of, 69
    anomalies of, 69, 186, 362
    external
        as nasal vascular supply, 79
        as tonsillar blood supply, 326
    internal, as nasal vascular supply, 79
    left common, anomalous, 186
    location within carotid sheath, 142
    neoplastic invasion of, 361
Carotid blowout, 142
Carotid body tumors, 228
Carotid space lesions, 357
Carpenter syndrome, 337
Cartilage
    arytenoid. *See* Arytenoid cartilage
    autogenous costal grafts of, 325
    nasal, 78, 79
Catabolism, postoperative, effect on serum potassium levels, 383
Catecholamines, as intraoperative tachycardia cause, 369
Catheters
    central venous, for total parenteral nutrition delivery, 392
    peripheral, for total parenteral nutrition delivery, 391
    urinary, in trauma patients, 285–286
Catlin, George, 58
Cat-scratch disease, in HIV-infected patients, 156
"Cauliflower ear", 34
Caustic chemicals, inhalation of, as pediatric airway obstruction cause, 323
Caustic ingestion
    as esophageal cancer and injury cause, 132, 218
    as esophagoscopy contraindication, 175
CD4 count, 153, 154
Cefixime, 161
Ceftriaxone, 161–162
Cefuroxime, 161–162
Cellulitis
    orbital, 373–375
    periorbital, 374
    preseptal, 373–374
Cementoblastoma, 203
Cementoma, 200
Central lines, for total parenteral nutrition delivery, 391
Central nervous system
    diseases of, as esophageal dysmotility cause, 134
    as respiratory alkalosis cause, 386

Central nervous system (*cont.*)
    retarded development of, choanal atresia-related, 332
    tumors of, as vertigo cause, 48, 56
Central pontine myelinosis, 383
Central venous pressure (CVP) monitoring, in trauma patients, 284
Cephalexin, 162
Cephalosporins, 159–160
    use with anterior packs, 288
    prophylactic use, in head and neck surgery patients, 164
    as septal abscess therapy, 292
Cerebellopontine angle
    anatomy of, 73
    neoplasms of, 362
    surgical approaches to, 74–75
    tumors of, 56, 61, 74, 76, 362
Cerebellum tumors, 56
Cerebrospinal fluid
    leaks of
        skull-base surgery-related, 75
        temporal bone fracture-related, 315, 317, 318, 320
    pressure increase of, respiratory acidosis-related, 385
Cerebrovascular accidents, 48, 59
    as skull-base surgery complication, 75
Cerumen
    impaction of
        as canal squeeze cause, 63
        cleaning of, 36
        as conductive hearing loss cause, 22, 23
    within tympanic membrane, as tinnitus cause, 58
Cervical spine, fractures of, 299
Chagas' disease, 134
CHARGE mnemonic, for choanal atresia, 332
Chemical exposure
    as cutaneous squamous cell carcinoma cause, 231
    as esophageal cancer cause, 218
Chemical face peels, 251, 252, 253
Chemodectoma, 228
Chemo-prevention, 242
Chemoreception, trigeminal, 346
Chemosis, blepharoplasty-related, 267
Chemotherapy
    adjuvant, 198–199, 241
    for cerebellopontine angle tumors, 76
    as epistaxis cause, 287
    for esophageal cancer, 220
    for head and neck cancer, **240–243**
    for laryngeal cancer, 212
    neoadjuvant, 240–241
    for oral cavity carcinoma, 198–199
    organ-preservation, 242–243
    for pharynx carcinoma, 198–199
    for sinonasal cancer, 207
    for skull base tumors, 76
    for tracheal cancer, 216
Cherubism, 200, 202
Cheselden, William, 426

Chicken pox virus, as Ramsay Hunt syndrome
 cause, 36
Chicken soup, as mucolytic agent, 104
Childbirth, maternal-fetal HIV transmission during,
 153
Children
 AIDS/HIV infection in, 153, 156
 airway obstruction in, **321–325**
 of allergic parents, allergy risk of, 350
 cardiopulmonary resuscitation in, 408
 cochlear implants in, 76
 endotracheal intubation in, 321, 323, 324–325,
  406, 407
 eye disorders in, 376
 foreign bodies in ears of, 36–37
 head and neck examination of, 6
 head and neck tumors in, 227
 head colds in, as air travel contraindication,
  63–64
 hearing aids for, 32
 hearing loss in, 20–21, 23, 336
  relationship to parental hearing loss, 337
 malignant hyperthermia in, 366
 mandibular fractures in, 307
 masseter muscle rigidity in, during anesthetic
  induction, 370
 midfacial growth in, 85
 nasal fractures in, 292
 obstructive sleep apnea in, 146
 otitis media in, 40, 167
 otoplasty in, 269
 parotid masses in, 192
 primary tracheal neoplasms in, 215
 rhinoplasty in, 85
 septoplasty in, 85
 sinusitis in, 98, 103, 112
 tinnitus in, 58
 tracheotomies in, 399
 upper respiratory infections in, general anesthesia
  and, 369–370
Chin lift, for airway management, 283
Chinese, nasopharyngeal carcinoma prevalence in,
 196
Chloramphenicol, 160, 161–162
Chlorhexidine, as taste disorder cause, 347
Chloroprocaine, 366, 367
Cholecystitis, as fever cause, 421
Cholesteatoma, 43–44
 acquired, 43, 44
 of cerebellopontine angle, 74
 in cleft palate patients, 340
 as conductive hearing loss cause, 23, 24
 congenital, 43, 332
 of external auditory canal, 35
 as facial paralysis cause, 125, 130
 of middle ear, 69
 of petrous apex, 69
 presurgical imaging of, 361
 temporal bone fracture-related, 315–316
 treatment of, 24
Cholesterol granuloma, 45, 69, 74
Chondritis, of auricle, 34–35

Chondrosarcoma
 of jaw, 200
 laryngeal, 208
 of petrous apex, 69
Chordoma, of petrous apex, 69
Chromium, as total parenteral nutrition component,
 391
Chromosomal abnormalities
 as genetic hearing loss cause, 336
 otolaryngologic considerations in, 337–338
Chromosome 18 deletion, 337
Chromosome 22q deletion, 334
Chronic obstructive pulmonary disease, 35
Chronotropic agents, as shock therapy, 418
Cilia, nasal, function of, 81
Cimetidine, interaction with theophylline, 165
Cinepharyngography, 173
Cineradiography, 171
Ciprofloxacin, 160–161
 interaction with theophylline, 165
Cisplatin, 241, 242
Clarithromycin, 160
Clark levels, of malignant melanoma, 234
Clavicle, fractures of, 290
Clavulanic acid, 161, 162
Cleft alveolus, 342, 343
Cleft lip/plate, 334, **338–344**
 genetic syndromes-related, 334
 incomplete, 339
 repair of, 340, 341–343
 submucous, 327
Cleft uvula, 334
Cleveland, Grover, 427, 428
Clindamycin, 160, 162, 164
Clomipramine, taste and smell effects of, 348
Clostridium infections, 160, 161
Coagulation defects
 assessment of, 395
 blood transfusion-related, 369
Cobalt, as total parenteral nutrition component, 391
Cocaine
 as anesthetic, 167, 170, 366, 367
 as intraoperative tachycardia cause, 369
 effect on nasal septum, 84
 toxic dose of, 366
 vasoconstrictive effect of, 167
Cochlea
 anatomy of, 10, 11
 sound stimuli transmission to, 10, 12
 traumatic injury to, 28
Cochlear implants, 25, 32–33, 72, 76, 429
Cochlear membrane, rupture of, 27
Cochlear reserve, 46
Cogan's syndrome, 27, 56–57
Colds, in children, as air travel contraindication, 63–64
Collagen
 sun exposure-related changes in, 251
 in wounds, 396
Collagen III antibodies, 85
Collagen vascular disease, 48, 238, 421, 423
Collar button tube, 329
Colloids, 382

Coloboma, 332
Colon cancer, of Ronald Reagan, 427
"Commando" procedure, in head and neck surgery, 199
Composite resection, in head and neck surgery, 199
Compression injury, as facial paralysis cause, 125
Computed tomography (CT), of head and neck, **354–365**
    for airway obstruction evaluation, 298, 324
    for brachial plexopathy evaluation, 364
    of carotid artery metastases, 361
    of carotid space schwannoma, 357
    for cerebrospinal fluid rhinorrhea evaluation, 363
    of congenital ear anomalies, 362
    of esophageal cancer, 219
    of ethmoid sinuses, 82
    for facial paralysis evaluation, 70–71, 126
    of jaw swelling, 203
    of juvenile angiofibroma, 365
    of laryngeal cancer, 210–211
    of masticator space abscess, 356
    of maxillofacial trauma, 311
    of orbital fractures, 373
    paranasal, 363–364, 380
    of parapharyngeal space, 354–355
    of pleomorphic adenoma, 356
    of retropharyngeal space abscess, 358
    of salivary gland tumors, 189
    of sinonasal tumors, 206
    for sinusitis evaluation, 100, 364
    of temporal bone trauma, 316–317, 362, 363
    for temporomandibular disease evaluation, 115
    for tinnitus evaluation, 60, 362
    of tracheal tumors, 215
    of vestibular lesions, 52
Concha
    bullosa, 95
    deeply cupped, protruding, 272
    numbness of, 73
Condylar fractures, 302, 307, 308
Congenital aural atresia, 36, 71–72, 76, 331
Congenital malformations, **329–333**
    as facial paralysis cause, 125
    multifactorial, 334
Congestive heart failure, distinguished from cardiogenic shock, 416
Conjunctivitis, 377
Conley, John, 429
Connective tissue disorders, esophageal dysmotility-related, 133
Continuous positive airway pressure (CPAP), as obstructive sleep apnea treatment, 147
Contralateral acoustic reflex neural pathway, 19
Converse technique, of otoplasty, 271
Conversion disorders, 152
Cooper, Astley Paston, 426
Copper, as total parenteral nutrition component, 391
Copper deficiency, total parenteral nutrition-related, 392
Cornea
    abrasion of, 377
    desiccation of, facial paralysis-related, 128

Coronoid process fractures, 302, 303, 307
Corti, Marquis Alfonso, 427
Corticosteroid therapy
    for allergic hypersensitivity, 166
    for Bell's palsy, 130
    intranasal, 164–165
    as oral candidiasis cause, 120
    for sensorineural hearing loss, 25, 28
    for sinusitis, 102, 104
    for rhinitis, 89
    for upper airway obstruction, 299
Cost-effectiveness, of otolaryngology, **378–380**
Cottle, Maurice, 79
Cough
    bronchoscopic evaluation of, 178–179
    esophageal cancer-related, 218
    hoarseness associated with, 151
COWS mnemonic, for nystagmus direction evaluation, 52
Coxsackievirus, as tonsillitis causal organism, 326
CPR (cardiopulmonary resuscitation), **408–413**
Cranial nerves
    innervation of external canal by, 62
    in neuro-otologic skull-base surgery, 75
    paralysis of, jugular foramen syndrome-related, 69
    VII. *See* Facial nerve
    VIII. *See* Acoustic nerve
Craniomandibular disorders, 113
Craniosynostosis, 337
Cribiform plate fractures, as nasogastric tube contraindication, 286
Cricoid split, anterior, 325
Cricopharyngeus muscle, 131, 132, 173
Cricothyroidectomy, 284
Cricothyroid node, 224
Cricothyroidotomy, 301
Cricothyrotomy, 401–402
Cri du chat, 337
Crocodile tears, 128
Cromolyn sodium, 166
Crossover, in hearing evaluations, 15–16
Croup, 162, 322, 323
Crouzon syndrome, 337
Cryoprecipitate, 393, 394
Cryptococcus neoformans, as sinusitis causal organism, 100
Crystalloids, 382, 415
Cultures, of ear, nose, and throat, 380
"Cup ear" deformity, 272–273, 332, 335
Cupulolithiasis, 57, 318
Cystic fibrosis, 338
Cystine, as metabolic acidosis cause, 387
Cysts
    arachnoid, of cerebellopontine angle, 74
    auricular, sebaceous, 68
    branchial, 329–330, 358–359
    bronchogenic, 215
    dentigerous, 194, 201
    dermoid, 330, 332
    ductal retention, 406
    epidermoid, 56, 69, 74

Cysts (*cont.*)
  esophageal, 219
  fissural, 204
  follicular, 201
  of jaw, 200, 201
  lymphoepithelial, in HIV-infected patients,
    155–156, 157
  median palatal, 200, 204
  odontogenic, 200
    calcifying, 203
  parotid, 139–140, 155–156
  periapical, 201
  preauricular, 331
  retention, 200, 201, 406
  of salivary glands, 189
  of thyroglossal duct, 136, 330, 332, 359, 360
  thyroid, 222, 224
Cytogenetic studies, indications for, 334
Cytomegalovirus infections
  blood transfusion transmission of, 394
  HIV infection-related, 154
  retinitis as, 153, 377
  sinusitis associated with, 100

"Danger triangle", 79
dB A scale, 25–26
Deafness. *See* Hearing loss
Death, trimodal distribution of, 283
Decibel, 15
Decibels Hearing Level (dB HL), 15
Decibels Sound Pressure Level (dB SPL), 15
Decompression sickness, 66
Decongestants
  use by divers, 67
  Mecca position for administration of, 103–104
  as rhinitis medicamentosa cause, 103
  as rhinitis therapy, 88, 89
  as sinusitis therapy, 102, 103–104
Deep space neck infections, **141–144**, 162
Defibrillation, 408, 409–410, 412
Delphian node, 224
Deltopectoral flap, 248
Dementia, AIDS-related, 153
Dental caries
  radiation therapy-related, 240
  salivary gland hypofunction-related, 119
Dental disease
  as deep space infection cause, 141
  in HIV-infected patients, 155
  as sinusitis cause, 100
  as sinusitis mimic, 99
Dental evaluation, pre-radiation therapy, 240
Dental occlusion
  angle classification of, 304
  relationship to temporomandibular disorders,
    117–118
Dentinosarcoma, ameloblastic, 200
Dentures
  in mandibular fracture fixation, 305
  use following mandibular reconstruction, 204
Depression, chemosensory distortions associated
  with, 349

Depressor-retractor muscles, mandibular, 303
Dermabrasion, 251, 252, 253
Dermoid cysts, 330, 332
Dermatochalasis, 262
Dermatologic disorders, HIV infection-related, 154
Dermatomyositis, 133
Diabetes mellitus
  as esophageal dysmotility cause, 134
  as facial paralysis cause, 125
  as hearing loss cause, 24
  as lactic acidosis cause, 388
  as metabolic acidosis cause, 387
  as olfactory disorders cause, 346
  as taste dysfunction cause, 347
Diaphragm, rupture of, 284
Diarrhea, 382, 390
Dicloxacillin, 162
Didanosine, use in HIV-infected patients, 163
Diphenylhydantoin, as fever cause, 421
Diplophonia, 150
Disc displacement, 115
Diuretics
  loop, ototoxicity of, 26
  as metabolic alkalosis cause, 388
  as shock therapy, 418
  as tinnitus cause, 59
Diverticula
  tracheal, 331
  Zenker's, 131, 219
Diverticulitis, as fever cause, 421
Diving, as ear injury cause, 62–63, 64–67
Dix-Hallpike maneuver, 49–50, 57
Dizziness, **47–53**
Doll's eye test, 51
Do not resuscitate (DNR) order, 412
Douglas, John H., 427
Down syndrome, 338, 369
Drainage, of deep space neck infections, 143
Dressler's syndrome, 421
Drooling
  management of, 140
  peritonsillar abscess-related, 142
Drugs. *See also* specific drugs
  for cardiac arrest management, 411
  as dizziness cause, 48
  ototoxicity of, 26, 165–166, 366
  as perinatal hearing loss cause, 336
  pyrogenic, 421, 422
  as respiratory alkalosis cause, 386
Dry eye syndrome, 267, 377
Duction testing, forced, 311
Dysgeusia, 346, 349
Dysosmia, 346, 349
Dysostosis, cleidocranial, 194
Dysautonomia, familial, 346
Dysphagia
  in elderly persons, 134
  esophageal tumor-related, 218
  hoarseness associated with, 151
  in immunocompromised patients, 135
  lusoria, 134
  neck penetrating trauma-related, 295

Dysphagia (*cont.*)
peritonsillar abscess-related, 142
Dysphonia, 150
spastic, 167
Dysplasia
"eye-ear-spine", 269
fibrous
of jaw, 200, 202, 204
of temporal bone and external ear canal, 68
Dystonia, facial, botulinum-A toxin treatment of, 167

Electroneuronography, 70
Ear. *See also* External ear; Inner ear; Middle ear
anatomy and physiology of, **9–12**
as organ of fertility, 426
Ear canal physical volume test, 18
Ear drops, 167
Ear infections. *See also* Otitis externa; Otitis media
chronic, tumors presenting as, 68
eustachian tube dysfunction-related, 10
terminology of, 39
Ear injuries, diving and flying-related, 62–68
Ear lobes, protruding, 272
Ear pain
flying and diving-related, 62–63, 64
oral and pharyngeal cancer-related, 195
Ear plugs, as canal squeeze cause, 63
Ear surgery, antibiotic prophylaxis in, 379–380
Ear tumors, presenting as chronic ear infections, 68
Ecchymosis
periorbital, 316
postauricular, 316
subconjunctival, 267
E COLI mnemonic, for auditory brainstem response
interpretation, 19
Ectropion, blepharoplasty-induced, 267
Edema
laryngeal, 152, 174, 175, 252
pulmonary, 300, 400
subglottic, 151
EENT (eyes, ears, nose, throat), definition of, 1
Elastosis, 275
Elderly persons, swallowing disorders in, 134
Elective lymph node dissection (ELND), 236
Electrocardiography (EKG)
in hyperkalemic patients, 383
in hypokalemic patients, 383
in trauma patients, 285
Electrolyte imbalances, total parenteral nutrition-
related, 392
Electrolyte management, **381–384**
in cardiac arrest patients, 411
Electromechanical dissociation, 411
Electromyography (EMG), 127, 171
Electroneuronography (ENoG), 127
Electronystagmography (ENG), 52, 318
Electronystagmometry, 28
Electro-olfactogram, 80
Electrophysiologic tests, for facial paralysis
evaluation, 126–127
Emergencies, ocular, 371

Emphysema
bronchoscopic evaluation of, 178–179
subcutaneous, 295, 297
Empyema, subarachnoid, 293
Enalapril, taste and smell effects of, 347
Encephalocele, nasal, 332
Encephalopathy, hepatic, 386
Endocrine disorders, as fever cause, 421
Endolymph, 11
Endolymphatic hydrops, trauma-induced, 318
Endolymphatic shunt, 70
Endoscope, 429
cleaning of, following use on HIV-infected
patients, 156
Endoscopic procedures
anesthesia for, 367
in facial plastic surgery, 280
functional endoscopic sinus surgery (FESS), 91,
108–110, 111
for sinusitis diagnosis, 99
Endotracheal tube, size selection, 406
Enophthalmos, midfacial trauma-related, 312
ENT (eyes, nose, throat), definition of, 1
Enteral nutrition, 390
with tracheotomy, 401
Enteroviruses, as tonsillitis causal organisms, 326
Epidermoid carcinoma/tumors, 189, 362
Epidermoid cysts, 56, 69, 74
Epidermolysis, selective photothermal, 253
Epiglottitis, 162, 322–323, 364
Epilepsy, 346, 347
Epinephrine
in cardioplumonary resuscitation, 411, 412
co-administration with lidocaine, 167, 170, 254
per milliliter of 1:200,000 solution, 368
racemic, as upper airway obstruction therapy, 299
Epiphora, 205
Epistaxis, 79, **286–290**
angiofibroma-related, 196, 205, 228
in critical care patients, 287
histiocytosis-related, 205
nasal septal trauma-related, 83
patron saint of, 426
polychondritis-related, 95
Epithelial tumors, esophageal, 217
Epithelium, nasal, 80–81
Epley maneuver, 53
Epstein-Barr virus
as hairy leukoplakia cause, 121
as nasopharyngeal cancer cause, 196
as oropharyngeal cancer cause, 194
as tonsillitis cause, 326
Erdman, J. F., 428
Erythromycin, 160
co-administration with sulfonamides, 161
interaction with theophylline, 161, 165
ototoxicity of, 26, 165
Erythroplakia, 195
Escherichia coli infections, 40, 159, 161
Esophageal cancer, **217–221**
nutritional therapy in, 390
as vocal cord paralysis cause, 152

Esophageal pain, differentiated from cardiac pain, 135

Esophageal reflux. *See* Gastroesophageal reflux disease

Esophageal rings, 133

Esophageal webs, 133, 219

Esophagectomy, 220, 221

Esophagography, barium, 134

Esophagoscopy, **172–175**
  of esophageal cancer, 219
  flexible, 175
  rigid, 175

Esophagus, **131–135**, 173
  anatomy of, 173
  atresia of, 173, 330, 331
  Barrett's, 219
  cervical lacerations to, 143
  embryology of, 172
  functional assessment of, 173
  inadvertent endotracheal placement in, 300
  nutcracker, 135
  penetrating trauma to, 295
  perforation of, 174–175, 295
  spasm of, 134
  strictures of, misdiagnosed as esophageal cancer, 219
  tumors of, **217–221**

Ethmoid area, surgical access to, 108–109

Ethmoid arteries, 93–94
  ligation of, in epistaxis management, 289, 290

Ethmoid bone
  anatomy of, 108
  fractures of, 311

Ethmoidectomy, 110–111
  blood units required for, 393

Ethmoid infundibulum, 90, 91

Ethmoid nerve, 94

Etidocaine, 366, 367

Eustachian tube
  closed, as normal position, 62
  dilatation of, muscles involved in, 67
  during diving, 62
  dysfunction of, 23, 43
    cleft palate-related, 340
    as conductive hearing loss cause, 23
    Down syndrome-related, 338
  first description of, 426
  during flying, 63–64
  functions of, 39–40
  middle ear aeration function of, 10
  size of, 40

Eustachio, Bartolomeo, 426

Exostoses, differentiated from auditory canal osteoma, 35

External ear. *See also* Auricle
  anatomic landmarks of, in otoplasty, 268
  anatomy and physiology of, 9, 268
  congenital anomalies of, 361–362
  diseases of, 34–37
  malformations of, classification of, 269
  pathologies of, as conductive hearing loss cause, 22
  protruding, 332

Eye, orbit and, **371–378**

Eyebrow
  in blepharoplasty, 263–264
  ideal position of, 280
  relationship to upper eyelid, 263

Eyebrow lifts, 280

Eyelid
  blepharoplasty of, **262–268**
  malignant tumors of, 377
  marginal lacerations of, 376
  Oriental, "westernization" of, 268
  upper anatomy of, 264–265

Eye movement, spontaneous abnormal, as oscillopsia cause, 55

Eyes, nose, throat (ENT), definition of, 1

Face
  anatomic divisions of, 293
  embryological development of, 77, 78
  fractures of, **309–314**
    epistaxis management in, 289
    as nasogastric tube contraindication, 286
    as upper airway obstruction cause, 297
  involuntary movements of, 129–130
  osseocutaneous retaining ligaments of, 275–276
  paralysis of. *See* Facial nerve, paralysis of
  penetrating trauma to, **293–296**
  plastic surgery of, 1, 280, 429
  skin resurfacing of, 251–253
  venous network of, 375
  wound repair of, 397

Facelift. *See* Rhytidectomy

Face peels, 251, 252, 253

Facial artery, 79

Facial nerve, 62, **123–130**
  anatomic segments of, 70, 123, 126, 138, 276–277, 279
  blood supply to, 123
  in congenital aural atresia surgery, 71–72
  distribution of, 247
  as nasal innervation, 80
  paralysis of
    as Bell's palsy, 36, 70–71, 125, 127, 130, 347
    common causes of, 125
    evaluation of, 125–127
    lesion sites in, 70
    medical treatment of, 128
    ocular complications of, 377
    parotid mass-related, 189–190
    parotid surgery-related, 192
    Ramsay Hunt syndrome-related, 36, 70, 125, 130, 155
    rhytidectomy-related, 277, 278
    skull-base surgery-related, 75
    surgical treatment of, 70–71
    temporal bone trauma-related, 315, 317, 320
  in parotid gland tumor excision, 191
  in reconstructive surgery, 247
  schwannoma of, 362
  severing of
    facial trauma-related, 294
    surgery-related, 128

Facial nerve (*cont.*)
surgical landmarks of, 123–124
surgical removal of, facial function following, 130
taste bud innervation by, 345
in temporal bone trauma, 125, 129, 315, 316, 319–320
traumatic injury to, 71, 125, 129, 294, 315, 316
suction lipectomy-related, 279
surgery-related, 128
weakness of, 263
Facial pain, sinusitis-related, 98
Falloppio, Gabriele, 426
Familial dysplastic nevus syndrome, 235–236
Farrior technique, of otoplasty, 271
Fasciculation, segmental, 130
Fasciocutaneous flaps, 249
Fat, pseudoherniation of, 262
Fat, dietary, surgical patients' daily requirements, 390
Fatty infiltration, chronic, as salivary gland enlargement cause, 138
Febrile nonhemolytic transfusion reaction, 395
Felbanate, effect on taste and smell, 348
Fernandez, Cesar, 429
Fertility, ear as organ of, 426
FESS (functional endoscopic sinus surgery), 91, 108–110, 111
Fetor oris, 327
Fever
catheter infection-related, 392
in critical care patients, **418–423**
distinguished from hyperthermia, 419
as fluid loss cause, 382–383
as intraoperative tachycardia cause, 369
otitis media-related, 40
peritonsillar abscess-related, 142
postoperative, 422, 423
of unknown origin, 106, 422–423
upper airway obstruction-related, 297
Fibrin glue, 394
Fibrinogen level, in hemostatic defects, 395
Fibroma
ameloblastic, 203
central cementifying, 203
odontogenic, 200
ossifying, 200, 202
Fibro-odontoma, 203
Fibrosarcoma
ameloblastic, 200, 203
laryngeal, 208
Fillers, injectable, use in skin resurfacing, 251, 253
Fine-needle aspiration biopsy
for jaw swelling evaluation, 203
of neck mass, 196
of parotid mass, 190
of thyroid nodule, 224
Fires, laser-related, in airway, 367
Fistula
branchial, 329
enterocutaneous, tracheotomy-related, 398
of labyrinthine window, 66

Fistula (*cont.*)
oral-nasal, cleft palate repair-related, 342
of oval window, 70
otic capsule fracture-related, 317–318
perilymphatic, 47–48, 55, 64, 65, 67, 318, 319, 320
of round window, 70
salivary, 192
tracheal-innominate, 400
tracheocutaneous, 398
tracheoesophageal, 134, 173, 301, 330–331, 399
Fistula test, 65
Fitzpatrick Skin Classification System, 251
Flail chest, 284, 384
Flaps, 199
in blepharoplasty, 265, 266
categories of, 245, 247–250
in cleft lip/palate repair, 342
differentiated from grafts, 245
pharyngeal, 199, 343
Fluid management, **381–384**
Fluoroquinolones, 160–161
Fluoroscopy, for pediatric airway obstruction evaluation, 324
5-Fluorouracil, 241
adverse effects of, 242
as basal cell carcinoma therapy, 231
Flying, as ear injury cause, 62–64, 65–67
Food, as anaphylactic shock cause, 352–353
Food allergies, 61, 86, 119
Forced duction testing, 311
Fordyce spots, 122
Foreign body
in airway, 215, 323
in children, 36–37, 323
conjunctival, 377
in ear, 36–37
as epistaxis cause, 286
esophageal, 131, 174, 219
in external auditory canal, 58, 61
mediastinal, 186
in neck, 294
as sinusitis cause, 97
within tympanic membrane, 58
Frankfort horizontal plane, 254
Frederick III, of Germany, 428–429
Frenzl lenses, 49
Frequency response, 29
Fresh frozen plasma, 393, 394
Frey's syndrome, 192
Frostbite, of external auricle, 35
Frozen sections, of salivary tumors, 193
Functional endoscopic sinus surgery (FESS), 91, 108–110, 111
Fungal infections
cutaneous, HIV infection-associated, 154
ketoconazole therapy for, 162
sinusitis as, 97, 104–105
Furnas technique, of otoplasty, 271
Furniture-making, as nasal and sinus cancer risk factor, 206

Galen, Claudius, 135, 426
Ganglioneuroma, 223
Garcia, Manuel, 425
Gardner's sydnrome, 194
Gasserian ganglion, in temporal bone fractures, 316
Gastroesophageal junction, 132
Gastroesophageal reflux disease, 132–133, 167, 405
    as laryngeal cancer risk factor, 209
Gastrointestinal disorders, as fever cause, 421
Genetic issues, in otolaryngology, **333–338**
Genioglossus muscle, 303
Geniohyoid muscle, 303
Genioplasty, advancement, as obstructive sleep
    apnea treatment, 147
Gentamicin, 162
    ototoxicity of, 55
Germ cell tumors, 186
Gilles approach, in zygomatic arch fracture repair,
    312–313
Gingival cancer, metastases of, 197
Gingivitis, 120, 122, 155
Glabella, 255
Glasgow Coma Scale, 285
Glaucoma, acute, 371, 377
Glioma
    nasal, 332
    as vertigo cause, 56
Globe, perforation of, 371, 373
Globus pharyngeus, 132
Glogau classifcation system, of skin aging, 252
Glomus jugulare, 45, 125, 228
Glomus tumors, 58, 69, 76
Glomus tympanicum, 45, 228
Glossectomy
    blood units required for, 393
    as obstructive sleep apnea treatment, 147
Glossopharyngeal nerve
    blocks of, 177
    taste bud innervation by, 345
Glottis
    anterior commissure cancer of, 213
    congenital malformations of, 331
Glucocorticoids, as fever therapy, 420
Glucopyrrolate, as intraoperative tachycardia cause,
    369
Goblet cells, 94
Gogh, Vincent van, 58
Goiter, 136, 222, 426
Goldenhar syndrome, 269
Gold therapy, as dysgeusia cause, 348
Gorlin's syndrome, 230
Gout, as fever cause, 421
Gracilis myogenous microvascular free flap, 250
Grafts, 245–246, 250
    autogenous, use in rhinoplasty, 261
    full-thickness, 245, 246, 397
    medial crural strut, 258
    split-thickness, 245, 246, 397
    for wound coverage, 397
Gram-negative sepsis, as respiratory alkalosis cause,
    385, 386
Grand (basal) lamella, 95

Grant, Ulysses S., 427–428
Granulation bodies, thyroid, 222
Granulation tissue, 396
Granuloma
    cholesterol, 45, 69, 74
    contact, of arytenoid cartilage, 152
    eosinophilic, 205
    intubation, 405
    pyogenic, 205
Graves' disease, 136, 222, 346
Gruber, Josef, 425
Guaifenesin, 104
Guillain-Barre syndrome, 125
Gums, examination of, 5
Gunfire, as hearing loss cause, 25

Haemophilus influenzae infections
    amoxicillin-resistant strains of, 380
    antibiotic therapy for, 159–161, 162
    otitis media as, 40, 41, 167
    septal abscess as, 292
    sinusitis as, 97
    tonsillitis as, 326
Hair cells, cochlear, 11, 25
Halitosis, 327
Haller cells, 95
Hand-Schuller-Christian disease, 205
Hanging, as neck blunt trauma cause, 295
H_1-antihistamines, sedating effects of, 165
Harris-Benedict equation, for basal metabolic rate
    calculation, 389
Hasbrouck, Ferdinand, 428
Hashimoto's thyroiditis, 85
Head and neck
    examination of, **3–7**
        for hoarseness evaluation, 151
        for sleep apnea evaluation, 145
    infections of, 160–161
        deep space, **141–144**
    radiology of, **354–365**
    vascular tumors of, **227–229**
Head and neck cancer, 429
    chemotherapy for, **240–243**
    cutaneous, **229–237**
    radiation therapy for, **237–240**
Head and neck cancer patients, anesthesia use in, 367
Head and neck surgery, 1
    antibiotic prophylaxis in, 163–164, 379
    "commando" procedure of, 199
    grafts and flaps in, 245–246
    reconstructive, 246, 247
Head colds, in children, as air travel
    contraindication, 63–64
Head mirror, use of, 4
Head trauma
    as recurrent meningitis cause, 317–318
    as retrobulbar hemorrhage cause, 373
    as taste and smell disorders cause, 346, 347, 349
Health care costs, direct and indirect, 378–379
Hearing
    frequency range of, 15
    normal, 15

Hearing aids, **29–33**
Hearing evaluation, **12–21**
  audiograms in, 14–17
  "gold standard" test of, 17–18
  in pediatric patients, 20–21
  for sensorineural hearing loss, 25
  tuning fork tests for, 13–14, 21–22,
    for tinnitus evaluation, 60
    versus audiogram, 17–18
Hearing loss
  acoustic neuroma-related, 72
  aminoglycosides-related, 59
  autoimmune, as dizziness cause, 47–48
  chemotherapy-related, 242
  in children, 20–21, 23, 336
    relationship to parental hearing loss, 337
  choanal atresia associated with, 332
  conductive, 12, **21–24**
    air-bone gap in, 16–17
    cleft palate-related, 340
    differentiated from sensorineural hearing loss,
      16
    evaluation of, 21–22
    glomus tumor-related, 69
    perilymphatic fistula-related, 65
    temporal bone trauma-related, 315, 316, 319
  Down syndrome-related, 338
  frequency-loss, 67
  hereditary, 24, 25, 26–27, 336–337
  ossicular dysfunction-related, 46
  ototoxic, 26, 59
  perinatal, 336
  postlingual, 32
  postnatal, 336
  prelingual, 32
  prenatal congenital, 336
  sensorineural, 13, **24–28**
    in children, 336
    differentiated from conductive hearing loss, 16,
      429
    evaluation of, 24
    hearing aid use in, 31
    hereditary, 24, 25, 26–27
    Meniere's disease-related, 53
    perilymphatic fistula-related, 65
    skull-base surgery-related, 75
    sudden, 27–28
    temporal bone trauma-related, 315, 316, 319
    sporadic, recurrence risk of, 337
    viral infection-related, 54–55
Heart disease, choanal atresia associated with, 332
Heart failure, fever-related, 419–420
Helium-oxygen treatment, of upper airway
    obstruction, 299
Hemangioma
  in children, 192, 227, 324
  of middle ear, 69
  parotid, 192
  sinonasal, 204
  strawberry, 227
  subglottic, 331
Hematemesis, 295

Hematologic disorders, as fever cause, 421
Hematoma
  auricular, untreated, 34
  blepharoplasty-related, 267
  of nasal septum, 83, 291
  neck trauma-related, 295
  otoplasty-related, 273
  parotid surgery-related, 192
  retrobulbar, blepharoplasty-related, 267
  rhytidectomy-related, 279
  subglottic, in infants, 322
  subperichondrial, 34
Hemiplegia, 75
Hemodialysis, as epistaxis cause, 287
Hemophilia, as epistaxis cause, 287
Hemoptysis
  bronchoscopic evaluation of, 178–179
  esophageal cancer-related, 218
  hoarseness associated with, 151
  neck penetrating trauma-related, 295
Hemorrhage
  during bronchoscopy, 178
  of central nervous system, as dizziness cause, 47
  as fever cause, 421
  as hypovolemic shock cause, 413
  intracranial, skull-base surgery-related, 75
  retrobulbar, 373
  subconjunctival, 377
  during trachcotomy, 399
  upper airway obstruction-related, 297
Hemostasis, primary, assessment of, 395
Hemothorax, in trauma patients, 284
Hemotympanum, 58
  flying or diving-related, 65–66
  idiopathic, 45
  temporal bone trauma-related, 316
Henry's law, 62
Hepatitis, 394, 421
Hereditary disorders, **333–338**. *See also* specific
    disorders
Hernia, hiatal, 134
Herpes infections, 163, 252
Herpes simplex infections, 119, 326
Herpes zoster infections, in AIDS patients, 155
Herpes zoster ophthalmicus, 377
Herpes zoster oticus. *See* Ramsay Hunt syndrome
Hetastarch, 382
Heterotopic tumors, esophageal, 217
Hexetidine, effect on taste, 347
Hiatus semilunaris, 90–91
High-fat diet, as metabolic acidosis cause, 387
Hilger facial nerve stimulator, 70
His, six hillocks of, 34
Histiocytoma, fibrous laryngeal, 208
Histiocytosis, 68, 125, 205
Histoplasmosis, 153, 156, 186
Hitselberger's sign, 73
Hoarseness, **149–152**
  esophageal cancer-related, 218
  laryngeal cancer-related, 211
  laryngitis-related, 162
  neck penetrating trauma-related, 295

Hoarseness (*cont.*)
  thyroidectomy-related, 225
  upper airway obstruction-related, 297
Hodgkin's disease, 186, 217
Home sleep studies, for obstructive sleep apnea
    evaluation, 145
Homografts, use in rhinoplasty, 261
Hopkins rod, 177, 429
Horseradish, as mucolytic agent, 104
House, Bill, 429
House, Howard, 429
Howarth, Walter, 429
Human immunodeficiency virus (HIV) infection
  blood transfusion-related, 394
  in utero transmission of, 153
  sinusitis associated with, 100
  wasting syndrome of, 153
Human papillomavirus, 194
  as cutaneous squamous cell carcinoma cause, 231
  as esophageal cancer cause, 218
  as sinonasal papilloma cause, 205
Human T-cell leukemia virus, 394
Humidification, as upper airway obstruction
    therapy, 298
Hürthle cell tumor, 223
Hyaluronate injections, as temporomandibular
    disorders treatment, 115
Hygroma, cystic, 227, 330
Hyoid bone
  in deep space neck infections, 141, 143
  low-lying, as obstructive sleep apnea risk factor,
    146
Hyoid suspension, as obstructive sleep apnea
    treatment, 147
Hyperadrenocorticoid states, as metabolic alkalosis
    cause, 388
Hyperbilirubinemia, as pediatric hearing loss risk
    factor, 21
Hypercalcemia, 137
Hypercapnia, total parenteral nutrition-related, 392
Hyperglycemia, total parenteral nutrition-related,
    391
Hypernatremia, in intensive care unit patients,
    383
Hyperparathyroidism, 137
Hypersensitivity reactions, 86, 350, 351
Hypertension
  decongestant rebound-related, 67
  as dizziness cause, 48
  skull-base surgery-related, 75
Hyperthermia
  distinguished from fever, 419
  malignant, 365–366, 369, 370, 419, 421
  treatment of, 420
Hyperthyroidism
  as fever cause, 421
  most common cause of, 136
  thyroid nodule-related, 224
Hypertrophy, obstructive adenoid, 327
Hyperventilation
  mechanical ventilation-related, 403
  psychogenic, 385, 386

Hyphema, 372
  as orbital fracture surgical repair
    contraindication, 373
Hypnotherapy, for tinnitus, 61
Hypnotics, as tinnitus cause, 59
Hypoglossal nerve, in submandibular resection, 138
Hypoglycemia
  as dizziness cause, 48
  total parenteral nutrition-related, 391
Hypokalemia
  as metabolic alkalosis cause, 388
  as respiratory acidosis cause, 385
Hypomagnesemia, as metabolic alkalosis cause, 388
Hyponatremia, 383, 386
Hypopharynx, 193–194
  cancer of, 197, 238
  foreign bodies in, in children, 323
  penetrating trauma to, 295
Hypoplasia, genital, choanal atresia associated, 332
Hyposmia, 346
Hypotension
  anaphylactic shock-related, 353
  metabolic acidosis-related, 386–387
  positive-pressure ventilation-related, 403
Hypothalamic disorders, as hyperthermia cause, 419
Hypothyroidism, 87, 347
Hypoventilation, mechanical ventilation-related,
    403
Hypovitaminoses, as epistaxis cause, 287
Hypovolemia, clinical indicators of, 382
Hypoxemia, as respiratory alkalosis cause, 386
Hypoxia
  as intraoperative tachycardia cause, 369
  as lactic acidosis cause, 388
  mechanical ventilation and, 403, 404
  upper airway obstruction treatment in, 301

Ileostomy, as metabolic acidosis cause, 387
Illicit drugs, as dizziness cause, 48
Imipenem, 160
Imipramine, as taste and smell disorders cause, 348
Immittance measurement, 18, 19, 20
Immune complexes, 351
Immunocompromised patients. *See also* Acquired
    immunodeficiency syndrome (AIDS); Human
    immunodeficiency virus (HIV) infections
  dysphagia in, 135
  hospitalized, rhinosinusitis in, 143
  odynophagia in, 135
  oral candidiasis in, 120
  sinusitis in, 100, 105
Immunoglobulin E, in allergic response, 350, 351,
    352
Immunology, of allergies, 350–353
Immunosuppression, as cutaneous squamous cell
    carcinoma cause, 231
Immunotherapy, 88, 105, 352
Incisions
  in nasal fracture reduction, 291, 292
  infections of, 422
  Lynch, in ethmoidectomy, 111
  in rhinoplasty, 257

Incisor teeth, relationship to esophageal landmarks, 173
Incudostapedial joint, in temporal bone trauma, 319
Incus
    anatomy of, 9
    in temporal bone trauma, 319
Indigo carmine/saccharin sodium test, 81–82
Infants
    airway obstruction in, 322
    cardiopulmonary resuscitation in, 408
    cleft lip/palate in, 339
    hearing aids for, 32
    nasal breathing by, 321
    otitis media in, 41
Infarcts, of central nervous system, as dizziness cause, 47
Infection
    as facial paralysis cause, 125
    as fever cause, 421
    mechanical ventilation-related, 403, 404
    as respiratory alkalosis cause, 386
    as rhinitis cause, 86
    as sensorineural hearing loss cause, 27, 28
    as third spacing cause, 383
    of wounds, 396, 397, 421
Infectious disease
    as fever of unknown origin cause, 423
    as jaw mass cause, 200
Infectious mononucleosis, 125
Inflammatory bowel disease, 421
Inflammatory disorders
    differential diagnosis of, 114
    as fever cause, 421
    as jaw mass cause, 200
Infundibulum, in sinus drainage, 107
Inhalants, adverse effects of, 61, 86
Injections, intramuscular, as fever cause, 421
Inner ear. *See also* Cochlea
    anatomy and physiology of, 10–12
    barotrauma to, 66–67
    congenital anomalies of, 361–362
    traumatic injury to, as dizziness cause, 47–48
    viral infections of, 54–55
Innominate artery
    anomalous, 186
    location in mediastinum, 182
    mediastinoscopy-related injury to, 184
    as tracheal blood supply source, 214
Inotropes, as shock therapy, 418
Intensive care unit (ICU) patients
    fever in, **418–423**
    sinusitis in, 101–102, 106
    tracheotomy in, 400, 401
Intercostal artery, as tracheal blood supply source, 214
Intermaxillary fixation. *See* Maxillomandibular fixation
Interposed abdominal counterpulsation, 412
Intracranial neoplasms, myoclonus associated with, 59
Intracranial pressure elevation
    mechanical ventilation-related, 403
    as respiratory acidosis cause, 385

Intraosseous carcinoma, 200, 203
Intravascular lines
    as fever cause, 422
    for total parenteral nutrition delivery, 391
Intravenous drug abusers, deep space neck infections in, 141
Intravenous fluids, electrolyte composition of, 382
Intubation
    endotracheal
        in children, 321, 323, 324–325, 406, 407
        complications of, 300–301, 403, 405–406
        for laser surgery, 367
        long-term, 405–406
        with RAE tubes, 367
        for resuscitation medications administration, 411
        safe time limit for, 407
        tube placement confirmation in, 368
        tube sizes for, 407
        in upper airway obstruction, 298, 299
    nasogastric, in trauma patients, 285, 286
    nasotracheal, 300
        in trauma patients, 283
    orotracheal, 299–300
        in trauma patients, 283
Iodine, as total parenteral nutrition component, 391
Iodine deficiency, total parenteral nutrition-related, 392
Ipratropium bromide, as rhinitis treatment, 89
Ipsilateral acoustic reflex neural pathway, 19
Iris constrictor mechanism, injury to, 371
Iritis, 377
Iron, as total parenteral nutrition component, 391
Irrigation
    of ear
        for foreign body removal, 36–37
        for impacted cerumen removal, 36
    sinonasal
        in HIV-infected patients, 155
        as sinusitis therapy, 102, 104
Ischemia, fever-related, 419–420
Ischemic heart disease, 416
Isoflurane, as intraoperative tachycardia cause, 369
Isoniazid, as lactic acidosis cause, 388
Isosporiasis, as AIDS indicator disease, 153
Isotretinoin, as head and neck cancer prophylaxis, 242
Itraconazole, 163

Jackson-Weiss syndrome, 337
Jacobsen's neurectomy, 192
Jacobson's nerve, 62
Jacobson's organ, 82
Jafek, Bruce W., 429
Janeway, Edward, 428
Jaw. *See also* Mandible; Maxilla
    cysts, tumors and lesions of, **200–204**
Jaw thrust technique, for airway management, 283
Joseph, Jacques, 429
Jugular bulb, dehiscent, presenting as middle ear tumor, 69
Jugular foramen, tumors of, 69

Jugular foramen syndrome, 69
Jugular vein
    anomalies of, as tinnitus cause, 362
    internal, 142

Kallmann's syndrome, 346–347
Kaposi's sarcoma, 153, 154, 156
    esophageal, 217
    of eyelids, 377
    of head and neck, 236
Kartagener's syndrome, 81
Keen, W. W., 428
Keloids, 36, 397
Keratitis
    exposure, facial nerve palsy-related, 377
    obturans, 35
Keratoacanthoma, 232
Keratocyst, odontogenic, 194, 200, 201, 203
Keratoses
    actinic, 229–230
        as skin resurfacing indication, 251, 252
    seborrheic, 229
Ketoacidosis, 375, 387
Ketoconazole, 162, 164
Kiesselbach's plexus, 287
Killian's triangle, 131
Kirchner, John, 429
KITTENS mnemonic, for neck mass differential
    diagnosis, 196
Klebsiella infections, as septic shock cause,
    415–416
Kussmaul's respirations, 387
Küstner, Otto, 350

Labyrinth
    membranous
        anatomy of, 10
        concussive injury to, 318
        vestibular, massive injury to, 318
Labyrinthectomy, 54, 70
Labyrinthine window, fistula of, in divers, 66
Labyrinthitis, 39, 47–48
Lacrimal collection system injury, 314, 376
Lacrimal duct, blockage of, 205
Lagophthalmos, 263, 267
Lag screws, in mandibular fracture fixation, 306
Laryngeal cancer, **208–213**
    hoarseness associated with, 150
    radiation therapy for, 238, 239
    relationship to lung cancer, 212
    staging system for, 210, 211–212
Laryngeal mirror, 5
Laryngeal nerve
    endotracheal intubation-related injury to, 301
    nonrecurrent, 225
    recurrent, injury to, 225, 399
    recurrent paralysis of, as pediatric airway
        obstruction cause, 323
    superior
        anesthesia of, 170
        injury to, 211, 225
        nerve block of, 177

Laryngeal tumors, cutaneous hemangioma-related,
    227
Laryngeal webs, congenital, 322
Laryngectomy
    blood units required for, 393
    first performance of, 429
    horizontal supraglottic, 212
    near-total, 212
    total, 213, 239
    voice rehabilitation following, 429
Laryngitis, 150, 162
Laryngocardiac reflex, 171
Laryngocele, 209
Laryngology, 425
Laryngomalacia, 322, 331
Laryngoscope, 171, 172
Laryngoscopy, **169–172**
    anesthesia use in, 169, 170, 171
    direct, 169, 171–172
        for laryngeal cancer evaluation, 211
    fiberoptic, 6, 7, 169
    indirect, 169
Laryngospasm, 171, 384
Larynx
    aerodynamic ability of, 171
    anatomic divisions of, 209
    dyskinesia of, 298
    edema of, 152, 174, 175, 252
    first visualization of, 425
    foreign bodies in, in children, 323
    fractures of, as airway obstruction cause, 297,
        323
    innervation of, 151
    lymphatic drainage of, 212
    obstruction of, 296
    papillomas of, 151
    polyps of, 151
    swallowing-related elevation of, 131–132
    trauma to
        blunt trauma, 295
        as endotracheal intubation contraindication,
            299
        intubation-related, 406
        mechanical ventilation-related, 405, 406
        penetrating trauma, 295
        stents for management of, 296
Laser, definition of, 253
Laser surgery
    anesthesia for, 367
    for skin resurfacing, 253
    as tracheal tumor treatment, 215
Latissimus dorsi myocutaneous free flap, 248, 250
Lavage. *See* Irrigation
Lead intoxication, 138
Leatherworking, as sinonasal cancer cause, 206
LeFort fractures, classification of, 309–310
Legionella infections, 160
Leiomyoma, esophageal, 217
Lentigo maligna melanoma, 234
Letterer-Siwe disease, 205
Leukemia
    ear involvement in, 68

Leukemia (*cont.*)
  as epistaxis cause, 287
  as facial paralysis cause, 125
  as fever of unknown origin cause, 423
  of temporal bone and external ear canal, 68
Leukoplakia, 121, 195
  hairy, 121
    in HIV-infected patients, 155
Levator veli palatini muscle
  in cleft lip/palate, 341
  in eustachian tube dilatation, 67
Levodopa, effect on taste and smell, 348
Lichen planus, 195
Lidocaine
  in cardiopulmonary resuscitation, 411
  co-administration with epinephrine, 167, 170, 254
  in laryngoscopy, 170
  pharmacology of, 167, 366
  as tinnitus therapy, 60
  toxic doses of, 367
Light reflex, otologic, 6
Lindsey, John, 429
Lingual nerve, in submandibular resection, 138
Lingual thyroid carcinoma, 223
Lip(s)
  cleft. *See* Cleft lip/palate
  examination of, 5
Lipectomy, suction, in facial rejuvenation, 279
Lipoma, 74, 217
Liposarcoma, malignant, 186
Lithium carbonate, effect on taste and smell, 348
Little's area, 287
Liver failure, as lactic acidosis cause, 388
Lobectomy, thyroid, 225
Local anesthetics, 366–367
  as anaphylactic shock cause, 352–353
  for rhinoplasty, 254
  toxic doses of, 366
Lop ear deformity, 335
Loré, John, 429
Lung
  contusions of, 284
  divisions of, 178
  edema of, 300, 400
  translobar biopsy of, 180
Lung cancer
  lymphatic drainage in, 183
  mediastinoscopic evaluation of, 181–187
  relationship to laryngeal cancer, 212
  resectability of, preoperative tests for, 184
  squamous cell, 170, 179
  staging of, 184–185
Lung tumors, as vocal cord paralysis cause, 152
Lyme disease, 125
Lymphadenopathy, thyroid, 222
Lymphangioma, 324, 330
Lymphatic drainage
  endolaryngeal, 212
  pulmonary, 183
Lymphatics, of nose and paranasal sinuses, 80
Lymph nodes
  elective dissection of, 236

Lymph nodes (*cont.*)
  in HIV-infected patients, 156
  malignancy of, imaging of, 360
  in malignant melanoma, 234
  mediastinoscopic biopsy of, 183–184, 185, 187
  ten classic groups of, 6
Lymphoepithelial disease, of salivary glands, 138, 139, 189
Lymphoma
  as AIDS indicator disease, 153
  as epistaxis cause, 287
  esophageal, 217
  as fever of unknown origin cause, 423
  mediastinoscopic evaluation of, 186
  non-Hodgkin's, in HIV-infected patients, 153, 156
Lymphoproliferative cancer, esophageal, 217
Lynch incision, in ethmoidectomy, 111
Lyre sign, of carotid body tumors, 228
Lysozyme, 81

Mackenzie, Morell, 425, 428, 429
Macroglossia, Down syndrome-related, 369
Macrolides, 160, 162
Magnetic resonance angiography (MRA)
  of carotid paraganglioma, 358
  of temporal bone trauma, 362
Magnetic resonance imaging (MRI)
  of acoustic neuroma, 73
  for brachial plexopathy evaluation, 364
  of branchial cysts, 359
  of carotid artery metastases, 361
  for cerebrospinal fluid rhinorrhea evaluation, 363
  of congenital ear malformations, 361–362
  for facial paralysis evaluation, 126
  of juvenile angiofibroma, 365
  of laryngeal cancer, 211
  of neck cancer, 360
  of paraganglioma, 357
  of parapharyngeal space, 354–355
  of pediatric airway obstruction, 324
  of rhabdomyosarcoma, 361
  of salivary gland tumors, 189
  of sinonasal tumors, 206
  for sinusitis evaluation, 100
  of temporal bone trauma, 316–317, 362
  for temporomandibular disease evaluation, 116
  for tinnitus evaluation, 60, 362
  of vestibular lesions, 52
Malar bone, fractures of, 310
Malignant melanoma. *See* Melanoma
Mallampati classification system, for posterior pharyngeal visualization, 368
Malleolar folds, anatomy of, 2
Malleus
  anatomy of, 9
  fractures of, 319
Mandible
  fractures of, 114, **302–309**
    body, 302, 303, 304, 306
    open reduction and fixation of, 305–306, 307, 308
    as pediatric airway obstruction cause, 323

Mandible (*cont.*)
  muscle groups of, 303
  hypermobility of, 114
  hypomobility of, 114
  osteomyelitis of, 356
  penetrating trauma to, 294
  reconstruction of, 204, 250
Mandibular angle plane, 294
Mandibular nerve, 304
  marginal, in submandibular resection, 138
Mandibular positioning devices, as obstructive sleep
    apnea treatment, 147
Mandibulectomy, blood units required for, 393
Manganese, as total parenteral nutrition component,
    391
Manganese deficiency, total parenteral nutrition-
    related, 392
Manubrium, anatomy of, 2
Marcus Gunn pupil, 371
Marfanoid habitus, 223
Masking
  in hearing evaluations, 15–16
  of tinnitus, 60
Masseter muscle, 303, 356
  in mandibular fractures, 304
  rigidity of, malignant hyperthermia-related, 370
  in temporomandibular disorders, 114
Mast cells, in allergic response, 350
Masticator space, 356
Mastoidectomy
  blood units required for, 393
  as conductive hearing loss treatment, 24
  as malignant otitis externa treatment, 35
Mastoiditis
  antibiotic therapy for, 162
  causal organisms of, 40, 155
  definition of, 39
  as facial paralysis cause, 125, 129
  Pneumocystis carinii, 155
Maxilla, fractures of, 114
Maxilla cancer, of Grover Cleveland, 427
Maxillary artery, ligation of, for epistaxis
    management, 290
Maxillectomy
  blood units required for, 393
  intraoral partial, performed on Grover Cleveland,
    428
Maxillofacial trauma, imaging evaluation of, 311–312
Maxillomandibular fixation, 305, 306
  in edentulous patients, 307
Maxillomandibular growth disorders, 114
Maximal stimulation test (MST), 127
Maximum surgical blood order schedule (MSBOS),
    393
Mecca position, 104
Mechanical ventilation, **402–407**
  failure of, as respiratory acidosis cause, 385
  indications for, 402
  as respiratory alkalosis cause, 386
  risks of, 385, 386, 403, 404, 405–406
  ventilator modes in, 402–403
  weaning from, 404

Mechanical ventilation patients, parenteral
    nutritional formula for, 391
Medial canthal tendon, disruption and repair of,
    313, 314
Medial crural strut graft, 258
Mediastinoscopy, **181–187**
Mediastinum
  divisions of, 182
  superior, vascular anomalies of, 186
Mediastinitis, 143
Medullary carcinoma, thyroid, 223, 224
Melanoma
  of auricle, 68
  clinical subdivisions of, 234
  cutaneous, 233–237
  in Franklin D. Roosevelt, 427
  metastatic, 208, 235, 236–237
  mucosal
    differentiated from cutaneous melanoma, 237
    esophageal, 217
    of oral cavity, 121
    sinonasal, 205
  staging of, 234–235
Melkersson-Rosenthal syndrome, 125
Ménière's disease, 53–54
  allergy and, 353
  as dizziness cause, 48
  as hearing loss cause, 24
  streptomycin therapy for, ototoxicity of, 166
  as tinnitus cause, 61
  vascular loop and, 57
Ménière's triad, 53–54
Meningioma
  of cerebellopontine angle, 74, 362
  as facial paralysis cause, 125
  of petrous apex, 69
  as vertigo cause, 56
Meningitis
  cerebrospinal fluid leak-related, 318, 320
  as fever cause, 421, 423
  as hearing loss cause, 21, 28, 336
  recurrent, head trauma-related, 317–318
  septal abscess-related, 293
  sinusitis-related, 101
  skull-base surgery-related, 75
Meniscal displacement, 115
Menstruation, as nasal congestion cause, 86
MEN syndromes (multiple endocrine neoplasia
    syndromes), 137, 223
Mental nerve, 304
Mepivacaine, 366, 367
Mercury intoxication, 138
Mesenchymal tumors, esophageal, 217
Metabolic disorders
  as facial paralysis cause, 125
  as fever cause, 421
Metastases, 74
  to esophagus, 217
  of head and neck cancer, 241
    as jaw mass cause, 200
    of laryngeal cancer, 208, 209–210
    mediastinoscopic evaluation of, 186

Metastases (*cont.*)
  of head and neck cancer (*cont.*)
    of melanoma, 235
    of oropharyngeal cancer, 196–197
    of sinonasal cancer, 207
Methimazole, effect on taste and smell, 348
Methionine, as metabolic acidosis cause, 387
Methotrexate, 241, 242
α-Methyldopa, as fever cause, 421
Metronidazole, 161, 162
  effect on taste and smell, 347–348
Microscopic surgery, 429
Microsomia, hemifacial, 269
Microtia, 36, 331
Microtia reconstruction otoplasty, 273
Midarm muscle circumference, 389
Middle ear
  anatomy and physiology of, 9–10
  congenital aural atresia-related anomalies of, 71
  diseases of, **43–47**
    as conductive hearing loss cause, 22–23
    effusions from, 41, 43, 61
    glomus tumors of, 69
    nitrous oxide use in, 367
    temporal bone fracture-related hemorrhage in,
      315, 319
Middle fossa approach, to cerebellopontine angle,
    74–75
Midface
  buttress system of, 309
  fractures of, **309–314**
Migraine, 48, 55–56, 99
Milia, 252, 267
Millard rotation-advancement repair, for cleft lip,
    341
Minutiae, in otolaryngology, **425–430**
Mirror
  head, 4
  laryngeal, 5
  nasopharyngeal, 5
Mitomycin-C, 241, 242
Mobius syndrome, 71, 125, 128
Moh's micrographic surgery, 230–231
Molluscum contagiosum, of eyelids and face, 377
Molybdenum deficiency, total parenteral nutrition-
    related, 392
Monitors, use in trauma patients, 285
Moraxella infections
  antibiotic therapy for, 159–161
  otitis media as, 40, 41
  sinusitis as, 97
  tonsillitis as, 326
Morocco, ear and nose disease prevention ritual in,
    426
Motion sickness, 56, 166
Mouthwash, as taste disorder cause, 347
Mucocele
  definition of, 101, 122
  of petrous apex, 69
  sinusitis-related, 100, 106
Mucociliary flow, measurement of, 81–82
Mucoepidermoid carcinoma, 189, 192, 208

Mucolytics, as sinusitis therapy, 102, 104
Mucormycosis, 168, 375
Mucositis, radiation therapy-related, 242
Mucous blanket, paranasal, 81, 94
Mucous clearance, from sinuses, 94
Mucous plugging, of tracheotomy, 399, 400
Mucous transport time (MTT), 82
Müller's maneuver, 145
Müller's muscle, 265
Multiple endocrine neoplasia (MEN) syndromes,
    137, 223
Multiple sclerosis, 24, 27, 59, 346
Multiple sleep latency test (MSLT), 145
Mumps, as parotitis cause, 138–139
Muscle relaxants, as temporomandibular disorder
    pain therapy, 116
Muscular dystrophy, 385
Mustardé technique, of otoplasty, 271
Mutations, autosomal dominant, 333–334
Myasthenia gravis, 346, 385
Mycobacterial infections, disseminated, 153
Mycoplasma infections, antibiotic therapy for, 160
Myeloma, as epistaxis cause, 287
Mylohyoid muscle, in mandibular fractures, 303,
    304
Myocardial infarction, as fever cause, 420, 421
Myoclonus, palatal, 59
Myofunctional pain dysfunction (MPD), 114
Myogenic pain, temporomandibular disorders-
    related, 114–115, 116–117
Myokymia, facial, 130
Myoma, esophageal, 217
Myopathy, as malignant hyperthermia cause, 366
Myringitis, 39
Myringoplasty, 24
Myringosclerosis, 39
Myringotomy, 41
  blood units required for, 393
  origin of, 426
  as otitis media-related hearing loss treatment, 23
Myringotomy tubes, use during air travel, 63
Myxoma, odontogenic, 200, 203

N0 neck, 199, 213
Nafcillin, 162
Naloxone, use in cardiopulmonary resuscitation,
    411
Narcotics
  as respiratory acidosis cause, 385
  as temporomandibular disorder pain therapy, 116
  as tinnitus cause, 59
Nare, anterior, 79
Nasal adhesions, postoperative, 85
Nasal aesthetic units, 256
Nasal base, rhinoplastic reduction of, 259
Nasal bones, 78
  fractures of, 290–292, 293
Nasal cartilage, 78, 79
Nasal cavity
  anatomy of, 108
  cancer of, 206
  cultures of, 380

Nasal congestion
  acute bacterial sinusitis-related, 98
  during menstruation, 86
  during pregnancy, 87
Nasal continuous positive airway pressure, as
    obstructive sleep apnea treatment, 147
Nasal culture, for sinusitis diagnosis, 99
Nasal cycle, 82
Nasal deformity, cleft lip/palate-related, 342, 343
Nasal hump, dorsal, rhinoplasty of, 254, 259
Nasal length, rhinoplastic reduction of, 259
Nasal lobules, volume reduction of, 259
Nasal obstruction
  iatrogenic, as pediatric airway obstruction cause,
    323
  measurement of, 82
Nasal reflex, 80
Nasal septum
  abnormalities of, **83–86**
  abscess of, 292–293
  anatomy of, 83
  cancer of, 206
  deviated, as rhinitis cause, 87
  hematoma of, 29
  orbital, 376
  surgery-related nasal adhesions of, 85
Nasal sill, relationship to sphenoid sinus, 95
Nasal sprays, as sinusitis therapy, 102
Nasal submucosal vascular plexus, 81
Nasal surgery, as obstructive sleep apnea treatment,
    148
Nasal tip
  deformities of, cleft lip/palate-associated,
    343
  poorly defined, rhinoplastic alteration, 254
  projection of, 255
    measurement of, 258
  in rhinoplasty, 257–258
  rotation of, 255
    upward, 258
  volume of, 255
Nasal tripod, 258
  fractures of, 310, 312
Nasal valve, 79
Nasal vestibule, 79
Nasion, 79, 255
Nasolabial angle, rhinoplastic alteration of, 259
Nasolabial fold, 275
Naso-orbito-ethmoid region, fractures of, 313
Nasopharyngeal airway, for airway management,
    283
Nasopharyngeal mirror, 5
Nasopharyngoscope, for tinnitus evaluation, 60
Nasopharyngoscopy, 156, 297
Nasopharynx, 194
  anatomy of, 193–194
  cultures of, 380
  obstruction of, 296
Nasopharynx cancer, 196
  of petrous apex, 69
  radiation treatment of, 238
  staging of, 197

Nausea
  chemotherapy-related, 242
  postoperative, 365
NAVEL mnemonic, for endotracheal resuscitation
    drug administration, 411
Neck. *See also* Head and neck; Head and neck
    cancer; Head and neck surgery
  anatomic divisions of, 294
  blunt trauma to, 295
  deep space infections of, **141–144**
  dissection of
    blood units required for, 393
    in cervical esophageal carcinoma, 220
    in oropharyngeal cancer, 199
    in salivary gland cancer, 193
  N0 cervical node status of, 199, 213
  oropharyngeal metastases of, 196, 197
  penetrating trauma to, **293–296**
  as sinonasal cancer metastases site, 207
Neck mass
  bronchoscopic evaluation of, 178–179
  congenital, differential diagnosis of, 329
  malignant, imaging of, 360
  midline anterior, preoperative imaging of, 332
  solitary, 196
Neck pain, whiplash-associated, 57
Neck veins, in hypovolemic shock, 414
Needlestick exposure, from HIV-positive patients,
    156
Neisseria gonorrhoeae infections, 160
Neomycin
  as external auditory canal treatment, 167
  ototoxicity of, 55
Nephrotic syndrome, 413
Nerve compression, as hoarseness cause, 151–152
Nerve excitability test (NET), 126
Nerve injury
  as hoarseness cause, 152
  pathophysiology of, 124–125
Nerve sheath tumors, of jugular foramen, 69
Neural transmission impairment, as sensorineural
    hearing loss cause, 25
Neurapraxia, 124
Neurectomy
  Jacobsen's, 192
  vidian, 89, 90
Neuritis, vestibular, 54
Neurodegenerative diseases, olfactory disorders
    associated with, 346
Neurofibromatosis, 73, 337
Neurogenic tumors, mediastinoscopic evaluation of,
    186
Neurolabyrinthitis, 48, 54
Neuroleptic malignant syndrome, 419
Neuroleptics, as dizziness cause, 48
Neurologic examination
  for dizziness evaluation, 49
  for sensorineural hearing loss evaluation, 25
  in trauma patients, 285
Neuroma
  acoustic, 72–73
    of cerebellopontine angle, 74, 362

Neuroma (*cont.*)
  acoustic (*cont.*)
    as dizziness and vertigo cause, 48, 56
    neurofibromatosus-related, 337
    radiosurgical treatment of, 75–76
    as sudden sensorineural hearing loss cause, 27, 28
    as taste dysfunction cause, 347
    as tinnitus cause, 60
  mucosal, 223
Neuro-otology, **68–76**, 429
Neuropathy, traumatic optic, 372
Neurotmesis, 125
Nevus
  familial dysplastic, 235–236
  flammeus, 227
Nickel exposure, as sinonasal cancer cause, 206
Nicotine, as respiratory alkalosis cause, 386
Nifedipine, effect on taste and smell, 347
Nitrogen balance, 390
Nitrous oxide, use in middle ear, 367
Nodules
  thyroid, 222, 223–224
  of vocal cords, 150, 152
Noise, as hearing loss cause, 24, 25
  occupational dB A scale for, 25–26
Nonsteroidal anti-inflammatory drugs
  as anaphylactic shock cause, 352–353
  as epistaxis cause, 287
  as fever therapy, 420
  ototoxicity of, 59
  as temporomandibular disorders therapy, 115, 116
Norepinephrine, as shock therapy, 418
Nose. *See also* Nasal entries
  aesthetic units of, 256
  anatomy and physiology of, **77–83**, 255–256
  basal view of, 255
  congenital malformations of, 332
  "danger triangle" of, 79
  dorsal profile of, 255
  embryological development of, 77, 78
  examination of, 3, 4
    in divers, 67
  external
    anatomy and development of, 77
    examination of, 4
  functions of, 80
  innervation of, 80
  internal
    anatomy and development of, 78–79
    examination of, 4
  inverting papillomas of, 84, 204–205, 207
  mucous blanket of, 81, 94
  obstruction of, 296
  polyps of, 353–354
    inverting papilloma misdiagnosed as, 204
  proportional relationship to face, 255
  soft triangle of, 257
  traumatic injury to, **290–293**
    as pediatric airway obstruction cause, 323
  tumors of, **204–208**
  vascular supply to, 79

Nose bleeds. *See* Epistaxis
Nutritional assessment and therapy, **389–392**
  of head and neck chemotherapy patients, 242
  of tracheotomy patients, 401
Nylén, Carl Olof, 429
Nystagmus
  benign positional, differentiated from static positional nystagmus, 52
  direction of, 52
  Dix-Hallpike maneuver associated with, 50
  positional, 49, 52
  temporal bone trauma-related, 316
Nystain, 163

Obesity, as obstructive sleep apnea risk factor, 147, 144
Obtundation, skull-base surgery-related, 75
Occlusion effect, of hearing aids, 31
Occupational exposure, as sinonasal cancer cause, 206
Odontoma, 200, 203
Odontosarcoma, 200, 203
Odynophagia
  esophageal candidiasis-related, 155
  hoarseness associated with, 151
  in immunocompromised patients, 135
  neck penetrating trauma-related, 295
Ofloxacin, 160–161
Ogura, Joseph, 429
Ohngren's line, 206
O'Reilly, Robert, 428
Olfaction, **345–349**
  disorders of, 346–349
Olfactory esthesioneuroblastoma, sinonasal, 205
Oncocytoma, of salivary glands, 189
Onodi cells, 95
Ontogenic tumors, adenomatoid, 200, 203
Open reduction and internal fixation (ORIF), of mandibular fractures, 305–306
  in children, 307
  in edentulous patients, 308
Ophthalmic artery, 79
Ophthalmologic examination, pre-blepharoplasty, 263
Ophthalmoscope, for tinnitus evaluation, 60
Optic nerve
  within Onodi cells, 95
  traumatic neuropathy of, 372
Oral cavity
  anatomic structures of, 193
  ENT procedures in, airway management during, 367
  examination of, 5
  flaps for, 248
  lesions of, **118–121**, 195
  lymphatic drainage of, 196–197
  trauma to, as endotracheal intubation contraindication, 299
  tumors of, 194 196
Oral cavity cancer, 120, 121, **193–200**
  metastases of, 196–197
  staging of, 197–198

Oral contraceptives, 87, 166
Orbicularis muscle
    blepharoplasty of, 262, 263
    in cleft lip/palate, 340–341
    hypertrophy of, 262
Orbit
    bones of, 311
    fractures of, 311–314
    injury to, 371
        evaluation by nonophthalmologists, 372
    venous network of, 375
Orbital compartments, fat compartments of, 266
Orbital exenteration, of advanced sinus cancers, 207
Orbital floor
    in blowout fracture repair, 312
    in orbital wall reconstruction, 313
Orbital septum, 376
Orbital wall, blowout fractures of, 311, 312, 314
    teardrop sign of, 312, 373
    timing of repair of, 378
Organ of Corti, 11, 427
Organ of Jacobson, 82
Organ perfusion, in trauma patients, 284
Organ-preservation chemotherapy, 242–243
Oropharyngeal airway, for airway management,
    283
Oropharyngeal examination, 4–5
Oropharynx, 194
    reconstruction of, flaps in, 248
Oscillopsia, 55
Osler-Weber-Rendu disease, 287
Osmotic demyelination syndrome, 383
Osseocutaneous retaining ligaments, 275–276
Ossicles, of middle ear, 9
    deformities of
        as conductive hearing loss cause, 23
        congenital aural atresia-related, 71
    discontinuity of, 23, 24, 46
    dysfunction of, signs and symptoms of, 46
    in temporal bone trauma, 315, 319
Ossicular chain
    fixation of, 46, 319
    lever action of, 10
    reconstruction of, 46
Ossiculoplasty, 24
Osteoblastoma, of jaw, 200
Osteoma
    of auditory canal, differentiated from exostoses,
        35
    of jaw, 194, 200
    of nose, 204
    of sinuses, 204
Osteomeatal complex
    anatomy of, 108
    definition of, 91, 96
    sinus drainage into, 91, 107
    sinusitis-related obstruction of, 103, 105
Osteomyelitis
    of petrous apex, 60
    sinusitis-related, 100, 106
Osteomyocutaneous flaps, 249
Osteosarcoma, as jaw mass cause, 200

Osteotomy
    LeFort I, as obstructive sleep apnea treatment,
        147
    in nasal fracture reduction, 292
    use in rhinoplasty, 260
Ostiomeatal, vs. osteomeatal, 96
Otalgia, 40, 195
Otic capsule, fractures of, incomplete healing of,
    317–318
Otic drops, 167
Otitis externa
    acute, antibiotic therapy for, 163
    allergic, 353
    definition of, 39
    malignant, 35
Otitis media, **39–43**
    acute, 40, 41
        antibiotic therapy for, 161, 167, 380
        HIV infection-related, 154
        vestibular lesion-related, 52
    adenotonsillar hypertrophy-related, 327
    allergic, 353
    causal organisms of, 40
    in children, 40, 167
    chronic, 40
        antibiotic therapy for, 161
        cleft palate-related, 340
        with effusion, 40, 41
        as facial paralysis cause, 125
        tympanic perforations associated with,
            37–38
    collar button tube use in, 429
    definition of, 39
    Down syndrome as risk factor for, 338
    with effusion, 23, 40, 41, 42
    eustachian tube dysfunction-related, 10
    as facial paralysis cause, 125, 129
    HIV infection-related, 154–155
    Pneumocystis carinii, 155
    as sensorineural hearing loss cause, 28
    serous, HIV infection-related, 154
    surgical treatment of, 41
    tymphanogram of, 22
    unilateral, 42
    untreated, 42
Otolaryngologist-head and neck surgeons, training
    of, 1–2
Otolaryngology
    cost-effectivness of, **378–380**
    definition of, 1
    minutiae in, **425–430**
    origin of, 425
    subdivisions of, 1
    subspecializations of, 2
Otologic history, 60
Otology
    fellowships in, 2
    history of, 425
    as otolaryngology subdivision, 1
Otomycosis, 35–36
Otoplasty, **268–274**
Otorhinolaryngology, origin of, 425

Otorrhea
  cerebrospinal fluid, temporal bone fracture-
    related, 316, 317
  otitis media-related, 40
Otosclerosis, 45–46
  as conductive hearing loss cause, 22, 23, 24
  family pedigree of, 337
  as tinnitus cause, 61
Otoscopic examination, 2
Otoscopy, pneumatic, 4
Otosyphilis, 27
Oval window
  fistula of, 70
  rupture of, 64–65
Oxygen therapy, for upper airway obstruction, 298
Ozena, 87–88

Packed red blood cells, 393, 394
  HIV transmission in, 153
Packs, for epistaxis management, 288, 289
Paclitaxel, 241, 242
Palate
  anatomy of, 339
  cleft. See Cleft lip/palate
  mobile, LeFort fracture-related, 310
  myoclonus of, 59
Palatoglossus muscle, 326
  in cleft lip/palate, 341
Palatopharyngeus muscle, 326
  in cleft lip/palate, 341
Palatoplasty, 342
Palliative treatment, for esophageal cancer patients,
    221
Pancreatitis, as fever cause, 421
Pancuronium, as intraoperative tachycardia cause,
    369
Panendoscopy, 196
Panic attacks, 48
Papillary-follicular carcinoma, thyroid, 223
Papilloma
  esophageal, 217
  laryngeal, 151
  respiratory, 215
  sinonasal, inverting, 84, 204–205, 207
  squamous, of oral cavity, 194
Papillomatosis
  juvenile, as laryngeal cancer cause, 209
  recurrent respiratory, as pediatric airway
    obstruction cause, 324
Paraganglioma
  of carotid space, 357
  of middle ear, 69
Paragangliomas. See Glomus tumors
Paraglottic space, 211
Parainfluenza virus, as tonsillitis cause, 326
Parapharyngeal space, 354–355
Parasymphyseal fractures, 302, 303, 304, 306
Parathyroid glands, 136–137
  accidental surgical removal of, 225–226
  adenoma of, 186
  carcinoma of, 226
  identification of, 225

Parenteral nutrition, 390–392
Parkinson's disease, 298, 346
Parotid duct, penetrating trauma to, 294
Parotid gland, 137, 138
  cysts of, 139–140, 155–156
  pleomorphic adenoma of, 355
  traumatic injury to, 140
  tumors of, 191–193
    facial nerve palsy-associated, 189–190
    malignant degeneration of, 192–193
Parotitis, 138–139
Pars flaccida, anatomy of, 2
Partial ossicular reconstruction prosthesis (PORP),
    46–47
Partial pressure of carbon dioxide (PCO$_2$), in
    mechanical ventilation, 404
Partial pressure of oxygen (PO$_2$), in mechanical
    ventilation, 404
Partial thromboplastin time (PTT), in epistaxis
    patients, 289
Passavant's ridge, 325
Patron saints, of otolaryngology, 426
"Pawn broker" sign, 185
PEA (pulseless electrical activity), 411
Pectoralis major flap, 248, 249
PEEP (positive end-expiratory pressure), 403–404
Pendred syndrome, 336
Penetrating trauma, to neck and face, **293–296**
Penicillamine, effect on taste and smell, 348
Penicillin-hypersensitive patients, cephalosporins
    use in, 160
Penicillins
  as anaphylactic shock cause, 352–353
  clinical spectrum of, 159
  interaction with oral contraceptives, 166
  as pharyngitis therapy, 162
Pentamidine, effect on taste and smell, 347–348
Periapical disease, 100
Pericarditis, as fever cause, 421
Perichondritis
  of auricle, 34–35
  of nasal septum, 83
Perilymph, 11
Perilymphatic fistula, 47–48, 55, 64, 65, 67, 318,
    319, 320
Periodontal disease, as sinusitis cause, 100
Periodontitis, in HIV-infected patients, 155
Peripheral nervous system, defects of, as respiratory
    acidosis cause, 384
Peritonitis, as third spacing cause, 383
Peritonsillitis, 427
Petrous apex, lesions of, 69
Peutz-Jeghers disease, 121
Pfeiffer syndrome, 337
Phantosomia, 346
Pharmacology, of otolaryngology, **164–168**. See
    also specific drugs
Pharyngectomy, pharynx resection following, 199
Pharyngitis, antibiotic therapy for, 161, 162
Pharynx
  anatomy of, 193–194
  lymphatic drainage of, 196–197

Pharynx (*cont.*)
  obstruction of, 296
  posterior, Mallampati classification of, 368, 369
  premalignant lesions of, 195
  resection of, following pharyngectomy, 199
Pharynx cancer, 194–195, 196–199
  metastases of, 196
  staging of, 197–198
Pheochromocytoma, 223, 419
Phobias, 48
Photoaging, of skin, 251
Photoglottography, 171
Photothermolysis, laser selective, 251
Physical therapy, as temporomandibular disorders
    therapy, 115
Pickwickian syndrome, 144, 145
Pierre Robin sequence, 334, 335
Pindborg tumor, 200, 203
Plasma, osmolality of, 382
Plastic surgery, facial, 1, 280, 429
Platelet count, 395
Platelets, 393, 394
Platysma ligament, 275–276
Platysma muscle, 276, 303
  in rhytidectomy, 278, 279
Plica sublingualis, 138
Pliny, 426
Plummer's disease, 136
Plummer-Vinson syndrome, 133, 194, 218
Pneumocephalus, 75, 318
Pneumococcus, amoxicillin-resistant strains of, 380
Pneumococcal infections
  antibiotic therapy for, 159, 160
  HIV infection-associated, 155
  septic shock as, 416
Pneumocystis carinii infections
  mastoiditis as, 155
  otitis media as, 155
  pneumonia as, as AIDS indicator disease, 153, 154
Pneumonia
  aspiration, enteral nutrition-related, 390
  as fever cause, 421, 422
  mechanical ventilation-related, 404, 422
  Pneumocystis carinii, 153, 154
Pneumothorax
  mechanical ventilation-related, 403
  as respiratory acidosis cause, 384
  total parenteral nutrition-related, 392
  in trauma patients, 284
Pneumotoscopy, for tinnitus evaluation, 60
Politzer, Adam, 425
Pollybeak deformity, 260
Polychondritis, 85
Polyenes, 163
Polymyositis, 133
Polyps
  esophageal, 217
  of large bowel, Gardner's syndrome-related, 194
  laryngeal, 151
  sinonasal, 353–354
    inverting papilloma misdiagnosed as, 204
  of vocal cords, 152

Polysomnography, for obstructive sleep apnea
    evaluation, 145
PORP (partial ossicular reconstruction prosthesis),
    46–47
Port-wine stain, 227
Positive airway pressure, inspiratory and expiratory
    (biPAP), 405
Positive end-expiratory pressure (PEEP), 403–404
Post-concussive syndrome, 318
Posterior fossa neoplasms, 362
Posterior packs, 289
Postnasal drip, hoarseness associated with, 150
Postoperative patients, urinary output in, 382
Posturography, 53
Potassium, postoperative serum levels of, 383
Potassium replacement therapy, 381
Pott's puffy tumor, 101
Prausnitz, Carl, 350
Pregnancy
  facial paralysis during, 125
  maternal-fetal HIV transmission during, 153
  nasal congestion during, 87
  otosclerosis during, 46
  as radiation therapy contraindication, 238
  respiratory alkalosis during, 385, 386
Presbycusis, 13, 24, 26
Presbyesophagus, 134
Presidents, of United States, otolaryngologic
    disorders in, 427–428
Pressure changes, as epistaxis cause, 287
Pressure-control ventilation, 402
Pressure equalization tubes (PET), 23, 47
Pressure-support ventilation, 402
Prilocaine, 366
Primary care physicians
  cost-effectiveness of otolaryngologic care by,
      380
  referrals by, 106, 380
Procainamide, as fever cause, 421
Procaine, 366, 367
Prominent ear deformities, 332
Propranolol, interaction with theophylline, 165
Protein, surgical patients' daily requirements,
    389–390
Proteus infections
  antibiotic therapy for, 159, 161, 162
  otitis media as, 40
Prothrombin time (PT), 395
  in epistaxis patients, 289
Protrusor muscle, mandibular, 303
Prussak's space, 37
Pseudohyponatremia, 383
Pseudomonas infections
  antibiotic therapy for, 159, 160–161, 162
  cholesteatoma-related, 44
  otitis externa as, 35
  otitis media as, 40
  as septic shock cause, 415–416
  sinusitis as, 100
  ventilator-associated pneumonia as, 422
Psychiatric disorders, taste and olfactory disorders
    associated with, 346, 347

Pterygoid muscles, 303, 356
   inflammation of, 377
   in mandibular fractures, 304
   in temporomandibular disorders, 114
Pterygoid plates, LeFort fractures of, 309–310
Ptosis
   in children, 376
   post-blepharoplasty, 267
Pulseless electrical activity (PEA), 411
Pupil, Marcus Gunn, 371
Pure-tone average, 15
Pyriform sinus cancer, 212, 213
Pyrogens, 419

Quality-adjusted life-years (QALY), 379
Quinidine
   as fever cause, 421
   ototoxicity of, 165
Quinine, ototoxicity of, 165, 166
Quinsy, 142, 326–327, 427

Raccoon sign, 316
Radiation exposure, as esophageal cancer risk
      factor, 218
Radiation therapy, **237–240**
   for basal cell carcinoma, 231
   combined with chemotherapy, 242
      for esophageal cancer, 221
      for head and neck cancer, 242–243
   for esophageal cancer, 220, 221
   external-beam, 237, 239–240
   for parotid tumors, 192
   for glomus tumors, 76
   for glottic cancer, 213
   as hyperparathyroidism cause, 137
   for laryngeal cancer, 212
   as laryngeal cancer risk factor, 209
   for oral cavity carcinoma, 198
   for sinonasal cancers, 207
   for tracheal cancer, 216
Radioiodine scanning, 224, 225
Radiology. See also X-rays
   of head and neck, **353–365**
Radiosurgery, as acoustic neuroma treatment, 75–76
Radix, 255
RAE tubes, 367
Ramsay Hunt syndrome, 36, 70, 125, 130
   in AIDS patients, 155
Ramus fractures, 302, 303, 307
Ranula, 140
RAST (radioallerogo sorbent test), 351, 352
Raynaud's disease, 133
Reagan, Ronald, 427
Reconstructive surgery
   facial, 1, 280, 429
   of head and neck, 246, 247
   mandibular, 204, 250
   tracheal, 176
Recurrent nerve, paralysis of, 211
Red eye, differential diagnosis of, 377
Reduction
   of mandibular fractures, 305–306, 307, 308

Reduction (*cont.*)
   of nasal fractures, 291–292
Referrals, to otolaryngologists, 380
   of sinusitis patients, 106
Referred pain, from sinuses, 98
Refractive errors, in children, 376
Reinke's space, 211
Reissner's membrane, 11
   rupture of, 27
Relative afferent pupillary deficit (RAPD), 371
REM sleep, obstructive sleep apnea during, 146
Renal failure, as lactic acidosis cause, 388
Renal infections, as fever cause, 421
Resonance theory, of Helmholz, 427
Respiratory arrest, tracheotomy-related, 400
Respiratory depression, as respiratory acidosis
      cause, 385
Respiratory disease, bronchoscopic evaluation of,
      178
Respiratory distress, in thyroidectomy patients, 225
Respiratory quotient (RQ), 391
Respiratory syncytial virus, 326
Respiratory tract infections
   Down syndrome as risk factor for, 338
   as tonsillectomy indication, 327
   upper
      in children, general anesthesia and, 369–370
      as taste and smell disorders cause, 346, 348
Resuscitation
   cardiopulmonary, **408–413**
   of shock victims, 415, 417–418
Retina
   detachment of, 376
   necrosis of, 377
   tears of, 373
Retinal artery, central occlusion of, 371
Retinitis, cytomegalovirus, 153
Retinoic acid (Retin-A), use in facial skin
      resurfacing, 251, 252
Retraction pocket, 43, 44
Retrobulbar abscess, 375
Retrobulbar hemorrhage, 373
Retrolabyrinthine approach, to cerebellopontine
      angle, 74
Retropharyngeal space, abscess of, 358
Reversed squeeze, 63
Reye's syndrome, 420
Rhabdomyosarcoma
   as facial paralysis cause, 125
   imaging of, 361
   laryngeal, 208
   of middle ear, 69
Rhinion, 255
Rhinitis, **86–90**
   adenotonsillar hypertrophy-related, 327
   allergic, 86, 87, 88, 89, 98
      perennial, 352
      seasonal, 352
   atrophic, 87–88
   bacterial, 84
   medicamentosa, 88–89, 103, 165
   nonallergic, 86, 87

Rhinitis (*cont.*)
  polychondritis-related, 85
  rebound, 103
  sinusitis-related, 99
  vasomotor, 88, 89, 353
Rhinology, 1, 2
Rhinomanometry, 81
Rhinometry, 82
Rhinophyma, 253
Rhinoplasty, **254–261**
  anesthesia in, 254
  blood units required for, 393
  in children, 85
  in cleft lip patients, 343
  closed, 261
  implant materials in, 261
  nasal anatomy and, 255–257
  open, 260–261
  techniques of, 254–261
Rhinorrhea, cerebrospinal fluid, 316, 317, 363
Rhinosinusitis
  in hospitalized immunocompromised patients,
    143
  as nasopharyngeal carcinoma cause, 196
Rhytidectomy, 253, **274–281**
  patient psychological evaluation for, 280–281
  types of, 278
Rim fractures, 311
Rings, esophageal, 133
Rinne tuning fork test, 13, 60
Roosevelt, Franklin D., 427
Rosacea, as skin resurfacing indication, 251
Rosen, Sam, 429
Round window
  fistula of, 70
  rupture of, 64–65
Royal College of Physicians, 429
Royal Society of England, 426
Royal Society of Surgeons, 429
Rule of 10's, for carotid body tumor malignancy,
  228

Saccule, receptor cells of, 12
Saethre-Chotzen syndrome, 337
Sagittal split, as obstructive sleep apnea treatment,
  147
Saints, patron, of otolaryngology, 426
Salicylates
  as anaphylactic shock cause, 352–353
  as lactic acidosis cause, 388
  as metabolic acidosis cause, 387
  ototoxicity of, 26, 59, 165
  as respiratory alkalosis cause, 386
Salivary gland cancer, **189–193**, 195, 238
Salivary glands. *See also* Parotid gland
  anatomy of, 137–138
  ectopic tissue of, pleomorphic adenoma of, 355,
    356
  histologic differences among, 190
  hypofunction of, 118–119
  infections of, as deep space neck infection cause,
    141

Salivary glands (*cont.*)
  origin of, 137
  radiation-related dysfunction of, 118
  tumors of, **189–193**
Salivary gland surgery, antibiotic prophylaxis for,
  379–380
Salpingopharyngeus muscle, in eustachian tube
  dilatation, 67
Sarcoid, appearance upon mediastinoscopy, 185
Sarcoidosis, 125, 186, 423
Sarcoma
  cutaneous, 236
  deep-tissue, 236
  esophageal, 217
  of jugular foramen, 69
  laryngeal, 208
  of temporal bone and external ear canal, 68
Saturation sound pressure, 29
Scala media, 11
Scala tympani, 11
Scala vestibuli, 11
Scars, hypertrophic, differentiated from keloids, 397
Schatzki's ring, 133, 219
Schirmer's test, 126, 263
Schuknecht, Harold, 429
Schwabach tuning fork test, 14
Schwannoma
  of carotid space, 357
  of facial nerve, 125, 362
Schwartze's sign, 45
Scleral show, blepharoplasty-related, 267
Scleritis, 377
Scleroderma, 85, 133
Scotoma, 55
Sea-level pressure, 62
Sedatives
  as obstructive sleep apnea cause, 146, 147
  preoperative use of, 365
  as respiratory acidosis cause, 385
  as tinnitus cause, 59
Seizures
  fever and, 420, 421
  as lactic acidosis cause, 388
  skull-base surgery-related, 75
Selenium, as total parenteral nutrition component,
  391
Selenium deficiency, total parenteral nutrition-
  related, 392
Sellion, differentiated from nasion, 255
Semicircular canals, receptor cells of, 12
Semilunar hiatus, in sinus drainage, 107
Sepsis
  gram-negative, 385, 386
  as intraoperative tachycardia cause, 369
  as lactic acidosis cause, 388
Septoplasty
  blood units required for, 393
  in children, 85
  as obstructive sleep apnea treatment, 148
  with rhinoplasty, 254
Septum. *See* Nasal septum
Serratia infections, 415–416

Serum sodium, relationship to blood glucose, 383
Sexual intercourse, as HIV transmission method, 153
SHDBGIFT mnemonic, for malignant hyperthermia management, 366
Shea, John, 429
Shock, **413–418**
  anaphylactic, 352–353
  cardiogenic, 413, 416, 417, 418
  controversial drug therapy for, 418
  definition of, 284
  gram-negative endotoxic, 415–416
  hemorrhagic, 284, 383, 413, 415
  hypovolemic, 413–415, 417, 418
  neurogenic, 413, 416–417
  septic, 142, 413, 415–416, 417, 418
Short process, anatomy of, 2
Sialadenitis, suppurative, 139
Sialography, 189
Sialometaplasia, necrotizing, 194
Silicosis, 185–186
Simmons, Blair, 429
Simonart's band, 339
Simon method, of nasal tip projection measurement, 258
Sinus cancer, 205–207
Sinuses
  anatomy and function of, **90–96**
  branchial, 330
  cavernous, venous network of, 375
  drainage of, 91, 107, 109
  embryological development of, 91, 92, 93
  ethmoid, 90, 92, 93
    as cancer site, 206
    limited computed tomography of, 82
    sinusitis of, 110–111, 364
  frontal, 90, 92
    imaging of, 82
    surgical dissection of, 108–109
  functional significance of, 94
  innervation of, 94
  maxillary, 90, 91–92, 94, 95
    aspiration of, 99
    as cancer site, 206
    imaging of, 82
    sinusitis of, 110
    surgically-facilitated drainage of, 109
  mucous blanket of, 81, 94
  paranasal, 93, 94
    imaging of, 363–364, 380
    lymphatics of, 80
    malignancy of, 99
  physical examination of, 6
  polyps of, 353–354
  posterior, surgical dissection of, 108
  pyriform, in endotracheal tube placement, 300
  referred pain from, 98
  sphenoid, 90, 93, 95
    as cancer site, 206
    sinusitis of, 364
  surgical dissection of, 108–109
  transillumination of, 6, 99
Sinuses (*cont.*)
  tumors of, **204–208**
  vascular supply of, 79
Sinusitis, **96–102**
  acute, 96–97, 98–99
  categories of, 96
  chronic, 97
  complications of, 100–101
    intracranial, 100, 101, 105–106
    orbital, 100, 101, 105, 375–376
  dental, 100
  endotracheal intubation-related, 301
  as epistaxis cause, 286
  ethmoid, 110–111
    computed tomographic detection of, 364
  as fever cause, 421
  fungal, 105
  in HIV-infected patients, 105, 155, 156–157
  as keratitis obturans cause, 35
  maxillary, surgical approach to, 110
  medical management of, **102–107**, 164, 166
    antibiotic therapy, 102–103, 380
    differentiated from otitis media treatment, 161–162
    of ethmoid sinusitis, 110–111
    failure of, 106
    immunotherapy, 105
    of maxillary sinusitis, 110
  as olfactory disorders cause, 346
  sphenoid, computed tomographic detection of, 364
  spontaneous resolution of, 102
  surgical management of, **107–112**
    functional endoscopic sinus surgery (FESS), 91, 108–110, 111
    indications for, 106
  as taste and smell disorders cause, 348
Sinus ostia, sinusitis-related obstruction of, 103
Sinus surgery, **107–112**
  fellowships in, 2
Sipple's syndrome, 223
Six-pack platelet transfusion, HIV transmission by, 153
Sjogren's syndrome, 85, 118
Skin
  aging of, as skin resurfacing indication, 251–252
  effect of radiation therapy on, 239
  types of, 251
Skin cancer. *See also* Basal cell carcinoma, cutaneous; Melanoma, cutaneous; Squamous cell carcinoma, cutaneous
  ultraviolet radiation B-related, 274
Skin grafts. *See* Grafts
Skin infections, as fever cause, 421
Skin resurfacing, **251–253**
Skin slough, rhytidectomy-related, 279–280
Skin tests, for allergy diagnosis, 351
Skull-base surgery, 2, 75, 429
Sleep apnea, **144–149**
  central, 144
  mixed, 144

Sleep apnea (*cont.*)
  obstructive, 144–149
    Down syndrome-related, 338
    as tonsillectomy indication, 327
    tracheotomy for, 401
SMAS (superficial musculo-aponeurotic system), 275, 277
Smell. *See* Olfaction
Smoking
  as laryngeal cancer cause, 208–209
  as oral cavity cancer cause, 194
  as pharynx cancer cause, 194
  by rhytidectomy patients, 280
Snap test, 263
Snoring, 144, 146, 148–149
Sodium fluoride therapy, for otosclerosis, 47
Sodium replacement therapy, 381
Soft palate cancer, metastases of, 197
Sound pressure, tinnitus masking effect of, 60
Spasm
  broncho-, 353
  esophageal, 134
  hemifacial, 129
Speculum
  for head and neck examination, 2
  nasal, 4
Speech. *See also* Voice
  frequency of, 150
  hypernasal, cleft palate repair-related, 342
  production of, 149, 151
Speech discrimination test, 17
Speech reception threshold (SRT) test, 17
Sphenopalatine artery, 93
  ligation of, for epistaxis management, 289
Sphenopalatine nerve, 94
Sphygmomanometer, 60
Spirometry, for upper airway obstruction evaluation, 298
Spironolactone, as metabolic acidosis cause, 387
Splints
  intranasal, 85
  postoperative use, in rhinoplasty patients, 260
  as temporomandibular disorders therapy, 115
Spondees, 17
Sputum cytology, 179–180
Squamous cell carcinoma
  of auricle, 68
  carotid space metastases of, 357
  cutaneous, 231–233
    actinic keratoses-related, 229–230
    staging and grading systems for, 232–233
  esophageal, 217, 218
  of glottic larynx, 239
  inverting papilloma-related, 204
  laryngeal, 208
  of middle ear, 69
  of nasal septum, 84
  of oral cavity, 121, 195
  pharyngeal, 195
  pulmonary, 170, 179
  sinonasal, 205, 206

Squamous cell carcinoma (*cont.*)
  as solitary neck mass, 196
  staging panendoscopy of, 380
  tracheal, 214
  of vocal cords, 152
"Squeeze effect", 62
Stab wounds, facial, as deep space neck infection cause, 142
Stafne's mandibular lingual cortical defect, 200
Stapedectomy, 24
Stapedial arch, fractures of, 319
Stapedius muscles, function of, 10, 19
Stapeotomy, 24
Stapes, anatomy of, 9
Staphylococcus aureus, methicillin-resistant, 161
Staphylococcal infections
  antibiotic therapy for, 159, 160, 161, 162
  deep space neck infections as, 141
  as fever cause, 422
  HIV infection-associated, 154
  septal abscess as, 292
  sialadenitis as, 139
  sinusitis as, 97
  tonsillitis as, 326
Starch-iodine test, 192
Stark, Anne, 429
Stay sutures, 399
Stenosis
  bronchoscopic evaluation of, 178–179
  esophageal, 173
  of first branchial groove, 331
  laryngeal, endotracheal intubation-related, 301
  subglottic, 322, 323, 325, 331, 405
  tracheal, 400
Stenson's duct, 137
Stents, in laryngeal trauma management, 296
Stereocilia, 11
  damage to, as sensorineural hearing loss cause, 25
Sternocleidomastoid muscle flap, 248
Steroid therapy
  as esophagoscopy contraindication, 174, 175
  for rhinitis, 88, 89
  for sensorineural hearing loss, 25, 27
Stevens-Johnson syndrome, 377
Stickler syndrome, 334, 337
Stomatitis, aphthous, 119
Strabismus, in children, 376
Strangulation attempts, as neck blunt trauma cause, 295
Streptococcal infections
  antibiotic therapy for, 159, 160, 161
  aphthous ulcers as, 119
  deep space neck infections as, 141
  group A β-hemolytic, 326
  otitis media as, 40, 41, 167
  septal abscess as, 292
  as septic shock cause, 416
  sinusitis as, 97
  tonsillitis as, 326
  ventilator-associated pneumonia as, 422
  of wounds, 396

Streptomycin, ototoxicity of, 55, 165, 166
Streptozocin, as lactic acidosis cause, 388
Stress, effect on threshold allergic response, 352
Stress management, by tinnitus patients, 61
Stress-related symptoms, differentiated from
 sinusitis, 99
Strictures, esophageal, misdiagnosed as esophageal
 cancer, 219
Stridor, 150
 bronchoscopic evaluation of, 178–179
 in children, 321–322
 hemangioma-related, 227
 neck penetrating trauma-related, 295
 upper airway obstruction-related, 297
Stroboscope, 170
Stroke. *See* Cerebrovascular accidents
Sturge-Weber syndrome, 227
Subclavian artery
 right, aberrant, 186
 as tracheal blood supply source, 214
Subcondylar fractures, 302–303, 304
Subglottic cancer, 384
Subglottic stenosis, 322, 323, 325, 331, 405
Submandibular glands, 138
 differentiated from submaxillary glands, 138
 traumatic injury to, 140
Submaxillary glands, differentiated from
 submandibular glands, 138
Suboccipital/retrosigmoid approach, to
 cerebellopontine angle, 75
Subspecialization certification, in otolaryngology, 2
Sulfonamides, 161, 162
 interaction with oral contraceptives, 166
Sun exposure. *See* Ultraviolet radiation
Superficial musculo-aponeurotic system (SMAS),
 275, 277
Supraglottis, congenital malformation of, 331
Suprasternal retractions, upper airway obstruction-
 related, 297
Surgery. *See also* specific surgical procedures
 blood units required for, 393
Surgical patients
 allergic tendencies of, 351
 metabolic alkalosis in, 388–389
 protein requirements of, 389–390
Sutures, stay, 399
Swallowing
 airway protection during, 131–132
 disorders of, as tonsillectomy indication, 327
Sympathomimetics, as rhinitis therapy, 88
Symphyseal fractures, 302, 303, 304, 306
Synchronized intermittent mechanical ventilation,
 402–403
Syphilis
 as dizziness cause, 52
 as hearing loss cause, 24, 25, 27, 28
 as rhinitis cause, 89
 as septal perforation cause, 83
Systemic disorders
 as dizziness cause, 48
 as facial paralysis cause, 125
 as lactic acidosis cause, 388

Systemic disorders (*cont.*)
 myoclonus-associated, 59
 as olfactory disorders cause, 346
Systemic lupus erythematosus, 27, 133, 423

Tachycardia
 hypovolemic shock-related, 414
 intraoperative, 369
Tags, auricular, 335–336
Tamponade, cardiac, 411
Tanzer's classification system, of external ear
 malformations, 269
Taste, **345–349**
 disorders of, 346, 347–349
 differentiated from olfactory disorders, 348
Taste papillae, 345
Taxotere, 242
Teardrop sign, of blowout fractures, 312, 373
Tectus abdominus myocutaneous free flap, 249
Teeth
 examination of, 5
 incisor, relationship to esophageal landmarks, 173
 involvement in mandibular fractures, 303, 305,
  307, 308
 universal lettering and numbering systems of, 304
Telecanthus, 313
"Telephone ear" deformity, 273
Temporal bone
 fractures of, 70, 315–318, 320
  classification of, 315
  complications of, 315–316
  as conductive hearing loss cause, 23
  as facial nerve injury cause, 125, 129
 neoplasms of, 68
 traumatic injury to, **314–320**
  as dizziness cause, 47–48
  as facial nerve injury cause, 315, 316, 317,
   319–320
  radiographic evaluation of, 362, 363
  as sensorineural hearing loss cause, 28
Temporalis muscle, 303, 356
 in mandibular fractures, 304
 in temporomandibular disorders, 114
Temporomandibular disorders, **113–118**
 differential diagnosis of, 113–114
Temporomandibular joint
 anatomy of, 113
 ankylosis of, maxillomandibular fixation-related,
  308
 internal displacement of, 115
Tension-related symptoms, differentiated from
 sinusitis, 99
Tensor tympani muscle
 in eustachian tube dilatation, 67
 function of, 10
Tensor veli palatini muscle
 in cleft lip/palate, 341
 in eustachian tube dilatation, 67
Teratoma
 comparison with dermoid cysts, 330
 as pediatric airway obstruction cause, 324
 thyroid, 222

Tetracaine, 366, 367
Tetracyclines
    interaction with oral contraceptives, 166
    limitations of, 160
Theophylline
    drug interactions of, 161, 165
    toxicity of, 165
Thiamazole, effect on taste and smell, 348
Third nerve, palsy of, 377
Third spacing, 383
Thoracic artery, internal, as tracheal blood supply
        source, 214
Thoracic cage disorders, 384
Thoracotomy, 184, 220–221
Threshold allergic response, 352
Throat, patron saint of, 426
Thrombocytopenia, dilutional, blood transfusion-
        related, 369
Thrombosis
    cavernous sinus, 293, 374
    deep venous, 421, 422
        total parenteral nutrition-related, 392
    venous sinus, sinusitis-related, 101
Thrush, 120
Thymitaq, 242
Thymoma, 186
Thyroglossal duct, cysts of, 136, 330, 332, 359, 360
Thyroid artery, inferior, as tracheal blood supply
        source, 214
Thyroidectomy, risks of, 225
Thyroid function tests, 224
Thyroid gland
    disorders of, **137–138**
        cancer, 224, 225
        cysts, 222, 224
        focal enlargement, 222
        nodules, 222, 223–224
        as olfactory disorders cause, 346
        tumors, 152, **222–226**
    ectopic, 332
    substernal, 186
Thyroid hormone, 136
Thyroiditis, 222
Thyroid replacement, post-thyroidectomy, 225
Thyroid surgery
    anesthesia in, 368
    antibiotic prophylaxis for, 379–380
Thyrotoxicosis, 369, 419
"Tics", facial, 129–130
Tinnitus, **58–61**
    acoustic neuroma-related, 72–73
    drug-related, 59
    glomus tumor-related, 69
    Meniere's disease-related, 53
    vascular anomalies-related, 362
Tobacco use. See also Smoking
    as esophageal cancer cause, 218
    as oral cancer cause, 194, 195
Tobramycin, ototoxicity of, 55
Tongue
    "geographic", 121
    lymphatic drainage of, 196–197

Tongue (cont.)
    physical examination of, 5
    retrodisplacement of, as pediatric airway
            obstruction cause, 323
Tongue blade, use in oral cavity examination, 5
Tongue cancer
    metastases of, 196–197
    radiation treatment of, 238
    of Ulysses S. Grant, 427
Tongue-retaining devices, as obstructive sleep apnea
        treatment, 147
Tonsil(s), **325–329**
    abscess of, 142
    cancer of
        radiation treatment of, 238
        of Ulysses S. Grant, 427–428
    function of, 326
    post-tonsillectomy regrowth of, 328
Tonsillar pillars, 326
Tonsillectomy
    complications of, 328
    contraindications to, 327
    in Down syndrome patients, 369
    endotracheal intubation during, 367
    indications for, 327
Tonsillitis, 141, 162, 326, 327
Tonsillolithiasis, 327
Topotecan, 242
TORP (total ossicular reconstruction prosthesis),
        46–47
Torus mandibulae, 121, 122
Torus palatinus, 121, 122
Total body water (TBW), 381
Total ossicular reconstruction prosthesis (TORP),
        46–47
Total parenteral nutrition, 390–392
Toxic shock syndrome, 417
Toxin ingestion, as metabolic acidosis cause, 387
Toxoplasmosis, in HIV-infected patients, 153, 154,
        156
Trace elements, 391
Trace mineral deficiencies, total parenteral
        nutrition-related, 392
Trachea
    anatomy of, 214
    arterial blood supply of, 214
    congenital malformations of, 331
    embryologic development of, 176
    fractures of, as upper airway obstruction cause, 297
    functions of, 176
    obstruction of, 296
    penetrating trauma to, 295
    physical examination of, 6
    reconstructive surgery of, 176
    resection of, 215–216
    stenosis of, tracheotomy-related, 400
    tumors of, **214–217**
        as intubation contraindication, 215
        secondary, 214
Tracheal button, 400
Tracheobronchial tree, epithelium of, 214
Tracheocutaneous fistula, 398

Tracheoesophageal fistula, 134, 173, 301, 330–331, 399
Tracheoesophageal puncture, 429
Tracheomalacia, 322, 331, 368
Tracheomegaly, 331
Tracheostomy
  in children, indications for, 324, 325
  differentiated from tracheotomy, 398
  as obstructive sleep apnea treatment, 148
Tracheotomy, **398–402**
  complications of, 399–400
  conversion from cricothyroidotomy, 301
  differentiated from tracheostomy, 398
  first, 426
Tracheotomy tubes
  displacement of, in pediatric patients, 399
  fenestrated, 400
  size determination of, 399
Tracheotomy valves, one-way, 400
Transconjunctival technique, in blepharoplasty, 265, 266
Transcutaneous pacing, 410
Transient ischemic attacks, 48, 56
Transillumination, of nasal sinuses, 6, 99
Transitional cell carcinoma, sinonasal, 205
Translabyrinthine approach, to cerebellopontine angle, 74
Trapezius myocutaneous flap, 248
Trauma, **283–286**
  acoustic, as sensorineural hearing loss cause, 25
  blunt, to neck, 295
  as cardiogenic shock cause, 416
  as epistaxis cause, 286
  as facial paralysis cause, 125
  "golden hour" in, 283
  as hearing loss cause, 24, 25, 28
  midfacial, **309–314**
  as mortality cause, 283
  nasal, 290–293
  penetrating, to neck and face, **293–296**
  as respiratory alkalosis cause, 386
  to temporal bone, **314–320**
  as third spacing cause, 383
Trauma surgery, antibiotic prophylaxis in, 379–380
Traumatic optic neuropathy, 372, 377–378
Traveling wave, 11
Treacher Collins syndrome, 269, 334, 337
Trench mouth, 122
Triamterine, as metabolic acidosis cause, 387
Triceps skinfold thickness, 389
Tricyclic antidepressants, as xerostomia cause, 118
Trigeminal nerve
  mandibular nerve branch of, 304
  as nasal and paranasal innervation, 80, 94
  in taste and smell disorders, 345–346
Trimethoprim, co-administration with sulfonamides, 161
Trimethoprim-sulfamethoxazole, 161
Trismus, peritonsillar abscess-related, 142
Trisomy 13, 337
Trisomy 21, 337
Tube cuff pressure, in tracheotomy, 399

Tuberculosis, 156, 179, 185–186
Tuning fork tests, 13–14, 21–22
  audiogram versus, 17–18
  for tinnitus evaluation, 60
Turbinate, corticosteroid injections in, as rhinitis therapy, 89
Turbinate surgery
  as nasal adhesion cause, 85
  as obstructive sleep apnea treatment, 148
  as rhinitis treatment, 89–90
Turbinectomy, inferior, 89–90
"Turkey gobbler", rhytidectomy for correction of, 278–279
Tympanic membrane
  abnormal signs on, 37
  anatomy of, 38
  area effect of, 10
  diseases of, 37–39
  foreign bodies within, 58
  innervation of, 62
  normal, 2–3
  in otitis media, 40
  perforation of, 37–38
    barotrauma-related, 66
    as conductive hearing loss, 23
    diagnosis of, 66
    ossicular discontinuity associated with, 46
    paper patching of, 38
    pressure differential required for, 64
    temporal bone trauma-related, 316, 319
Tympanocentesis, 41
Tympanograms, classification of, 18
Tympanography, 22
Tympanometry, 18, 40
Tympanoplasty, 24, 429
Tympanostomy tubes
  complications of, 42
  indications for, 41
  as otitis media-related hearing loss treatment, 23
Type and crossmatch, 393
Type and screen, 393

Ulcers, aphthous, 119
Ultrasonography
  of branchial cleft cysts, 359
  endoscopic, of esophageal cancer, 219
  for thyroid nodule evaluation, 224
Ultraviolet radiation, cutaneous effects of
  actinic keratoses, 229
  basal cell carcinoma, 230
  squamous cell carcinoma, 231
  xeroderma pigmentosum, 233
Ultraviolet radiation A, as cutaneous actinic damage cause, 274–275
Ultraviolet radiation B, as skin cancer cause, 274
Umbo, anatomy of, 2
Uncinate process, 90
Universal numbering and lettering systems, for teeth, 304
Upper gastrointestinal studies, for pediatric airway obstruction evaluation, 324
Urban, Jack, 429

Uremia, as metabolic acidosis cause, 387
Ureterosigmoidostomy, as metabolic acidosis cause, 387
Urinary output, in postoperative patients, 382
Urinary tract infections, as fever cause, 421, 422
Usher's syndrome, 26, 336
Utricle, receptor cells of, 12
U-triple-P (uvulopalatopharyngoplasty), 147, 148
Uvula
  bifid, 327
  cleft, 334
Uvular muscle, in cleft lip/palate, 341
Uvulopalatopharyngoplasty (U-triple-P), 147, 148
Uvulopalatoplasty, 148–149

Vagus nerve
  location within carotid sheath, 142
  taste bud innervation by, 345
Valium, use in cardiopulmonary resuscitation, 411
Valsalva, Antonio, 426
Valsalva maneuver, 426
  use by divers, 64–65
Valvular heart disease, as cardiogenic shock cause, 416
Vancomycin, 161–162
  ototoxicity of, 165
Van der Woude syndrome, 334
Vascular anomalies, of superior mediastinum, 186
Vascular disorders
  as fever of unknown origin cause, 423
  as sudden sensorineural hearing loss cause, 27
Vascular injuries, to neck, 295
Vascular loops, as vertigo cause, 57
Vascular rings, esophageal, 219
Vascular tumors
  esophageal, 217
  of head and neck, **227–229**
  resection of, blood units required for, 393
Vasculature, sinonasal, 79, 81, 93–94
Vasculitides
  of central nervous system, as dizziness cause, 48
  as fever cause, 421
Vasoconstriction, cocaine-related, 167
Vasodilators, as shock therapy, 418
Velopharyngeal dysfunction, 340
Velopharyngeal incompetence, 343
Velopharyngeal insufficiency, 327, 340, 342
Veloplasty, Schweckendiek's primary, 342
Venous hum, 58
Ventilation
  mechanical. See Mechanical ventilation
  transtracheal needle, 301
Verrucous carcinoma, 208, 428
Vertebrobasilar insufficiency, 56
Vertigo
  acoustic neuroma-related, 73
  alternobaric, 64
  aminoglycosides-related, 59
  benign paroxysmal positional, 48, 49–50, 53, 57
  common causes of, 49
  control of, 48
  in divers, 64

Vertigo (cont.)
  Ménière's disease-related, 53, 54
  migraine-related, 56
  temporal bone trauma-related, 315, 318
  whiplash (cervical), 57
Vestibular ablation, chemical, 70
Vestibular disorders, 48, **53–57**
Vestibular end organs, 10, 12
Vestibular lesions, 51–52
Vestibular nerve section, 69
Vestibular reflexes, 12
Vestibulocochlear nerve. See Acoustic nerve
Vestibulo-ocular reflex, vestibular injury-related impairment of, 55
Videolaryngoscopy, 170
Videolaryngostroboscopy, 170
Vienna, role in history of otolaryngology, 425
Viral infections. See also specific viral infections
  cutaneous, HIV infection-related, 154
  as hoarseness cause, 151
  of inner ear, 54–55
  of middle ear, 40
  as sensorineural hearing loss cause, 27, 28
  as vertigo cause, 48
Virchow, Rudolf, 428–429
Vision loss, blepharoplasty-related, 267
Visual tracking system, electronystagmographic evaluation of, 52
Vitamin K deficiency, 391, 392
Vocal cords
  biopsy of, 170
  endotracheal intubation-related injury to, 406
  endotracheal intubation-related tethering of, 405
  "fixed" (immobile), 211
  in hysterical aphonia, 152
  lesions of, direct laryngoscopic treatment of, 171–172
  neoplastic disorders of, 152
  nodules of, 150, 152
  paralysis of, 150, 151–152
    bronchoscopic evaluation of, 178–179
    endotracheal intubation-related, 406
    in infants, 322
    thyroidectomy-related, 225
    upper airway obstruction-related, 297
  polyps of, 152
  "stripping" of, 172
Voice, upper airway obstruction-related changes in, 297
Voice abuse
  as hoarseness cause, 151
  lesions caused by, 152
Volatile chemical inhalation, as olfactory disorders cause, 346
Volume expanders, 382
Vomeronasal organ, 82
Vomiting
  chemotherapy-related, 242
  postoperative, 365
von Recklinghausen disease, 73
V-Y pushback (Oxford) method, of cleft palate repair, 342

5 W's, of postoperative fever, 422
Waardenburg's syndrome, 26, 337
Waldeyer's ring, 325
Ward, Paul, 429
Warfarin, as epistaxis cause, 287
Warm water irrigation. *See* Irrigation
Warthin's tumor, 189
Washington, George, 427
Water loss, fever-related, 420
Weber tuning fork test, 13, 22, 60
Webs
  congenital laryngeal, 322
  esophageal, 133, 219
  pharyngoesophageal, 218
Weerda classification system, of external ear
    malformations, 269
Wegener's granulomatosis, 27, 83–84
Welch, William M., 428
Wermer's syndrome, 223
Wharton's duct, 138
Wheezing, bronchoscopic evaluation of, 178–179
White noise, 60
Whooping cough, patron saint of, 426
Willis, Thomas, 426
Wolf-Hirschhorn chromosomal abnormality, 337
Wood dust, as sinonasal cancer cause, 206
Wounds
  dehiscence of, 397
  healing of, **396–398**
  infections of, 396, 397, 421
  postoperative, as third spacing cause, 383
Wrist, fractures of, 290

Xeroderma pigmentosum, 233
Xerostomia, 118–119

Xerostomia (*cont.*)
  benign lymphoepithelial disease-related, 139
  pharmacological treatment of, 164
  radiation therapy-related, 239, 240
X-linked genetic disorders, 333
X-linked inheritance, of hearing loss, 336
X-rays
  of blowout fractures, 373
  chest
    of esophageal cancer, 218
    for upper airway obstruction evaluation, 298
  for facial paralysis evaluation, 126
  of mandibular fractures, 305
  of maxillofacial trauma, 311, 312
  of nasal fractures, 293
  of nose, 82
  panoramic view
    for jaw swelling evaluation, 202–203
    of mandibular fractures, 305
  of paranasal sinuses, 380
  for pediatric airway obstruction evaluation, 324
  of sinuses, 82, 99, 363–364, 380
  for sinusitis evaluation, 99
  for temporomandibular disease evaluation, 115
  of tracheal tumors, 215
  in trauma patients, 286

Zenker's diverticulum, 131, 219
Zidovudine, 156, 163
Zinc, as total parenteral nutrition component, 391
Zona pellucida, of soft palate, 339
Z-plasty, 342
Zygomatic arch fractures, 310, 312–313
l nutrition component, 391
Zona pellucid